The Vitamins

Fundamental Aspects in Nutrition and Health

Third Edition

The Vitamins

Fundamental Aspects in Nutrition and Health

Third Edition

Gerald F. Combs, Jr., Ph.D.

Professor Emeritus
Division of Nutritional Sciences
Cornell University
Ithaca, New York

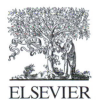

AMSTERDAM • BOSTON • HEIDELBERG • LONDON
NEW YORK • OXFORD • PARIS • SAN DIEGO
SAN FRANCISCO • SINGAPORE • SYDNEY • TOKYO

Academic press is an imprint of Elsevier

ELSEVIER

Elsevier Academic Press

30 Corporate Drive, Suite 400, Burlington, MA 01803, USA

525 B Street, Suite 1900, San Diego, California 92101-4495, USA

84 Theobald's Road, London WC1X 8RR, UK

This book is printed on acid-free paper. ∞

Library of Congress Cataloging-in-Publication Data

The vitamins : fundamental aspects in nutrition and health / editor, Gerald F. Combs. — 3rd ed.
     p.; cm.
  Includes bibliographical references and index.
  ISBN-13: 978-0-12-183493-7 (hardcover : alk. paper) 1. Vitamins. 2. Nutrition.
  [DNLM: 1. Vitamins. 2. Nutrition Physiology. QU 160 C731v 2008] I. Combs, Gerald F.
  QP771.C645 2008
  612.3'99—dc22
                              2007026776

British Library Cataloguing in Publication Data
A catalogue record for this book is available from the British Library

ISBN 13: 978-0-12-183493-7

For all information on all Elsevier Academic Press publications
visit our Web site at www.books.elsevier.com

Printed in the United States of America
07 08 09 10 9 8 7 6 5 4 3 2 1

To Henry

Contents

Preface   xi
Preface to the Second Edition   xiii
Preface to the First Edition   xv
How to Use This Book   xvii

PART I. PERSPECTIVES ON THE VITAMINS IN NUTRITION

Chapter 1 What Is a Vitamin?   3
  I.   Thinking about Vitamins   3
  II. Vitamin: A Revolutionary Concept   4
  III. An Operating Definition of a Vitamin   4
  IV. The Recognized Vitamins   5
       Study Questions   6

Chapter 2 Discovery of the Vitamins   7
  I.   The Emergence of Nutrition as a Science   8
  II.   The Process of Discovery in Nutritional
        Science   8
  III. The Empirical Phase of Vitamin Discovery   9
  IV.   The Experimental Phase of Vitamin
        Discovery   12
  V.   The Vitamine Theory   15
  VI.   Elucidation of the Vitamins   18
  VII. Vitamin Terminology   30
  VIII. Other Factors Sometimes Called
        Vitamins   31
  IX.   The Modern History of the Vitamins   31
        Study Questions and Exercises   32
        Recommended Reading   32

Chapter 3 Chemical and Physiological Properties of the Vitamins   35
  I.   Chemical and Physical Properties
        of the Vitamins   36
  II.   Vitamin A   42
  III. Vitamin D   45
  IV.   Vitamin E   47
  V.   Vitamin K   49
  VI.   Vitamin C   51
  VII. Thiamin   52

  VIII. Riboflavin   53
  IX.   Niacin   54
  X.   Vitamin B_6 55
  XI.   Biotin   56
  XII.   Pantothenic Acid   56
  XIII. Folate   57
  XIV.   Vitamin B_{12} 59
  XV.   General Properties of the Vitamins   60
  XVI.   Physiological Utilization of the Vitamins   64
  XVII. Metabolism of the Vitamins   69
  XVIII. Metabolic Functions of the Vitamins   72
         Study Questions and Exercises   73
         Recommended Reading   73

Chapter 4 Vitamin Deficiency   75
  I.   The Concept of Vitamin Deficiency   76
  II.   The Many Causes of Vitamin
        Deficiencies   78
  III. Clinical Manifestations of Vitamin
        Deficiencies   79
  IV.   Vitamin Deficiency Diseases:
        Manifestations of Biochemical Lesions   86
        Study Questions and Exercises   92
        Recommended Reading   92

PART II. CONSIDERING THE INDIVIDUAL VITAMINS

Chapter 5 Vitamin A   95
  I.   Significance of Vitamin A   96
  II.   Sources of Vitamin A   97
  III. Absorption of Vitamin A   99
  IV.   Transport of Vitamin A   102
  V.   Metabolism of Vitamin A   109
  VI.   Excretion of Vitamin A   113
  VII. Metabolic Functions of Vitamin A   113
  VIII. Vitamin A Deficiency   130
  IX.   Vitamin A Toxicity   135
  X.   Case Studies   139
        Study Questions and Exercises   141
        Recommended Reading   141

Chapter 6   Vitamin D   **145**
    I.   Significance of Vitamin D   146
    II.   Sources of Vitamin D   147
    III.   Enteric Absorption of Vitamin D   150
    IV.   Transport of Vitamin D   151
    V.   Metabolism of Vitamin D   154
    VI.   Metabolic Functions of Vitamin D   157
    VII.   Vitamin D Deficiency   169
    VIII.   Vitamin D Toxicity   175
    IX.   Case Studies   176
      Study Questions and Exercises   177
      Recommended Reading   177

Chapter 7   Vitamin E   **181**
    I.   Significance of Vitamin E   182
    II.   Sources of Vitamin E   182
    III.   Absorption of Vitamin E   184
    IV.   Transport of Vitamin E   185
    V.   Metabolism of Vitamin E   189
    VI.   Metabolic Functions of Vitamin E   191
    VII.   Vitamin E Deficiency   206
    VIII.   Pharmacologic Uses of Vitamin E   207
    IX.   Vitamin E Toxicity   208
    X.   Case Studies   210
      Study Questions and Exercises   211
      Recommended Reading   212

Chapter 8   Vitamin K   **213**
    I.   The Significance of Vitamin K   214
    II.   Sources of Vitamin K   214
    III.   Absorption of Vitamin K   216
    IV.   Transport of Vitamin K   217
    V.   Metabolism of Vitamin K   218
    VI.   Metabolic Functions of Vitamin K   221
    VII.   Vitamin K Deficiency   227
    VIII.   Vitamin K Toxicity   229
    IX.   Case Studies   230
      Study Questions and Exercises   232
      Recommended Reading   232

Chapter 9   Vitamin C   **235**
    I.   The Significance of Vitamin C   236
    II.   Sources of Vitamin C   236
    III.   Absorption of Vitamin C   239
    IV.   Transport of Vitamin C   240
    V.   Metabolism of Vitamin C   241
    VI.   Metabolic Functions of Vitamin C   243
    VII.   Vitamin C Deficiency   254
    VIII.   Pharmacological Uses of Vitamin C   257
    IX.   Vitamin C Toxicity   258
    X.   Case Studies   260
      Study Questions and Exercises   262
      Recommended Reading   263

Chapter 10   Thiamin   **265**
    I.   The Significance of Thiamin   266
    II.   Sources of Thiamin   266
    III.   Absorption of Thiamin   268
    IV.   Transport of Thiamin   269
    V.   Metabolism of Thiamin   269
    VI.   Metabolic Functions of Thiamin   270
    VII.   Thiamin Deficiency   274
    VIII.   Thiamin Toxicity   278
    IX.   Case Studies   278
      Study Questions and Exercises   280
      Recommended Reading   280

Chapter 11   Riboflavin   **281**
    I.   The Significance of Riboflavin   282
    II.   Sources of Riboflavin   282
    III.   Absorption of Riboflavin   283
    IV.   Transport of Riboflavin   284
    V.   Metabolism of Riboflavin   285
    VI.   Metabolic Functions of Riboflavin   287
    VII.   Riboflavin Deficiency   288
    VIII.   Riboflavin Toxicity   293
    IX.   Case Study   293
      Study Questions and Exercises   294
      Recommended Reading   294

Chapter 12   Niacin   **295**
    I.   The Significance of Niacin   296
    II.   Sources of Niacin   296
    III.   Absorption of Niacin   298
    IV.   Transport of Niacin   298
    V.   Metabolism of Niacin   299
    VI.   Metabolic Functions of Niacin   303
    VII.   Niacin Deficiency   304
    VIII.   Pharmacologic Uses of Niacin   307
    IX.   Niacin Toxicity   309
    X.   Case Study   309
      Study Questions and Exercises   310
      Recommended Reading   311

Chapter 13   Vitamin B_6   **313**
    I.   The Significance of Vitamin B_6 314
    II.   Sources of Vitamin B_6 314
    III.   Absorption of Vitamin B_6 316
    IV.   Transport of Vitamin B_6 316
    V.   Metabolism of Vitamin B_6 317
    VI.   Metabolic Functions of Vitamin B_6 318
    VII.   Vitamin B_6 Deficiency   323
    VIII.   Pharmacologic Uses of Vitamin B_6 326
    IX.   Vitamin B_6 Toxicity   327
    X.   Case Studies   327
      Study Questions and Exercises   329
      Recommended Reading   329

Chapter 14   Biotin   **331**
   I. The Significance of Biotin   331
   II. Sources of Biotin   332
   III. Absorption of Biotin   334
   IV. Transport of Biotin   334
   V. Metabolism of Biotin   335
   VI. Metabolic Functions of Biotin   336
   VII. Biotin Deficiency   338
   VIII. Biotin Toxicity   341
   IX. Case Study   341
     Study Questions and Exercises   343
     Recommended Reading   344

Chapter 15   Pantothenic Acid   **345**
   I. The Significance of Pantothenic Acid   345
   II. Sources of Pantothenic Acid   346
   III. Absorption of Pantothenic Acid   347
   IV. Transport of Pantothenic Acid   347
   V. Metabolism of Pantothenic Acid   348
   VI. Metabolic Functions of
     Pantothenic Acid   350
   VII. Pantothenic Acid Deficiency   352
   VIII. Pantothenic Acid Toxicity   353
   IX. Case Study   353
     Study Questions and Exercises   354
     Recommended Reading   354

Chapter 16   Folate   **355**
   I. The Significance of Folate   356
   II. Sources of Folate   356
   III. Absorption of Folate   358
   IV. Transport of Folate   360
   V. Metabolism of Folate   362
   VI. Metabolic Functions of Folate   365
   VII. Folate Deficiency   375
   VIII. Pharmacologic Uses of Folate   377
   IX. Folate Toxicity   377
   X. Case Study   378
     Study Questions and Exercises   379
     Recommended Reading   379

Chapter 17   Vitamin B_{12}   **381**
   I. The Significance of Vitamin B_{12} 382
   II. Sources of Vitamin B_{12} 382
   III. Absorption of Vitamin B_{12} 383
   IV. Transport of Vitamin B_{12} 385
   V. Metabolism of Vitamin B_{12} 386
   VI. Metabolic Functions of Vitamin B_{12} 387
   VII. Vitamin B_{12} Deficiency   388
   VIII. Vitamin B_{12} Toxicity   395
   IX. Case Study   395
     Study Questions and Exercises   397
     Recommended Reading   397

Chapter 18   Quasi-vitamins   **399**
   I. Is the List of Vitamins Complete?   400
   II. Choline   401
   III. Carnitine   406
   IV. *myo*-Inositol   413
   V. Pyrroloquinoline Quinone   418
   VI. Ubiquinones   420
   VII. Flavonoids   422
   VIII. Non-Provitamin A Carotenoids   425
   IX. Orotic Acid   428
   X. *p*-Aminobenzoic Acid   429
   XI. Lipoic Acid   429
   XII. Ineffective Factors   430
   XIII. Unidentified Growth Factors   431
     Study Questions and Exercises   431
     Recommended Reading   432

**PART III.   USING CURRENT KNOWLEDGE
         OF THE VITAMINS**

Chapter 19   Sources of the Vitamins   **437**
   I. Vitamins in Foods   437
   II. Vitamin Contents of Feedstuffs   441
   III. Predicting Vitamin Contents   441
   IV. Vitamin Bioavailability   448
   V. Vitamin Losses   449
   VI. Vitamin Supplementation and
     Fortification of Foods   451
   VII. Vitamins in Human Diets   454
   VIII. Vitamin Supplements   457
   IX. Vitamin Labeling of Foods   459
   X. Vitamins in Livestock Feeds   461
     Study Questions and Exercises   466
     Recommended Reading   467

Chapter 20   Assessing Vitamin Status   **469**
   I. General Aspects of Nutritional
     Assessment   469
   II. Assessment of Vitamin Status   471
   III. Vitamin Status of Human
     Populations   474
     Study Questions and Exercises   483
     Recommended Reading   484

Chapter 21   Quantifying Vitamin Needs   **485**
   I. Dietary Standards   485
   II. Determining Dietary Standards
     for Vitamins   486
   III. Factors Affecting Vitamin Requirements   487
   IV. Vitamin Allowances for Humans   494
   V. Vitamin Allowances for Animals   498
     Study Questions and Exercises   502
     Recommended Reading   502

Chapter 22   Vitamin Safety   **503**
    I. Uses of Vitamins above Required Levels   503
   II. Hazards of Excessive Vitamin Intakes   504
 III. Signs of Hypervitaminoses   505
 IV. Safe Intakes of Vitamins   510
      Study Questions and Exercises   513
      Recommended Reading   514

Appendices
Appendix A   Vitamin Terminology: Past and Present   515
Appendix B   Original Reports for Case Studies   519

Appendix C   A Core of Current Vitamin Research
             Literature   521
Appendix D   Vitamin Contents of Foods   527
Appendix E   Vitamin Contents of Feedstuffs   561

Index   **565**

Online companion site:
http://books.elsevier.com/companions/9780121834937

Preface

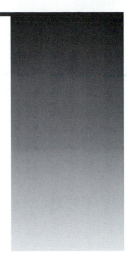

I am delighted to have the chance of producing a third edition of *The Vitamins*. Because the previous editions were well received, I have not changed the basic format in writing this edition. *The Vitamins* remains a book designed for use in an academic course on the topic; thus, I retained its conceptual orientation. But the book is also intended to serve as a ready reference for nutritionists, dieticians, food scientists, clinicians, and other professionals in the biomedical and health communities. For this reason, I have expanded its depth of coverage in several areas, particularly those related to the health effects associated with vitamin status and/or use. In so doing, I also increased the documentation provided by footnoting important findings with citations from the primary literature. I made such revisions to each chapter based on recent research findings. Therefore, it is of interest to note that generally the chapters I expanded most were those to which I had made the most significant changes in preparing the second edition: vitamin A (5), vitamin D (6), vitamin E (7), vitamin C (8), and folate (16). To this list I add the chapters on quasi-vitamins (19) and quantifying vitamin requirements (20). I revised the coverage of the quasi-vitamins with an expanded discussion of flavonoids and a new section on non-provitamin A carotenoids (lycopene, xanthophylls, etc.) both of which areas are the subject of interesting current research. I completed the vitamin requirements chapters with expanded information about the Dietary Reference Intakes (DRIs), not all of which had been published by the time the second edition went to press.

I appreciate the supportive efforts of my editors, Chuck Crumley, Mara Conner, and Julie Ochs. Working with each has been a pleasure.

There is a saying that "to teach is to learn twice." I find that to be the case for writing a book of this nature; it is, after all, a form of teaching. So it is that I have taken from this effort an understanding about the vitamins much deeper than I could otherwise have gained. Certainly, that justifies the weekends and evenings spent wading through the stacks and stacks and stacks of scientific papers, books, and reviews filling my study. I enjoyed this work. I hope you will find it useful.

G. F. Combs, Jr.
Grand Forks, North Dakota
October 2006

The companion Web site containing an image collection, links, errata, and author information to complement the text can be found at http://books.elsevier.com/companions/9780121834937.

Preface to the Second Edition

Since writing the first edition of *The Vitamins*, I have had a chance to reflect on that work and on the comments I have received from Cornell students and from various other instructors and health professionals who have used it at other institutions. This, of course, has been an appropriately humbling experience that has focused my thinking on ways to improve the book. In writing the second edition I have tried to make those improvements, but I have not changed the general format, which I have found to facilitate using the book as a classroom text.

Those familiar with the first edition will find the revision to be expanded and more detailed in presentation in several ways. The most important changes involve updating to include new information that has emerged recently, particularly important findings in the areas of molecular biology and clinical medicine. This has included the addition of key research results, many in tabular form, and the expansion of the footnote system to include citations to important research papers. The reference lists following each chapter have been expanded, but these citations include mainly key research reviews, as in the first edition. While each chapter has been expanded in these ways, the most significant changes were made in the chapters on vitamin A (5), vitamin D (6), vitamin E (7), vitamin C (8), and folate (16), which areas have experienced the most rapid recent developments. Some smaller changes have been made in the structures of the vitamin chapters (5–18): each has been given an internal table of contents; an overview of the general significance of the vitamin in nutrition and health has been included; the topics of deficiency and toxicity are discussed under separate headings.

Perhaps the most striking aspect of the second edition will be its professional layout. That reflects the contributions of the editors and staff at Academic Press. They have made of this revision a book that is not only more handsome but also, I believe, easier to use than was the first edition which I laid out on my own computer. I am grateful to Charlotte Brabants and Chuck Crumley, who handled *The Vitamins,* for their professionalism and for their patience. I am also grateful to my wife, Dr. Barbara Combs, for her suggestions for the design and use of a teaching text in a discussion-based learning environment, as well as for her understanding in giving up so many weekends and evenings to my work on this project

The Vitamins remains a book intended for use by nutrition instructors, graduate students in nutrition, dietetics, food science and medicine, clinicians, biomedical scientists, and other health professionals. It can be used as a teaching text or as a desk reference. It is my hope that it will be used—that it will become one of those highly annotated, slightly tattered, note-stuffed volumes that can be found on many bookshelves.

G. F. Combs, Jr.
Ithaca, New York
August 1997

Preface to the First Edition

I have found it to be true that one learns best what one has to teach. And because I have had no formal training either in teaching or in the field of education in general, it was not for several years of my own teaching that I began to realize that the good teacher must understand more than the subject matter of his or her course. In my case, that realization developed, over a few years, with the recognition that individuals learn in different ways and that the process of learning itself is as relevant to my teaching as the material I present. This enlightenment has been for me invaluable because it has led me to the field of educational psychology from which I have gained at least some of the insights of the good teacher. In fact, it led me to write this book.

In exploring that field, I came across two books that have influenced me greatly: *A Theory of Education*[1] by another Cornell professor, Joe Novak, and *Learning How to Learn*[2] by Professor Novak and his colleague Bob Gowin. I highly recommend their work to any scientific "expert" in the position of teaching within the area of his or her expertise. From those books and conversations with Professor Novak, I have come to understand that people think (and, therefore, learn) in terms of *concepts*, not facts. Therefore, for the past few years I have experimented in offering my course at Cornell University, "The Vitamins," in ways that are more concept-centered than I (or others, for that matter) have used previously. While I regard this experiment as an ongoing activity, it has already resulted in my shifting away from the traditional lecture format to one based on open classroom discussions aimed at involving the students, each of whom, I have found, brings a valuable personal perspective to discussions. I have found this to be particularly true for discussions concerning the vitamins; while it is certainly possible in modern societies to be misinformed about nutrition, it is virtually impossible to be truly naive. In other words, every person brings to the study of the vitamins some relevant conceptual framework and it is, thus, the task of the teacher to build upon that framework by adding new concepts, establishing new linkages and modifying existing ones where appropriate.

It quickly became clear to me that my own notes, indeed, all other available reference texts on the subject of the vitamins, were insufficient to support a concept-centered approach to the subject. Thus, I undertook to write a new type of textbook on the vitamins, one that would be maximally valuable in this kind of teaching. In so doing, I tried to focus on the key concepts and to make the book itself useful in a practical sense. Because I find myself writing in virtually any book that I really use, I gave this text margins wide enough for the reader to do the same. Because I have found the technical vocabularies of many scientific fields to present formidable barriers to learning, I have listed what I regard as the most important technical terms at the beginning of each chapter and have used each in context. Because I intend this to be an accurate synopsis of present understanding but not a definitive reference to the original scientific literature, I have cited only current major reviews that I find useful to the student. Because I have found the discussion of real-world cases to enhance learning of the subject, I have included case reports that can be used as classroom exercises or student assignments. I have designed the text for use as background reading for a one-semester upper-level college course within a nutrition-related curriculum.

---

[1] Cornell University Press, Ithaca, NY, 1977, 324 pp.

[2] Cambridge University Press, New York, 1984, 199 pp.

In fact, I have used draft versions in my course at Cornell as a means of refining it for this purpose.

While *The Vitamins* was intended primarily for use in teaching, I recognize that it will also be useful as a desk reference for nutritionists, dieticians and many physicians, veterinarians, and other health professionals. Indeed, I have been gratified by the comments I have received from colleagues to that effect.

It is my hope that *The Vitamins* will be read, reread, written in, and thought over. It seems to me that a field as immensely fascinating as the vitamins demands nothing less.

G. F. Combs, Jr.
Ithaca, New York
August 1991

How to Use This Book

The Vitamins is intended as a teaching text for an upper-level college course within a nutrition or health-related curriculum; however, it will also be useful as a desk reference or as a workbook for self-paced study of the vitamins. It has several features that are designed to enhance its usefulness to students as well as instructors.

To the Student

Before reading each chapter, take a few moments to go over the **Anchoring Concepts** and **Learning Objectives** listed on the chapter title page. *Anchoring Concepts* are the ideas fundamental to the subject matter of the chapter; they are the concepts to which the new ones presented in the chapter will be related. The *Anchoring Concepts* identified in the first several chapters should already be very familiar to you; if they are not, then it will be necessary for you to do some background reading or discussion until you feel comfortable in your understanding of these basic ideas. You will find that most chapters are designed to build on the understanding gained through previous chapters; in most cases, the *Anchoring Concepts* of a chapter relate to the *Learning Objectives* of previous chapters. Pay attention to the *Learning Objectives*; they are the key elements of understanding that the chapter is intended to support. Keeping the *Learning Objectives* in mind as you go through each chapter will help you maintain focus on the key concepts. Next, read through the **Vocabulary** list and *mark* any terms that are unfamiliar or about which you feel unsure. Then, as you read through the text, look for them; you should be able to get a good feel for their meanings from the contexts of their uses. If this is not sufficient for any particular term, then you should consult a good medical or scientific dictionary.

As you go through the text, note what information the layout is designed to convey. First, note that the major sections of each chapter are indicated with a bold heading above a bar, and that the wide left margin contains key words and phrases that relate to the major topic of the text at that point. These features are designed to help you *scan* for particular information. Also note that the footnoted information is largely supplementary but not essential to the understanding of the key concepts presented. Therefore, the text may be read at two levels: at the basic level, one should be able to ignore the footnotes and still get the key concepts; at the more detailed level, one should be able to pick up more of the background information from the footnotes.

Chapters 5–17 are each followed by a **Case Study** comprised of one or more clinical case reports abstracted from the medical literature. For each case, use the associated questions to focus your thinking on the features that relate to vitamin functions. As you do so, try to ignore the obvious connection with the subject of the chapter; put yourself in the position of the attending physician who was called upon to diagnose the problem without prior knowledge that it involved any particular nutrient, much less a certain vitamin. You may find the additional case studies in Appendix B similarly interesting.

Take some time and go through the **Study Questions and Exercises** at the end of each chapter. These, too, are designed to direct your thinking back to the key concepts of each chapter and to facilitate integration of those concepts with those you already have. To this end, you are asked in this section of several chapters to prepare a *concept map* of the subject matter. Many people find the *concept map* to be a powerful learning tool; therefore, if you have had no previous experience with this device, then it will be well worth your while to consult *Learning How to Learn*.[1]

At the end of each chapter is a reading list. With the exception of Chapter 2, which lists papers of landmark significance to the discovery of the vitamins, the reading lists consist of key reviews in prominent scientific journals. Thus, while primary research reports are not cited in the text, you should be able to trace research papers on topics of specific interest through the reviews that are listed.

Last, but certainly not least, have *fun* with this fascinating aspect of the field of nutrition!

To the Instructor

I hope you will find this format and presentation useful in your teaching of the vitamins. To that end, some of my experiences in using *The Vitamins* as a text for my course at Cornell may be of interest to you.

I have found that *every* student comes to the study of the vitamins with *some* background knowledge of the subject, although those backgrounds are generally incomplete, frequently with substantial areas of no information and misinformation. This is true for upper-level nutrition majors and for students from other fields, the difference being largely one of magnitude. This is also true for instructors, most of whom come to the field with specific expertise that relates to only a subset of the subject matter. In addition, I have found that, by virtue of having at least *some* background on the subject and being motivated by any of a number of reasons to learn more, *every* student brings to the study of the vitamins a unique perspective that may not be readily apparent to the instructor.

I am convinced that meaningful learning is served when both instructor and students come to understand each others' various perspectives. This has two benefits in teaching the vitamins. First, it is in the instructor's interest to know the students' ideas and levels of understanding concerning issues of vitamin need, vitamin function, and the like, such that these can be built upon and modified as may be appropriate. Second, I have found that many upper-level students have interesting experiences (through personal or family histories, their own research, information from other courses, etc.) that can be valuable contributions to classroom discussions, thus mitigating

against the "instructor knows all" notion, which we all know to be false. To identify student perspectives, I have found it useful to assign on the first class period for submission at the second class a written autobiographical sketch. I distribute one I wrote for this purpose, and I ask each student to write "as much or as little" as he or she cares to, recognizing that I will distribute copies of whatever is submitted to each student in the class. The biographical sketches that I see range from a few sentences that reveal little of a personal nature to longer ones that provide many good insights about their authors; I have found *every one* to help me get to know my students personally and to get a better idea of their understandings of the vitamins and of their expectations of my course. The exercise serves the students in a similar manner, thus promoting a group dynamic that facilitates classroom discussions.

I have come to use *The Vitamins* in my teaching as the text from which I make regular reading assignments, usually a chapter at a time, as preparation for each class, which I generally conduct in an open discussion format. Long ago, I found it difficult, if not impossible, to cover in a traditional lecture format all of the information about the vitamins I deemed important for a nutritionist to know. Thus, I have put that information in this text and have shifted more of the responsibility for learning to the student for gleaning it from reading. I use my class time to assist the student by providing discussions of issues of particular interest or concern. Often, this means that certain points were not clear upon reading or that the reading itself stimulated questions not specifically addressed in the text. Usually, these questions are nicely handled by eliciting the views and understandings of other students and by my giving supplementary information. Therefore, my class preparation involves the collation of research data that will supplement the discussion in the text and the identification of questions that I can use to initiate discussions. In developing my questions, I have found it useful to prepare my own concept maps of the subject matter and to ask rather simple questions about the linkages between concepts, for example, "How does the mode of enteric absorption of the tocopherols relate to what we know about its physiochemical properties?" If you are unfamiliar with concept mapping, then I strongly recommend your consulting *Learning*

---

[1] Novak, J. D., and Gowin, D. B. (1984). *Learning How to Learn*. Cambridge University Press, New York, 199 pp.

How to Learn and experimenting with the technique to determine whether it can assist you in your teaching.

I have found it useful to give weekly written assignments for which I use the **Study Questions and Exercises** or **Case Studies**. In my experience, regular assignments keep students focused on the topic and prevent them from letting the course slide until exam time. More importantly, I believe there to be learning associated with the thought that necessarily goes into these written assignments. In order to support that learning, I make a point of going over each assignment briefly at the beginning of the class at which it is due, and of returning it by the *next* class with my written comments on *each* paper. You will find that the *Case Studies* I have included are abstracted from actual clinical reports; however, I have presented them without some of the pertinent clinical findings (e.g., responses to treatments) that were originally reported, in order to make of them learning exercises. I have found that students do well on these assignments and that they particularly enjoy the *Case Studies*. For that reason, I have included in the revised edition additional case studies in Appendix B; I encourage you to use them in class discussions.

I evaluate student performance on the basis of class participation, weekly written assignments, a review of a recent research paper, and either one or two examinations (i.e., either a final or a final plus a midterm). In order to allow each student to pursue a topic of specific individual interest, I ask them to review a research paper published within the last year, using the style of *Nutrition Reviews*. I evaluate each review for its critical analysis as well as on the importance of the paper that was selected, which I ask them to discuss. This assignment has also been generally well received. Because many students are inexperienced in research and thus feel uncomfortable in criticizing it, I have found it helpful to conduct in advance of the assignment a discussion dealing with the general principles of experimental design and statistical inference. Because I have adopted a concept-oriented teaching style, I long ago abandoned the use of short-answer questions (e.g., "Name the species that require dietary sources of vitamin C") on examinations. Instead, I use brief case descriptions and actual experimental data and ask for diagnostic strategies, development of hypotheses, design of means of hypothesis testing, interpretation of results and the like. Many students may prefer the more traditional short-answer test; however, I have found that such inertia can be overcome by using examples in class discussions or homework assignments.

The Vitamins has been of great value in enhancing my teaching of the course by that name at Cornell. Thus, it is my sincere wish that it will assist you similarly in your teaching. I have been helped very much by the comments on the previous editions, which I have received both from my students and from instructors and others who have used this book. Please let me know how it meets your needs.

G. F. Combs, Jr.

PERSPECTIVES ON THE VITAMINS IN NUTRITION

I

What Is a Vitamin?

1

Imagination is more important than knowledge.
— A. Einstein

I.	Thinking about Vitamins	3
II.	Vitamin: A Revolutionary Concept	4
III.	An Operating Definition of a Vitamin	4
IV.	The Recognized Vitamins	5
	Study Questions	6

Vocabulary

Vitamine
Vitamin
Vitamer
Provitamin

Anchoring Concepts

1. Certain factors, called *nutrients*, are necessary for normal physiological function of animals, including humans. Some nutrients cannot be synthesized adequately by the host and must, therefore, be obtained from the external chemical environment; these are referred to as *dietary essential nutrients*.
2. *Diseases* involving physiological dysfunction, often accompanied by morphological changes, can result from insufficient intake of dietary essential nutrients.

Learning Objectives

1. To understand the classic meaning of the term *vitamin* as it is used in the field of nutrition.
2. To understand that the term *vitamin* describes both a concept of fundamental importance in nutrition and any member of a rather heterogeneous array of nutrients, any one of which may not fully satisfy the classic definition.
3. To understand that some compounds are vitamins for one species and not another; and that some are vitamins only under specific dietary or environmental conditions.
4. To understand the concepts of a *vitamer* and a *provitamin*.

I. Thinking about Vitamins

Among the nutrients required for the many physiologic functions essential to life are the vitamins. Unlike other classes of nutrients, the vitamins do not serve structural functions, nor does their catabolism provide significant energy. Instead, their various uses each tend to be highly specific, and, for that reason, the vitamins are required in only small amounts in the diet. The common food forms of most vitamins require some metabolic activation to their functional forms.

Although the vitamins share these general characteristics, they show few close chemical or functional similarities, their categorization as vitamins being strictly empirical. Consider also that, whereas several vitamins function as enzyme cofactors (vitamins A, K, and C, thiamin, niacin, riboflavin, vitamin B_6, biotin, pantothenic acid, folate, and vitamin B_{12}), not all enzyme cofactors are vitamins.[1] Some vitamins function as biological antioxidants (vitamins E and C), and several function as cofactors in metabolic oxidation–reduction reactions (vitamins E, K, and C, niacin, riboflavin, and pantothenic acid). Two vitamins (vitamins A and D) function as hormones; one of them (vitamin A) also serves as a photoreceptive cofactor in vision.

---

[1] Other enzyme cofactors are biosynthesized (e.g., heme, coenzyme Q, and lipoic acid).

II. Vitamin: A Revolutionary Concept

Everyday Word or Revolutionary Idea?

The term *vitamin*, today a common word in everyday language, was born of a revolution in thinking about the interrelationships of diet and health that occurred at the beginning of the twentieth century. That revolution involved the growing realization of two phenomena that are now so well understood that they are taken for granted even by the layperson:

1. Diets are sources of many important nutrients.
2. Low intakes of specific nutrients can cause certain diseases.

In today's world, each of these concepts may seem self-evident; but in a world still responding to and greatly influenced by the important discoveries in microbiology made in the nineteenth century, each represented a major departure from contemporaneous thinking in the area of health. Nineteenth-century physiologists perceived foods and diets as being sources of only five types of nutrients: *protein, fat, carbohydrate, ash,*[2] and *water*. After all, these accounted for very nearly 100% of the mass of most foods. With this view, it is understandable that, at the turn of the century, experimental findings that now can be seen as indicating the presence of hitherto unrecognized nutrients were interpreted instead as substantiating the presence of natural antidotes to unidentified disease-causing microbes.

Important discoveries in science have ways of directing, even entrapping, one's view of the world; resisting this tendency depends on critical and constantly questioning minds. That such minds were involved in early nutrition research is evidenced by the spirited debates and frequent polemics that ensued over discoveries of apparently beneficial new dietary factors. Still, the systematic development of what emerged as nutritional science depended on a new intellectual construct for interpreting such experimental observations.

Vitamin or Vitamine?

The elucidation of the nature of what was later to be called *thiamin* occasioned the proposition of just such a new construct in physiology.[3] Aware of the impact of what was a departure from prevailing thought, its author, the Polish biochemist Casimir Funk, chose to generalize from his findings on the chemical nature of that "vital amine" to suggest the term **vitamine** as a generic descriptor for many such *accessory factors* associated with diets. That the factors soon to be elucidated comprised a somewhat chemically heterogeneous group, not all of which were nitrogenous, does not diminish the importance of the introduction of what was first presented as the *vitamine theory*, later to become a key concept in nutrition: the vitamin.

The term *vitamin* has been defined in various ways. While the very concept of a vitamin was crucial to progress in understanding nutrition, the actual definition of a vitamin has evolved in consequence of that understanding.

III. An Operating Definition of a Vitamin

For the purposes of the study of this aspect of nutrition, a vitamin is defined as follows:

A **vitamin** …

- Is an *organic compound* distinct from fats, carbohydrates, and proteins
- Is a *natural component of foods* in which it is usually present in minute amounts
- Is essential, also usually in minute amounts, for *normal physiological function* (i.e., maintenance, growth, development, and/or production)
- Causes, by its absence or underutilization, a *specific deficiency syndrome*
- Is *not synthesized by the host* in amounts adequate to meet normal physiological needs

This definition will be useful in the study of vitamins, as it effectively distinguishes this class of nutrients from others (e.g., proteins and amino acids, essential

---

[2] The residue from combustion (i.e., minerals).

[3] This is a clear example of what T. H. Kuhn called a "scientific revolution" (*The Structure of Scientific Revolutions*, 1968), that is, the discarding of an old paradigm with the invention of a new one.

fatty acids, and minerals) and indicates the needs in various normal physiological functions. It also points out the specificity of deficiency syndromes by which the vitamins were discovered. Furthermore, it places the vitamins in that portion of the chemical environment on which animals (including humans) must depend for survival, thus distinguishing vitamins from hormones.

Some Caveats

It will quickly become clear, however, that, despite its usefulness, this operating definition has serious limitations, notably with respect to the last clause, for many species can indeed synthesize at least some of the vitamins. Four examples illustrate this point:

> *Vitamin C*   Most animal species have the ability to synthesize ascorbic acid. Only those few that lack the enzyme L-gulonolactone oxidase (e.g., the guinea pig, humans) cannot; only for them can ascorbic acid properly be called *vitamin C*.
>
> *Vitamin D*   Individuals exposed to modest amounts of sunlight can produce cholecalciferol, which functions as a hormone. Only individuals without sufficient exposure to ultraviolet light (e.g., livestock raised in indoor confinement, people spending most of their days indoors) require dietary sources of *vitamin D*.
>
> *Choline*   Most animal species have the metabolic capacity to synthesize choline; however, some (e.g., the chick, the rat) may not be able to employ that capacity if they are fed insufficient amounts of methyl-donor compounds. In addition, some (e.g., the chick) do not develop that capacity fully until they are several weeks of age. Thus, for the young chick and for individuals of other species fed

diets providing limited methyl groups, *choline* is a vitamin.

> *Niacin*   All animal species can synthesize nicotinic acid mononucleotide (NMN) from the amino acid tryptophan. Only those for which this metabolic conversion is particularly inefficient (e.g., the cat, fishes) and others fed low dietary levels of tryptophan require a dietary source of *niacin*.

With these counterexamples in mind, the definition of a vitamin can be understood as having specific connotations to animal species, stage of development, diet or nutritional status, and physical environmental conditions.[4]

The *vitamin caveat*:

- Some compounds are vitamins for one species and not another.
- Some compounds are vitamins only under specific dietary or environmental conditions.

IV. The Recognized Vitamins

Thirteen substances or groups of substances are now generally recognized as vitamins (see Table 1-1); others have been proposed.[5] In some cases, the familiar name is actually the generic descriptor for a family of chemically related compounds having qualitatively comparable metabolic activities. For example, the term *vitamin E* refers to those analogs of tocol or tocotrienol[6] that are active in preventing such syndromes as fetal resorption in the rat and myopathies in the chick. In these cases, the members of the same vitamin family are called **vitamers**. Some carotenoids can be metabolized to yield the metabolically active form of vitamin A; such a precursor of an actual vitamin is called a **provitamin**.

---

[4] For this reason it is correct to talk about vitamin C for the nutrition of humans but ascorbic acid for the nutrition of livestock.

[5] These include such factors as inositol, carnitine, bioflavonoids, pangamic acid, and laetrile, for some of which there is evidence of vitamin-like activity (see Chapter 19).

[6] Tocol is 3,4-dihydro-2-methyl-2-(4,8,12-trimethyltridecyl)-6-chromanol; tocotrienol is the analog with double bonds at the 3', 7', and 11' positions on the phytol side chain. See Chapter 7.

Table 1.1   The vitamins: their vitamers, provitamins, and functions

Group	Vitamers	Provitamins	Physiological functions
Vitamin A	Retinol Retinal Retinoic acid	β-Carotene Cryptoxanthin	Visual pigments; epithelial cell differentiation
Vitamin D	Cholecalciferol (D_3) Ergocalciferol (D_2)		Calcium homeostasis; bone metabolism
Vitamin E	α-Tocopherol γ-Tocopherol		Membrane antioxidant
Vitamin K	Phylloquinones (K_1) Menaquinones (K_2) Menadione (K_3)		Blood clotting; calcium metabolism
Vitamin C	Ascorbic acid Dehydroascorbic acid		Reductant in hydroxylations in the formation of collagen and carnitine, and in the metabolism of drugs and steroids
Vitamin B_1	Thiamin		Coenzyme for decarboxylations of 2-keto acids (e.g., pyruvate) and transketolations
Vitamin B_2	Riboflavin		Coenzyme in redox reactions of fatty acids and the tricarboxylic acid (TCA) cycle
Niacin	Nicotinic acid Nicotinamide		Coenzyme for several dehydrogenases
Vitamin B_6	Pyridoxol Pyridoxal Pyridoxamine		Coenzyme in amino acid metabolism
Folic acid	Folic acid Polyglutamyl folacins		Coenzyme in single-carbon metabolism
Biotin	Biotin		Coenzyme for carboxylations
Pantothenic acid	Pantothenic acid		Coenzyme in fatty acid metabolism
Vitamin B_{12}	Cobalamin		Coenzyme in the metabolism of propionate, amino acids, and single-carbon units

Study Questions

1. What are the key features that define a vitamin?

2. What are the fundamental differences between vitamins and other classes of nutrients? between vitamins and hormones?

3. Using key words and phrases, list briefly what you know about each of the recognized vitamins.

Discovery of the Vitamins

2

When science is recognized as a framework of evolving concepts and contingent methods for gaining new knowledge, we see the very human character of science, for it is creative individuals operating from the totality of their experiences who enlarge and modify the conceptual framework of science.

—J. D. Novak

I.	The Emergence of Nutrition as a Science	8
II.	The Process of Discovery in Nutritional Science	8
III.	The Empirical Phase of Vitamin Discovery	9
IV.	The Experimental Phase of Vitamin Discovery	12
V.	The Vitamine Theory	15
VI.	Elucidation of the Vitamins	18
VII.	Vitamin Terminology	30
VIII.	Other Factors Sometimes Called Vitamins	31
IX.	The Modern History of the Vitamins	31
	Study Questions and Exercises	32
	Recommended Reading	32

Anchoring Concepts

1. A scientific theory is a plausible explanation for a set of observed phenomena; because theories cannot be tested directly, their acceptance relies on a preponderance of supporting evidence.
2. A scientific hypothesis is a tentative supposition that is assumed for the purposes of argument or testing and is, thus, used in the generation of evidence by which theories can be evaluated.
3. An empirical approach to understanding the world involves the generation of theories strictly by observation, whereas an experimental approach involves the undertaking of operations (experiments) to test the truthfulness of hypotheses.
4. Physiology is that branch of biology dealing with the processes, activities, and phenomena of life and living organisms, and biochemistry deals with the molecular bases for such phenomena. The field of nutrition, derived from both of these disciplines, deals with the processes by which animals or plants take in and utilize food substances.

Learning Objectives

1. To understand the nature of the process of discovery in the field of nutrition.
2. To understand the impact of the vitamine theory, as an intellectual construct, on that process of discovery.
3. To recognize the major forces in the emergence of nutrition as a science.
4. To understand that the discoveries of the vitamins proceeded along indirect lines, most often through the seemingly unrelated efforts of many people.
5. To know the key events in the discovery of each of the vitamins.
6. To become familiar with the basic terminology of the vitamins and their associated deficiency disorders.

Vocabulary

Accessory factor
Anemia
Animal model
Animal protein factor
Ascorbic acid
Beriberi
Biotin
Black tongue disease
β-Carotene
Cholecalciferol
Choline
Dermatitis
Ergocalciferol
Fat-soluble A
Filtrate factor
Flavin
Folic acid

Germ theory
Hemorrhage
Lactoflavin
Model
Niacin
Night blindness
Ovoflavin
Pantothenic acid
Pellagra
Polyneuritis
Prothrombin
Provitamin
Purified diet
Pyridoxine
Repeatability
Relevance
Retinen
Riboflavin
Rickets
Scurvy
Thiamin
Vitamin
Vitamin A
Vitamin B
Vitamin B_2
Vitamin B complex
Vitamin B_6
Vitamin B_{12}
Vitamin C
Vitamin D
Vitamin E
Vitamin K
Vitamine
Vitamine theory
Water-soluble B
Xerophthalmia

I. The Emergence of Nutrition as a Science

In the span of only five decades commencing at the very end of the nineteenth century, the vitamins were discovered. Their discoveries were the result of the activities of hundreds of people who can be viewed retrospectively as having followed discrete branches of intellectual growth. Those branches radiated from ideas originally derived inductively from observations in the natural world, each starting from the recognition of a relationship between diet and health. Subsequently, branches were pruned through repeated analysis and deduction, a process that both produced and proceeded from the fundamental approaches used in experimental nutrition today. Once pruned, the limb of discovery may appear straight to the naive observer. Scientific discovery, however, does not occur that way; rather, it tends to follow a zig-zag course, with many participants contributing many branches. In fact, the contemporaneous view of each participant may be that of a thicket of tangled hypotheses and facts. The seemingly straightforward appearance of the emergent limb of discovery is but an illusion achieved by discarding the dead branches of false starts and unsupported hypotheses, each of which can be instructive about the process of scientific discovery.

With the discovery of the vitamins, therefore, nutrition moved from a largely observational activity to one that relied increasingly on hypothesis testing through experimentation; it moved from empiricism to science. Both the process of scientific discovery and the course of the development of nutrition as a scientific discipline are perhaps best illustrated by the history of the discovery of the vitamins.

II. The Process of Discovery in Nutritional Science

Empiricism and Experiment

History shows that the process of scientific discovery starts with the synthesis of general ideas about the natural world from observations of particulars in it — an *empirical phase*. In the discovery of the vitamins, this initial phase was characterized by the recognition of associations between diet and human diseases, namely, night blindness, scurvy, beriberi, rickets, and pellagra, each of which was long prevalent in various societies. The next phase in the process of discovery involves the use of these generalizations to generate hypotheses that can be tested experimentally — the *experimental phase*. In the discovery of the vitamins, this phase necessitated the development of two key tools of modern experimental nutrition: the **animal model** and the **purified diet**. The availability of both of these tools proved to be necessary for the discovery of each vitamin; in cases where an animal model was late to be developed (e.g., for pellagra), the elucidation of the identity of the vitamin was substantially delayed.

III. The Empirical Phase of Vitamin Discovery

The major barrier to entering the empirical phase of nutritional inquiry proved to be the security provided by prescientific attitudes about foods that persisted through the nineteenth century. Many societies had observed that human populations in markedly contrasting parts of the world tend to experience similar health standards despite the fact that they subsist on very different diets. These observations were taken by nineteenth-century physiologists to indicate that health was not particularly affected by the kinds of foods consumed. Foods were thought important as sources of the only nutrients known at the time: *protein, available energy, ash,* and *water*. While the "chemical revolution" led by the French scientist Antoine Lavoisier, started probing the elemental components and metabolic fates of these nutrients, the widely read ideas of the German chemist Justus von Liebig[1] resulted in protein being regarded as the only real essential nutrient, supporting both tissue growth and repair as well as energy production. In the middle part of the century, attention was drawn further from potential relationships of diet and health by the major discoveries of Pasteur, Liebig, Koch, and others in microbiology. For the first time, several diseases, first anthrax and then others, could be understood in terms of a microbial etiology. By the end of the century, **germ theory**, which proved to be of immense value in medicine, directed hypotheses for the etiologies of most diseases. The impact of this understanding as a barrier to entering the inductive phase of nutritional discovery is illustrated by the case of the Dutch physician Christian Eijkman, who found a water-soluble factor from rice bran to prevent a beriberi-like disease in chickens (now known to be the vitamin thiamin) and concluded that he had found a "pharmacological antidote" against the beriberi "microbe" presumed to be present in rice.

Diseases Linked to Diet

Nevertheless, while they appeared to have little effect on the prevailing views concerning the etiology of human disease, by the late 1800s, several empirical associations had been made between diet and disease.

Diseases empirically associated with diet:

Scurvy	Corneal Ulceration
Beriberi	Rickets
Night Blindness	Pellagra

Scurvy

For several centuries it has been known that **scurvy**, the disease involving sore gums, painful joints, and multiple hemorrhages, could be prevented by including in the diet green vegetables or fruits. Descriptions of cases in such sources as the Eber papyrus (ca. 1150 B.C.) and the writings of Hippocrates (ca. 420 B.C.) are often cited to indicate that scurvy was prevalent in those ancient populations. Indeed, signs of the disease are said to have been found in the skeletal remains of primitive humans. Scurvy was common in northern Europe during the Middle Ages, a time when local agriculture provided few sources of vitamin C that lasted through the winter. Scurvy was very highly prevalent among seamen, who subsisted for months at a time on dried and salted foods. The Portuguese explorer Vasco da Gama reported losing more than 60% of his crew of 160 sailors in his voyage around the Cape of Good Hope in 1498. In 1535–1536, the French explorer Jacques Cartier reported that signs of scurvy were shown by all but three of his crew of 103 men (25 of whom died) during his second Newfoundland expedition. In 1593, the British admiral Richard Hawkins wrote that, during his career, he had seen some 10,000 seamen die of the disease.

Although the link between scurvy and preserved foods was long evident, the first report of a cure for the disease appears to have been Cartier's description of the rapidly successful treatment of his crew with an infusion of the bark of Arborvitae (*Thuja occidentalis*) prepared by the indigenous Hurons of Newfoundland. By 1601, the efficacy of regular consumption of citrus fruits or juices was recognized as a means of preventing the disease. In that year, the English privateer Sir James Lancaster introduced regular issues of such foods on the ships of the East India Company. However, recognizing the perishability of citrus fruits, and viewing

---

[1] In his widely read book *Animal Chemistry, or Organic Chemistry in Its Application to Physiology and Pathology*, Liebig argued that the energy needed for the contraction of muscles, in which he was able to find no carbohydrate or fat, must come only from the breakdown of protein. Protein, therefore, was the only true nutrient.

scurvy as a "putrid" disease in which affected tissues became alkaline, the prestigious College of Physicians in London stated that other acids could act as substitutes. Hence, British ship's surgeons were supplied with vitriol (sulfuric acid).

Against this background, a British naval surgeon, James Lind, later to be called the founder of modern naval hygiene, conducted what are now recognized as the first controlled clinical trials when, in 1746, he undertook to compare various therapies recommended for scurvy in British sailors at sea. Those experiments involved 12 sailors with scurvy, whom he assigned in pairs to a two-week regimen including lemons and oranges, dilute sulfuric acid, vinegar, or other putative remedies. Lind's results were clear: the pair treated with lemons and oranges recovered almost completely within six days, whereas no other treatment showed improvement. In 1753, he published his now-classic *Treatise on Scurvy*, which had great impact on the medical thought of the time as it detailed past work on the subject, most of which was anecdotal, and presented the results of his experiments. Although Lind believed that citrus contained "a saponaceous, attenuating and resolving virtue [detergent action]" that helped free skin perspiration that had become clogged by sea air, the power of his results, which came from the controlled nature of his experiment, established the value of fresh fruits in treating the disease. Accordingly, by 1804 the British navy had made it a regular practice to issue daily rations of lemon juice to all seamen—a measure that gave rise to the term *limey*[2] as a slang expression for a British seaman. In the early part of the nineteenth century, there remained no doubt of a dietary cause and cure of scurvy; still, it would be more than a century before its etiology and metabolic basis would be elucidated. Outbreaks of scurvy continued in cases of food shortages: in British prisons, during the California gold rush, among troops in the Crimean War, among prisoners in the American Civil War, and among citizens during the Siege of Paris (1871).

Beriberi

It is said that signs consistent with **beriberi** (e.g., initial weakness and loss of feeling in the legs leading to heart failure, breathlessness and, in some cases, edema) are described in ancient Chinese herbals (ca. 2600 B.C.). Certainly, beriberi, too, has been a historic disease prevalent in many Asian populations subsisting on diets in which polished (i.e., "white" or dehulled) rice is the major food. For example, in the 1860s, the Japanese navy experienced the disease affecting 30 to 40% of its seamen. Interesting clinical experiments conducted with sailors in the 1870s by Dr. Kanehiro Takaki, a British trained surgeon who later became director general of the Japanese Naval Medical Service, first noted an association between beriberi and diet: Japanese sailors were issued lower protein diets than their counterparts in European navies, which had not seen the disease. Takaki conducted an uncontrolled study at sea in which he modified sailors' rations to increase protein intake by including more meat, condensed milk, bread, and vegetables at the expense of rice. This cut both the incidence and severity of beriberi dramatically, which he interpreted as confirmation of the disease being caused by insufficient dietary protein. The adoption of Takaki's dietary recommendations by the Japanese navy was effective — eliminating the disease as a shipboard problem by 1880 — despite the fact that his conclusion, reasonable in the light of contemporaneous knowledge, later proved to be incorrect.

Rickets

Rickets, the disease of growing bones, manifests itself in children as deformations of the long bones (e.g., bowed legs, knock knees, curvatures of the upper and/or lower arms), swollen joints, and/or enlarged heads and is generally associated with the urbanization and industrialization of human societies. Its appearance on a wide scale was more recent and more restricted geographically than that of either scurvy or beriberi. The first written account of the disease is believed to be that of Daniel Whistler, who wrote on the subject in his medical thesis at Oxford University in 1645. A complete description of the disease was published shortly thereafter (in 1650) by the Cambridge professor Francis Glisson, so it is clear that by the middle of the seventeenth century rickets had become a public health problem in England. However, rickets appears not to have affected earlier societies, at least on such a scale. Studies in the late 1800s by the English physician T. A. Palm showed that the mummified remains of Egyptian dead bore no signs of the disease. By the

---

[2] It is a curious fact that lemons were often called *limes*, a source of confusion to many writers on this topic.

latter part of the nineteenth century, the incidence of rickets among children in London exceeded one-third; by the turn of the twentieth century, estimates of prevalence were as high as 80% and rickets had become known as the "English disease." Noting the absence of rickets in southern Europe, Palm in 1890 was the first to point out that rickets was prevalent only where there is relatively little sunlight (e.g., in the northern latitudes). He suggested that sunlight exposure prevented rickets; but others held that the disease had other causes, for example, heredity or syphilis. Through the turn of the twentieth century, much of the Western medical community remained either unaware or skeptical of a food remedy that had long been popular among the peoples of the Baltic and North Sea coasts and that had been used to treat adult rickets in the Manchester Infirmary by 1848: cod liver oil. Not until the 1920s would the confusion over the etiology of rickets become clear.

Pellagra

Pellagra, the disease characterized by lesions of the skin and mouth, and by gastrointestinal and mental disturbances, also became prevalent in human societies fairly recently. There appears to have been no record of the disease, even in folk traditions, before the eighteenth century. Its first documented description, in 1735, was that of the Spanish physician Gaspar Casal, whose observations were disseminated by the French physician François Thiery, whom he met some years later after having been appointed as physician to the court of King Philip V. In 1755, Thiery published a brief account of Casal's observations in the *Journal de Vandermonde*; this became the first published report on the disease. Casal's own description was included in his book on the epidemic and endemic diseases of northern Spain, *Historia Natural y Medico de el Principado de Asturias*, which was published in 1762, three years after his death. Casal regarded the disease popularly called *mal de la rosa* as a peculiar form of leprosy. He associated it with poverty and with the consumption of spoiled corn (maize).

In 1771, a similar dermatological disorder was described by the Italian physician Francesco Frapolli. In his work, *Animadversiones in Morbum Volgo Pelagrum*, he reported the disease to be prevalent in northern Italy. In that region corn, recently introduced from America, had become a popular crop, displacing rye as the major grain. The local name for the disease was *pelagra*, meaning rough skin. There is some evidence that it had been seen as early as 1740. At any rate, by 1784, the prevalence of *pelagra* (now spelled *pellagra*) in that area was so great that a hospital was established in Legano for its treatment. Success in the treatment of pellagra appears to have been attributed to factors other than diet, for example, rest, fresh air, water, sunshine. Nevertheless, the disease continued to be associated with poverty and the consumption of corn-based diets.

Following the finding of pellagra in Italy, the disease was reported in France by Hameau in 1829. It was not until 1845 that the French physician Roussel associated pellagra with Casal's *mal de la rosa* and proposed that these diseases, including a similar disease called *flemma salada*,[3] were related or identical. To substantiate his hypothesis, Roussel spent seven months of 1847 in the area where Casal had worked in northern Spain[4] investigating *mal de la rosa* cases; on his return, he presented to the French Academy of Medicine evidence in support of his conclusion. Subsequently, pellagra, as it had come to be called, was reported in Romania by Theodari in 1858 and in Egypt by Pruner Bey in 1874. It was a curiosity not to be explained for years that pellagra was never endemic in the Yucatán Peninsula where the cultivation of corn originated; the disease was not reported there until 1896.

It is not known how long pellagra had been endemic in the United States; however, it became common early in the twentieth century. In 1912, J. W. Babcock examined the records of the state hospital of South Carolina and concluded that the disease had occurred there as early as 1828. It is generally believed that pellagra also appeared during or after the American Civil War (1861–1865) in association with food shortages in the southern states. It is clear

---

[3] Literally meaning "salty phlegm," *flemma salada* involved gastrointestinal signs, delirium, and a form of dementia. It did not, however, occur in areas where maize was the major staple food; this and disagreement over the similarities of symptoms caused Roussel's proposal of a relationship between these diseases to be challenged by his colleague Arnault Costallat. From Costallat's letters describing *flemma salada* in Spain in 1861, it is apparent that he considered it to be a form of acrodynia, then thought to be due to ergot poisoning.

[4] Casal practiced in the town of Oviedo in the Asturias of northern Spain.

from George Searcy's 1907 report to the American Medical Association that the disease was endemic at least in Alabama. By 1909, it had been identified in more than 20 states, several of which had empaneled Pellagra Commissions, and a national conference on the disease was held in South Carolina.

Since it first appeared, pellagra was associated with poverty and with the dependence on corn as the major staple food. Ideas arose early on that it was caused by a toxin associated with spoiled corn; yet, by the turn of the twentieth century, other hypotheses were also popular. These included the suggestion of an infectious agent with, perhaps, an insect vector.

Ideas Prevalent by 1900

Thus, by the beginning of the twentieth century, four different diseases had been linked with certain types of diet. Further more, by 1900 it was apparent that at least two, and possibly three, diseases could be cured by changes in diet (see Table 2-1).

Other diseases, in addition to those listed in Table 2-1, were known since ancient times to respond to what would now be called diet therapy. An example is the disease of **night blindness**, that is, impaired dark adaptation, one of the first recorded medical conditions. The writings of ancient Greek, Roman, and Arab physicians show that animal liver was known to be effective in both the prevention and cure of the disease. In fact, the use of liver for the prevention of night blindness became part of the folk cultures of most seafaring communities. Corneal ulceration, now known to be a related condition resulting in permanent blindness, was recognized in the eighteenth and nineteenth centuries in association with protein-energy malnutrition as well as such diseases as meningitis, tuberculosis, and typhoid fever. In Russia, it occurred during long Lenten fasts. Then, in 1881,

Table 2-1. Diet–disease relationships recognized by 1900

Disease	Associated diet	Recognized prevention
Scurvy	Salted (preserved) foods	Fresh fruits and vegetables
Beriberi	Polished rice based	Meats, vegetables
Rickets	Few "good" fats	Eggs, cod liver oil
Pellagra	Corn based	None

cod liver oil was found effective in curing both night blindness and early corneal lesions (Bitot's spots), and by the end of the century cod liver oil, as well as meat and milk, were used routinely in Europe to treat both conditions.

Unfortunately, much of this knowledge was overlooked, and its significance was not fully appreciated by a medical community galvanized by the new germ theory of disease. Alternative theories for the etiologies of these diseases were popular. Thus, as the twentieth century began, it was widely held that scurvy, beriberi, and rickets were each caused by a bacterium or bacterial toxin rather than by the simple absence of something required for normal health. Some held that rickets might also be due to hypothyroidism, while others thought it to be brought on by lack of exercise or excessive production of lactic acid. These theories died hard and had lingering deaths. In explanation of the lack of interest in the clues presented by the diet–disease associations outlined above, Harris (1955, p. 6) mused:

> *Perhaps the reason is that it seems easier for the human mind to believe that ill is caused by some positive evil agency, rather than by any mere absence of any beneficial property.*

Limitations of Empiricism

In actuality, the process of discovery of the vitamins had moved about as far as it could in its empirical phase. Further advances in understanding the etiologies of these diseases would require the rigorous testing of the various hypotheses, that is, entrance into the deductive phase of nutritional discovery. That movement, however, required tools for productive scientific experimentation — tools that had not been available previously.

IV. The Experimental Phase of Vitamin Discovery

In a world where one cannot examine all possible cases (i.e., use strictly inductive reasoning), natural truths can be learned only by inference from premises already known to be true (i.e., through deduction). Both the inductive and deductive approaches may be linked; that is, probable conclusions derived from observation may be used as hypotheses for testing deductively in the process of scientific experimentation.

Requirements of Nutrition Research

In order for scientific experimentation to yield informative results, it must be both *repeatable* and *relevant*. The value of the first point, **repeatability**, should be self-evident. Inasmuch as natural truths are held to be constant, nonrepeatable results cannot be construed to reveal them. The value of the second point, **relevance**, becomes increasingly important when it is infeasible to test a hypothesis in its real-world context. In such circumstances, it becomes necessary to employ a representation of the context of ultimate interest, a construct known in science as a **model**. Models are born of practical necessity, but they must be developed carefully in order to serve as analogs of situations that cannot be studied directly.

Defined Diets Provided Repeatability

Repeatability in nutrition experimentation became possible with the use of *diets of defined composition*. The most useful type of defined diet that emerged in nutrition research was the **purified diet**. Diets of this type were formulated using highly refined ingredients (e.g., isolated proteins, refined sugars and starches, refined fats) for which the chemical composition could be reasonably well known. It was the use of defined diets that facilitated experimental nutrition; such diets could be prepared over and over by the same or other investigators to yield comparable results. Results obtained through the use of defined diets were repeatable and, therefore, predictable.

Appropriate Animal Models Provided Relevance

Relevance in nutrition research became possible with the identification of **animal models**[5] appropriate to diseases of interest in human medicine or to physiological processes of interest in human medicine or animal production. The first of these was discovered quite by chance by keen observers studying human disease. Ultimately, the use of animal models would lead to the discovery of each of the vitamins, as well as to the elucidation of the nutritional roles and metabolic functions of each of the approximately 40 nutrients. The careful use of appropriate animal models made possible studies that would otherwise be infeasible or unthinkable in human subjects or in other animal species of interest.

Major Forces in the Emergence of Nutritional Science

- Recognition that certain diseases were related to diet
- Development of appropriate animal models
- Use of defined diets

An Animal Model for Beriberi

The analytical phase of vitamin discovery, indeed modern nutrition research itself, was entered with the finding of an animal model for beriberi in the 1890s. In 1886, Dutch authorities sent a commission led by Cornelius Pekalharing to their East Indian colony (now Indonesia) to find the cause of beriberi, which had become such a problem among Dutch soldiers and sailors as to interrupt military operations in Atjeh, Sumatra. Pekalharing took an army surgeon stationed in Batavia (now Jakarta), Christian Eijkman, whom he had met when both were on study leaves (Pekalharing from his faculty post at the University of Utrecht and Eijkman as a medical graduate from the University of Amsterdam) in the laboratory of the great bacteriologist, Robert Koch. The team, unaware of Takaki's work, expected to find a bacterium as the cause and was therefore disappointed, after eight months of searching, to uncover no such evidence. They concluded:

> *Beriberi has been attributed to an insufficient nourishment and to misery: but the destruction of the peripheral nervous system on such a large scale is not caused by hunger or grief. The true cause must be something coming from the outside, but is it a poison or an infection?*
> (Carpenter, 2000, p. 33)

---

[5] In nutrition and other biomedical research, an animal model consists of the experimental production in a conveniently managed animal species of biochemical and/or clinical changes that are comparable to those occurring in another species of primary interest but that may be infeasible, unethical, or uneconomical to study directly. Animal models are, frequently, species with small body weights (e.g., rodents, chicks, rabbits); however, they may also be larger species (e.g., monkeys, sheep), depending on the target problem and species they are selected to represent. In any case, background information on the biology and husbandry should be available. The selection and/or development of an animal model should be based primarily on representation of the biological problem of interest without undue consideration of the practicalities of cost and availability.

But looking for a poison, they observed, would be very difficult, whereas they had techniques for looking for a microorganism that had been successful for other diseases. Thus, they tried to culture organisms from blood smears from patients and to create the disease in monkeys, rabbits, and dogs by inoculations of blood, saliva, and tissues from patients and cadavers. When single injections produced no effects, they used multiple-injection regimens. Despite the development of abscesses at the point of some injections, it appeared that multiple inoculations could produce some nerve degeneration in rabbits and dogs. Pekalharing concluded that beriberi was, indeed, an infectious disease but an unusual one requiring repeated reinfection of the host. Before returning to Holland, Pekalharing persuaded the Dutch military to allow Eijkman to continue working on the beriberi problem.

The facilities used by Pekalharing's commission at the military hospital at Batavia became a new Laboratory for Bacteriology and Pathology of the colonial government, with Eijkman named as director with one assistant. His efforts in 1888 to infect rabbits and monkeys with Pekalharing's micrococcus were altogether unsuccessful, causing him to posit that beriberi must require a long time before the appearance of signs. The following year, he started using chickens as his animal model. Later in the year, he noted that many of these animals, regardless of whether they had been inoculated, lost weight and started walking with a staggering gait. Some developed difficulty standing and died. Eijkman noted on autopsy no abnormalities of the heart, brain, or spinal cord, but observed microscopic degeneration of the peripheral nerves, particularly in the legs. The latter findings were signs he had observed in people dying of beriberi. But he was unable to culture any consistent type of bacteria from the blood of affected animals. It would have been easy for Eijkman to dismiss the thought that this avian disease, which he called polyneuritis, might be related to beriberi.

Serendipity or a Keen Eye?

After persisting in his flock for some five months, the disease suddenly disappeared. Eijkman reviewed his records and found that in June, shortly before the chickens had started to show paralysis, a change in their diet had been occasioned by failure of a shipment of feed-grade brown (unpolished) rice to arrive. His assistant had instead, used, white (polished) rice

from the hospital kitchen. It turned out that this extravagance had been discovered a few months earlier by a new hospital superintendent, who had ordered it stopped. When Eijkman again fed the chickens brown rice, he found that the affected animals recovered completely within days.

With this clue, Eijkman immediately turned to the chicken as the animal model for his studies. He found that the chicks showed signs of **polyneuritis** within days of being fed polished rice and that their signs disappeared even more quickly if they were then fed unpolished rice. It was clear that there was something associated with rice polishings that protected chickens from the disease. After discussing these results, Eijkman's colleague, Adolphe Verdeman, the physician inspector of prisons in the colony, surveyed the use of polished and unpolished rice and the incidence of beriberi among inmates. His results (summarized in Table 2-2), later to be confirmed in similar epidemiological investigations by other groups, showed the advantage enjoyed by prisoners eating unpolished rice: they were much less likely to contract beriberi.

This kind of information, in conjunction with his experimental findings with chickens, allowed Eijkman to investigate by means of bioassay the beriberi-protective factor apparently associated with rice husks.

Antiberiberi Factor Announced

Eijkman used this animal model in a series of investigations in 1890–1897 and found that the antipolyneuritis factor could be extracted from rice hulls with water or alcohol, that it was dialyzable, but that it was rather easily destroyed with moist heat. He concluded that the water-soluble factor was a "pharmacological antidote" to the "beriberi microbe," which, though still not identified, he thought to be present in the rice kernel proper. Apparently, Gerrit Grijns, who continued Eijkman's work in Batavia when Eijkmann went back to Holland suffering

Table 2-2. Beriberi in Javanese prisons ca. 1890

Diet	Population	Cases	Prevalence (cases/ 10,000 people)
Polished rice	150,266	4,200	279.5
Partially polished rice	35,082	85	24.2
Unpolished rice	96,530	86	8.9

from malaria in 1896, came to interpret their findings somewhat differently. Grijns went on to show that polyneuritis could be prevented by including mung bean (*Vigna radiata*) in the diet; this led to mung beans being found effective in treating beriberi. In 1901, Grijns suggested for the first time that beriberi-producing diets "lacked a certain substance of importance in the metabolism of the central nervous system." Subsequently, Eijkman came to share Grijn's view; in 1906, the two investigators published a now-classic paper in which they wrote:

> There is present in rice polishings a substance different from protein, and salts, which is indispensable to health and the lack of which causes nutritional polyneuritis. (*Arch für Hygiene*. **58**, 150–170)

V. The Vitamine Theory

Defined Diets Revealed Needs for Accessory Factors

The announcement of the antiberiberi factor constituted the first recognition of the concept of the vitamin, although the term itself was yet to be coined. At the time of Eijkman's studies, but a world removed and wholly separate, others were finding that animals would not survive when fed "synthetic" or "artificial" diets formulated with purified fats, proteins, carbohydrates, and salts, that is, containing all of the nutrients then known to be constituents of natural foods. Such a finding was first reported by the Swiss physiologist, Nicholai Lunin, in 1888, who found that the addition of milk to a synthetic diet supported the survival of mice. Lunin concluded:

> A natural food such as milk must, therefore, contain besides these known principal ingredients small quantities of other and unknown substances essential to life. (Harris, 1955, p. 14)

Lunin's finding was soon confirmed by several other investigators. By 1912, Rhömann in Germany, Socin in Switzerland, Pekalharing in The Netherlands, and Hopkins in Great Britain had each demonstrated that the addition of milk to purified diets corrected the impairments in growth and survival that were otherwise produced in laboratory rodents. The German physiologist Stepp took another experimen-

tal approach. He found it possible to extract from bread and milk factors required for animal growth. Although Pekalharing's 1905 comments, in Dutch, lay unnoticed by many investigators (most of whom did not read that language), his conclusions about what Hopkins had called the **accessory factor** in milk alluded to the modern concept of a vitamin:

> If this substance is absent, the organism loses the power properly to assimilate the well known principal parts of food, the appetite is lost and with apparent abundance the animals die of want. Undoubtedly this substance not only occurs in milk but in all sorts of foodstuffs, both of vegetable and animal origin. (Harris, 1955, p. 16)

Perhaps the most important of the early studies with defined diets were those of the Cambridge biochemist Frederick Gowland Hopkins.[6] His studies demonstrated that the growth-promoting activities of accessory factors were independent of appetite and that such factors prepared from milk or yeast were biologically active in very small amounts.

Two Lines of Inquiry

Therefore, by 1912, two independently developed lines of inquiry had revealed that foods contained beneficial factor(s) in addition to the nutrients known at the time. That these factor(s) were present and active in minute amounts was apparent from the fact that almost all of the mass of food was composed of the known nutrients.

Two Lines of Inquiry Leading to the Discovery of the Vitamins

- The study of substances that prevent deficiency diseases
- The study of accessory factors required by animals fed purified diets

Comments by Hopkins in 1906 indicate that he saw connections between the accessory factors and the deficiency diseases. On the subject of the accessory growth factors in foods he wrote:

> No animal can live on a mixture of pure protein, fat and carbohydrate, and even when

---

[6] Sir Frederick Gowland Hopkins, Professor of Biochemistry at Cambridge University, is known for his pioneering work in biochemistry, which involved not only classic work on accessory growth factors (for which he shared, with Christian Eijkman, the 1929 Nobel Prize in Medicine), but also the discoveries of glutathione and tryptophan.

the necessary inorganic material is carefully supplied the animal still cannot flourish. The animal is adjusted to live either on plant tissues or the tissues of other animals, and these contain countless substances other than protein, carbohydrates and fats. In diseases such as rickets, and particularly scurvy, we have had for years knowledge of a dietetic factor; but though we know how to benefit these conditions empirically, the real errors in the diet are to this day quite obscure.... They are, however, certainly of the kind which comprises these minimal qualitative factors that I am considering.
(Hopkins, F. G. [1906]. *Analyst.* **31**, 395–403)

Hopkins demonstrated the presence of a factor(s) in milk that stimulated the growth of animals fed diets containing all of the then-known nutrients (Fig. 2-1).

The Lines Converge

Eijkman and Grijns's discovery had stimulated efforts by investigators in several countries to isolate the antiberiberi factor in rice husks. Umetaro Suzuki of Imperial University Agricultural College in Tokyo succeeded in preparing a concentrated extract from rice bran for the treatment of polyneuritis and beriberi. He called the active fraction "oryzanin," but he could not achieve its purification in crystalline form.

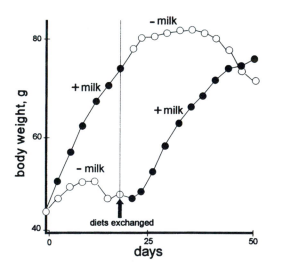

Fig. 2-1. Evidence of an accessory factor in milk necessary for the growth of puppies (From Hopkins [1906]. *Analyst* **21**, 395–403).

Casimir Funk, a Polish-born chemist schooled in Switzerland, Paris, and Berlin, and then working in the Lister Institute in London, concluded from the various conditions in which it could be extracted and then precipitated that the antipolyneuritis factor in rice husks was an organic base and, therefore, nitrogenous in nature. When he appeared to have isolated the factor, Funk coined a new word for it, with the specific intent of promoting the new concept in nutrition to which Hopkins had alluded. Having evidence that the factor was an organic base and, therefore, an *amine*, Funk chose the term **vitamine**[7] because it was clearly *vital*, that is, pertaining to life.

Funk's Theory

In 1912, Funk published his landmark paper presenting the **vitamine theory**; in this paper he proposed, in what some have referred to as a leap of faith, four different vitamines. That the concept was not a new one, and that not all of these factors later proved to be amines (hence, the change to **vitamin**[8]), are far less important than the focus the newly coined term gave to the diet–health relationship. Funk (1912) was not unaware of the importance of the term itself; he wrote:

I must admit that when I chose the name "vitamine" I was well aware that these substances might later prove not all to be of an amine nature. However, it was necessary for me to use a name that would sound well and serve as a "catch-word." (Funk, C. [1912]. *J. State Med.* **20**, 341–368)

Funk's Vitamines

- Antiberiberi vitamine
- Antirickets vitamine
- Antiscurvy vitamine
- Antipellagra vitamine

Impact of the New Concept

The vitamine theory opened new possibilities in nutrition research by providing a new intellectual construct for interpreting observations of the natural world. No longer was the elucidation of the etiologies of diseases to be constrained by the germ theory.

---

[7] Harris (1955) reported that the word *vitamine* was suggested to Funk by his friend, Dr. Max Nierenstein, Reader in Biochemistry, at the University of Bristol.

[8] The dropping of the *e* from *vitamine* is said to have been the suggestion of J. C. Drummond.

Thus, Funk's greatest contribution involves not the data generated in his laboratory, but rather the theory produced from his thoughtful review of information already in the medical literature of the time. This fact caused Harris (1955, p. 13) to write:

> *The interpreter may be as useful to science as the discoverer. I refer here to any man[9] who is able to take a broad view of what has already been done by others, to collect evidence and discern through it all some common connecting link.*

The real impact of Funk's theory was to provide a new concept for interpreting diet-related phenomena. As the educational psychologist Novak[10] observed more recently:

> *As our conceptual and emotional frameworks change, we see different things in the same material.*

Still, by 1912 it was not clear whether the accessory factors were the same as the vitamines. Until 1915, there was considerable debate concerning whether the growth factor for the rat was a single or multiple entity (it was already clear that there was more than one vitamine). Some investigators were able to demonstrate it in yeast and not butter; others found it in butter and not yeast. Some showed it to be identical with the antipolyneuritis factor; others showed that it was clearly different.

More Than One Accessory Factor

The debate was resolved by the landmark studies of the American investigator Elmer McCollum and his volunteer assistant Marguerite Davis at the University of Wisconsin in 1913–1915. Using diets based on casein and lactose, they demonstrated that at least two different additional growth factors were required to support normal growth of the rat. One factor could be extracted with ether from egg or butterfat (but not olive or cottonseed oils) but was nonsaponifiable; it appeared to be the same factor shown earlier by the German physiologist Wilhelm Stepp and by Thomas Osborne and Lafayette Mendel at Yale University in the same year, to be required to sustain growth of the rat. The second factor was extractable with water

and prevented polyneuritis in chickens and pigeons. McCollum called these factors **fat-soluble A** and **water-soluble B**, respectively (Table 2-3).

Accessory Factors Prevent Disease

Subsequent studies conducted by McCollum's group showed that the ocular disorders (i.e., **xerophthalmia**[11]) that developed in rats, dogs, and chicks fed fat-free diets could be prevented by feeding them cod liver oil, butter, or preparations of fat-soluble A, which then became known as the *antixerophthalmic factor*. Shortly, it was found that the so-called water-soluble B material was not only required for normal growth of the rat, but also prevented polyneuritis in the chick. Therefore, it was clear that water-soluble B was identical to or at least contained Funk's antiberiberi vitamine; hence, it became known as *vitamine B*.

Accessory Factors Same as Vitamines

With these discoveries, it became apparent that the biological activities of the accessory factors and the vitamines were likely to be due to the same compounds. Thus, the concept of a vitamine was, generalized to include nonnitrogenous compounds, and the antipolyneuritis vitamine became **vitamin B**.

Elucidation of the Vitamins

So it was, through the agencies of several factors, a useful new intellectual construct, the use of defined diets, and the availability of appropriate animal models, that nutrition emerged as a scientific discipline. By 1915, thinking about diet and health had been forever changed, and it was clear that the earlier notions about the required nutrients had been incomplete.

Table 2-3. McCollum's rat growth factors

Factor	Found in:	Not found in:
Fat-soluble A	Milk fat, egg yolk	Lard, olive oil
Water-soluble B	Wheat, milk, egg yolk	Polished rice

---

[9] Harris's word choice reveals him as a product of his times. Because it is clear that the process of intellectual discovery to which Harris refers does not recognize gender, it is more appropriate to read this word as *person*.

[10] Novak, J. D. (1977). *A Theory of Education*. Cornell University Press, Ithaca, N.Y., p. 22.

[11] Xerophthalmia, from the Greek *xeros* ("dry") and *ophthalmos* ("eye"), involves dryness of the eyeball owing to atrophy of the periocular glands, hyperkeratosis of the conjunctiva, and, ultimately, inflammation and edema of the cornea, which leads to infection, ulceration, and blindness.

Therefore, it should not be surprising to find, by the 1920s, mounting interest in the many questions generated by what had become sound nutritional research. That interest and the further research activity it engendered resulted, over the brief span of only five decades, in the development of a fundamental understanding of the identities and functions of about 40 nutrients, one-third of which are considered vitamins.

Crooked Paths to Discovery

The paths leading to the discovery of the vitamins wandered from Java with the findings of Eijkman in the 1890s to England with Funk's theory in 1912 to the United States with the recognition of fat-soluble A and water-soluble B in 1915. By that time, the paths had already branched, and for the next four decades, they would branch again and again as scientists from many laboratories and many nations would pursue many unexplained responses to diet among many types of animal models. Some of these pursuits appeared to fail, but, in the aggregate, all laid the groundwork of understanding on which the discoveries of those factors now recognized to be vitamins were based. When viewed in retrospect, the path to that recognition may seem deceptively straight, but it most definitely was not linear. The way was branched and crooked; in many cases, progress was made by several different investigators traveling in apparently different directions. The following recounts the highlights of the exciting search for the elucidation of the vitamins.

VI. Elucidation of the Vitamins

New Animal Model Reveals New Vitamin: "C"

Eijkman's report of polyneuritis in the chicken and an animal model for beriberi stimulated researchers Axel Holst and Theodor Frölich at the University of Christiana in Oslo who were interested in *shipboard beriberi*, a common problem among Norwegian seamen. Working with pigeons, they found a beriberi diet to produce the polyneuritis described by Eijkman; however, they considered that condition very different from the disease of sailors. In 1907, they attempted to produce the disease in another experimental animal species, the common Victorian household pet, the guinea pig. Contrary to their expectations, they failed to produce by feeding that species a cereal-based diet anything resembling beriberi; instead, they observed the familiar signs of scurvy. Eijkman's work suggested to them that, like beriberi, scurvy, too, might be due to a dietary deficiency. Having discovered, quite by chance, one of the few possible animal species in which scurvy could be produced,[12] Holst and Frölich had produced something of tremendous value — an animal model of scurvy.[13]

This finding led Henriettte Chick and E. M. Hume, in the 1910s, to use the guinea pig to develop a bioassay for the determination of the antiscorbutic activity in foods, and Zilva and colleagues at the Lister Institute to isolate from lemons the crude factor that had come to be known as **vitamin C**. It was soon found that vitamin C could reduce the dye 2,6-dichloroindophenol; but the reducing activity determined with that reagent did not always correlate with the antiscorbutic activity determined by bioassay. Subsequently, it was found that the vitamin was reversibly oxidized, but that both the reduced and oxidized forms had antiscorbutic activity.

In 1932, Albert Szent-Györgi, a Hungarian scientist working in Hopkins's laboratory at Cambridge University, and Glen King at the University of Pittsburgh established that the antiscorbutic factor was identical with the reductant *hexuronic acid*,[14] now called **ascorbic acid**. Szent-Györgi had isolated it in crystalline form from adrenal cortex whereas King had isolated it from cabbage and citrus juice.[15] After Szent-Györgi returned to Hungary to take a

---

[12] Their finding was, indeed, fortuitous, as vitamin C is now known to be an essential dietary nutrient only for the guinea pig, primates, fishes, some fruit-eating bats, and some passiform birds. Had they used the rat, the mouse, or the chick in their study, vitamin C might have remained unrecognized for, perhaps, quite a while.

[13] In fact, scorbutic signs had been observed in the guinea pig more than a decade earlier, when a U.S. Department of Agriculture pathologist noted in an annual report *"When guinea pigs are fed with cereals (bran and oats mixed), without any grass, clover, or succulent vegetables, such as cabbage, a peculiar disease, chiefly recognizable by subcutaneous extravasation of blood, carries them off in four to eight weeks"* (Smith, A. H. [1918]. *Lancet.* **2**, 813–815). That this observation was not published for wider scientific audience meant that it failed to influence the elucidation of the etiology of scurvy.

[14] It is said that, when Szent-Györgi first isolated the compound, he was at a loss for a name for it. Knowing it to be a sugar, but otherwise ignorant of its identity, he proposed the name *ignose*, which was disqualified by an editor who did not appreciate the humor of the Hungarian chemist. Ultimately, the names *ascorbic acid* and *vitamin C,* by which several groups had come to refer to the antiscorbutic factor, were adopted.

[15] The reports of both groups (King and Waugh, 1932; Svirbely and Szent-Györgi, 1932) appeared within two weeks of one another. In fact, Svirbely had recently joined Szent-Györgi's group, having come from King's laboratory. In 1937, King and Szent-Györgi shared the Nobel Prize for their work in the isolation and identification of vitamin C.

professorship, he was joined by an American-born Hungarian, J. Svirbely, who had been working in King's laboratory. Szent-Györgi had isolated about 500 grams of crystalline hexuronic acid from peppers and then 25 grams of the vitamin from adrenal glands, making samples available to other laboratories. On April 1, 1932, King and Waugh reported that their crystals protected guinea pigs from scurvy. Two weeks later, Svirbely and Szent-Györgi reported virtually the same results. The following year, the chemical structure of ascorbic acid was elucidated by the groups of Haworth in Birmingham and Karrer in Zurich, both of which also achieved its synthesis.

Fat-Soluble A: Actually Two Factors

Pursuing the characterization of fat-soluble A, by 1919 McCollum's group[16] and others had found that, in addition to supporting growth for the rat, the factor also prevented xerophthalmia and night blindness in that species. In 1920, J. C. Drummond called the active lipid **vitamin A**.[17] This factor was present in cod liver oil, which at the turn of the century had been shown to prevent both xerophthalmia and night blindness, which C. Bitot some 40 years earlier had concluded had the same underlying cause.

Vitamin A Prevents Rickets?

Undoubtedly influenced by the recent recognition of vitamin A, Edward Mellanby, who had worked with Hopkins, undertook to produce a dietary model of rickets. For this study he used puppies, which the Scottish physician Findley found developed rickets if kept indoors.[18] Mellanby fed a low-fat diet based on oatmeal with limited milk intake to puppies that he kept indoors; the puppies developed the marked skeletal deformities characteristic of rickets. When he found that these deformities could be prevented by feeding cod liver oil or butterfat without allowing the puppies outdoors, he concluded that rickets, too, was caused by a deficiency of vitamin A, which McCollum had discovered in those materials.

New Vitamin: "D"

McCollum, however, suspected that the antirachitic factor present in cod liver oil was different from vitamin A. Having moved to the Johns Hopkins University in Baltimore, he conducted an experiment in which he subjected cod liver oil to aeration and heating (100°C for 14 hours), after which he tested its antixerophthalmic and antirachitic activities with rat and chick bioassays, respectively. He found that heating had destroyed the antixerophthalmic (vitamin A) activity, but that cod liver oil had retained antirachitic activity. McCollum called the heat-stable factor **vitamin D**.

β-Carotene, a Provitamin

At about the same time (1919), H. Steenbock in Wisconsin pointed out that the vitamin A activities of plant materials seemed to correlate with their contents of yellow pigments. He suggested that the plant pigment *carotene* was responsible for the vitamin A activity of such materials. Yet, the vitamin A activity in organic extracts of liver was colorless. Therefore, Steenbock suggested that carotene could not be vitamin A, but that it may be converted metabolically to the actual vitamin. This hypothesis was not substantiated until 1929, when von Euler and Karrer in Stockholm demonstrated growth responses to carotene in rats fed vitamin A-deficient diets. Furthermore, Moore in England demonstrated in the rat a dose–response relationship between dietary β-carotene and hepatic vitamin A concentration. This showed that β-carotene is, indeed, a **provitamin**.

Vitamin A Linked to Vision

In the early 1930s, the first indications of the molecular mechanism of the visual process were produced by George Wald of Harvard University but working in Germany at the time, who isolated the chromophore **retinen** from bleached retinas.[19] A decade later, Morton in Liverpool found that the chromophore was

---

[16] In 1917, McCollum moved to the newly established School of Public Health at Johns Hopkins University.

[17] In 1920, J. C. Drummond proposed the use of the names *vitamin A* and *vitamin B* for McCollum's factors, and the use of the letters C, D, etc., for any vitamins subsequently to be discovered.

[18] Exposing infants to sunlight has been a traditional practice in many cultures and had been a folk treatment for rickets in northern Europe.

[19] For this and other discoveries of the basic chemical and physiological processes in vision, George Wald was awarded, with Haldan K. Hartline (of the United States) and R. Grant (of Sweden), the Nobel Prize in 1967.

the aldehyde form of vitamin A, that is, *retinaldehyde*. Just after Wald's discovery, Karrer's group in Zurich elucidated the structures of both β-carotene and vitamin A. In 1937, Holmes and Corbett succeeded in crystallizing vitamin A from fish liver. In 1942, Baxter and Robeson crystallized *retinol* and several of its esters; in 1947, they crystallized the 13-*cis*-isomer. Isler's group in Basel achieved the synthesis of retinol in the same year and that of β-carotene three years later.

The Nature of Vitamin D

McCollum's discovery of the antirachitic factor he called vitamin D in cod liver oil, which was made possible through the use of animal models, was actually a *rediscovery*, as that material had been long recognized as an effective medicine for rickets in children. Still, the nature of the disease was the subject of considerable debate, particularly after 1919, when Huldschinsky, a physician in Vienna, demonstrated the efficacy of ultraviolet light in healing rickets. This confusion was clarified by the findings in 1923 of Goldblatt and Soames, who demonstrated that when livers from rachitic rats were irradiated with ultraviolet light, they could cure rickets when fed to rachitic, nonirradiated rats. The next year, Steenbock's group demonstrated the prevention of rickets in rats by ultraviolet irradiation of either the animals themselves *or* their food. Furthermore, the light-produced antirachitic factor was associated with the fat-soluble portion of the diet.[20]

Vitamers D

The ability to produce vitamin D (which could be bioassayed using both rat and chick animal models) by irradiating lipids led to the finding that large quantities of the vitamin could be produced by irradiating plant sterols. This led Askew's and Windaus's groups, in the early 1930s, to the isolation and identification of the vitamin produced by irradiation of *ergosterol*. Steenbock's group, however, found that, while the rachitic chick responded appropriately to irradiated products of cod liver oil or the animal sterol *cho-*

lesterol, that animal did *not* respond to the vitamin D so produced from ergosterol. On the basis of this apparent lack of equivalence, Wadell suggested in 1934 that the irradiated products of ergosterol and cholesterol were different. Subsequently, Windaus's group synthesized 7-dehydrocholesterol and isolated a vitamin D-active product of its irradiation. In 1936, they reported its structure, showing it to be a side-chain isomer of the form of the vitamin produced from plant sterols. Thus, two forms of vitamin D were found: **ergocalciferol** (from ergosterol), which was called vitamin D_2[21]; and **cholecalciferol** (from cholesterol), which was called vitamin D_3. While it was clear that the vitamers D had important metabolic roles in calcification, insights concerning the molecular mechanisms of the vitamin would not come until the 1960s. Then, it became apparent that neither vitamer was metabolically active per se; each is converted *in vivo* to a host of metabolites that participate in a system of calcium homeostasis that continues to be of great interest to the biomedical community.

Multiple Identities of Water-Soluble B

By the 1920s, it was apparent that the antipolyneuritis factor, called water-soluble B and present in such materials as yeasts, was not a single substance. This was demonstrated by the finding that fresh yeast could prevent both beriberi and pellagra. However, the antipolyneuritis factor in yeast was unstable to heat, while such treatment did not alter the efficacy of yeast to prevent dermititic lesions (i.e., **dermatitis**) in rodents. This caused Goldberger to suggest that the so-called vitamin B was actually at least *two* vitamins: the antipolyneuritis vitamin and a new antipellagra vitamin.

In 1926, the heat-labile antipolyneuritis/beriberi factor was first crystallized by Jansen and Donath working in the Eijkman Institute (which replaced Eijkman's simple facilities) in Batavia. They called the factor *aneurin*. Their work was facilitated by the use of the small rice bird (*Munia maja*) as an animal model in which they developed a rapid bioassay for antipolyneuritic activity.[22] Six years later, Windaus's

---

[20] This discovery, that by ultraviolet irradiation it was possible to induce vitamin D activity in such foods as milk, bread, meats, and butter, led to the widespread use of this practice, which has resulted in the virtual eradication of rickets as a public health problem.

[21] Windaus's group had earlier isolated a form of the vitamin he had called vitamin D_1, which had turned out to be an irradiation-breakdown product, *lumisterol*.

[22] The animals, which consumed only 2 grams of feed daily, showed a high (98+%) incidence of polyneuritis within 9 to 13 days if fed white polished rice. The delay of onset of signs gave them a useful bioassay of antipolyneuritic activity suitable for use with small amounts of test materials. This point is not trivial, in as much as there is only about a teaspoon of thiamin in a ton of rice bran. The bioassay of Jansen and Donath was sufficiently responsive for 10 mcg of active material to be curative.

group isolated the factor from yeast, perhaps the richest source of it. In the same year (1932), the chemical structure was determined by R. R. Williams, who named it **thiamin**, that is, the vitamin containing sulfur (*thios*, in Greek). Noting that deficient subjects showed high blood levels of pyruvate and lactate after exercise, in 1936 Rudolph Peters of Oxford University for the first time used the term *biochemical lesion* to describe the effects of the dietary deficiency. Shortly thereafter, methods of synthesis were achieved by several groups, including those of Williams, Andersag, and Westphal, and Todd. In 1937, thiamin diphosphate (thiamin pyrophosphate) was isolated by Lohmann and Schuster, who showed it to be identical to the *cocarboxylase* that had been isolated earlier by Auhagen. That many research groups were actively engaged in the research on the antipolyneuritis/beriberi factor is evidence of intense international interest due to the widespread prevalence of beriberi.

The characterization of thiamin clarified the distinction of the antiberiberi factor from the antipellagra activity. The latter was not found in maize (corn), which contained appreciable amounts of thiamin. Goldberger called the two substances the A-N (antineuritic) factor and the P-P (pellagra-preventive) factor. Others called these factors vitamins F (for Funk) and G (for Goldberger), respectively; but these terms did not last.[23] By the mid-1920s the terms *vitamin B₁* and *vitamin B₂* had been rather widely adapted for these factors, respectively; this practice was codified in 1927 by the Accessory Food Factors Committee of the British Medical Research Council.

Vitamin B₂: A Complex of Several Factors

That the thermostable second nutritional factor in yeast, which by that time was called **vitamin B₂**, was not a single substance was not immediately recognized, giving rise to considerable confusion and delay in the elucidation of its chemical identity (identities). Efforts to fractionate the heat-stable factor were guided almost exclusively by bioassays with experi-

mental animal models. Yet, different species yielded discrepant responses to preparations of the factor. When such variation in responses among species was finally appreciated, it became clear that vitamin B₂ actually included *several* heat-stable factors. Vitamin B₂, as then defined, was indeed a complex.

Components of the Vitamin B₂ Complex

- The P-P factor (preventing pellagra in humans and pellagra-like diseases in dogs, monkeys, and pigs)
- A growth factor for the rat
- A pellagra-preventing factor for the rat
- An antidermatitis factor for the chick

Vitamin B₂ Complex Yields Riboflavin

The first substance in the vitamin B₂ complex to be elucidated was the heat-stable, water-soluble, rat growth factor, which was isolated by Kuhn, György, and Wagner-Jauregg at the Kaiser Wilhelm Institute in 1933. Those investigators found that thiamin-free extracts of autoclaved yeast, liver, or rice bran prevented the growth failure of rats fed a thiamin-supplemented diet. They also noted that a yellow-green fluorescence in each extract promoted rat growth, and that the intensity of fluorescence was proportional to the effect on growth. This observation enabled them to develop a rapid chemical assay that, in conjunction with their bioassay, they exploited to isolate the factor from egg white in 1933. They called it **ovoflavin**. The same group then isolated by the same procedure a yellow-green fluorescent growth-promoting compound from whey (which they called **lactoflavin**). This procedure involved the adsorption of the active factor on fuller's earth,[24] from which it could be eluted with base.[25] At the same time, Ellinger and Koschara at the University of Düsseldorf isolated similar substances from liver, kidney, muscle, and yeast, and Booher in the United States isolated the factor from whey. These water-soluble growth factors became designated as **flavins**.[26] By 1934, Kuhn's

---

[23] In fact, the name *vitamin F* was later used, with some debate as to the appropriateness of the term, to describe essential fatty acids. The name *vitamin G* has been dropped completely.

[24] Floridin, a nonplastic variety of kaolin containing an aluminum magnesium silicate. The material is useful as a decolorizing medium. Its name comes from an ancient process of cleaning or *fulling* wool, in which a slurry of earth or clay was used to remove oil and particulate dirt.

[25] By this procedure the albumen from 10,000 eggs yielded about 30 milligrams of riboflavin.

[26] Initially, the term *flavin* was used with a prefix that indicated the source material; for example, ovoflavin, hepatoflavin, and lactoflavin designated the substances isolated from egg white, liver, and milk, respectively.

group had determined the structure of the so-called flavins. These substances were thus found to be identical; because each contained a ribose-like (ribotyl) moiety attached to an isoalloxazine nucleus, the term **riboflavin** was adopted. Riboflavin was synthesized by Kuhn's group (then at the University of Heidelberg) and by Karrer's group at Zurich in 1935. As the first component of the vitamin B_2 complex, it is also referred to as vitamin B_2. However, that should not be confused with the earlier designation of the pellagra-preventive (P-P) factor.

Vitamin B_2 Complex Yields Niacin

Progress in the identification of the P-P factor was retarded by two factors: the pervasive influence of the germ theory of disease and the lack of an animal model. The former made acceptance of evidence suggesting a nutritional origin of the disease a long and difficult undertaking. The latter precluded the rigorous testing of hypotheses for the etiology of the disease in a timely and highly controlled manner. These challenges were met by Joseph Goldberger, a U.S. Public Health Service bacteriologist who, in 1914, was put in charge of the Service's pellagra program.

Pellagra: An infectious disease?

Goldberger's first study[27] is now a classic. He studied a Jackson, Mississippi, orphanage in which pellagra was endemic. He noted that, whereas the disease was prevalent among the inmates it was absent among the staff, including the nurses and physicians who cared for patients; this suggested to him that pellagra was not an infectious disease. Noting that the food available to the professional staff was much different from that served to the inmates (the former included meat and milk not available to the inmates), Goldberger suspected that an unbalanced diet was responsible for the disease. He secured funds to supply meat and milk to inmates for a two-year period of study. The results were dramatic: pellagra soon disappeared, and no new cases were reported for the duration of the study. However, when funds expired at the end of the study and the institution was forced to return to

its former meal program, pellagra reappeared. While the evidence from this uncontrolled experiment galvanized Goldberger's conviction that pellagra was a dietary disease, it was not sufficient to affect a medical community that thought the disease likely to be an infection.

Over the course of two decades, Goldberger undertook to elucidate the dietary basis of pellagra. Among his efforts to demonstrate that the disease was not infectious was the exposure, by ingestion and injection, of himself, his wife, and 14 volunteers to urine, feces, and biological fluids from *pellagrins*.[28] He also experimented with 12 male prisoners who volunteered to consume a diet (based on corn and other cereals, but containing no meat or dairy products) that he thought might produce pellagra: within five months, half of the subjects had developed dermatitis on the scrotum and some also showed lesions on their hands.[29] The negative results of these radical experiments, plus the finding that therapy with oral supplements of the amino acids cysteine and tryptophan was effective in controlling the disease, led by the early 1920s to the establishment of a dietary origin of pellagra. Further progress was hindered by the lack of an appropriate animal model. Although pellagra-like diseases had been identified in several species, most proved not to be useful as biological assays (indeed, most of these later proved to be manifestations of deficiencies of other vitamins of the B_2 complex and to be wholly unrelated to pellagra in humans).

The identification of a useful animal model for pellagra came from Goldberger's discovery in 1922 that maintaining dogs on diets essentially the same as those associated with human pellagra resulted in the animals developing a necrotic degeneration of the tongue called **black tongue disease**. This animal model for the disease led to the final solution of the problem.

Impact of an Animal Model for Pellagra

This finding made possible experimentation that would lead rather quickly to an understanding of the etiology to the disease. Goldberger's group soon

---

[27] See the list of papers of key historical significance in the section Recommended Reading at the end of this chapter.

[28] People suffering from pellagra.

[29] Goldberger conducted this study with the approval of prison authorities. As compensation for participation, volunteers were offered release at the end of the six-month experimental period, which each exercised immediately upon the conclusion of the study. For that reason, Goldberger was unable to demonstrate to a doubting medical community that the unbalanced diet had, indeed, produced pellagra.

found that yeast, wheat germ, and liver would prevent canine black tongue and produce dramatic recoveries in pellagra patients. By the early 1930s, it was established that the human pellagra and canine black tongue curative factor was heat-stable and could be separated from the other B_2 complex components by filtration through fuller's earth, which adsorbed only the P-P factor. Thus, the P-P factor became known as the **filtrate factor**. In 1937, Elvehjem isolated *nicotinamide* from liver extracts that had high antiblack tongue activity and showed that nicotinamide and *nicotinic acid* each cured canine black tongue. Both compounds are now called **niacin**. In the same year, several groups went on to show the curative effect of nicotinic acid against human pellagra.

It is ironic that the antipellagra factor was already well known to chemists of the time. Some 70 years earlier, the German chemist Huber had prepared nicotinic acid by the oxidation of nicotine with nitric acid. Funk had isolated the compound from yeast and rice bran in his search for the antiberiberi factor; however, because it had no effect on beriberi, for two decades nicotinic acid remained an entity with unappreciated biological importance. This view changed in the mid-1930s when Warburg and Christian isolated nicotinamide from the hydrogen-transporting coenzymes I and II,[30] giving the first clue to its importance in metabolism. Within a year, Elvehjem had discovered its nutritional significance.

B_2 Complex Yields Pyridoxine

During the course of their work leading to the successful isolation of riboflavin, Kuhn and colleagues noticed an anomalous relationship between the growth-promoting and fluorescence activities of their extracts: the correlation of the two activities diminished at high levels of the former. Furthermore, the addition of nonfluorescent extracts was necessary for the growth-promoting activity of riboflavin. They interpreted these findings as evidence for a second component of the heat-stable complex — one that was removed during the purification of riboflavin. These factors were also known to prevent dermatoses in

the rat, an activity called *adermin*; however, the lack of a critical assay that could differentiate between the various components of the B_2 complex led to considerable confusion.

In 1934, György proffered a definition of what he called *vitamin B_6 activity*[31] as the factor that prevented what had formerly been called *acrodynia* or *rat pellagra*, which was a symmetrical florid dermatitis spreading over the limbs and trunk with redness and swelling of the paws and ears. His definition effectively distinguished these signs from those produced by riboflavin deficiency, which involves lesions on the head and chest and inflammation of the eyelids and nostrils. The focus provided by György's definition strengthened the use of the rat in the bioassay of vitamin B_6 activity by clarifying its end point. Within two years, his group had achieved partial purification of **vitamin B_6** and in 1938 (only four years after the recognition of the vitamin), five research groups achieved the isolation of vitamin B_6 in crystalline form. The chemical structure of the substance was quickly elucidated as 3-hydroxy-4,5-bis-(hydroxymethyl)-2-methylpyridine. In 1939, Folkers achieved the synthesis of this compound, which György called **pyridoxine**.

B_2 Complex Yields Pantothenic Acid

In the course of studying the growth factor called vitamin B_2, Norris and Ringrose at Cornell described, in 1930, a pellagra-like syndrome of the chick. The lesions could be prevented with aqueous extracts of yeast or liver, which was then recognized to contain the B_2 complex. In studies of B_2 complex-related growth factors for chicks and rats, Jukes and colleagues at Berkeley found positive responses to a thermostable factor that, unlike pyridoxine, was not adsorbed by fuller's earth from an acid solution. They referred to it as their *filtrate factor*.

At the same time and quite independently, the University of Texas microbiologist R. J. Williams was pursuing studies of the essential nutrients for *Saccharomyces cerevisiae* and other yeasts. His group found a potent growth factor that they could isolate from a wide variety of plant and animal tissues.[32]

---

[30] Nicotinamide adenine dinucleotide (NAD) and nicotinamide adenine dinucleotide phosphate (NADP), respectively.

[31] György defined vitamin B_6 activity as "that part of the vitamin B-complex responsible for the cure of a specific dermatitis developed by rats on a vitamin-free diet supplemented with vitamin B_1, and lactoflavin."

[32] The first isolation of pantothenic acid employed 250 kilograms of sheep liver. The autolysate was treated with fuller's earth; the factor was adsorbed to Norite and eluted with ammonia. Brucine salts were formed and were extracted with chloroform–water, after which the brucine salt of pantothenic acid was converted to the calcium salt. The yield was 3 grams of material with about 40% purity.

They called it **pantothenic acid**, meaning "found everywhere," and also referred to the substance as *vitamin B₃*. Later in the decade, Snell's group found that several lactic and propionic acid bacteria require a growth factor that had the same properties. Jukes recognized that his filtrate factor, Norris's chick antidermatitis factor, and the unknown factors required by yeasts and bacteria were identical. He showed that both his filtrate factor and pantothenic acid obtained from Williams could prevent dermatitis in the chick. Pantothenic acid was isolated and its chemical structure was determined by Williams's group in 1939. The chemical synthesis of the vitamin was achieved by Folkers the following year.

The various factors leading to the discovery of pantothenic acid are presented in Table 2-4.

A Fat-Soluble, Antisterility Factor: Vitamin E

Interest in the nutritional properties of lipids was stimulated by the resolution of fat-soluble A into vitamins A and D by the early 1920s. Several groups found that supplementation with the newly discovered vitamins A, C, and D and thiamin markedly improved the performance of animals fed purified diets containing adequate amounts of protein, carbohydrate, and known required minerals. But H. M. Evans and Katherine Bishop, at the University of California, observed that rats fed such supplemented diets seldom reproduced normally. They found that fertility was abnormally low in both males (which showed testicular degeneration) and females (which

Table 2-4. Factors leading to the discovery of pantothenic acid

Factor	Bioassay
Filtrate factor	Chick growth
Chick antidermatitis factor	Prevention of skin lesions and poor feather development in chicks
Pantothenic acid	Growth of *S. cerevisiae* and other yeasts

showed impaired placental function and failed to carry their fetuses to term).[33] Dystrophy of skeletal and smooth muscles (i.e., those of the uterus) was also noted. In 1922, these investigators reported that the addition of small amounts of yeast or fresh lettuce to the purified diet would restore fertility to females and prevent infertility in animals of both sexes. They designated the unknown fertility factor as *factor X*. Using the prevention of *gestation resorption* as the bioassay, Evans and Bishop found factor X activity in such unrelated materials as dried alfalfa, wheat germ, oats, meats, and milk fat, from which it was extractable with organic solvents. They distinguished the new fat-soluble factor from the known fat-soluble vitamins by showing that single droplets of wheat germ oil administered daily completely prevented gestation resorption, whereas cod liver oil, known to be a rich source of vitamins A and D, failed to do so.[34] In 1924, Sure at the University of Arkansas confirmed this work, concluding that the fat-soluble factor was a new vitamin, which he called **vitamin E**.

A Classic Touch in Coining *Tocopherol*

Evans was soon able to prepare a potent concentrate of vitamin E from the unsaponifiable lipids of wheat germ oil; others prepared similar vitamin E-active concentrates from lettuce lipids. By the early 1930s, Olcott and Mattill at the University of Iowa had found that such preparations, which prevented the gestation resorption syndrome in rats, also had chemical antioxidant properties that could be assayed *in vitro*.[35] In 1936, Evans isolated from unsaponifiable wheat germ lipids allophanic acid esters of three alcohols, one of which had very high biological vitamin E activity. Two years later, Fernholz showed that the latter alcohol had a phytyl side chain and a hydroquinone moiety, and proposed the chemical structure of the new vitamin. Evans coined the term *tocopherol*, which he derived from the Greek words *tokos* ("childbirth") and *pherein* ("to bear");[36] he used the suffix *-ol* to indicate that the factor is an alcohol. He also named

---

[33] The vitamin E-deficient rat carries her fetuses quite well until a fairly late stage of pregnancy, at which time they die and are resorbed by her. This syndrome is distinctive and is called *gestation resorption*.

[34] In fact, Evans and Bishop found that cod liver oil actually increased the severity of the gestation resorption syndrome, a phenomenon now understood on the basis of the antagonistic actions of high concentrations of the fat-soluble vitamins.

[35] Although the potencies of the vitamin preparations in the *in vivo* (rat gestation resorption) and *in vitro* (antioxidant) assays were not always well correlated.

[36] Evans wrote in 1962 that he was assisted in the coining of the name for vitamin E by George M. Calhoun, professor of Greek and a colleague at the University of California. It was Calhoun who suggested the Greek roots of this now-familiar name.

the three alcohols α-, β-, and γ-tocopherol. In 1938, the synthesis of the most active vitamer, α-tocopherol, was achieved by the groups of Karrer, Smith, and Bergel. A decade later another vitamer, δ-tocopherol, was isolated from soybean oil; not until 1959 were the *tocotrienols* described.[37]

Antihemorrhagic Factor: Vitamin K

In the 1920s, Henrik Dam, at the University of Copenhagen, undertook studies to determine whether cholesterol was an essential dietary lipid. In 1929, Dam reported that chicks fed diets consisting of food that had been extracted with nonpolar solvents to remove sterols developed subdural, subcutaneous, or intramuscular **hemorrhages, anemia**, and abnormally long blood-clotting times. A similar syndrome in chicks fed ether-extracted fish meal was reported by McFarlane's group, which at the time was attempting to determine the chick's requirements for vitamins A and D. They found that nonextracted fish meal completely prevented the clotting defect. Holst and Holbrook found that cabbage prevented the syndrome, which they took as evidence of an involvement of vitamin C. By the mid-1930s Dam had shown that the clotting defect was also prevented by a fat-soluble factor present in green leaves and certain vegetables and distinct from vitamins A, C, D, and E. He named the fat-soluble factor **vitamin K**.[38]

At that time, Herman Almquist and Robert Stokstad at the University of California found that the hemorrhagic disease of chicks fed a diet based on ether-extracted fish meal and brewers' yeast, polished rice, cod liver oil, and essential minerals was prevented by a factor present in ether extracts of alfalfa and also produced during microbial spoilage of fish meal and wheat bran. Dam's colleague, Schønheyder, discovered the reason for prolonged blood-clotting times of vitamin K-deficient animals. He found that the clotting defect did not involve a deficiency of tissue thrombokinase or plasma fibrinogen, or an accumulation of plasma anticoagulants; he also determined

that affected chicks showed relatively poor thrombin responses to exogenous thromboplastin. The latter observation suggested inadequate amounts of the clotting factor **prothrombin**, a factor already known to be important in the prevention of hemorrhages.

In 1936, Dam partially purified chick plasma prothrombin and showed its concentration to be depressed in vitamin K-deficient chicks. It would be several decades before this finding was fully understood.[39] Nevertheless, the clotting defect in the chick model served as a useful bioassay tool. When chicks were fed foodstuffs containing the new vitamin, their prothrombin values were normalized; hence, clotting time was returned to normal and the hemorrhagic disease was cured. The productive use of this bioassay led to the elucidation of the vitamin and its functions.

Vitamers K

Vitamin K was first isolated from alfalfa by Dam in collaboration with Paul Karrer at the University of Zurich in 1939. They showed the active substance, which was a yellow oil, to be a quinone. The structure of this form of the vitamin (called *vitamin K_1*) was elucidated by Doisy's group at the University of St. Louis, as well as by Karrer's, Almquist's, and Feiser's groups in the same year. Soon Doisy's group isolated a second form of the vitamin from putrified fish meal; this vitamer (called *vitamin K_2*) was crystalline. Subsequent studies showed this vitamer to differ from vitamin K_1 by having an unsaturated isoprenoid side chain at the 3-position of the naphthoquinone ring. In addition, putrified fish meal was found to contain several vitamin K_2-like substances with polyprenyl groups of differing chain lengths. Syntheses of vitamins K_2 were later achieved by Isler's and Folker's groups. A strictly synthetic analog of vitamers K_1 and K_2, consisting of the methylated head group alone (i.e., 2-methyl-1,4-naphthoquinone), was shown by Ansbacher and Fernholz to have high antihemorrhagic activity in the chick bioassay. It is, therefore, referred to as *vitamin K_3*.

---

[37] The tocotrienols differ from the tocopherols only by the presence of three conjugated double bonds in their phytyl side chains.

[38] Dam cited the fact that the next letter of the alphabet that had not previously been used to designate a known or proposed vitamin-like activity was also the first letter in the German or Danish phrase *koagulation faktor* and was, thus, a most appropriate designator for the antihemorrhagic vitamin. The phrase was soon shortened to *K factor* and, hence, *vitamin K*.

[39] It should be remembered that, at the time of this work, the biochemical mechanisms involved in clotting were incompletely understood. Of the many proteins now known to be involved in the process, only prothrombin and fibrinogen had been definitely characterized. It would not be until the early 1950s that the remainder of the now-classic clotting factors would be clearly demonstrated and that, of these, factors VII, IX, and X would be shown to be dependent on vitamin K. While these early studies effectively established that vitamin K deficiency results in impaired prothrombin activity, that finding would be interpreted as indicative of a vitamin K-dependent activation of the protein to its functional form.

Bios Yields Biotin

During the 1930s, independent studies of a yeast growth factor (called *bios IIb*[40]), a growth- and respiration-promoting factor for *Rhizobium trifolii* (called *coenzyme R*), and a factor that protected the rat against hair loss and skin lesions induced by raw egg white feeding (called *vitamin H*[41]) converged in an unexpected way. Kögl's group isolated the yeast growth factor from egg yolk and named it **biotin**. In 1940, György, du Vigneaud, and colleagues showed that vitamin H prepared from liver was remarkably similar to Kögl's egg yolk biotin. Owing to some reported differences in physical characteristics between the two factors, the egg yolk and liver substances were called, for a time, α-biotin and β-biotin,[42] respectively. These differences were later found to be incorrect, and the chemical structure of biotin was elucidated in 1942 by du Vigneaud's group at Cornell Medical College[43]; Karl Folkers achieved its complete synthesis in the following year.

A summary of the factors leading to the discovery of biotin is presented in Table 2-5.

Table 2-5. Factors leading to the discovery of biotin

Factor	Bioassay
Bios IIb	Yeast growth
Coenzyme R	*Rhizobium trifolii* growth
Vitamin H	Prevention of hair loss and skin lesions in rats fed raw egg white

Antianemia Factors

The last discoveries that led to the elucidation of new vitamins involved findings of anemias of dietary origin. The first of these was reported in 1931 by Lucy Wills's group as a *tropical macrocytic anemia*[44] observed in women in Bombay, India, which was often a complication of pregnancy. They found that the anemia could be treated effectively by supplementing the women's diet with an extract of autolyzed yeast.[45] Wills and associates found that a macrocytic anemia could be produced in monkeys by feeding them food similar to that consumed by the women in Bombay. Further more, the monkey anemia could be cured by oral administration of yeast or liver extract, or by parenteral administration of extract of liver; these treatments also cured human patients. The antianemia activity in these materials thus became known as the *Wills factor*.

Vitamin M?

Elucidation of the Wills factor involved the convergence of several lines of research, some of which appeared to be unrelated. The first of these came in 1935 from the studies of Day and colleagues at the University of Arkansas Medical School, who undertook to produce riboflavin deficiency in monkeys. They fed their animals a cooked diet consisting of polished rice, wheat, washed casein, cod liver oil, a mixture of salts, and an orange; quite unexpectedly,

---

[40] Bios IIb was one of three essential factors for yeasts that had been identified by Wilders at the turn of the century in response to the great controversy that raged between Pasteur and Liebig. In 1860, Pasteur had declared that yeast could be grown in solutions containing only water, sugar, yeast ash (i.e., minerals), and ammonium tartrate; he noted, however, the growth-promoting activities of *albuminoid materials* in such cultures. Liebig challenged the possibility of growing yeast in the absence of such materials. Although Pasteur's position was dominant through the close of the century, Wilders presented evidence that proved that cultivation of yeast actually did require the presence of a little wort, yeast water, peptone, or beef extract. (Wilders showed that an inoculum the size of a bacteriological loopful, which lacked sufficient amounts of these factors, was unsuccessful, whereas an inoculum the size of a pea grew successfully.) Wilders used the term *bios* to describe the new activity required for yeast growth. For three decades, investigators undertook to characterize Wilders's bios factors. By the mid-1920s, three factors had been identified: *bios I,* which was later identified as meso-inositol; *bios IIa,* which was replaced by pantothenic acid in some strains and by β-alanine plus leucine in others; and *bios IIb,* which was identified as biotin.

[41] György used the designation *H* after the German word *haut,* meaning "skin."

[42] The substances derived from each source were reported as having different melting points and optical rotations, giving rise to these designations. Subsequent studies, however, have been clear in showing that such differences are not correct, nor do these substances show different biological activities in microbiological systems. Thus, the distinguishing of biotin on the basis of source is no longer valid.

[43] du Vigneaud was to receive a Nobel Prize in Medicine for his work on the metabolism of methionine and methyl groups.

[44] A *macrocytic anemia* is one in which the number of circulating erythrocytes is below normal, but the mean size of those present is greater than normal (normal range, 82 to 92 μm^3). Macrocytic anemias occur in such syndromes as pernicious anemia, sprue, celiac disease, and macrocytic anemia of pregnancy. Wills's studies of the macrocytic anemia in her monkey model revealed megaloblastic arrest (i.e., failure of the large, nucleated, embryonic erythrocyte precursor cell type to mature) in the erythropoietic tissues of the bone marrow and a marked reticulocytosis [i.e., the presence of young red blood cells in numbers greater than normal (usually <1%), occurring during active blood regeneration]; both signs were eliminated coincidentally on the administration of extracts of yeast or liver.

[45] Wills's yeast extract was not particularly potent, as they needed to administer 4 grams of it two to four times daily to cure the anemia.

they found them to develop anemia, leukopenia,[46] ulceration of the gums, diarrhea, and increased susceptibility to bacillary dysentery. They found that the syndrome did not respond to thiamin, riboflavin, or nicotinic acid; however, it could be prevented by feeding daily 10 grams of brewers' yeast or 2 grams of a dried hog liver–stomach preparation. Day named the protective factor in brewers' yeast *vitamin M* (for monkey).

Factors U and R and Vitamin B$_c$

In the late 1930s, three groups (Robert Stokstad's at the University of California, Leo Norris's at Cornell, and Albert Hogan's at the University of Missouri) reported syndromes characterized by anemia in chicks fed highly purified diets. The anemias were found to respond to dietary supplements of yeast, alfalfa, and wheat bran. Stokstad and Manning called this unknown factor *factor U*; Baurenfeind and Norris called it *factor R*. Shortly thereafter, Hogan and Parrott discovered an antianemic substance in liver extracts; they called it *vitamin B$_c$*.[47] At the time (1939) it the extent to which these factors may have been related was unclear.

Yeast Growth Related to Anemia?

At the same time, the microbiologists Snell and Peterson, who were studying the bios factors required by yeasts, reported the existence of an unidentified water-soluble factor that was necessary for the growth of *Lactobacillus casei*. This factor was present in liver and yeast, from which it could be prepared by adsorption to and then elution from Norit (a carbon-based filtering agent); for a while, they called it the *yeast Norit factor*, but it quickly became known as the *L. casei factor*. Hutchings and colleagues at the University of Wisconsin further purified the factor from liver and found it to stimulate chick growth; this suggested a possible identity of the bacterial and chick factors. The factor from liver was found to stimulate the growth of both *L. helveticus* and *Streptococcus faecalis* R,[48] whereas the yeast-derived

factor was twice as potent for *L. helveticus* as it was for *S. faecalis*. Thus, it became popular to refer to these as the liver *L. casei* factor and the yeast (or fermentation) *L. casei* factor.

Snell's group found that many green leafy materials were potent sources of something with the microbiological effects of the *Norit eluate factor*; that is, extracts promoted the growth of both *S. faecalis* and *L. casei*. They named the factor, by virtue of its sources, **folic acid**. In 1943, a fermentation product was isolated that stimulated the growth of *S. faecalis* but not *L. casei*; this was called the *SLR factor* and, later, *rhizopterin*.

Who's on First?

It was far from clear in the early 1940s whether any of these factors were at all related, as folic acid appeared to be active for both microorganisms and animals, whereas concentrates of vitamin M, factors R and U, and vitamin B$_c$ appeared to be effective only for animals. Clues to solving the puzzle came from the studies of Mims and associates at the University of Arkansas Medical School, who showed that incubation of vitamin M concentrates in the presence of rat liver enzymes caused a marked increase in the folic acid activity (i.e., assayed using *S. casei* and *S. lactis* R.) of the preparation. Subsequent work showed such "activation" enzymes to be present in both hog kidney and chick pancreas. Charkey, of the Cornell group, found that incubation of their factor R preparations with rat or chick liver enzymes produced large increases in their folic acid potencies for microorganisms. These studies indicated for the first time that at least some of these various substances may be related.

Derivatives of Pteroylglutamic Acid

The real key to solving what was clearly the most complicated puzzle in the discovery of the vitamins came in 1943 with the isolation of pteroylglutamic acid from liver by Stokstad's group at the Lederle Laboratories of American Cyanamid, Inc., and by Piffner's group at Parke-Davis, Inc. Stokstad's group

---

[46] Leukopenia refers to any situation in which the total number of leukocytes (i.e., white blood cells) in the circulating blood is less than normal, which is generally about 5000 per mm^3.

[47] Hogan and Parrott used the subscript *c* to designate this factor as one required by the chick.

[48] *Streptococcus faecalis* was then called *S. lactis* R.

achieved the synthesis of the compound in 1946. Soon it was found that pteroylmonoglutamic acid was, indeed, the substance that had been variously identified in liver as factor U, vitamin M, vitamin B$_c$, and the liver *L. casei* factor. The yeast *L. casei* factor was found to be the diglutamyl derivative (pteroyldiglutamic acid) and that the liver-derived vitamin B$_c$ was the hexaglutamyl derivative (pteroylhexaglutamic acid). Others of these factors (the *SLR factor*) were subsequently found to be single-carbon metabolites of pteroylglutamic acid. These various compounds thus became known generically as **folic acid**.

A summary of the factors leading to the discovery of folic acid is presented in Table 2-6.

Antipernicious Anemia Factor

The second nutritional anemia that was found to involve a vitamin deficiency was the fatal condition of human patients that was first described by J. S. Combe in 1822 and became known as *pernicious anemia*.[49] The first real breakthrough toward understanding the etiology of pernicious anemia did not come until 1926, when Minot and Murphy

Table 2-6. Factors leading to the discovery of folic acid

Factor	Bioassay
Wills factor	Cure of anemia in humans
Vitamin M	Prevention of anemia in monkeys
Vitamin B$_c$	Prevention of anemia in chicks
Factor R	Prevention of anemia in chicks
Factor U	Prevention of anemia in chicks
Yeast Norit factor	Growth of *Lactobacillus casei*
Lactobacillus casei factor	Growth of *Lactobacillus casei*
SLR factor	Growth of *Rhizobium* species
Rhizopterin	Growth of *Rhizobium* species
Folic acid	Growth of *Streptococcus faecalis* and *Lactobacillus casei*

found that lightly cooked liver, which the prominent hematologist G. H. Whipple had found to accelerate the regeneration of blood in dogs made anemic by exsanguination, was highly effective as therapy for the disease.[50,51] This indicated that liver contained a factor necessary for hemoglobin synthesis.

Intrinsic and Extrinsic Factors

Soon, studies of the antipernicious anemia factor in liver revealed that its enteric absorption depended on yet another factor in the gastric juice, which W. B. Castle in 1928 called the *intrinsic factor* to distinguish it from the *extrinsic factor* in liver. Biochemists then commenced a long endeavor to isolate the antipernicious anemia factor from liver. The isolation of the factor was necessarily slow and arduous for the reason that the only bioassay available was the hematopoietic response of human pernicious anemia patients, which were frequently not available. No animal model had been found; and a bioassay could not be replaced by a chemical reaction or physical method because, as is now known, this most potent vitamin is active at exceedingly low concentrations. Therefore, it was most important to the elucidation of the antipernicious anemia factor when, in 1947, Mary Shorb of the University of Maryland found that it was also required for the growth of *Lactobacillus lactis* Dorner.[52] Through Shorb's microbiological assay, isolation of the factor, by that time named **vitamin B$_{12}$** by the Merck group, proceeded rapidly.

Animal Protein Factors

At about the same time, animal growth responses to factors associated with animal proteins or manure were reported as American animal nutritionists sought to eliminate expensive and scarce animal byproducts from the diets of livestock. Norris's group at Cornell attributed responses of this time to an **animal protein factor**; the factor in liver necessary for rat

[49] Pernicious anemia is also called *Addison's anemia* after T. Addison, who described it in great detail in 1949, and *Biemer's anemia* after A. Biemier, who reported the disease in Zurich in 1872 and coined the term *pernicious anemia*.

[50] Minot and Murphy treated 45 pernicious anemia patients with 120 to 240 grams of lightly cooked liver per day. The patients' mean erythrocyte count increased from 1.47×10^6 per milliliter before treatment to 3.4×10^6 per milliliter and 4.6×10^6 per milliliter after one and two months of treatment, respectively.

[51] Whipple, Minot, and Murphy shared the 1934 Nobel Prize in Medicine for the discovery of whole liver therapy for pernicious anemia.

[52] For a time, this was referred to as the *LLD factor*.

growth was called *factor X* by Cary and *zoopherin*[53] by Zucker and Zucker. Soon it became evident that these factors were probably identical. Stokstad's group found the factor in manure and isolated an organism from poultry manure that would synthesize a factor that was effective both in promoting chick growth and in treating pernicious anemia. That the antipernicious anemia factor was produced microbiologically was important in that it led to an economical means of industrial production of vitamin B_{12}.

Vitamin B_{12} Isolated

By the late 1940s, Combs[54] and Norris, using chick growth as their bioassay procedure, were fairly close to the isolation of vitamin B_{12}. However, in 1948, Folkers at Merck, using the *Lactobacillus lactis* Dorner assay, succeeded in first isolating the antipernicious anemia factor in crystalline form. This achievement was accomplished in the same year by Lester Smith's group at the Glaxo Laboratories in England (who found their pink crystals to contain cobalt), assaying their material on pernicious anemia patients in relapse.[55] The elucidation of the complex chemical structure of vitamin B_{12} was finally achieved in 1955 by Dorothy Hodgkin's group at Oxford with the use of X-ray crystallography. In the early 1960s several groups accomplished the partial synthesis of the vitamin; it was not until 1970 that the *de novo* synthesis of vitamin B_{12} was finally achieved by Woodward and Eschenmoser.

A summary of the factors leading to the discovery of vitamin B_{12} is presented in Table 2-7.

Vitamins Discovered in Only Five Decades

Beginning with the concept of a vitamin, which emerged with Eijkman's proposal of an antipolyneuritis factor in 1906, the elucidation of the vitamins continued through the isolation of vitamin B_{12} in potent form in 1948 (see Table 2-8). Thus, the identification of the presently recognized vitamins was achieved within a period of only 42 years! For some

vitamins (e.g., pyridoxine) for which convenient animal models were available, discoveries came rapidly; for others (e.g., niacin, vitamin B_{12}) for which animal models were late to be found, the pace of scientific progress was much slower. These paths of discovery were marked by nearly a dozen Nobel Prizes (Table 2-9).

Table 2-7. Factors leading to the discovery of vitamin B_{12}

Factor	Bioassay
Extrinsic factor	Cure of anemia in humans
LLD factor	Growth of *Lactobacillus lactis* Dorner
Vitamin B_{12}	Growth of *Lactobacillus lactis* Dorner
Animal protein factor	Growth of chicks
Factor X	Growth of rats
Zoopherin	Growth of rats

Table 2-8. Timelines for the discoveries of the vitamins

Vitamin	Proposed	Isolated	Structure determined	Synthesis achieved
Thiamin	1906	1926	1932	1933
Vitamin C	1907	1926	1932	1933
Vitamin A	1915	1937	1942	1947
Vitamin D	1919	1932	1932 (D_2)	1932
			1936 (D_3)	1936
Vitamin E	1922	1936	1938	1938
Niacin	1926	1937	1937	1867[a]
Vitamin B_{12}	1926	1948	1955	1970
Biotin	1926	1939	1942	1943
Vitamin K	1929	1939	1939	1940
Pantothenic acid	1931	1939	1939	1940
Folate	1931	1939	1943	1946
Riboflavin	1933	1933	1934	1935
Vitamin B_6	1934	1936	1938	1939

[a]Much of the chemistry of niacin was known before its nutritional roles were recognized.

---

[53] The term *zoopherin* carries the connotation: "to carry on an animal species."

[54] Characterization of the animal protein factor was the subject of the author's father's doctoral thesis in Norris's laboratory at Cornell in the late 1940s.

[55] Friedrich (1988) has pointed out that it should be no surprise that vitamin B_{12} was first isolated in industrial laboratories, because the task required industrial-scale facilities to handle the enormous amounts of starting material that were needed. For example, the Merck group used a ton of liver to obtain 20 milligrams of crystalline material.

Table 2-9. Nobel prizes awarded for research on vitamins

Year awarded	Recipients	Discovery
	Prizes in Medicine and Physiology	
1929	Christian Eijkman and Frederick G. Hopkins	Discovery of the antineuritic vitamin; discovery of the growth-stimulating vitamins
1934	George H. Whipple, George R. Minot, and William P. Murphy	Discoveries concerning liver therapy against pernicious anemia
1937	Albert von Szent-Györgi and Charles G. King	Discoveries in connection with the biological combustion, with special reference to vitamin C, and the catalysis of fumaric acid
1943	Henrik Dam and Edward A. Doisy	Discovery of vitamin K; discovery of the chemical nature of vitamin K
1953	Fritz A. Lipmann	Discovery of coenzyme A and its importance in intermediary metabolism
1955	Hugo Theorell	Discoveries relating to the nature and mode of action of oxidizing enzymes
1964	Feordor Lynen and Konrad Bloch	Discoveries concerning the mechanism and regulation of cholesterol and fatty acid metabolism
	Prizes in Chemistry	
1928	Adolf Windaus	Studies on the constitution of the sterols and their connection with the vitamins
1937	Paul Karrer and Walter N. Haworth	Researches into the constitution of carbohydrates and vitamin C
		Researches into the constitution of carotenoids, flavins, and vitamins A and B
1938	Richard Kuhn	Work on carotenoids and vitamins
1967	George Wald, H. K. Hartline, and R. Grant	Discoveries of the basic chemical and physiological processes in vision

VII. Vitamin Terminology

The terminology of the vitamins can be as daunting as that of any other scientific field. Many vitamins carry alphabetic or alphanumeric designations, yet the sequence of such designations has an arbitrary appearance by virtue of its many gaps and inconsistent application to all of the vitamins. This situation notwithstanding, the logic underlying the terminology of the vitamins becomes apparent when it is viewed in terms of the history of vitamin discovery. The familiar designations in use today are, in most cases, the surviving terms coined by earlier researchers on the paths to vitamin discovery. Thus, because McCollum and Davis used the letters A and B to distinguish the lipid-soluble antixerophthalmic factor from the water-soluble antineuritic and growth activity that was subsequently found to consist of several vitamins, such chemically and physiologically unrelated substances as thiamin, riboflavin, pyridoxine, and cobalamins (in fact, all water-soluble vitamins except ascorbic acid, which was designated before the **vitamin B complex** was partitioned) are all called B vitamins. In the case of folic acid, certainly the name survived its competitors by virtue of its relatively attractive sound (e.g., versus *rhizopterin*). Therefore, in most cases the accepted designations for the vitamins, have relevance only to the history and chronology of their discovery, and not to their chemical or metabolic similarities. The discovery of the vitamins left a path littered with designations of "vitamins," "factors," and other terms, most of which have been discarded (see Appendix A for a complete listing).

VIII. Other Factors Sometimes Called Vitamins

Several other factors have, at various times or under certain conditions, been called vitamins. Many remain today only as historic markers of once incompletely explained phenomena, which are now better understood. Today some would appear to satisfy, for at least some species, the operating definition of a vitamin, although, in practice, that term is restricted to those factors required by higher organisms.[56] Therefore, these can be referred to as *quasi-vitamins* (see Table 2-10). At various times, of course, other factors have been represented as vitamins; however, no solid evidence supports such claims. These pseudofactors (see Table 2-11) are not to be confused with the vitamins.

IX. The Modern History of the Vitamins

Subsequent to the recognition of the vitamins and the discovery of their identities, it became apparent that much more information would be needed in order to use these substances fully to improve human and animal health and to optimize the efficiency of producing food animals. Thus, recent research interest in the vitamins has centered on certain foci (see Table 2-12). This information, much of which is still emerging today, will be the subject of the following chapters.

Table 2-11. Pseudofactors that are not vitamins

Substance	Purported biological activity
Laetrile	A cyanogenic glycoside; unsubstantiated claims of antitumorigenicity
Gerovital	Unsubstantiated antiaging elixir
Orotic acid	Normal metabolic intermediate of pyrimidine biosynthesis with hypocholesterolemic activity
Pangamic acid	Ill-defined substance(s), originally derived from apricot pits, with unsubstantiated claims for a variety of health benefits

Table 2-10. Quasi-vitamins

Substance	Biological activity
Choline	Component of the neurotransmitter acetylcholine and the membrane structural component phosphatidylcholine; essential for normal growth and bone development in young poultry; can spare methionine in many animal species and, can thus, be essential in diets that provide limited methyl groups
p-Aminobenzoic acid	Essential growth factor for several microbes, in which it functions as a provitamin of folic acid; reported to reverse diet- or hydroquinone-induced achromotrichia in rats, and to ameliorate rickettsial infections
myo-Inositol	Component of phosphatidylinositol; prevents diet-induced lipo-dystrophies due to impaired lipid transport in gerbils and rats. Essential for some microbes, gerbils, and certain fishes
Bioflavonoids	Reported to reduce capillary fragility and inhibit *in vitro* aldolase reductase (has role in diabetic cataracts) and o-methyltransferase (inactivates epinephrine and norepinephrine)
Ubiquinones	Group includes a component of the mitochondrial respiratory chain; are antioxidants and can spare vitamin E in preventing anemia in monkeys and in maintaining sperm motility in birds
Lipoic acid	Cofactor in oxidative decarboxylation of α-keto acids; essential for growth of several microbes, but inconsistent effects on animal growth
Carnitine	Essential for transport of fatty acyl-CoA from cytoplasm to mitochondria for β oxidation; synthesized by most species except some insects, which require a dietary source for growth
Pyrroloquinoline quinone	Component of certain bacterial and mammalian metallo-oxidoreductases; deprivation impairs growth, causes skin lesions in mice

---

[56] Organic growth-promoting substances required only by microorganisms are frequently called *nutrilites*.

Table 2-12. Foci of current vitamin research

Focus	Research activities
Analytical and physical chemistry	Determining chemical and biological potencies and stabilities (to storage, processing ,and cooking) of the vitamins, their various vitamers and chemical derivatives; developing analytical methods for measuring vitamin contents of food
Biochemistry and molecular biology	Elucidating the molecular mechanisms of vitamin action, including roles in gene expression; elucidating pathways of vitamin metabolism; determining the interactions with other nutrients and/or factors (e.g., disease, oxidative stress) that affect vitamin functions and needs
Nutritional surveillance and epidemiology	Determining vitamin intakes and status of populations and at-risk subgroups; elucidating relationships of vitamin intake/status and disease risks
Medicine	Determining roles of vitamins in etiology and/or management of chronic (e.g., cancer, heart disease), congenital (e.g., neural tube defects), and infectious diseases; determining vitamin needs over the life cycle
Agriculture and international development	Developing smallholder farming/gardening systems and other food-based approaches that support nutritional adequacy with respect to vitamins and other nutrients
Food technology	Developing food-processing techniques that retain vitamins in food; and methods for the effective vitamin fortification of foods

Study Questions and Exercises

1. How did the *vitamin theory* influence the interpretation of findings concerning diet and health associations?

2. For each vitamin, list the key empirical observations that led to its initial recognition.

3. In what general ways were animal models employed in the discovery of the vitamins? What ethical issues must be addressed in this type of research?

4. Which vitamins were discovered as results of efforts to use chemically defined diets for raising animals? How would you go about developing such a diet?

5. Which vitamins were discovered primarily through human experimentation? What ethical issues must be addressed in this type of research?

6. Prepare a concept map illustrating the interrelationships of the various prevalent ideas and the many goals, approaches, and outcomes that resulted in the discovery of the vitamins.

Recommended Reading

General History of the Vitamins

Carpenter, K. J. (1986). *The History of Scurvy and Vitamin C.* Cambridge University Press, Cambridge, 288 pp.

Carpenter, K. J. (2000). *Beriberi, White Rice and Vitamin B: A Disease, a Cause, and a Cure.* University of California Press, Los Angeles, 282 pp.

Carpenter, K. J. (2003). "A Short History of Nutritional Science: Part 1 (1785–1885)." *J. Nutr.* **133**, 638.

Carpenter, K. J. (2003). "A Short History of Nutritional Science: Part 2 (1885–1912)." *J. Nutr.* **133**, 975.

Carpenter, K. J. (2003). "A Short History of Nutritional Science: Part 3 (1912–1944)." *J. Nutr.* **133**, 3023.

Carpenter, K. J. (2003). "A Short History of Nutritional Science: Part 4 (1945–1985)." *J. Nutr.* **133**, 3331.

Györgi, P. (1954). "Early experiences with riboflavin — a retrospect." *Nutr. Rev.* **12,** 97.

Harris, L. J. (1955). *Vitamins in Theory and Practice*, pp. 1–39. Cambridge University Press, Cambridge.

Lepkovsky, S. (1954). "Early Experiences with Pyridoxine — A retrospect." *Nutr. Rev.* **12,** 257.

Roe, D. A. (1973). *A Plague of Corn: The Social History of Pellagra.* Cornell University Press, Ithaca, N.Y.

Sebrell, W. H., Jr. (1981). "History of Pellagra." *Fed. Proc.* **40,** 1520.

Wald, G. (1968). "Molecular Basis of Visual Excitation." *Science* **162,** 230–239.

Wolf, G. (2001) "The Discovery of the Visual Function of Vitamin A." *J. Nutr.* **131,** 1647–1650.

Papers of Key Historical Significance

Vitamin concept	Funk, C. (1912). *J. State Med.* **20,** 341.
Vitamin A	McCollum, E. V., and Davis, M. (1913). *J. Biol. Chem.* **15,** 167.
	Osborne, T. B., and Mendel, L. B. (1917). *J. Biol. Chem.* **31,** 149.
	Wald, G. (1933). "Vitamin A in the retina." *Nature (London)* **132,** 316.
	Steenbock, H. (1919). *Science* **50,** 352.
Vitamin D	McCollum, E. V., Simmonds, N., and Pitz, W. (1916). *J. Biol. Chem.* **27,** 33.
Vitamin E	Evans, H. M., and Bishop, K. S. (1922). *Science* **56,** 650.
	Olcott, H. S., and Mattill, H. A. (1931). *J. Biol. Chem.* **93,** 65–70.
Vitamin K	Dam, H. (1929). *Biochem. Z.* **215,** 475.
Ascorbic acid	Holst, A., and Frolich, T. (1907). *J. Hyg. (Camb.)* **7,** 634.
	King, C. G., and Waugh, W. A. (1932). *Science* **75,** 357.
	Svirbely, J. L., and Szent-Györgi, A. (1932). Nature (*London*) **129,** 576.
Thiamin	Eijkman, C. (1890). *Med. J. Dutch East Indies* **30,** 295.
	Eijkman, C. (1896). *Med. J. Dutch East Indies* **36,** 214.
Riboflavin	Kuhn, P., Györgi, P., and Wagner-Juregg, T. (1933). *Ber.* **66,** 317.
Niacin	Elvehjem, C., Madden, R., Strong, F., and Wolley, D. (1937). *J. Am. Chem. Soc.* **59,** 1767.
	Goldberger, J. (1922). *J. Am. Med. Assoc.* **78,** 1676.
	Warburg, O., and Christian, W. (1936). *Biochem. Z.* **43,** 287.
Vitamin B_6	Györgi, P. (1934). *Nature (London)* **133,** 498.
Biotin	Kögl, F., and Tonnis, B. (1936). *Z. Physiol. Chem.* **242,** 43.
Pantothenic acid	Norris, L. C., and Ringrose, A. T. (1930). *Science* **71,** 643.
	Williams, R. J., Lyman, C., Goodyear, G., Truesdail, J., and Holaday, D. (1933). *J. Am. Chem. Soc.* **55,** 2912.
Folate	Jukes, T. H. (1939). *J. Am. Chem. Soc.* **61,** 975.
	Mimms, V., Totter, J. R., and Day, P. L. (1944). *J. Biol. Chem.* **155,** 401.
Vitamin B_{12}	Castle, W. B. (1929). *Am. J. Med. Sci.* **178,** 748.
	Minot, G. R., and Murphy, W. P. (1926). *J. Am. Med. Assoc.* **87,** 470.
	Wills, L., Contab, M. A., and Lond, B. S. (1931). *Br. Med. J.* **1,** 1059.
	Shorb, M. S. (1948). *Science* **107,** 398.

Chemical and Physiological Properties of Vitamins

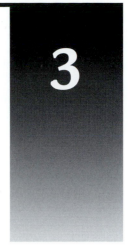

3

La vie est une fonction chimique.
— A. L. Lavoisier

I.	Chemical and Physical Properties of the Vitamins	36
II.	Vitamin A	42
III.	Vitamin D	45
IV.	Vitamin E	47
V.	Vitamin K	49
VI.	Vitamin C	51
VII.	Thiamin	52
VIII.	Riboflavin	53
IX.	Niacin	54
X.	Vitamin B_6	55
XI.	Biotin	56
XII.	Pantothenic Acid	56
XIII.	Folate	57
XIV.	Vitamin B_{12}	59
XV.	General Properties of the Vitamins	60
XVI.	Physiological Utilization of the Vitamins	64
XVII.	Metabolism of the Vitamins	69
XVIII.	Metabolic Functions of the Vitamins	72
	Study Questions and Exercises	73
	Recommended Reading	73

Anchoring Concepts

1. The chemical composition and structure of a substance determine both its physical properties and chemical reactivity.
2. The physicochemical properties of a substance determine the ways in which it acts and is acted on in biological systems.
3. Substances tend to be partitioned between hydrophilic regions (plasma, cytosol, and mitochondrial matrix space) and hydrophobic regions (membranes, bulk lipid droplets) of biological systems on the basis of their relative solubilities; overcoming such partitioning requires actions of agents (micelles, binding or transport proteins) that serve to alter their effective solubilities.
4. Isomers and analogs of a given substance may not have equivalent biological activities.

Learning Objectives

1. To understand that the term *vitamin* refers to a family of compounds, that is, structural analogs, with qualitatively similar biological activities but often with different quantitative potencies.
2. To become familiar with the chemical structures and physical properties of vitamins.
3. To understand the relationship between the physicochemical properties of vitamins and their stabilities, and how these properties affect their means of enteric absorption, transport, and tissue storage.
4. To become familiar with the general nature of vitamin metabolism.

Vocabulary

Adenosylcobalamin
Ascorbic acid
β-Carotene
β-Ionone nucleus
Binding proteins
Bioavailability
Biopotency
Biotin
Carotenoid
Cholecalciferol
6-Chromanol nucleus
Chylomicrons
Coenzyme A
Cobalamin
Corrin nucleus
Cyanocobalamin

Dehydroascorbic acid
Ergocalciferol
Flavin adenine dinucleotide (FAD)
Flavin mononucleotide (FMN)
Folacin
Folic acid
HDL
Isoalloxazine nucleus
Isoprenoid
LDL
Lipoproteins
Menadione
Menaquinone
Methylcobalamin
Micelle
NAD(H)
NADP(H)
Naphthoquinone nucleus
Niacin
Nicotinamide
Nicotinic acid
Pantothenic acid
Phylloquinone
Portomicron
Pteridine
Pteroylglutamic acid
Pyridine nucleus
Pyridoxal
Pyridoxamine
Pyridoxine
Pyridoxol
Pyrimidine ring
Retinal
Retinoic acid
Retinoid
Retinol
Riboflavin
Steroid
Tetrahydrofolic acid
Tetrahydrothiophene (thiophane) nucleus
Thiamin
Thiamin pyrophosphate

Thiazole ring
Tocol
Tocopherol
Tocotrienol
Ureido nucleus
Vitamin A
Vitamin B_2
Vitamin B_6
Vitamin B_{12}
Vitamin C
Vitamin D
Vitamin D_2
Vitamin D_3
Vitamin E
Vitamin K
Vitamin K_1
Vitamin K_2
Vitamin K_3
VLDL

I. Chemical and Physical Properties of the Vitamins

Classifying the Vitamins According to Their Solubilities

The vitamins are organic, low-molecular-weight substances that have key roles in metabolism. Few of the vitamins are single substances; almost all are families of chemically related substances (i.e., *vitamers*) sharing qualitatively (but not necessarily quantitatively) biological activities. Thus, the vitamers comprising a vitamin family may vary in biopotency, and the common vitamin name is actually a generic descriptor for all of the relevant vitamers. Otherwise, vitamin families are chemically heterogeneous; therefore, it is convenient to consider their physical properties (Table 3-1), which offer an empirical means of classifying the vitamins broadly.

The vitamins are frequently described according to their solubilities, that is, as being either fat soluble or water soluble.[1] This way of classifying the vitamins

(Text continued on page 42)

---

[1] The concept of solubility refers to the interactions of solutes and solvents; a material is said to be soluble if it can disperse on a molecular level within a solvent. Solvents such as water, which can either donate or accept electrons, are said to be *polar*, whereas solvents (e.g., many organic solvents) incapable of such interactions are called *nonpolar*. Compounds that themselves are polar or that have charged or ionic character are soluble in polar solvents such as water (the compounds are *hydrophilic*) but are insoluble in nonpolar organic solvents (*lipophobic*). Molecules that do not contain polar or ionizable groups tend to be insoluble in water (*hydrophobic*) but soluble in nonpolar organic solvents (*lipophilic*). Some large molecules (e.g., phospholipids, fatty acids, bile salts) that have local areas of charge or ionic bond density as well as other areas without charged groups exhibit both polar and nonpolar character. Such molecules, called *amphipaths*, have both hydrophilic and lipophilic internal regions; they tend to align along the interfaces of mixed polar/nonpolar phases. Amphipathic molecules are important in facilitating the dispersion of hydrophobic substances in aqueous environments; they do this by surrounding those substances, forming the submicroscopic structure called the mixed **micelle**.

Table 3-1. Physical properties of vitamins

Vitamin	Vitamer	MW	Solubility Organic[a]	Solubility H₂O	Absorption maximum (nm)	Molar absorptivity ε	Absorptivity A¹% 1cm	Fluorescence Excitation nm	Fluorescence Emission nm	Melting point (°C)	Color/form
Vitamin A	all-*trans*-retinol	286.4	+	−	325	52,300	1845	325	470	62–64	Yellow/crystal
	11-*cis*-retinol	286.4	+	−	319	34,900	1220				
	13-*cis*-retinol	286.4	+	−	328	48,300	1189				
	Retinal	284.4	+	−	373		1548			61–64	Orange/crystal
	all-*trans*-retinoic acid	300.4	+	sl[b]	350	45,300	1510			180–182	Yellow/crystal
	13-*cis*-retinoic acid	300.4	+	sl[b]	354	39,800	1325			180–182	Yellow/crystal
	all-*trans*-retinyl acetate	312.0	+	sl[b]	326		1550			57–58	Yellow/crystal
	all-*trans*-retinyl palmitate	508.0	+	sl[b]	325–328		975			28–29	Yellow/crystal
Provitamin A	β-carotene	536.9	+	−	453	2,592	139			183	Purple/crystal
	α-carotene	536.9	+	−	444	2,800				187	Purple/crystal
Vitamin D	Vitamin D₂	396.7	+	−	264	18,300	459	no fluorescence		115–118	White/crystal
	Vitamin D₃	384.6	+	−	265	19,400	462	no fluorescence		84–85	White/crystal
	25(OH) vitamin D₃	400.7	+	−	265	18,000	449	no fluorescence			
	1α,25(OH)₂ vitamin D₃	416.6	+	−	264	19,000	418	no fluorescence			
Vitamin E	α-Tocopherol	430.7	+	−	292	3,265	75.8	295	320	2.5	Yellow/oil
	β-Tocopherol	416.7	+	−	296	3,725	89.4	297	322		Yellow/oil
	γ-Tocopherol	416.7	+	−	298	3,809	91.4	297	322	−2.4	Yellow/oil
	δ-Tocopherol	402.7	+	−	298		91–92	297	322		Yellow/oil
	α-Tocopheryl acetate	472.8	+	−	286	1,891–2,080	40–44	290	323		Yellow/oil
	α-Tocopheryl succinate	530.8	+	−	286	2,044	38.5	285	310		
	α-Tocotrienol	424.7	+	−	292	3,652	86.0				

(Continued)

Table 3-1. Physical properties of vitamins—Cont'd

Vitamin	Vitamer	MW	Solubility Organic[a]	Solubility H₂O	Absorption maximum (nm)	Molar absorptivity ε	Absorptivity A¹% 1cm	Fluorescence Excitation nm	Fluorescence Emission nm	Melting point (°C)	Color/form
	β-Tocotrienol	410.6	+	–	296	3,540	86.2	290	323		Yellow/oil
	γ-Tocotrienol	410.6	+	–	298	3,737	91.0	290	324		Yellow/oil
	δ-Tocotrienol	396.6	+	–	298	3,403	85.8	292	324		Yellow/oil
Vitamin K	Vitamin K₁	450.7	+	–	242	17,900	396	no fluorescence			Yellow/oil
					248	18,900	419				
					260	17,300	383				
					269	17,400	387				
					325	3,100	68				
	Vitamin K₂₍₂₀₎	444.7	+	–	248	19,500	439	no fluorescence		35	Yellow/crystals
	Vitamin K₂₍₃₀₎	580.0	+	–	243	17,600	304	no fluorescence		50	Yellow/crystals
					248	18,600	320				
					261	16,800	290				
					270	16,900	292				
	Vitamin K₂₍₃₅₎	649.2	+	–	243	18,000	278	no fluorescence		54	Yellow/crystals
					248	19,100	195				
					261	17,300	266				
					270	30,300	467				
					325–328	3,100	48				
	Vitamin K₃	172.2	+	–						105–107	Yellow/crystals
Vitamin C	Ascorbic acid	176.1	–	+	245	12,200	695	no fluorescence		190–192	White/crystals
	Calcium ascorbate	390.3	–	+							White/crystals
	Sodium ascorbate	198.1	–	xs[e]						218[c]	White/crystals
	Ascorbyl palmitate	414.5	–	+							White/crystals
Thiamin	Thiamin disulfide	562.7	–	sl[b]				no fluorescence		177	Yellow/crystals
	Thiamin HCl	337.3	–	xs[e]						246–250	White/crystals
	Thiamin mononitrate	327.4	–	+						196–200[c]	White/crystals
	Thiamin monophosphate	344.3	–								

	Thiamin pyrophosphate	424.3	–							220–222[c]	
	Thiamin triphosphate	504.3	–							228–232[c]	
Riboflavin[d]	Riboflavin	376.4	–	+	260, 375, 450	27,700, 10,600, 12,200	736, 282, 324	360, 465	521	278[c]	Orange-yellow/crystal
	Riboflavin-5'-phosphate	456.4			260	27,100	594	440–500	530		Orange-yellow/crystal
	FAD	785.6			260, 375, 450	37,000, 9,300, 11,300	471, 118, 144	440–500	530		
Niacin	Nicotinic acid	123.1	–	+	260	2,800	227	no fluorescence		237	White/crystal
	Nicotinamide	122.1	–	xs[e]	261	5,800	478	no fluorescence		128–131	White/crystal
Vitamin B_6	Pyridoxal HCl	203.6	–	+	390, 318	200, 8,128	9.8, 399	330[f], 310	382, 365[g]	165[c]	White/crystal
	Pyridoxine	169.2			254, 324	3,891, 7,244	230, 428	320, 332	380, 400	160	
	Pyridoxol HCl	205.6	–	+	253, 290, 292, 325	3,700, 8,400, 7,720, 7,100	180, 408, 375, 345			206–208	White/crystal
	Pyridoxamine di-HCl	241.1			253	4,571	190	320	370[g]	226–227	
	Pyridoxal 5'-phosphate	247.1			328, 330, 388	7,763, 2,500, 4,900	322, 101, 198	337, 365, 360, 330	400[h], 423[h], 430[g], 410[f]		
Biotin	*d*-Biotin	244.3	–	+	204	(very weak)		no fluorescence		232–233	Colorless/crystal
Pantothenic acid	Pantothenic acid	219.2	–	xs[e]	204	(very weak)		no fluorescence			Clear/oil
	Calcium pantothenate	467.5	–	–	no chromophore			no fluorescence		195–196[c]	White/crystal
	D-pantothenol	205.3		sl[b]	no chromophore			no fluorescence			Clear/oil

(Continued)

Table 3-1. Physical properties of vitamins—Cont'd

Vitamin	Vitamer	MW	Solubility Organic[a]	H$_2$O	Absorption maximum (nm)	Molar absorptivity ε	Absorptivity A$^{1\%}$ 1cm	Fluorescence Excitation nm	Emission nm	Melting point (°C)	Color/form
Folate	Folic acid	441.1			282	27,000	612	363	450–460[g]		
					350	7,000	159				
	Tetrahydrofolate	445.4			297	27,000	606	305–310	360[h]		
	10-formyl FH$_4$	473.5			288	18,200	384	313	360[f]		
	5-formyl FH$_4$	473.5			287	31,500	665	314	365[f]		
	5-methyl FH$_4$	459.5			290	32,000	697				
	5-formimino FH$_4$	472.5			285	35,400	749	308	360[f]		
	5,10-methenyl FH$_4$	456.4			352	25,000	548	370	470[h]		
	5,10-methylene FH$_4$	457.5			294	32,000	700				
Vitamin B$_{12}$	Cyanocobalamin	1355.4	–	xs[e]	278	8,700	115	no fluorescence			Dark red/crystal
					261	27,600	204				
					551	8,700	64				
	Hydroxyl-cobalamin (B$_{12a}$)	1346.4	–	+	279	19,000	141	no fluorescence			Dark red/crystal
					325	11,400	85				
					359	20,600	153				
					516	8,900	66				
					537	9,500	71				

Compound	MW	a	e	λ (nm)	ε	E	Color/form
Aquacobalamin (B₁₂ᵦ)	1347.0	−	+	274	20,600	153	Red/crystal
				317	6,100	45	
				351	26,500	197	
				499	8,100	60	
Nitrocobalamin (B₁₂c)	1374.6	−	+	352	21,000	153	Red/crystal
				357	19,100	139	
				528	8,400	60	
				535	8,700	63	
Methylcobalamin	1344.4	−	+	266	19,900	148	Red/crystal
				342	14,400	107	
				522	9,400	70	
Adenosylcobalamin cobamide	1579.6	−	+	288	18,100	115	Yellow-orange/crystal
				340	12,300	78	
				375	10,900	60	
				522	8,00	51	

[a]In organic solvents, fats, and oils.
[b]sl, Slightly soluble.
[c]Decomposes at this temperature.
[d]Fluoresces.
[e]xs, Freely soluble.
[f]Neutral pH.
[g]Alkaline pH.
[h]Acidic pH.

recapitulates the history of their discovery, calling to mind McCollum's fat-soluble A and water-soluble B. The water-soluble vitamins tend to have one or more **polar** or ionizable groups (carboxyl, keto, hydroxyl, amino, or phosphate), whereas the fat-soluble vitamins have predominantly aromatic and aliphatic characters.

Fat-soluble vitamins: appreciably soluble in nonpolar solvents

Vitamin A	Vitamin D
Vitamin E	Vitamin K

Water-soluble vitamins: appreciably soluble in polar solvents

Thiamin	Folate	Vitamin B_6
Niacin	Vitamin C	Pantothenic acid
Biotin	Riboflavin	Vitamin B_{12}

The fat-soluble vitamins have some traits in common, in that each is composed either entirely or primarily of five-carbon **isoprenoid** units (i.e., related to *isoprene*, 2-methyl-1,3-butadiene) derived initially from acetyl-CoA in those plant and animal species capable of their biosynthesis. In contrast, the water-soluble vitamins have, in general, few similarities of structure. The routes of their biosyntheses in capable species do not share as many common pathways.

Vitamin Nomenclature

The nomenclature of the vitamins is in many cases rather complicated, reflecting both the terminology that evolved nonsystematically during the course of their discovery, and more recent efforts to standardize the vocabulary of the field. Current standards for vitamin nomenclature policy were established by the International Union of Nutritional Sciences in 1978.[2] This policy distinguishes between generic descriptors used to describe families of compounds having vitamin activity (e.g., *vitamin D*) and to modify such terms as *activity* and *deficiency*, and trivial names

used to identify specific compounds (e.g., *ergocalciferol*). These recommendations have been adopted by the Commission on Nomenclature of the International Union of Pure and Applied Chemists, the International Union of Biochemists, and the Committee on Nomenclature of the American Institute of Nutrition. The last-named organization publishes the policy every few years.[3]

II. Vitamin A

Essential features of the chemical structure:

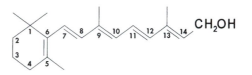

1. Substituted β-ionone nucleus [4-(2,6,6-trimethyl-2-cyclohexen-1-yl)-3-buten-2-one]
2. Side chain composed of three isoprenoid units joined head to tail at the 6-position of the β-ionone nucleus
3. Conjugated double-bond system among the side chain and 5,6-nucleus carbon atoms

Chemical structures of the vitamin A group:

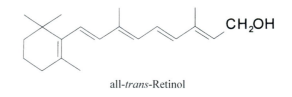

all-*trans*-Retinol

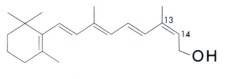

13-*cis*-Retinol

[2] Anonymous. (1978). *Nutr. Abstr. Rev.* **48A,** 831–835.
[3] Anonymous. (1990). *J. Nutr.* 120, 12–19.

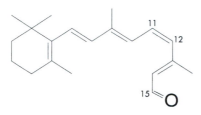

11-*cis*-Retinal

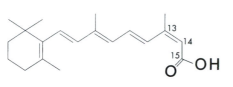

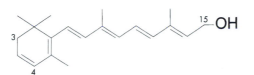

13-*cis*-Retinoic acid

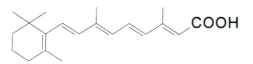

all-*trans*-3-Dehydroretinol
(sometimes called *vitamin A₂*)

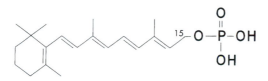

all-*trans*-Retinoic acid

all-*trans*-Retinyl phosphate

Chemical structures of provitamins A:

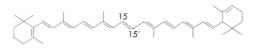

α-Carotene

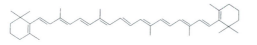

β-Carotene

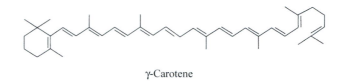

γ-Carotene

Vitamin A Nomenclature

Vitamin A is the generic descriptor for compounds with the qualitative biological activity of retinol. These compounds are formally derived from a monocyclic parent compound containing five carbon–carbon double bonds and a functional group at the terminus of the acyclic portion. Owing to their close structural similarities to retinol, they are called **retinoids**.

The Vitamin A-active retinoids occur in nature in three forms:

The alcohol … **retinol**
The aldehyde … **retinal** (also *retinaldehyde*)
The acid … **retinoic acid**

All three basic forms are found in two variants: with the **β-ionone nucleus** (vitamin A₁) or the dehydrogenated β-ionone nucleus (vitamin A₂). However, because the former is both quantitatively and qualitatively more important as a source of vitamin A activity, the term *vitamin A* is usually taken to mean vitamin A₁. Some compounds of the class of polyisoprenoid plant pigments called **carotenoids**, owing to their relation to the carotenes, yield retinoids on metabolism and, thus, also have vitamin A activity; these are called *provitamin A carotenoids* and include **β-carotene**, which is actually a tail-conjoined retinoid dimer.

Chemistry of Vitamin A

Vitamin A is insoluble in water, but soluble in ethanol and freely soluble in organic solvents including fats and oils. Of the 16 stereoisomers of vitamin A made possible by the four side-chain double bonds, most of the potential *cis* isomers are sterically hindered; thus, only a few isomers are known. In solution, retinoids and carotenoids can undergo slow conversion by light, heat, and iodine through *cis–trans* isomerism of the side-chain double bonds (e.g., in aqueous solution all-*trans*-retinol spontaneously isomerizes to an equilibrium mixture containing one-third *cis* forms).

Contrary to what might be expected by their larger number of double bonds, carotenoids in both plants and animals occur almost exclusively in the all-*trans* form. These conjugated polyene systems absorb light and, in the case of the carotenoids, appear to quench free radicals weakly. For the retinoids, the functional group at position 15 determines specific chemical reactivity. Thus, retinol can be oxidized to retinal and retinoic acid or esterified with organic acids; retinal can be oxidized to retinoic acid or reduced to retinol; and retinoic acid can be esterified with organic alcohols. Retinol and retinal each undergo color reactions with such reagents as antimony trichloride, trifluoroacetic acid, and trichloroacetic acids, which were formerly used as the basis of their chemical analyses by the Carr-Price reaction.

Most forms of vitamin A are crystallizable but have low melting points (e.g., retinol, 62–64°C; retinal, 65°C). Both retinoids and carotenoids have strong absorption spectra. Vitamin A and the provitamin A carotenoids are very sensitive to oxygen in air, especially in the presence of light and heat; therefore, isolation of these compounds requires the exclusion of air (e.g., sparging with an inert gas) and the presence of a protective antioxidant (e.g., α-tocopherol). The esterified retinoids and carotenoids in native plant matrices are fairly stable.

Vitamin A Biopotency

Of the estimated 600 carotenoids in nature, only about 50 have been found to have provitamin A activity, that is, those that can be cleaved metabolically to yield at least 1 molecule of retinol. Five or six of these are common in foods. While the chemical properties of each determine its **biopotency** (Table 3-2), dietary and physiological factors can affect the physiological utilization of each, referred to as its **bioavailability**.

To accommodate differences in biopotency, the reporting of vitamin A activity from its various forms in foods requires some means of standardization. Two systems are used for this purpose: *international units* (Ius) and *retinol equivalents* (REs).

In the calculation of RE values, corrections are made for the conversion efficiency of carotenoids to retinol. It is assumed that the retinol intermediate is completely absorbed (i.e., has an absorption efficiency is 100%). Although 1 mole of β-carotene can, in theory,

Reporting food vitamin A activity

1 retinol equivalent (RE) =	1 μg all-*trans*-retinol
	= 2 μg all-*trans*-β-carotene in dietary supplements
	= 12 μg all-*trans*-β-carotene in foods
	= 24 μg other provitamin A carotenoids in foods

For pharmaceutical applications:

1 USP[a] unit (or IU[b])	= 0.3 μg all-*trans*-retinol
	= 0.344 μg all-*trans*-retinyl acetate
	= 0.55 μg all-*trans*-retinyl palmitate

[a]United States Pharmacopeia.
[b]International Unit

be converted (by cleavage of the C-15 = C-15′ bond) to 2 moles of retinal, the physiological efficiency of this process appears to be much less; until recently, this has been assumed to be about 50%. When considered with a presumed 33% efficiency of intestinal absorption, this yielded a factor of one-sixth to calculate RE values from the β-carotene and, assuming an additional 50% discount, one of one-twelfth for other provitamin A carotenoids. Therefore, older recommendations used equivalency ratios of 6:1 and 12:1 in setting RE values for β-carotene in supplements and foods, respectively. However, recent work has shown that purified β-carotene in oils and nutritional supplements is utilized much more efficiently, at about half that of retinol, but that β-carotene in fruits and dark green, leafy vegetables is utilized much less well. While the relevant data

Table 3-2. Relative biopotencies of vitamin A and related compounds

Compound	Relative biopotency[a]
all-*trans*-Retinol	100
all-*trans*-Retinal	100
cis-Retinol isomers	23–75
Retinyl esters	10–100
3-Dehydrovitamin A	30
β-Carotene	50
α-Carotene	26
γ-Carotene	21
Cryptoxanthin	28
Zeaxanthin	0

[a]Most relative biopotencies were determined by liver storage bioassays with chicks and/or rats. In the case of 3-dehydrovitamin A, biopotency was assessed using liver storage by fish. In each case, the responses were standardized to that of all-*trans*-retinol.

are sparse,[4] in 2001 the IOM[5] revised its estimates of the vitamin A biopotency of carotenoids to the figures presented above.

III. Vitamin D

Essential features of the chemical structure:

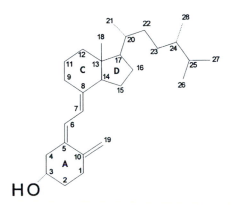

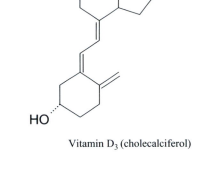

Vitamin D$_3$ (cholecalciferol)

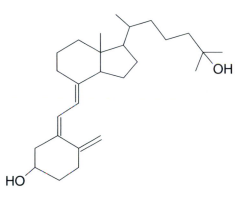

25-OH-Vitamin D$_3$

1. Side-chain-substituted, open-ring **steroid**[6]
2. *cis*-Triene structure
3. Open positions on carbon atoms at positions 1 (ring) and 25 (side chain)

Chemical structures of the vitamin D group:

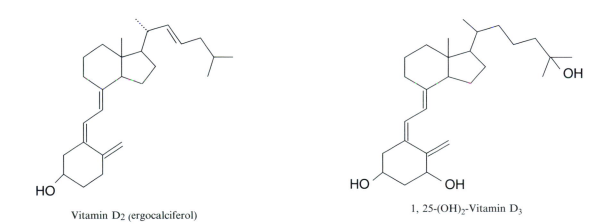

Vitamin D$_2$ (ergocalciferol)

1, 25-(OH)$_2$-Vitamin D$_3$

---

[4] In fact, the 2001 estimate was based on a single report (Sauberlich, H. E., Hodges, R. E., Wallace, D. L., Kolder, H., Canham, J. E., Hood, J., Raica, W., Jr., and Lowry, L. K. [1974]. *Vitamins Hormones* **32**, 251–275) of the efficacy of β-carotene in correcting impaired dark adaptation in two volunteers.

[5] Institute of Medicine, U.S. National Academy of Sciences.

[6] Steroids are four-ringed compounds related to the sterols, which serve as hormones and bile acids.

Vitamin D Nomenclature

Vitamin D is the generic descriptor for all steroids exhibiting qualitatively the biological activity of **cholecalciferol**. These compounds contain the intact A, C, and D steroid rings,[7] being ultimately derived *in vivo* by photolysis of the B ring of 7-dehydrocholesterol. That process frees the A ring from the rigid structure of the C and D rings, yielding conformational mobility in which the A ring undergoes rapid interconversion between two chair configurations.

Vitamin D-active compounds also have either of two types of isoprenoid side chains attached to the steroid nucleus at C-17 of the D ring. One side chain contains nine carbons and a single double bond. Vitamin D-active compounds with that structure are derivatives of **ergocalciferol**, which is also called **vitamin D_2**. This vitamer can be produced synthetically by the photolysis of plant sterols. The other type of side chain consists of eight carbons and contains no double bonds. Vitamin D-active compounds with that structure are derivatives of **cholecalciferol**, also called **vitamin D_3**, which is produced metabolically through a natural process of photolysis of 7-dehydrocholesterol on the surface of skin exposed to ultraviolet irradiation (e.g., sunlight). The metabolically active forms of vitamin D are ring- (at C-1) and side chain-hydroxylated derivatives of vitamins D_2 and D_3.

Vitamin D Chemistry

Unlike the ring-intact steroids, vitamin D-active compounds tend to exist in extended conformations (shown above) due to the 180° rotation of the A ring about the 6,7 single bond (in solution, the stretched and closed conformations are probably in a state of equilibrium favoring the former). The hydroxyl group on C-3 is thus in the β position (i.e., above the plane of the A ring) in the closed forms and in the α position (i.e., below the plane of the A ring) in the stretched forms. Rotation about the 5,6 double bond can also occur by the action of light or iodine to interconvert the biologically active 5,6-*cis*

compounds to 5,6-*trans* compounds, which show little or no vitamin D activity.

Vitamins D_2 and D_3 are white to yellowish powders that are insoluble in water; moderately soluble in fats, oils, and ethanol; and freely soluble in acetone, ether, and petroleum ether. Each shows strong ultraviolet (UV) absorption, with a maximum at 264 nm. Vitamin D is sensitive to oxygen, light, and iodine. Heating or mild acidity can convert it to the 5,6-*trans* and other inactive forms. Whereas the vitamin is stable in dry form, in organic solvents and most plant oils (owing to the presence of α-tocopherol, which serves as a protective antioxidant), its thermal and photolability can result in losses during such procedures as saponification with refluxing. Therefore, it is often necessary to use inert gas environments, light-tight sealed containers, and protective antioxidants in isolating the vitamin. In solution, both vitamins D_2 and D_3 undergo reversible, temperature-dependent isomerization to pre-vitamin D (*see* Chapter 6, Fig. 6-1), forming an equilibrium mixture with the parent vitamin (Fig. 3-1). For example, at 20°C a mixture of 93% vitamin D and 7% pre-vitamin D is established within 30 days, whereas at 100°C a mixture of 72% vitamin D and 28% pre-vitamin D is established within only 30 min.[8] Vitamin D_3 is extremely sensitive to photodegradation of the 5,6-*trans* isomer as well as to B-ring analogs referred to as suprasterols.

Vitamin D Biopotency

The vitamers D vary in biopotency in two ways. First, those vitamers that require metabolic activation (e.g., cholecalciferol and ergocalciferol) are less biopotent than those that are more proximal to the points of metabolic functioning (e.g., 25-OH-vitamin D). Second, because some species (avians) distinguish between ergocalciferol- and cholecalciferol-based vitamers (greatly in favor of the latter), vitamers D_3 have much greater biopotencies for those species. A summary of the relative biopotencies of the vitamers D is presented in Table 3-3.

---

[7] Steroids contain a polycyclic hydrocarbon cyclopentanaperhydrophenanthrene nucleus consisting of three six-carbon rings (referred to as the A, B, and C rings) and a five-carbon ring (the D ring).

[8] This designation connotes the light-rotational properties of the vitamer and comes from the Latin *rectus*, meaning right.

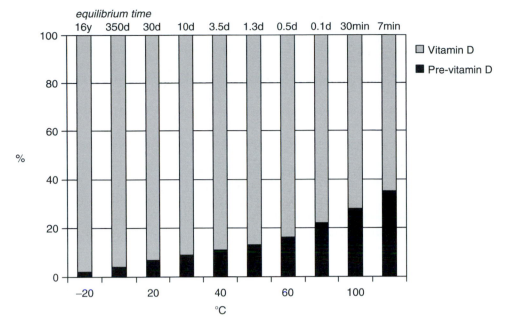

Fig. 3-1. Thermal isomerization of vitamin D.

Table 3-3.   Relative biopotencies of vitamin D-active compounds

Compound	Relative biopotency[a]
Vitamin D$_2$ (ergocalciferol)	100,[b] 10[c]
Vitamin D$_3$ (cholecalciferol)	100
Dihydrotachysterol[d]	5–10
25-OH-Cholecalciferol[e]	200–500
1,25-(OH)$_2$-Cholecalciferol[e]	500–1000
1α-OH-Cholecalciferol[f]	500–1000

[a]Results of rickets prevention bioassays in chicks and/or rats.
[b]Biopotencies of vitamins D$_2$ and D$_3$ are equivalent for mammalian species.
[c]Biopotency of vitamin D$_2$ is very low for chicks, which cannot use this vitamer effectively.
[d]A sterol generated by the irradiation of ergosterol.
[e]Normal metabolite of vitamin D$_3$; the analogous metabolite of vitamin D$_2$ is also formed and is comparably active in nonavian species.
[f]A synthetic analog.

IV. Vitamin E

Essential features of the chemical structure:

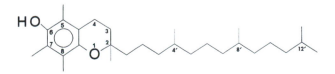

1. Side-chain derivative of a methylated **6-chromanol nucleus** (3,4-dihydro-2*H*-1-benzopyran-6-ol)
2. Side chain consists of three isoprenoid units joined head to tail
3. Free hydroxyl or ester linkage on C-6 of the chromanol nucleus

Chemical structures of the vitamin E group:

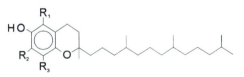

Tocopherols

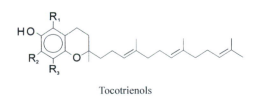

Tocotrienols

Vitamer	R_1	R_2	R_3
α-Tocopherol/α-tocotrienol	CH_3	CH_3	CH_3
β-Tocopherol/β-tocotrienol	CH_3	H	CH_3
γ-Tocopherol/γ-tocotrienol	H	CH_3	CH_3
δ-Tocopherol/δ-tocotrienol	H	H	CH_3
Tocol/tocotrienol	H	H	H

Vitamin E Nomenclature

Vitamin E is the generic descriptor for all tocol and tocotrienol derivatives that exhibit qualitatively the biological activity of α-tocopherol. These compounds are isoprenoid side-chain derivatives of 6-chromanol. The term **tocol** is the trivial designation for the derivative with a side chain consisting of three fully saturated isopentyl units; **tocopherol** denotes generically the mono-, di-, and trimethyl tocols regardless of biological activity. **Tocotrienol** is the trivial designation of the 6-chromanol derivative with a similar side chain containing three double bonds. Individual tocopherols and tocotrienols are named according to the position and number of methyl groups on their chromanol nuclei.

Because the tocopherol side chain contains two chiral center carbons (C-4′, C-8′) in addition to the one at the point of its attachment to the nucleus (C-2), eight stereoisomers are possible. However, only one stereoisomer occurs naturally: the $R,^9R,R$-form. The chemical synthesis of vitamin E produces mixtures of other stereoisomers, depending on the starting materials. For example, through the early 1970s the commercial synthesis of vitamin E used as the source of the side-chain isophytol isolated from natural sources (which has the R-configuration at both the 4- and 8-carbons); tocopherols so produced were racemic at only the C-2 position. Such a mixture of $2RS^{10}$-α-tocopherol was then called *dl*-α-tocopherol; its acetate ester was the form of commerce and was adopted as the international standard on which the biological activities of other forms of the vitamin are still based. In recent years, however, the commercial synthesis of vitamin E has turned away from using isophytol in favor of a fully synthetic side chain. Therefore, synthetic preparations of vitamin E presently available are mixtures of all eight possible stereoisomers, that is, $2RS,4′RS,8′RS$ compounds, which are designated more precisely with the prefix all-*rac*-. The acetate esters of vitamin E are used in medicine and animal feeding, whereas the unesterified (i.e., free alcohol) forms are used as antioxidants in foods and pharmaceuticals. Other forms (e.g., α-tocopheryl hydrogensuccinate, α-tocopheryl polyethylene glycol-succinate) are also used in multivitamin preparations.

Vitamin E Chemistry

The tocopherols are light yellow oils at room temperature. They are insoluble in water but are readily soluble in nonpolar solvents. Being monoethers of a hydroquinone with a phenolic hydrogen (in the hydroxyl group at position C-6 in the chromanol nucleus) with the ability to accommodate an unpaired electron within the resonance structure of the ring (undergoing transition to a semi-stable chromanoxyl radical before being converted to tocopheryl quinone), they are good quenchers of free radicals and thus serve as antioxidants. They are easily oxidized, however, and can be destroyed by peroxides, ozone, and permanganate in a process catalyzed by light and accelerated by polyunsaturated fatty acids and metal salts. They are very resistant to acids and (only under anaerobic conditions) to bases. Tocopheryl esters, by virtue of the blocking of the C-6 hydroxyl group, are very stable in air and are, therefore, the forms of choice as food/feed supplements. Because tocopherol is liberated by the saponification of its esters, extraction and isolation of vitamin E call for the use of protective antioxidants (e.g., propyl gallate, ascorbic acid), metal chelators, inert gas environments, and subdued light. The UV absorption spectra of tocopherols and their acetates in ethanol have maxima of 280–300 nm (α-tocopherol, 292 nm); however, their extinction coefficients are not great (70–91).[11] Because their fluorescence is significant

---

[9] This designation connotes the light-rotational properties of the vitamer and comes from the Latin *sinister*, meaning left.

[10] From Mulder, F. J., de Vries, E. J., and Borsje, B. (1971). *J. Assoc. Off. Anal. Chem.* **54**, 1168–1174.

(excitation, 294 nm; emission, 330 nm) particularly in polar solvents (e.g., diethyl ether or alcohols), this property has analytical utility.

Vitamin E Biopotency

The vitamers E vary in biopotency (Table 3-4), mainly according to the positions and numbers of their nucleus methyl groups, the most biopotent being the trimethylated (α) form.

V. Vitamin K

Essential features of the chemical structure:

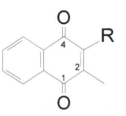

1. Derivative of 2-methyl-1,4-naphthoquinone
2. Ring structure has a hydrophobic constituent at the 3-position and can be alkylated with an isoprenoid side chain

Chemical structures of the vitamin K group:

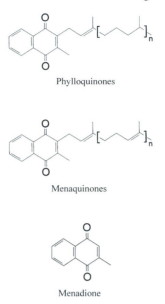

Phylloquinones

Menaquinones

Menadione

Vitamin K Nomenclature

Vitamin K is the generic descriptor for 2-methyl-1,4-naphthoquinone and all of its derivatives exhibiting qualitatively the biological (antihemorrhagic) activity of phylloquinone. Naturally occurring forms of the vitamin have an unsaturated isoprenoid side chain at C-3 of the **naphthoquinone nucleus**; the type and

Table 3-4. Relative biopotencies of vitamin E-active compounds

Trivial designation	Systematic name	Biopotency (IU/mg)[a]
R,R,R-α-Tocopherol[b]	2R,4′R,8′R-5,7,8-Trimethyltocol	1.49
R,R,R-α-Tocopheryl acetate	2R,4′R,8′R-5,7,8-Trimethyltocyl acetate	1.36
all-rac-α-Tocopherol[c]	2RS,4′RS,8′RS-5,7,8-Trimethyltocol	1.1
all-rac-α-Tocopheryl acetate	2RS,4′RS,8′RS-5,7,8-Trimethyltocylacetate	1.0
R,R,R-β-Tocopherol	2R,4′R,8′R-5,8-Dimethyltocol	0.12
R,R,R-γ-Tocopherol	2R,4′R,8′R-5,7-Dimethyltocol	0.05
R-α-Tocotrienol	trans-2R-5,7,8-Trimethyltocotrienol	0.32
R-β-Tocotrienol	trans-2R-5,8-Dimethyltocotrienol	0.05
R-γ-Tocotrienol	trans-2R-5,7-Dimethyltocotrienol	—

[a]International units per milligram of material, based chiefly on rat gestation-resorption bioassay data.
[b]Formerly called d-α-tocopherol.
[c]Formerly called dl-α-tocopherol; this form remains the international standard despite the fact that it has not been produced commercially for several years.

---

[11] UV absorption can nevertheless be useful for checking the quality of α-tocopherol standards: solutions containing 90% α-tocopherol show ratios of the absorption at the A_{min} (255 nm) and A_{max} (292 nm) of <0.18 (Balz, M. K., Schulte, E., and Thier, H. P. (1996). *Z. Lebensm. U.-Forsch* **202,** 80–81.

number of isoprene units (not carbon atoms) form the basis of the characterization of the side chain and, hence, the designation of the vitamer. The **phylloquinone** group includes forms with phytyl side chains and side chains that are further alkylated, thus consisting of several saturated isoprenoid units. The vitamers of this group have only one double bond in their side chains (i.e., on the proximal isoprene unit). These vitamers are synthesized by green plants. They are properly referred to as *phylloquinones*[12] and are abbreviated as *K*. The **menaquinone** group also includes vitamers with side chains consisting of variable numbers of isoprenoid units; however, each isoprene unit has a double bond. These vitamers are synthesized by bacteria. They are abbreviated as *MK*[13] and were formerly referred to as **vitamin K_2**. For each of these groups of vitamers, a numeric system is used to indicate side-chain length; for example, the abbreviations K-*n* and MK-*n* are used for the phylloquinones and menaquinones, respectively, to indicate specific vitamers with side chains consisting of *n* isoprenoid units (Table 3-5). The compound 2-methyl-1,4-naphthoquinone (i.e., without a side chain) is called **menadione**.[14] It does not exist naturally, but has biological activity by virtue of the fact that animals can alkylate it to produce such metabolites as MK-4. Menadione is the compound of commerce; it is made in several forms (e.g., menadione sodium bisulfite complex, menadione dimethylpyrimidinol bisulfite).

Vitamin K Chemistry

Phylloquinone (K_1) is a yellow oil at room temperature, but the other vitamers K are yellow crystals.

The vitamers K, MK, and most forms of menadione are insoluble in water, slightly soluble in ethanol, and readily soluble in ether, chloroform, fats, and oils. The vitamers K are sensitive to light and alkali, but are relatively stable to heat and oxidizing environments. Their oxidation proceeds to produce the 2,3-epoxide form. Being naphthoquinones, they can be reduced to the corresponding naphthohydroquinones (e.g., with sodium hydrogen sulfite), which can be reoxidized with mild oxidizing agents. The vitamers K show the characteristic UV spectra of the naphthoquinones; that is, their oxidized forms have four strong absorption bands in the 240- to 270-nm range. The reduced (hydroquinone) forms show losses of the band near 270 nm and increases of the band around 245 nm. Extinction decreases with increasing side-chain length.

Vitamin K Biopotency

The biopotency of vitamers K (Table 3-6) depends on both the nature and length of their isoprenoid side chains. In general, the menaquinones (K-2) tend to have greater biopotencies than the corresponding phylloquinone analogs, and members of each series with four or five isoprenoid side chains are the most biopotent. The reported biopotencies of the menadiones tend to be variable. This may be due, at least in part, to varying stabilities of the preparations tested as well as to whether the vitamin K antagonist sulfaquinoxaline was used in the assay diet.

Table 3-5.   Systems of vitamin K nomenclature

Chemical name	IUPAC[a] system[b]	IUNS[c] system	Traditional
2-Methyl-3-phytyl-1,4-naphthoquinone	Phylloquinone (K)	Phytylmenaquinone (PMQ)	K_1
2-Methyl-3-multiprenyl-1,4-naphthoquinone (*n*)	Menaquinone-*n* (MK-*n*)	Prenylmenaquinone-*n* (MQ-*n*)	$K_{2(n)}$
2-Methyl-1,4-naphthoquinone	Menadione	Menaquinone	K_3

[a]International Union of Pure and Applied Chemists.
[b]Preferred system.
[c]International Union of Nutritional Sciences.

---

[12] These vitamers were formerly called the *phytylmenaquinones*, or **vitamin K_1**; the latter term is still encountered.
[13] Formerly referred to as the *prenylmenaquinones*.
[14] Formerly referred to as **vitamin K_3**.

Table 3-6. Relative biopotencies of vitamin K-active compounds

Compound	Biopotency[a] (%)
Phylloquinones (formerly K₁)	
K-1[b]	5
K-2	10
K-3	30
K-4	100
K-5	80
K-6	50
Menaquinones (formerly K₂)	
MK-2[b]	15
MK-3	40
MK-4	100
MK-5	120
MK-6	100
MK-7	70
Forms of menadione (formerly K₃)	
Menadione	40–150
Menadione sodium bisulfite complex	50–150
Menadione dimethylpyrimidinol bisulfite	100–160

[a]Relative biopotency is based on chick prothrombin/clotting time bioassays using phylloquinone (K-1) as the standard.
[b]For both the phylloquinones (K) and menaquinones (MK), the number of side-chain isoprenoid units (each containing five carbons) is indicated after the hyphens.

VI. Vitamin C

Essential features of the chemical structure:

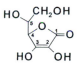

1. 6-Carbon lactone
2. 2,3-Endiol structure

Chemical structure of vitamin C:

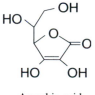

Ascorbic acid

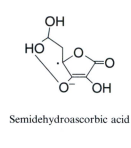

Semidehydroascorbic acid

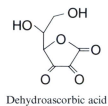

Dehydroascorbic acid

Vitamin C Nomenclature

Vitamin C is the generic descriptor for all compounds exhibiting qualitatively the biological activity of ascorbic acid. The terms *L-ascorbic acid* and **ascorbic acid** are both trivial designators for the compound 2,3-didehydro-L-threo-hexano-1,4-lactone, which was formerly known as *hexuronic acid*. The oxidized form of this compound is called *L-dehydroascorbic acid* or **dehydroascorbic acid**.

Vitamin C Chemistry

Ascorbic acid is a dibasic acid (with pK_a values of 4.1 and 11.8) because both enolic hydroxyl groups can dissociate. It forms salts, the most important of which are the sodium and calcium salts, the aqueous solutions of which are strongly acidic. A strong reducing agent, ascorbic acid is oxidized under mild conditions to dehydroascorbic acid via the radical intermediate semidehydroascorbic acid (sometimes called *monodehydroascorbic acid*). The semiquinoid ascorbic acid radical is a strong acid ($pK_a = -0.45$); after the loss of a proton, it becomes a radical anion that, owing to resonance stabilization, is relatively inert but disproportionates to ascorbic acid and dehydroascorbic acid. Thus, the three forms (ascorbic acid, semidehydroascorbic acid, and dehydroascorbic acid) compose a reversible redox system. Thus, it is an effective quencher of free radicals such as singlet oxygen ($^1O_2$). It reduces ferric (Fe^{3+}) to ferrous (Fe^{2+}) iron (and other metals analogously) and the superoxide radical ($O_2\bullet^-$) to H_2O_2 and is oxidized to monodehydroascorbic acid in the process. Ascorbic acid complexes with disulfides (e.g., oxidized glutathione, cystine) but does not reduce those disulfide bonds.

Dehydroascorbic acid is not ionized in environments of weakly acidic or neutral pH; therefore, it is relatively hydrophobic and is better able to penetrate membranes than ascorbic acid. In aqueous solution, dehydroascorbic acid is unstable and is degraded by hydrolytic ring opening to yield 2,3-dioxo-L-gulonic acid. Dehydroascorbic acid reacts with several amino acids to form brown-colored products, a reaction contributing to the spoilage of food.

Vitamin C Biopotency

Several synthetic analogs of ascorbic acid have been made. Some (e.g., 6-deoxy-L-ascorbic acid) have biological activity, whereas others (e.g., D-isoascorbic acid and L-glucoascorbic acid) have little or no activity. Several esters of ascorbic acid are converted to the vitamin *in vivo* and thus have good biological activity (e.g., ascorbyl-5,6-diacetate, ascorbyl-6-palmitate, 6-deoxy-6-chloro-L-ascorbic acid; see Table 3-7). Esters of the C-2 position show variable vitamin C activity among different species.

Table 3-7.   Relative biopotencies of vitamin C-active substances

Compound	Relative biopotency (%)
Ascorbic acid	100
Ascorbyl-5,6-diacetate	100
Ascorbyl-6-palmitate	100
6-Deoxy-6-chloro-L-ascorbic acid	70–98
Dehydroascorbic acid	80
6-Deoxyascorbic acid	33
Ascorbic acid 2-sulfate	±[a]
Isoascorbic acid	5
L-Glucoascorbic acid	3

[a]This form is active in fishes, which have an intestinal sulfohydrase that liberates ascorbic acid; it is inactive in guinea pigs, rhesus monkeys, and humans, which lack the enzyme.

VII.   Thiamin

Essential features of the chemical structure:

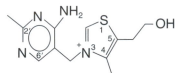

Chemical structure of thiamin

1. Conjoined pyrimidine and thiazole rings
2. Thiazole ring contains a quaternary nitrogen, an open C-2, and a phosphorylatable alkyl group on C-5
3. Amino group on C-4 of the pyrimidine ring

Chemical structure of thiamin:

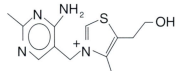

Thiamin (free base)

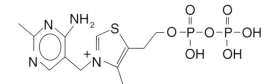

Thiamin pyrophosphate

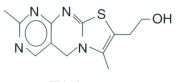

Thiochrome

Thiamin Nomenclature

The term **thiamin** is the trivial designation of the compound 3-[(4-amino-2-methyl-5-pyrimidinyl)methyl]-5-(2-hydroxyethyl)-4-methylthiazolium, formerly known as *vitamin B₁*, *aneurine*, and *thiamine*.

Thiamin Chemistry

Free thiamin is unstable because of its quaternary nitrogen; in water it is cleaved to the thiol form. For this reason the hydrochloride and mononitrate forms are used in commerce. Thiamin hydrochloride (actually, thiamin chloride hydrochloride) is a colorless crystal that is very soluble in water (1 g/ml, thus making it a very suitable form for parenteral administration), soluble in methanol and glycerol, but practically insoluble in acetone, ether, chloroform, and benzene. The protonated salt has two positive charges: one associated with the **pyrimidine ring** and one associated with the **thiazole ring**. The mononitrate form is more stable than the hydrochloride form, but it is less soluble in water (27 mg/ml). It is used in food/feed supplementation and in dry pharmaceutical preparations.

Free thiamin is easily oxidized to thiamin disulfide and other derivatives, including thiochrome, a yellow biologically inactive product with strong blue fluorescence that can be used for the quantitative determination of thiamin. The thiazole hydroxyethyl group can be phosphorylated *in vivo* to form thiamin mono-, di-, and triphosphates. Thiamin diphosphate, also called **thiamin pyrophosphate**, is the metabolically active form sometimes referred to as *cocarboxylase*. Thiamin antagonists of experimental significance include pyrithiamin (the analog consisting of a pyridine moiety replacing the thiazole ring) and oxythiamin (the analog consisting of a hydroxyl group replacing the C-4 amino group on the pyrimidine ring).

VIII. Riboflavin

Essential features of the chemical structure:

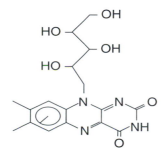

1. Substituted isoalloxazine nucleus
2. D-Ribityl side chain
3. Reducible nitrogen atoms in nucleus

Chemical structures of riboflavin and its nucleotide forms:

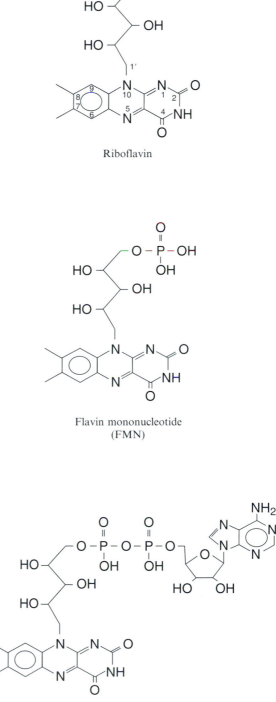

Riboflavin

Flavin mononucleotide
(FMN)

Flavin adenine dinucleotide
(FAD)

Riboflavin Nomenclature

Riboflavin is the trivial designation of the compound 7,8-dimethyl-10-(1′-D-ribityl)isoalloxazine, formerly known as **vitamin B$_2$**, vitamin G, lactoflavine, or riboflavine. The metabolically active forms are commonly called **flavin mononucleotide (FMN)** and **flavin adenine dinucleotide (FAD)**. Despite their acceptance each is a misnomer, as FMN is not a nucleotide and FAD is not a dinucleotide. More properly, these compounds should be called *riboflavin monophosphate* and *riboflavin adenine diphosphate*, respectively.

Riboflavin Chemistry

Riboflavin is a yellow tricyclic molecule that is usually phosphorylated (to FMN and FAD) in biological systems. In FAD, the isoalloxazine and adenine nuclear systems are arranged one above the other and are nearly coplanar. The flavins are light sensitive, undergoing photochemical degradation of the ribityl side chain, which results in the formation of such breakdown products as lumiflavin and lumichrome. Therefore, the handling of riboflavin must be done in the dark or under subdued red light.

Riboflavin is moderately soluble in water (10–13 mg/dl) and ethanol, but insoluble in ether, chloroform, and acetone. It is soluble but unstable under alkaline conditions. Because riboflavin cannot be extracted with the usual organic solvents, it is extracted with chloroform as lumiflavin after photochemical cleavage of the ribityl side chain. Flavins show two absorption bands at ~370 nm and ~450 nm with fluorescence emitting at 520 nm.

The catalytic functions of riboflavin are carried out primarily at positions N-1, N-5, and C-4 of the **isoalloxazine nucleus**. In addition, the methyl group at C-8 participates in covalent bonding with enzyme proteins. The flavin coenzymes are highly versatile redox cofactors because they can participate in either one- or two-electron redox reactions, thus serving as switching sites between obligate two-electron donors [e.g., NAD(H), succinate] and obligate one-electron acceptors (e.g., iron–sulfur proteins, heme proteins). They serve this function by undergoing reduction through a two-step sequence involving a radical anion intermediate. Because the latter can also react with molecular oxygen, flavins can also serve as cofactors in the two-electron reduction of O$_2$ to H$_2$O, and in the reductive four-electron activation and cleavage of O$_2$ in the monooxygenase reactions. In these redox reactions, riboflavin undergoes changes in its molecular shape (i.e., from a planar oxidized form to a folded reduced form). Differences in the affinities of the associated apoprotein for each shape affect the redox potential of the bound flavin.

Riboflavin antagonists include analogs of the isoalloxazine ring (e.g., diethylriboflavin, dichlororiboflavin) and the ribityl side chain (e.g., D-araboflavin, D-galactoflavin, 7-ethylriboflavin).

IX. Niacin

Essential features of the chemical structure:

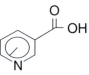

1. **Pyridine nucleus** substituted with a β-carboxylic acid or a corresponding amine
2. Pyridine nitrogen must be able to undergo reversible oxidation/reduction (i.e., quaternary pyridinium ion to/from tertiary amine)
3. Pyridine carbons adjacent to the nuclear nitrogen atom must be open

Chemical structures of niacin:

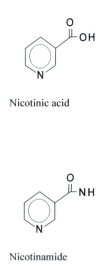

Nicotinic acid

Nicotinamide

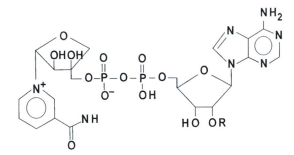

Nicotinamide adenine dinucleotide (NAD$^+$), R = H
Nicotinamide adenine dinucleotide phosphate (NADP$^+$), R = PO$_3$H$_2$

Niacin Nomenclature

Niacin is the generic descriptor for pyridine 3-carboxylic acid and derivatives exhibiting qualitatively the biological activity of nicotinamide.[15]

Niacin Chemistry

Nicotinic acid and **nicotinamide** are colorless crystalline substances. Each is insoluble or only sparingly soluble in organic solvents. Nicotinic acid is slightly soluble in water and ethanol; nicotinamide is very soluble in water and moderately soluble in ethanol. The two compounds have similar absorption spectra in water, with an absorption maximum at ~262 nm.

Nicotinic acid is amphoteric and forms salts with acids as well as bases. Its carboxyl group can form esters and anhydrides and can be reduced. Both nicotinic acid and nicotinamide are very stable in dry form, but in solution nicotinamide is hydrolyzed by acids and bases to yield nicotinic acid.

The coenzyme forms of niacin are the pyridine nucleotides, **NAD(H)** and **NADP(H)**. In each of these compounds, the electron-withdrawing effect of the N-1 atom and the amide group of the oxidized pyridine nucleus enables the pyridine C-4 atom to react with many nucleophilic agents (e.g., sulfite, cyanide, and hydride ions). It is the reaction with hydride ions (H$^-$) that is the basis of the enzymatic hydrogen transfer by the pyridine nucleotides; the reaction involves the transfer of two electrons in a single step.[16] The hydride transfer of nonenzymatic reactions of the pyridine nucleotides, plus those catalyzed by the pyridine

nucleotide-dependent dehydrogenases, is stereospecific with respect to both coenzyme and substrate. At least for reactions of the former type, this stereospecificity results from a specific intramolecular association between the adenine residue and the pyridine nucleus.

Several substituted pyridines are antagonists of niacin in biological systems: pyridine-3-sulfonic acid, 3-acetylpyridine, isonicotinic acid hydrazine,[17] and 6-aminonicotinamide.

X. Vitamin B$_6$

Essential features of the chemical structure:

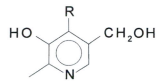

1. Derivative of 3-hydroxy-2-methyl-5-hydroxypyridine
2. Phosphorylatable 5-hydroxymethyl group
3. Substituent at ring carbon para to the pyridine nitrogen must be metabolizable to an aldehyde

Chemical structures of vitamin B$_6$:

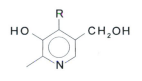

General structure of
vitamin B$_6$

R	Name
CH$_2$OH	pyridoxine
CHO	pyridoxal
COOH	pyridoxic acid
CH$_2$NH$_2$	pyridoxamine

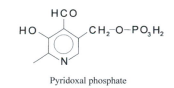

Pyridoxal phosphate

---

[15] This compound is sometimes referred to as *niacinamide,* which, because its use would suggest that nicotinic acid should be called niacin, invites confusion and is not recommended.

[16] It has been argued that the enzyme-catalyzed oxidation of NADH occurs in two steps with the intermediate formation of the NAD radical. Such a radical has been demonstrated, but it spontaneously dimerizes to an enzymatically inactive form (NAD)$_2$, thus making it unlikely that such a mechanism plays a significant role in the redox functions of the pyridine nucleotides.

[17] Also called *isoniazid,* this compound (4-pyridinecarboxylic acid hydrazide) is used as an antituberculous and antiactinomycotic agent.

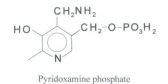

Pyridoxamine phosphate

Vitamin B₆ Nomenclature

Vitamin B₆ is the generic descriptor for all 3-hydroxy-2-methylpyridine derivatives exhibiting the biological activity of pyridoxine in rats. The term **pyridoxine** is the trivial designation of one vitamin B₆-active compound (i.e., 3-hydroxy-4,5-bis(hydroxymethyl)-2-methylpyridine), which was formerly called *adermin* or **pyridoxol**. The biologically active analogs of pyridoxine are the aldehyde **pyridoxal** and the amine **pyridoxamine**.

Vitamin B₆ Chemistry

Vitamers B₆ are colorless crystals at room temperature. Each is very soluble in water, weakly soluble in ethanol, and either insoluble or sparingly soluble in chloroform. Each is fairly stable in dry form and in solution.

Pyridoxine is oxidized *in vivo* and under mild oxidizing conditions *in vitro* to yield pyridoxal. The prominent feature of the chemical reactivity of pyridoxal is the ability of its aldehyde group to react with primary amino groups (e.g., of amino acids) to form Schiff bases.[18] The electron-withdrawing effect of the resulting Schiff base labilizes the other bonds on the bound carbon, thus serving as the basis of the catalytic roles of pyridoxal and pyridoxamine.

XI. Biotin

Essential features of the chemical structure:

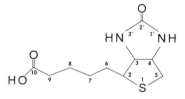

1. Conjoined ureido and tetrahydrothiophene nuclei
2. Ureido 3' nitrogen is sterically hindered, preventing substitution
3. Ureido 1' nitrogen is poorly nucleophilic

Chemical structure of biotin:

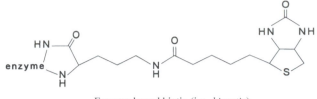

Enzyme-bound biotin (i.e., *biocytin*)

Biotin Nomenclature

Biotin is the trivial designation of the compound *cis*-hexahydro-2-oxo-1*H*-thieno[3,4-*d*]imidazole-4-pentanoic acid, formerly known as *vitamin H* or *coenzyme R*.

Biotin Chemistry

Biotin is a white crystalline substance that, in dry form, is fairly stable to air, heat, and light. In solution, however, it is sensitive to degradation under strongly acidic or basic conditions. Its structure consists of a planar **ureido nucleus** and a folded **tetrahydrothiophene (thiophane) nucleus**, which results in a boat configuration with a plane of symmetry passing through the S-1, C-2', and O positions in such a way as to elevate the sulfur atom above the plane of the four carbons. The molecule has three asymmetric centers; however, of the eight possible stereoisomers, only the (+)-isomer (called *d*-biotin) has biological activity. Biotin is covalently bound to its enzymes by an amide bond to the ε-amino group of a lysine residue and C-2 of the thiophane nucleus. This bond is flexible, allowing the coenzyme to move between the active centers of some enzymes. The biotin molecule is activated by polarization of the O and N-1' atoms of the ureido nucleus. This leads to increased nucleophilicity at N-1', which promotes the formation of a covalent bond between the electrophilic carbonyl phosphate formed from bicarbonate and ATP, and allows biotin to serve as a transport agent for CO_2.

XII. Pantothenic Acid

Essential features of the chemical structure:

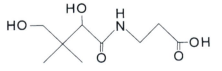

1. Formal derivative of pantoic acid and alanine
2. Optically active

---

[18] This reaction can occur with tris(hydroxymethyl)amino methane (i.e., Tris) and may thus affect the results of biochemical studies of vitamin B₆ in which this common buffering agent is employed.

Chemical structure of pantothenic acid:

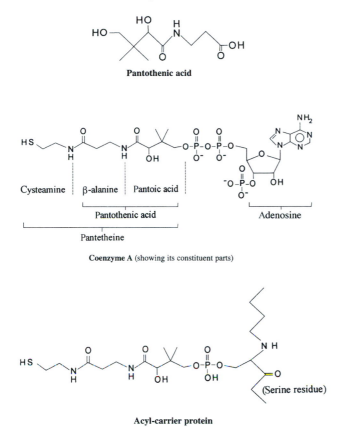

Pantothenic acid

Coenzyme A (showing its constituent parts)

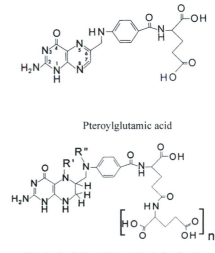

Acyl-carrier protein

Pantothenic Acid Nomenclature

Pantothenic acid is the trivial designation for the compound dihydroxy-β,β-dimethylbutyryl-β-alanine, which was formerly known as *pantoyl-β-alanine*. It has two metabolically active forms: **coenzyme A**, in which the vitamin is linked via a phosphodiester group with adenosine-3′,5′-diphosphate; and acyl-carrier protein, in which it is linked via a phosphodiester to a serinyl residue of the protein.

Pantothenic Acid Chemistry

Pantothenic acid is composed of β-alanine joined to 2,4-dihydroxy-3,3-dimethylbutyric acid via an amide linkage. The molecule has an asymmetric center, and only the *R*-enantiomer, usually called D-(+)*pantothenic acid*, is biologically active and occurs naturally. Pantothenic acid is a yellow, viscous oil. Its calcium and other salts, however, are colorless crystalline substances; calcium pantothenate is the main product of commerce. Neither form is soluble in organic solvents, but each is soluble in water and etha-

nol. Aqueous solutions of pantothenic acid are unstable to heating under acidic or alkaline conditions, resulting in the hydrolytic cleavage of the molecule (to yield β-alanine and 2,4-dihydroxy-3,3-dimethylbutyrate).[19] The analog panthenol (in which the carboxyl group is replaced by an hydroxymethyl group) is fairly stable in solution. In dry form, the salts are stable to air and light, but they (particularly sodium pantothenate) are hygroscopic.

XIII. Folate

Essential features of the chemical structure:

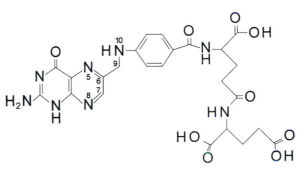

1. Pteridine derivative
2. Variable degree of hydrogenation of pteridine nucleus
3. Single-carbon units can bind nitrogens at position 5 and/or 10
4. One or more glutamyl residues linked via peptide bonds

Chemical structures of the folate group:

Pteroylglutamic acid

Tetrahydrofolic acid (and its derivatives)

---

[19] This reaction is often used in the chemical determination of pantothenic acid by quantifying colorimetrically the β-alanine released on alkaline hydrolysis using reagents such as 1,2-naphthoquinone 4-sulfonic acid or ninhydrin.

Key members of the folate family are listed in Table 3-8.

Folate Nomenclature

Folate is the generic descriptor for **folic acid** (pteroylmonoglutamic acid) and related compounds exhibiting the biological activity of folic acid. The terms **folacin**, *folic acids*, and **folates** are used only as general terms for this group of heterocyclic compounds based on the *N*-[(6-pteridinyl)methyl]-*p*-aminobenzoic acid skeleton conjugated with one or more L-glutamic acid residues. Folates can consist of a mono- or polyglutamyl conjugate; these are named for the number of glutamyl residues (n), using such notations as PteGlu$_n$.[20] The reduced compound tetrahydropteroylglutamic acid is called **tetrahydrofolic acid**; its single-carbon derivatives are named according to the specific carbon moiety bound.

Folate Chemistry

The folates include a large number of chemically related species, each differing with respect to the various substituents possible at three sites on the **pteroylglutamic acid** basic structure. Each is a formal derivative of **pteridine**.[21] With three known reduction states of the **pyrazine nucleus**, six different single-carbon substituents on N-5 and/or N-10, and as many as eight glutamyl residues on the benzene ring, more than 170 different folates are theoretically possible.[22] Not all of these occur in nature; but it has been estimated that as many as 100 different forms are found in animals. The compound called *folic acid* (i.e., pteroylmonoglutamic acid) is probably not present in living cells, being rather an artifact of isolation of the vitamin. The folates from most natural sources usually have a single carbon unit at N-5 and/or N-10; these forms participate in the metabolism of the *single-carbon pool*. The single-carbon units that may be transported and stored by folates can vary in oxidation state from the methyl (e.g., 5-CH$_3$-FH$_4$) to the formyl (e.g., 5-HCO-FH$_4$, 10-HCO-FH$_4$). Intracellular folates contain poly-γ-glutamyl chains usually of 2 to 8 glutamyl residues, sometimes extending to 12 in bacteria. Tissues contain enzymes called *conjugases* that hydrolytically remove glutamyl residues to release the monoglutamyl form (i.e., folic acid). While the actual biochemical role of the polyglutamyl side chain is not presently clear, it appears that the folylpolyglutamates are the actual coenzyme forms active intracellularly and that the monoglutamates, which can pass through membranes, are transport forms.

The folates have an asymmetric center at C-6. This introduces stereospecificity in the orientation of hydrogen atoms on reduction of the pteridine system; that is, they add to carbons 6 and 7 in positions below the plane of the pyrazine ring. The UV absorption spectra of the folates are characterized by the independent contributions of the pterin and 4-aminobenzoyl moieties; most have absorption maxima in the region of 280–300 nm.

Folic acid (pteroylmonoglutamic acid) is an orange-yellow crystalline substance that is soluble in water but insoluble in ethanol or less polar organic solvents. It is unstable to light, to acidic or alkaline conditions, to reducing agents, and,

Table 3-8. Key members of the folate family

Vitamer	Abbreviation	R′ (at N-5)	R″ (at N-10)
Tetrahydrofolic acid	FH$_4$	H	H
5-Methyltetra-hydrofolic acid	5-CH$_3$–FH$_4$	CH$_3$	H
5,10-Methenyltetra-hydrofolic acid	5,10-CH$^+$–FH$_4$	-CH$^+$– (bridge)	
5,10-Methylenetetra-hydrofolic acid	5,10-CH$_2$=FH$_4$	-CH$_2$= (bridge)	
5-Formyltetra-hydrofolic acid	5-HCO–FH$_4$	HCO	H
10-Formyltetra-hydrofolic acid	10-HCO–FH$_4$	H	HCO
5-Forminontetra-hydrofolic acid	5-HCNH–FH$_4$	HCNH	H

---

[20] Although they are still frequently used, the abbreviations using PteGlu to indicate pteroylglutamic acid are not suggested by current IUPAC-IUNS recommendations for vitamin nomenclature.

[21] More specifically, the folates are pterins, namely, 2-amino-4-hydroxypteridines. The pteridines are yellow compounds first isolated from butterfly wings, for which they were named (i.e., *pteron* is the Greek word meaning "wing"); many are folate antagonists.

[22] This estimate is low, as bacteria are known to have as many as 12 residues in their polyglutamyl chains.

except in dry form, to heat. It is reduced *in vivo* enzymatically (or *in vitro* with a reductant such as dithionite) first to 7,8-dihydrofolic acid (FH$_2$) and then to FH$_4$; both of these compounds are unstable in aerobic environments and must be protected by the presence of an antioxidant (e.g., ascorbic acid, 2 mercaptoethanol).

Two derivatives of folic acid, each having an amino group in the place of the hydroxyl at C-4, are folate antagonists of biomedical use: *aminopterin* (4-amino-folic acid) and *methotrexate* (4-amino-N^{10}-methylfolic acid). Aminopterin is used as a rodenticide; methotrexate is an antineoplastic agent.

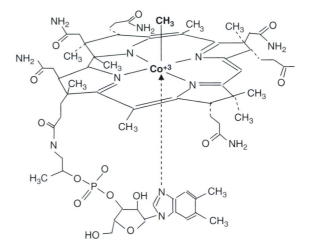

Methylcobalamin

XIV. Vitamin B$_{12}$

Essential features of the chemical structure:

1. Cobalt (Co)-centered corrin nucleus
2. Cobalt α position (below the plane of the corrin ring as shown) may be open or occupied by a side-chain heterocyclic nitrogen, or solvent
3. Cobalt β position (above the plane of the corrin ring as shown) may be occupied by a hydroxo, aqua, methyl, 5-deoxyadenosyl, CN⁻, Cl⁻, Br⁻, nitro, sulfito, or sulfato group[23]

Chemical structures of vitamin B$_{12}$:

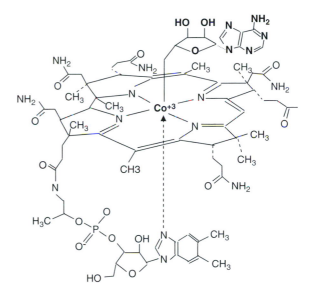

5'-Deoxyadenosylcobalamin

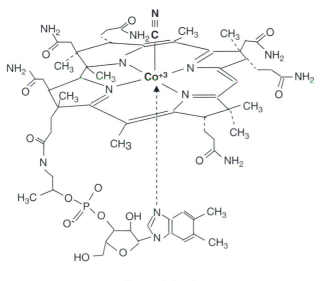

Cyanocobalamin

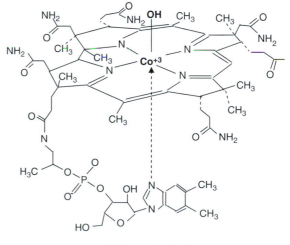

Hydroxocobalamin

---

[23] Only the first four liganded forms of vitamin B$_{12}$ are found in biological systems.

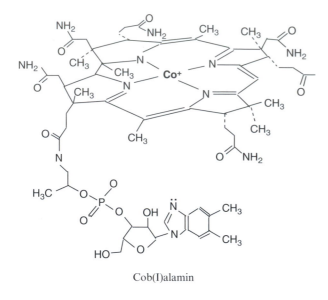

Cob(I)alamin

Vitamin B₁₂ Nomenclature

Vitamin B₁₂ is the generic descriptor for all corrinoids (i.e., compounds containing the **corrin nucleus**) exhibiting the qualitative biological activity of **cyanocobalamin**. Cyanocobalamin is the trivial designation of the vitamin B₁₂-active corrinoid (also called **cobalamin**) with a cyano ligand (CN⁻) at the β position of the cobalt atom. The analogs containing methyl-, 5′-deoxyadenosyl-, hydroxo- (OH) groups at that position are called **methylcobalamin, adenosylcobalamin**, and *hydroxocobalamin* (formerly vitamin B₁₂ᵦ), respectively. Those, as well as a form with an unliganded, reduced cobalt center, *cob(I)alamin*, are found intracellularly. Other analogs with vitamin B₁₂ activity include *aquacobalamin* (formerly vitamin B₁₂ₐ) and *nitritocobalamin* (formerly vitamin B₁₂ᶜ), which contain aqua- (H₂O) and nitrite groups, respectively.

Vitamin B₁₂ Chemistry

Vitamin B₁₂ is an octahedral cobalt complex consisting of a porphyrin-like, cobalt-centered macroring (called a *corrin ring* or *nucleus*), a nucleotide, and a second cobalt-bound group (e.g., CH₃, H₂O, CN⁻). The corrin nucleus consists of four reduced pyrrole nuclei linked by three methylene bridges and one direct bond. The triply ionized cobalt atom (i.e., Co³⁺) can form up to six coordinate bonds, is tightly bound to the four pyrrole nitrogen atoms, and can also bond a nucleotide and a small ligand below and above, respectively, the plane of the ring system. The cobalt atom is removed *in vitro* only with difficulty, resulting in loss of biological activity.

The corrinoids are red, red-orange, or yellow crystalline substances that show intense absorption spectra above 300 nm owing to the π–π transitions of the corrin nucleus. They are soluble in water and are fairly stable to heat but decompose at temperatures above ~210°C without melting.

Vitamin B₁₂ reacts with ascorbic acid, resulting in the reduction and subsequent degradation of the former, which releases its cobalt atom as the free ion. Cobalamins with relatively strongly bound ligands (e.g., cyano-, methyl-, and adenosylcobalamin) are less reactive and are, therefore, more stable in the presence of ascorbic acid. The cobalamins are unstable to light. Cyanocobalamin undergoes a photoreplacement of the CN⁻ ligand with water; the organocobalamins (methyl- and adenosylcobalamin) undergo photoreduction of the cobalt–carbon bond, resulting in the loss of the ligand and the reduction of the corrin cobalt. The vitamin can bind to proteins in the vitamin B₁₂ enzymes through an imidazole nitrogen of an histidyl residue on the protein, which serves as the ligand to the lower axial position of the cobalt atom instead of the dimethylbenzimidazole grouping.

XV. General Properties of the Vitamins

Multiple Forms of Vitamins

Few of the vitamins are biologically active without metabolic conversion to another species and/or binding to a specific protein. Thus, any consideration of the vitamins in nutrition involves, for each vitamin group, a number of vitamers and metabolites; some of these are important in the practical sense for food and diet supplementation (Table 3-9), whereas others are important in the physiological sense as they participate in metabolism.

Vitamin Stability

For the use of vitamins as food/feed additives, in diet supplements, and as pharmaceuticals, stability is a prime concern. In general, the fat-soluble vitamins, vitamin C, thiamin, riboflavin, and biotin are poorly stable to oxidation. They must be protected from heat, oxygen, metal ions (particularly Fe⁺⁺ and Cu⁺⁺), polyunsaturated lipids undergoing peroxidation, and ultraviolet light; antioxidants are frequently used in their formulations. For vitamins

Table 3-9.   The most important forms of the vitamins

Vitamin	Representative	Metabolically active forms	Important dietary forms
Vitamin A	Retinol	Retinol Retinal Retinoic acid	Retinyl palmitate and acetate, provitamins (β-carotene, other carotenoids)
Vitamin D	Cholecalciferol	25-OH-Cholecalciferol 1,25-(OH)$_2$-Cholecalciferol	Cholecalciferol, ergocalciferol
Vitamin E	α-Tocopherol	α-, β-, γ-, δ-Tocopherols	R,R,R-α-Tocopherol; all-rac-α-tocopheryl acetate
Vitamin K	Phylloquinone	Phylloquinones (K) Menaquinones (MK)	K, MK, menadione, menadione sodium bisulfite complex
Vitamin C	Ascorbic acid	Ascorbic acid Dehydroascorbic acid	L-Ascorbic acid, sodium ascorbate
Thiamin	Thiamin	Thiamin pyrophosphate	Thiamin; thiamin pyrophosphate, disulfide, HCl, mononitrate
Riboflavin	Riboflavin	FMN, FAD	FMN, FAD, flavoproteins, riboflavin
Niacin	Nicotinamide	NAD, NADP	NAD, NADP, nicotinamide, nicotinic acid
Vitamin B$_6$	Pyridoxine	Pyridoxal 5′-phosphate Pyridoxamine 5′-phosphate	Pyridoxal HCl, pyridoxal and pyridoxamine 5′-phosphates
Biotin	d-Biotin	d-Biotin	Biocytin, d-biotin
Pantothenic acid	Pantothenic acid	Coenzyme A	Calcium pantothenate, coenzyme A, acyl-CoAs
Folate	Pteroylglutamic acid	Pteroylpolyglutamates	Pteroyl poly- and monoglutamates
Vitamin B$_{12}$	Cyanocobalamin	Methylcobalamin 5′-Deoxyadenosylcobalamin	Cyano-, aqua-, hydroxo-, methyl-, and 5′-deoxyadenosylcobalamins

A and E, the more stable esterified forms are used for these purposes. Because of the instabilities of their naturally occurring vitamers, the amounts of the fat-soluble vitamins in natural foods and feedstuffs are highly variable, being greatly affected by the conditions of food production and processing. Niacin, vitamin B$_6$, pantothenic acid, folate, and vitamin B$_{12}$ tend to be more stable under most practical conditions (Table 3-10). Some vitamins can undergo degradation by reacting to factors in foods during sample storage and/or preparation: ascorbic acid with plant ascorbic acid oxidase; thiamin with sulfites or with plant or microbial thiaminases; folates with nitrites; and pantothenic acid with microbial pantothenases.

Vitamin Analysis

A variety of methods is available for the quantitative determination of the vitamins (Table 3-11). Because many vitamers are bound to proteins or other factors in biological specimens and foods, their extraction necessitates disruption of those complexes and separation from interfering substances. This must be done in ways that both are quantitative and can accommodate the intrinsic characteristics of each vitamer. Accordingly, conditions of sample extraction and clean-up must stabilize the vitamin(s) of interest in order to yield accurate results. Chromatographic separations have proven useful for determining vitamins A, D, E, K, C, thiamin, riboflavin, niacin, and vitamin B$_6$. They depend on separation by phase-partitioning (liquid-liquid,[24] or gas-liquid[25]) of vitamers for specificity, ascertained by comparison to authentic standards, and a suitable means of detection (e.g., ultraviolet–visible absorption, fluorescence, electrochemical reactivity) for sensitivity. Microbiological assays are available for thiamin, riboflavin, niacin, vitamin B$_6$, pantothenic acid, biotin, folate, and vitamin B$_{12}$. These methods are based on the absolute

---

[24] High-performance liquid chromatography (HPLC).
[25] Gas-liquid chromatography (GLC).

Table 3-10.   Stabilities of the vitamins

Vitamin	Vitamer	Unstable to:						To enhance stability:
		UV	Heat[a]	O_2	Acid	Base	Metals[b]	
Vitamin A	Retinol	+		+	+		+	Keep in the dark, sealed
	Retinal			+	+		+	Keep sealed
	Retinoic acid							Good stability
	Dehydroretinol			+				Keep sealed
	Retinyl esters							Good stability
	β-Carotene	+		+				Keep in the dark, sealed
Vitamin D	D_2	+	+	+	+		+	Keep cool, in the dark, sealed
	D_3	+	+	+	+	+	+	Keep cool, in the dark, sealed
Vitamin E	Tocopherols		+	+	+	+	+	Keep cool, at neutral pH
	Tocopheryl esters				+	+		Good stability
Vitamin K	K	+		+		+	+	Avoid reductants[c]
	MK	+		+		+	+	Avoid reductants[c]
	Menadione	+				+	+	Avoid reductants[c]
Vitamin C	Ascorbic acid			+[b]		+	+	Keep sealed, at neutral pH
Thiamin	Disulfide form		+	+	+	+	+	Keep at neutral pH[c]
	Hydrochloride[d]		+	+	+	+	+	Keep sealed, at neutral pH[c]
Riboflavin	Riboflavin	+[e]	+			+	+	Keep in the dark, at pH 1.5–4[c]
Niacin	Nicotinic acid							Good stability
	Nicotinamide							Good stability
Vitamin B_6	Pyridoxal	+	+					Keep cool
	Pyridoxol-HCl			+		+		Good stability
Biotin	Biotin			+		+		Keep sealed, at neutral pH
Pantothenic acid	Free acid[f]	+		+		+		Cool, neutral pH
	Calcium salt[d]			+				Keep sealed, at pH 6–7
Folate	FH_4	+	+	+	+[g]		+	Good stability[c]
Vitamin B_{12}	Cyano-B_{12}	+			+[h]		+[i]	Good stability[c]

[a] That is, 100°C.
[b] In solution with Fe^{3+} and Cu^{2+}.
[c] Unstable to reducing agents.
[d] Slightly hygroscopic.
[e] Especially in alkaline solution.
[f] Very hygroscopic.
[g] pH < 5.
[h] pH < 3.
[i] pH > 9.

requirement of certain microorganisms for particular vitamins for multiplication, which can be measured turbidimetrially or by the evolution of CO_2 from substrate provided in the growth media. Some forms of vitamins A, E, and C can be measured by chemical colorimetric reactions; however, only the dye reduction methods for ascorbic acid have appropriate specificity and reliability to be recommended.[26] Competitive protein-binding assays have been developed for biotin, folate, and vitamin B_{12}.[27] A radioimmunoassay and an enzyme-linked immunoabsorbent assay have been developed for pantothenic acid.

---

[26] *Vitamin A*: The Carr-Price method, which uses the time-sensitive production of a blue complex of retinol and antimony trichloride, is no longer recommended due to its lack of specificity and negative bias. *Vitamin E*: The Fe^{++}-dependent reduction of a fat-soluble dye such as bathophenanthroline by vitamin E is not recommended due to its lack of specificity, although many interfering substances can be partitioned into aqueous solvents during sample preparation. *Vitamin C*: The reaction of ascorbic acid with the dye 2,4-dinitrophenolindolphenol remains a useful method due to the fact that most interfering substances can be partitioned into organic solvents during sample preparation.

[27] Biotin and avidin; folate and folate-binding protein; vitamin B_{12} and R proteins.

Table 3-11.   Methods of vitamin analysis

| Vitamin | Sample preparation | Instrumental analysis | | Microbiological assay |
		Analyte separation	Analyte detection	
Vitamin A	Direct solvent extraction; alkaline HPLC[b] hydrolysis,[a] extraction into organic solvents	UV absorption		
Vitamin D	Alkaline hydrolysis with extraction into organic solvents	HPLC	UV absorption	
Vitamin E	Alkaline hydrolysis with extraction into organic solvents	HPLC	fluorescence, UV absorption	
Vitamin K	Direct solvent extraction; supercritical fluid extraction[c]; enzymatic hydrolysis	HPLC	UV absorption	
Vitamin C	Acid hydrolysis	HPLC, IEC,[d] MECC[e]	UV absorption	
Thiamin	Acid hydrolysis; enzymatic hydrolysis[g]	IEC, GLC,[f] HPLC	fluorescence, UV absorption, FID[i]	*Lactobacillus viridescens* (12706)[h]
Riboflavin	Acid hydrolysis	HPLC, MECC	fluorescence, UV absorption	*Lactobacillus casei* subsp. *rhamnsus* (7469)
				Enterococcus fecalis (10100)
Niacin	Alkaline hydrolysis	IEC, HPLC GLC, MECC	UV absorption, FID	*Lactobacillus plantarum* (8014)[j]
				Leuconostoc mesenteroides subsp. *mesenteroides* (9135)
Vitamin B$_6$	Acid hydrolysis	HPLC, IEC, GLC MECC	fluorescence, UV absorption, FID	*Saccharomyces carlbergensis* (9080)
				Kloectra apiculata (8714)
Pantothenic acid	Alkaline hydrolysis; enzymatic hydrolysis	GLC	FID	*Lactobacillus plantarum* (8014)[k]
Folate	Enzymatic hydrolysis[j]	IEC		*Lactobacillus casei* subsp. *rhamnsus* (7469)[l]
				Enterococcus hirae (8043)[k]
Biotin	Acid hydrolysis; enzymatic hydrolysis[k]			*Lactobacillus plantarum* (8014)
Vitamin B$_{12}$	Direct solvent extraction	MECC	UV absorption	*Lactobacillus delbrueckii*, subsp. *lactis* (4797)

[a]Saponification.
[b]High-performance liquid chromatography.
[c]Supercritical fluids are gases held above its critical temperature and critical pressure, which confers solvating properties similar to organic solvents with very low viscosities and very high diffusivities.
[d]Ion-exchange chromatography.
[e]Micellar electrokinetic capillary electrophoresis.
[f]Gas-liquid chromatography.
[g]Thiaminase or other phosphatase.
[h]American Type Culture Collection number.
[i]Flame ionization detection (used with GLC separation).
[j]Responds to nicotinic acid only.
[k]Responds to free vitamer only.
[l]Responds to all vitamers; yields "total" folate activity.
[m]Folyl conjugase.
[n]Papain.

XVI. Physiological Utilization of the Vitamins

Vitamin Bioavailability

Because not all vitamins in foods are completely utilized by the body, a measurement of the gross amounts of vitamins in foods (yielded by analysis) is insufficient to understand the actual nutritional value of those vitamin sources. This results from several factors (Table 3-12): differing losses, dietary effects, physiological effects and health status, as well as differing biopotencies. The actual rate and extent to which a vitamin is absorbed and utilized at the cellular level are referred to as its *bioavailability*. This concept differs from that of biopotency, which refers only to properties intrinsic to particular vitamers. Bioavailability refers to the integrated effects of those and other physiological and dietary factors. Some authors have used the term *bioefficacy* with a similar connotation.

Bioavailability

The concept of bioavailability, as applied to the vitamins and other essential nutrients, refers to the portion of ingested nutrient that is absorbed, retained, and metabolized through normal pathways in a form or forms that can be utilized for normal physiologic functions.

Vitamin Absorption

The means by which the vitamins are absorbed are determined by their chemical and associated physical properties. The fat-soluble vitamins (and hydrophobic substances such as carotenoids and cholesterol), which are not soluble in the aqueous environment of the alimentary canal, are associated with and dissolved in other lipid materials. In the upper portion of the gastrointestinal tract, they are dissolved in the bulk lipid phases of the emulsions that are formed of dietary fats[28] by the mechanical actions of mastication and gastric

Table 3-12. Several factors determining vitamin bioavailability

Factor	Description
	Extrinsic factors
Differing biopotencies	Different vitamers can have inherent differences in biopotencies, e.g., ergocalciferol is markedly less biopotent for the chick in comparison with cholecalciferol.
Losses	Some vitamins in foods show significant losses during storage, processing, and/or cooking, e.g., the vitamin C content of potatoes can drop by one-third within 1 month of storage.
Dietary effects	The composition of meals and diets can affect the absorption of some vitamins by affecting intestinal transit time and/or the enteric formation of mixed micelles; e.g., vitamin A and provitamin A carotenoids are absorbed very poorly from very low-fat diets.
	Intrinsic factors
Physiological effects	Age-related differences in gastrointestinal function can affect the absorption and postabsorptive utilization of certain vitamins; e.g., the absorption of vitamin B_{12} is reduced in many older persons who experience loss of gastric parietal cell function.
Health status	Some illnesses can affect the absorption and postabsorptive utilization of certain vitamins; e.g., folate absorption is impaired in patients with sprue.

---

[28] While it follows that the fat-soluble vitamins cannot be well absorbed from low-fat diets, the minimum amount of fat required is not clear. One recent study (Roodenburg, A. J., Leenen, R., van het Hof, K. H., Weststrate, J. A., and Tilburg, L. B. [2000]. *Am. J. Clin. Nutr.* **71**, 1187–1193) found that 3 grams of fat per meal was sufficient for optimal absorption of some pro-vitamin A carotenoids (α- and β-carotenes) but another study (Brown, M. J., Ferruzzi, M. G., Nguyen, M. L., Cooper, D. A., Eldridge, A. L., Schwartz, S. J., and White, W. S. [2004]. *Am. J. Clin. Nutr.* **80**, 396–403) found that 29.5 grams of fat per meal were insufficient.

churning. Emulsion oil droplets, however, are generally too large (e.g., 1000 Å) to gain the intimate proximity to the absorptive surfaces of the small intestine that is necessary to facilitate the diffusion of these substances into the hydrophobic environment of the brush border membranes of intestinal mucosal cells. However, *lipase*, which is present in the intestinal lumen, having been synthesized in and exported from the pancreas via the pancreatic duct, binds to the surface of emulsion oil droplets, where it catalyzes the hydrolytic removal of the α- and α′-fatty acids from triglycerides, which make up the bulk of the lipid material in these large particles.

The products of this process (i.e., free fatty acids and β-monoglycerides) have strong polar regions or charged groups and thus will dissolve to some extent monomerically in this aqueous environment. However, they also have long-chain hydrocarbon nonpolar regions; therefore, when certain concentrations (*critical micellar concentrations*) are achieved, these species and bile salts, which have similar properties, combine spontaneously to form small particles called *mixed micelles*. Mixed micelles thus contain free fatty acids, β-monoglycerides, and bile salts in which the nonpolar regions of each are associated interiorly and the polar or charged regions of each are oriented externally and are associated with the aqueous phase. The core of the mixed micelle is hydrophobic and thus serves to solubilize the fat-soluble vitamins and other nonpolar lipid substances. Because they are small (10–50 Å in diameter), mixed micelles can gain close proximity to microvillar surfaces of intestinal mucosa, thus facilitating the diffusion of their contents into and across those membranes. Because the enteric absorption of the fat-soluble vitamins depends on micellar dispersion, it is impaired under conditions of lipid malabsorption. Only one fat-soluble vitamer (phylloquinone) is known to be absorbed by active transport.

The water-soluble vitamins, which are soluble in the polar environment of the intestinal lumen, can be taken up by the absorptive surface of the gut more directly. Some (vitamin C, thiamin, niacin, vitamin B_6, biotin, pantothenic acid, folate, and vitamin B_{12}) are absorbed as the result of passive diffusion; others are absorbed via specific carriers as a means of overcoming concentration gradients unfavorable to simple diffusion. Several (vitamin C, vitamin B_{12}, thiamin, niacin, and folate) are absorbed via carrier-dependent mechanisms at low doses[29] and by simple diffusion (albeit at lower efficiency) at high doses.

The absorption of at least three water-soluble vitamins (vitamin C, riboflavin, and vitamin B_6) appears to be regulated in part by the dietary supply of the vitamin in a feedback manner. Thus, it has been questioned whether high doses of one vitamin/vitamer may antagonize the absorption of related vitamins. There is some evidence for such mutual antagonisms among the fat-soluble vitamins, as well as in the case of α-tocopherol, a high intake of which antagonizes the utilization of the related γ-vitamer.

A summary of modes of enteric absorption of the vitamins is presented in Table 3-13.

Vitamin Transport

The mechanisms of postabsorptive transport of the vitamins also vary according to their particular physical and chemical properties (Table 3-14). Again, therefore, the problem of solubility in the aqueous environments of the blood plasma and lymph is a major determinant of ways in which the vitamins are transported from the site of absorption (the small intestine) to the liver and peripheral organs. The fat-soluble vitamins, because they are insoluble in these transport environments, depend on carriers that are soluble there. These vitamins, therefore, are associated with the lipid-rich **chylomicrons**[30] that are elaborated in intestinal mucosal cells, largely of reesterified

---

[29] These processes show apparent K_m values in the range of 0.1–300 μM.

[30] Chylomicrons are the largest (approximately 1 μm in diameter) and the lightest of the blood lipids. They consist mainly of triglyceride with smaller amounts of cholesterol, phospholipid, protein, and the fat-soluble vitamins. They are normally synthesized in the intestinal mucosal cells and serve to transport lipids to tissues. In mammals, these particles are secreted into the lymphatic drainage of the small intestine (hence, their name). However, in birds, fishes, and reptiles, they are secreted directly into the renal portal circulation; therefore, in these species they are referred to as *portomicrons*. In either case, they are cleared from the plasma by the liver, and their lipid contents are either deposited in hepatic stores (e.g., vitamin A) or are released back into the plasma bound to more dense particles called *lipoproteins*.

Table 3-13. Enteric absorption of the vitamins[a]

Vitamer	Digestion	Site	Enterocytic metabolism	Efficiency (%)	Conditions of potential malabsorption
Micelle-dependent diffusion					
Retinol	—	D, J	Esterification	80–90	Pancreatic insufficiency (pancreatitis, selenium deficiency, cystic fibrosis, cancer), β-carotene cleavage, biliary atresia, obstructive jaundice, celiac disease, very low-fat diet
Retinyl esters	Deesterified	D, J	Reesterification		
		D, J	Esterification	50–60	Pancreatic or biliary insufficiency
Vitamins D	—	D, J	—	~50	Pancreatic or biliary insufficiency
Tocopherols	—	D, J	—	20–80	Pancreatic or biliary insufficiency
Tocopherol esters	Deesterified[b]	D, J	—	20–80	Pancreatic or biliary insufficiency
MKs	—	D, J	—	10–70	Pancreatic or biliary insufficiency
Menadione	—	D, J	—	10–70	Pancreatic or biliary insufficiency
Active transport					
Phylloquinone	—	D, J	—	~80	Pancreatic or biliary insufficiency
Ascorbic acid	—	I	—	70–80	D-Isoascorbic acid
Thiamin	—	D	Phosphorylation		Pyrithiamin, excess ethanol
Thiamin di-P	Dephosphorylation[b]	D	Phosphorylation		Pyrithiamin, excess ethanol
Riboflavin	—	J	Phosphorylation		
FMN, FAD	Hydrolysis[b]	J	Phosphorylation		
Flavoproteins	Hydrolysis[b]	J	Phosphorylation		
Folylmono-glu	—	J	Glutamation		Celiac sprue
Folylpoly-glu	Hydrolysis[b]	J	Glutamation		Celiac sprue
Vitamin B$_{12}$	Hydrolysis[b]	I	Adenosinylation, methylation	>90	Intrinsic factor deficiency (pernicious anemia)
Facilitated diffusion[c]					
Nicotinic acid	—	J		>90[d]	
Nicotinamide	—	J		~100[d]	
Niacytin	Hydrolysis[b]	J			
NAD(P)	Hydrolysis[b]	J			
Biotin	—	J			Biotinidase deficiency, consumption of raw egg white (avidin)
Biocytin	Hydrolysis[b]	J			Biotinidase deficiency, consumption of raw egg white (avidin)
Pantothenate	—				
Coenzyme A	Hydrolysis[b]				
Simple diffusion					
Ascorbic acid[e]	—	D, J, I	—	<50	
Thiamin[e,f]	—	J	Phosphorylation		
Nicotinic acid	—	J	—		
Nicotinamide	—	J	—		
Pyridoxol	—	J	Phosphorylation		
Pyridoxal	—	J	Phosphorylation		
Pyridoxamine	—	J	Phosphorylation		
Biotin	—	D, J	—	>95	Consumption of raw egg white (avidin)
Pantothenate	—		—		
Folylmono-glu[e]	—	J	Glutamation		
Vitamin B$_{12}$[e]	—	D, J	Adenosinylation, methylation	~1	

[a]*Abbreviations:* D, duodenum; J, jejunum; I, ileum; thiamin di-P, thiamin diphosphate; folylmono-glu, folylmonoglutamate; folylpoly-glu, folylpolyglutamate.
[b]Yields vitamin in absorbable form.
[c]Na$^+$-dependent saturable processes.
[d]Estimate may include contribution of simple diffusion.
[e]Simple diffusion important only at high doses.
[f]Symport with Na$^+$.

Table 3-14.   Postabsorptive transport of vitamins in the body

Vehicle	Vitamin	Form transported	Distribution
Lipoprotein bound			
Chylomicrons[a]	Vitamin A	Retinyl esters	Lymph[a]
	Vitamin A	β-Carotene	Lymph
	Vitamin D	Vitamin D[b]	Lymph
	Vitamin E	Tocopherols	Lymph
	Vitamin K	K, MK, menadione	Lymph
VLDL[c]/HDL[d]	Vitamin E	Tocopherols	Plasma
	Vitamin K	Mainly MK-4	Plasma
Associated nonspecifically with proteins			
Albumin	Riboflavin	Free riboflavin	Plasma
	Riboflavin	Flavin mononucleotide	Plasma
	Vitamin B_6	Pyridoxal	Plasma
	Vitamin B_6	Pyridoxal phosphate	Plasma
Immunoglobulins[e]	Riboflavin	Free riboflavin	Plasma
Bound to specific binding proteins			
Retinol BP (RBP)	Vitamin A	Retinol	Plasma
Cellular RBP (CRBP)	Vitamin A	Retinol	Intracellular
Cellular RBP, type II (CRBPII)	Vitamin A	Retinol	Enterocytic
Interstitial RBP (IRBP)	Vitamin A	Retinol	Interstitial spaces
Cellular retinal BP (CRALBP)	Vitamin A	Retinal	Intracellular
Cellular retinoic acid BP (CRABP)	Vitamin A	Retinoic acid	Intracellular
Transcalciferin	Vitamin D	D_2; D_3; 25-OH-D; 1,25-$(OH)_2$-D; 24,25-$(OH)_2$-D	Plasma
Vitamin D receptor	Vitamin D	1,25-$(OH)_2$-D	Enterocytes
Vitamin E BP	Vitamin E	Tocopherols	Intracellular
Riboflavin BP	Riboflavin	Riboflavin	Plasma
Flavoproteins	Riboflavin	Flavin mononucleotide	Intracellular
	Riboflavin	Flavin adenine dinucleotide	Intracellular
Transcobalamin I	Vitamin B_{12}	Vitamin B_{12}	Intracellular
Transcobalamin II	Vitamin B_{12}	Methylcobalamin	Plasma
Transcobalamin III	Vitamin B_{12}	Vitamin B_{12}	Plasma
Erythrocyte carried			
Erythrocyte membranes	Vitamin E	Tocopherols	Blood
Erythrocytes	Vitamin B_6	Pyridoxal phosphate	Blood
	Pantothenic acid	Coenzyme A	Blood
Free in plasma			
—	Vitamin C	Ascorbic acid	Plasma
—	Thiamin	Free thiamin	Plasma
—	Thiamin	Thiamin pyrophosphate	Plasma
—	Riboflavin	Flavin mononucleotide	Plasma
—	Pantothenic acid	Pantothenic acid	Plasma
—	Biotin	Free biotin	Plasma
—	Niacin	Nicotinic acid	Plasma
—	Niacin	Nicotinamide	Plasma
—	Folate	Pteroylmonoglutamates[f]	Plasma

[a]In mammals, lipids are absorbed into the lymphatic circulation, where they are transported to the liver and other tissues as large lipoprotein particles called *chylomicra* (singular, *chylomicron*); in birds, reptiles, and fishes lipids are absorbed directly into the hepatic portal circulation and the analogous lipoprotein particle is called a **portomicron**.
[b]Representation of vitamin D without a subscript is meant to refer to both major forms of the vitamin: ergocalciferol (D_2) and cholecalciferol (D_3).
[c]VLDL, Very low-density lipoprotein.
[d]HDL, High-density lipoprotein.
[e]For example, IgG, IgM, and IgA.
[f]Especially 5-CH_3-tetrahydrofolic acid.

triglycerides from free fatty acids and β-monoglycerides that have just been absorbed. As the lipids in these particles are transferred to other **lipoproteins**[31] in the liver, some of the fat-soluble vitamins (vitamins E and K) are also transferred to those carriers. Others (vitamins A and D) are transported from the liver to peripheral tissues by specific **binding proteins** of hepatic origin (see Table 3-14). Some of the water-soluble vitamins are transported by protein carriers in the plasma and therefore are not found free in solution. Some (riboflavin, vitamin B_6) are carried via weak, nonspecific binding to albumin and may thus be displaced by other substances (e.g., ethanol) that also bind to that protein. Others are tightly associated with certain immunoglobulins (riboflavin) or bind to specific proteins involved in their transport (riboflavin, vitamins A, D, E, and B_{12}). Several vitamins (e.g., vitamin C, thiamin, niacin, riboflavin, pantothenic acid, biotin, and folate) are transported in free solution in the plasma.

Tissue Distribution of the Vitamins

The retention and distribution of the vitamins among the various tissues also vary according to their general physical and chemical properties (Table 3-15). In general, the fat-soluble vitamins are well retained; they tend to be stored in association with tissue lipids. For that reason, lipid-rich tissues such as adipose and liver frequently have appreciable stores of the fat-soluble vitamins. Storage of these vitamins means that animals may be able to accommodate widely variable intakes without consequence by mobilizing their tissue stores in times of low dietary intakes.

In contrast, the water-soluble vitamins tend to be excreted rapidly and not retained well. Few of this group are stored to any appreciable extent. The notable exception is vitamin B_{12}, which, under normal circumstances, can accumulate in the liver in amounts adequate to satisfy the nutritional needs of the host for periods of years.

Table 3-15. Tissue distribution of the vitamins

Vitamin	Predominant storage form(s)	Depot(s)
Vitamin A	Retinyl esters (e.g., palmitate)	Liver
Vitamin D	D_3; 25-OH-D	Plasma, adipose, muscle
Vitamin E	α-Tocopherol	Adipose, adrenal, testes, platelets, other tissues
Vitamin K[a]	K: K-4, MK-4	Liver
	MK: MK-4	All tissues
	Menadione: MK-4	All tissues
Vitamin C	Ascorbic acid	Adrenals, leukocytes
Thiamin	Thiamin pyrophosphate[b]	Heart, kidney, brain, muscle
Riboflavin	Flavin adenine dinucleotide[b]	Liver, kidney, heart
Vitamin B_6	Pyridoxal phosphate[b]	Liver,[c] kidney,[c] heart[c]
Vitamin B_{12}	Methylcobalamin	Liver,[d] kidney,[c] heart,[c] spleen,[c] brain[c]
Niacin	No appreciable storage	—
Biotin	No appreciable storage[b]	—
Pantothenic acid	No appreciable storage	—
Folate	No appreciable storage	—

[a]The predominant form of the vitamin is shown for each major form of dietary vitamin K consumed.
[b]The amounts in the body are composed of the enzyme-bound coenzyme.
[c]Small amounts of the vitamin are found in these tissues.
[d]Predominant depot.

---

[31] As the name would imply, a *lipoprotein* is a lipid–protein combination with the solubility characteristics of a protein (i.e., soluble in the aqueous environment of the blood plasma) and, hence, involved in lipid transport. Four classes of lipoproteins, each defined empirically on the basis of density, are found in the plasma: chylomicrons/portomicrons, high-density lipoproteins (**HDLs**), low-density lipoproteins (**LDLs**), and very low-density lipoproteins (**VLDLs**). The latter three classes are also known by names derived from the method of electrophoretic separation, i.e., α-, β-, and pre-β-lipoproteins, respectively.

XVII. Metabolism of the Vitamins

Some Vitamins Have Limited Biosynthesis

By definition, the vitamins as a group of nutrients are obligate factors in the diet (i.e., the chemical environment) of an organism. Nevertheless, some vitamins do not quite fit that general definition by virtue of being biosynthesized regularly by certain species or by being biosynthesized under certain circumstances by other species (see "Some Caveats" in Chapter 1). The biosynthesis of such vitamins (Table 3-16) thus depends on the availability, either from dietary or metabolic sources, of appropriate precursors (e.g., adequate free tryptophan is required for niacin production; the presence of 7-dehydrocholesterol in the surface layers of the skin is required for its conversion to vitamin D_3; flux through the gulonic acid pathway is needed to produce ascorbic acid), as well as the presence of the appropriate metabolic and/or chemical catalytic activities (e.g., the several enzymes involved in the tryptophan–niacin conversion; exposure to UV light for the photolysis of 7-dehydrocholesterol to produce vitamin D_3; the several enzymes of the gulonic acid pathway, including L-gulonolactone oxidase, for the formation of ascorbic acid).

Most Vitamins Require Metabolic Activation

Whereas a few of the vitamins function in biological systems without some sort of metabolic activation or linkage to a cofunctional species (e.g., an enzyme), most require such metabolic conversions (Table 3-17).

Direct-Acting Vitamins
Vitamin E
Vitamin C

Some vitamers K (some forms of vitamin K, e.g., MK-4), are metabolically active per se, although most other forms undergo some dealkylation/realkylation in order to be converted to metabolically active vitamers)

The metabolic transformation of dietary forms of the vitamins into the forms that are active in metabolism may involve substantive modification of a vitamin's chemical structure and/or its combination with another metabolically important species. Thus, some vitamins are *activated* to their functional species; factors that may affect their metabolic (i.e., enzymatic) activation can have profound influences on their nutritional efficacy.

Vitamin Binding to Proteins

Some vitamins, even some of those requiring metabolic activation, are biologically active only when bound to a protein (Table 3-18). In most cases, this happens when the vitamin serves as the prosthetic group of an enzyme, remaining bound to the enzyme protein during catalysis.[32] In other cases, this involves a vitamer binding to a specific nuclear receptor to elicit transcriptional modulation of one or more protein products (Table 3-19).

Table 3-16. Vitamins that can be biosynthesized

Vitamin	Precursor	Route	Conditions increasing dietary need
Niacin	Tryptophan	Conversion to NMN via picolinic acid	Low 3-OH-anthranilic acid oxidase activity
			High picolinic acid carboxylase activity
			Low dietary tryptophan
			High dietary leucine[a]
Vitamin D_3	7-Dehydrocholesterol	UV photolysis	Insufficient sunlight/UV exposure
Vitamin C	Glucose	Gulonic acid pathway	L-Gulonolactone oxidase deficiency

[a]The role of leucine as an effector of the conversion of tryptophan to niacin is controversial (see Chapter 12).

---

[32] Vitamins of this type are properly called *coenzymes*; those that participate in enzymatic catalysis but are not firmly bound to enzyme protein during the reaction are, more properly, *cosubstrates*. This distinction, however, does not address mechanism, but only tightness of binding. For example, the associations of NAD and NADP with certain oxidoreductases are weaker than those of FMN and FAD with the flavoprotein oxidoreductases. Therefore, the term *coenzyme* has come to be used to describe enzyme cofactors of both types.

Table 3-17. Vitamins that must be activated metabolically

Vitamin	Active form(s)	Activation step	Condition(s) increasing need
Vitamin A	Retinol	Retinal reductase	Protein insufficiency
		Retinol hydrolase	
	11-*cis*-Retinol	Retinyl isomerase	
	11-*cis*-Retinal	Alcohol dehydrogenase	Zinc insufficiency
Vitamin D	1,25-$(OH)_2$-D	Vitamin D 25-hydroxylase	Hepatic failure
		25-OH-D 1-hydroxylase	Renal failure, lead exposure, estrogen deficiency, anticonvulsant drug therapy
Vitamin K	All forms	Dealkylation of Ks, MKs	Hepatic failure
		Alkylation of Ks, MKs, menadione	
Thiamin	Thiamin-diP[a]	Phosphorylation	High carbohydrate intake
Riboflavin	FMN, FAD	Phosphorylation	
		Adenosylation	
Vitamin B_6	Pyridoxal-P	Phosphorylation	High protein intake
		Oxidation	
Niacin	NAD(H), NADP(H)	Amidation (nicotinic acid)	Low tryptophan intake
Pantothenic acid	Coenzyme A	Phosphorylation	
		Decarboxylation	
		ATP condensation	
		Peptide bond formation	
	ACP[b]	Phosphorylation	
		Peptide bond formation	
Folate	C_1-FH$_4$[c]	Reduction	
		Addition of C_1	
Vitamin B_{12}	Methyl-B_{12}	Cobalamin methylation	Folate deficiency
		CH_3 group insufficiency	
	5′-Deoxyadenosyl-B_{12}	Adenosylation	

[a]Thiamin-diP, Thiamin pyrophosphate.
[b]ACP, Acyl carrier protein.
[c]C_1-FH$_4$, Tetrahydrofolic acid.

Table 3-18. Vitamins that must be linked to enzymes and other proteins

Vitamin	Form(s) linked
Biotin	Biotin
Vitamin B_{12}	Methylcobalamin, adenosylcobalamin
Vitamin A	11-*cis*-Retinal
Thiamin	Thiamin pyrophosphate
Riboflavin	FMN, FAD
Niacin	NAD, NADP
Vitamin B_6	Pyridoxal phosphate
Pantothenic acid	Acyl carrier protein
Folate	Tetrahydrofolic acid (FH$_4$)

Vitamin Excretion

In general, the fat-soluble vitamins, which tend to be retained in hydrophobic environments, are excreted with the feces via the enterohepatic circulation (Table 3-20). Exceptions include vitamins A and E, which to some extent have water-soluble metabolites (e.g., short-chain derivatives of retinoic acid; and the so-called *Simon's metabolites, carboxylchromanol mbetabolites*, of vitamin E), and menadione, which can be metabolized to a polar salt; these vitamin metabolites are excreted in the urine. In contrast, the water-soluble vitamins are generally excreted in the urine, both

Table 3-19. Vitamins that have nuclear receptor proteins

Vitamin	Form(s) linked	Receptor
Vitamin A	all-*trans*-Retinoic acid	Retinoic acid receptors (RARs)
	9-*cis*-Retinoid acid	Retinoid X receptors (RXRs)
Vitamin D	1,25-$(OH)_2$-vitamin D_3	Vitamin D receptor (VDR)

Table 3-20. Excretory forms of the vitamins

Vitamin	Urinary form(s)	Fecal form(s)
Vitamin A	Retinoic acid Acidic short-chain forms	Retinoyl glucuronides Intact-chain products
Vitamin D		$25,26\text{-}(OH)_2\text{-}D$ $25\text{-}(OH)_2\text{-}D\text{-}23,26\text{-lactone}$
Vitamin E		Tocopheryl quinone Tocopheronic acid and its lactone
Vitamin K (K, MK, and menadione)		Vitamin K-2,3-epoxide $2\text{-}CH_3\text{-}3(5'\text{-Carboxy-}3'\text{-}CH_3\text{-}2'\text{-pentenyl})$- 1,4-naphthoquinone $2\text{-}CH_3\text{-}3(3'\text{-Carboxy-}3'\text{-methylpropyl})$- 1,4-naphthoquinone Other unidentified metabolites
Menadione	Menadiol phosphate Menadiol sulfate	Menadiol glucuronide
Vitamin C[a]	Ascorbate-2-sulfate Oxalic acid 2,3-Diketogulonic acid	
Thiamin	Thiamin Thiamin disulfide Thiamin pyrophosphate Thiochrome 2-Methyl-4-amino-5-pyrimidine carboxylic acid 4-Methyl-thiazole-5-acetic acid 2-Methyl-4-amino-5-hydroxymethyl pyrimidine 5-(2-Hydroxyethyl)-4-methylthiazole 3-(2'-Methyl-4-amino-5'-pyrimidinylmethyl)- 4-methylthiazole-5-acetic acid 2-Methyl-4-amino-5-formylaminomethylpyrimidine Several other minor metabolites	
Riboflavin	Riboflavin 7 (and 8)-hydroxmethylriboflavin 8β-sulfonylriboflavin Riboflavinyl peptide ester 10-Hydroxyethylflavin Lumiflavin 10-Formylmethylflavin 10-Carboxymethylflavin Lumichrome	
Niacin	N^1-Methylnicotinamide Nicotinuric acid Nicotinamide-N^1-oxide N^1-Methylnicotinamide-N^1-oxide N^1-Methyl-4-pyridone-3-carboxamide N^1-Methyl-2-pyridone-5-carboxamide	
Vitamin B_6	Pyridoxol, pyridoxal, pyridoxamine, and phosphates 4-Pyridoxic acid and its lactone 5-Pyridoxic acid	
Biotin	Biotin; bis-*nor*-biotin Biotin *d*- and *l*-sulfoxide	
Pantothenic acid	Pantothenic acid	
Folate	Pteroylglutamic acid 5-Methyl-pteroylglutamic acid 10-HCO-FH_4, pteridine Acetaminobenzoylglutamic acid	Intact folates
Vitamin B_{12}	Cobalamin	Cobalamin

[a]Substantial amounts are also oxidized to CO_2 and are excreted across the lungs.

in intact forms (riboflavin, pantothenic acid) and as water-soluble metabolites (vitamin C, thiamin, niacin, riboflavin, pyridoxine, biotin, folate, and vitamin B_{12}).

XVIII. Metabolic Functions of the Vitamins

Vitamins Serve Five Basic Functions

The 13 families of nutritionally important substances called *vitamins* comprise two to three times that number of practically important vitamers and function in metabolism in five general and not mutually exclusive ways. The type of metabolic function of any particular vitamer or vitamin family, of course, is dependent on its tissue/cellular distribution and its chemical reactivity, both of which are direct or indirect functions of its chemical structure. For example, the antioxidative function of vitamin E reflects the ability of that vitamin to form semistable radical intermediates; its lipophilicity allows vitamin E to discharge this antioxidant function within the hydrophoblic regions of biomembranes, thus protecting polyunsaturated membrane phospholipids. Similarly, the redox function of riboflavin is due to its ability to undergo reversible reduction/oxidation involving a radical anion intermediate. These functions (summarized in Table 3-21), and the fundamental aspects of their significance in nutrition and health, are the subjects of Chapters 5–17.

Vitamins function as:

- Antioxidants
- Gene transcription elements
- H^+/e^- donors/acceptors
- Hormones
- Coenzymes

Table 3-21. Metabolic functions of the vitamins

Vitamin	Activities
Antioxidants	
Vitamin E	Protects polyunsaturated membrane phospholipids and other substances from oxidative damage via conversion of tocopherol to tocopheroxyl radical and, then, to tocopheryl quinone
Vitamin C	Protects cytosolic substances from oxidative damage
Hormones	
Vitamin A	Signals coordinate metabolic responses of several tissues
Vitamin D	Signals coordinate metabolism important in calcium homeostasis
H^+/e^- donors/acceptors (cofactors)	
Vitamin K	Converts the epoxide form in the carboxylation of peptide glutamyl residues
Vitamin C	Oxidizes dehydroascorbic acid in hydroxylation reactions
Niacin	Interconverts $NAD^+/NAD(H)$ and $NADP^+/NADP(H)$ couples in several dehydrogenase reactions
Riboflavin	Interconverts $FMN/FMNH/FMNH_2$ and $FAD/FADH/FADH_2$ systems in several oxidases
Pantothenic acid	Oxidizes coenzyme A in the synthesis/oxidation of fatty acids
Coenzymes	
Vitamin A	Rhodopsin conformational change following light-induced bleaching
Vitamin K	Vitamin K-dependent peptide-glutamyl carboxylase
Vitamin C	Cytochrome *P*-450-dependent oxidations (drug and cholesterol metabolism, steroid hydroxylations)
Thiamin	Cofactor of α-keto acid decarboxylases and transketolase
Niacin	NAD(H)/NADP(H) used by more than 30 dehydrogenases in the metabolism of carbohydrates (e.g., glucose-6-phosphate dehydrogenase), lipids (e.g., α-glycerol-phosphate dehydrogenase), protein (e.g., glutamate dehydrogenase); Krebs cycle, rhodopsin synthesis (alcohol dehydrogenase)

Table 3-21. Metabolic functions of the vitamins—Cont'd

Vitamin	Activities
Riboflavin	FMN: L-Amino-acid oxidase, lactate dehydrogenase, pyridoxine (pyridoxamine); 5′-phosphate oxidase
	FAD: D-Amino-acid and glucose oxidases, succinic and acetyl-CoA dehydrogenases; glutathione, vitamin K, and cytochrome reductases
Vitamin B_6	Metabolism of amino acids (aminotransferases, deaminases, decarboxylases, desulfhydratases), porphyrins (δ-aminolevulinic acid synthase), glycogen (glycogen phosphorylase), and epinephrine (tyrosine decarboxylase)
Biotin	Carboxylations (pyruvate, acetyl-CoA, propionyl-CoA, 3-methylcrotonyl-CoA carboxylases) and transcarboxylations (methylmalonyl-CoA carboxymethyltransferase)
Pantothenic acid	Fatty acid synthesis/oxidation
Folate	Single-carbon metabolism (serine–glycine conversion, histidine degradation, purine synthesis, methyl group synthesis)
Vitamin B_{12}	Methylmalonyl-CoA mutase, N^5-CH_3-FH_4:homocysteine methyltransferase

Study Questions and Exercises

1. Prepare a concept map of the relationships between the chemical structures, the physical properties, and the modes of absorption, transport and tissue distributions of the vitamins.

2. For each vitamin, identify the key feature(s) of its chemical structure. How is/(are) this/(these) feature(s) related to the stability and/or biologic activity of the vitamin?

3. Discuss the general differences between the fat-soluble and water-soluble vitamins and the implications of those differences in diet formulation and meal preparation.

4. Which vitamins would you suspect might be in shortest supply in the diets of livestock? in your own diet? Explain your answer in terms of the physicochemical properties of the vitamins.

5. Which vitamins would you expect to be stored well in the body? unstable in foods or feeds?

6. What factors would you expect to influence the absorption of specific vitamins?

Recommended Reading

Vitamin Nomenclature

Anonymous. (1987). Nomenclature policy: Generic descriptors and trivial names for vitamins and related compounds. *J. Nutr.* **120,** 12–19.

Vitamin Chemistry and Analysis

Ball, G. F. M. (1998). *Bioavailability and Analysis of Vitamins in Foods*. Chapman & Hall, New York, 569 pp.

Eitenmiller, R. R., and Landen, W. O. Jr. (1999). *Vitamin Analysis for the Health and Food Sciences*. CRC Press, New York, 518 pp.

Friedrich, W. (1988). *Vitamins*. Walter de Gruyter, New York.

Rucker, R. B., Suttie, J. W., McCormick, D. B., and Machlin, L. J. (eds.). (2001). *Handbook of Vitamins*. Marcel Dekker, New York, 600 pp.

Vitamin Deficiency

4

These diseases … were considered for years either as intoxication by food or as infectious diseases, and twenty years of experimental work were necessary to show that diseases occur which are caused by a deficiency of some essential substance in the food.

— C. Funk

I.   The Concept of Vitamin Deficiency   76
II. The Many Causes of Vitamin Deficiencies   78
III. Clinical Manifestations of Vitamin Deficiencies 79
IV. Vitamin Deficiency Diseases:
     Manifestations of Biochemical Lesions   86
     Study Questions and Exercises   92
     Recommended Reading   92

Anchoring Concepts

1. A *disease* is an interruption or perversion of function of any of the organs with characteristic signs and/or symptoms caused by specific biochemical and morphological changes.
2. *Deficient intakes* of essential nutrients can cause disease.

Learning Objectives

1. To understand the concept of *vitamin deficiency*.
2. To understand that deficient intakes of vitamins lead to *sequences of lesions* involving changes starting at the biochemical level, progressing to affect cellular and tissue function and, ultimately, resulting in morphological changes.
3. To appreciate the range of possible morphological changes in organ systems that can be caused by vitamin deficiencies.
4. To get an overview of *specific clinical signs and symptoms* of deficiencies of each vitamin in animals, including humans, as background for further study of the vitamins.
5. To appreciate the relationships of clinical manifestations of vitamin deficiencies and lesions in the biochemical functions of those vitamins.

Vocabulary

Achlorhydria
Achromotrichia
Acrodynia
Age pigments
Alopecia
Anemia
Anorexia
Arteriosclerosis
Ataxia
Beriberi
Bradycardia
Brown bowel disease
Brown fat disease
Cage layer fatigue
Capillary fragility
Cardiomyopathy
Cataract
Cervical paralysis
Cheilosis
Chondrodystrophy
Cirrhosis
Clinical signs
Clubbed down
Convulsion
Cornification
Curled toe paralysis
Dermatitis
Desquamation
Dystrophy
Edema
Encephalomalacia
Encephalopathy
Exudative diathesis
Fatty liver and kidney syndrome

Geographical tongue
Glossitis
Hyperkeratosis
Hypovitaminosis
Inflammation
Keratomalacia
Leukopenia
Lipofuscinosis
Malabsorption
Mulberry heart disease
Myopathy
Necrosis
Nephritis
Neuropathy
Night blindness
Nyctalopia
Nystagmus
Opisthotonos
Osteomalacia
Osteoporosis
Pellagra
Peripheral neuropathy
Perosis
Photophobia
Polyneuritis
Retrolental fibroplasia
Rickets
Scurvy
Steatitis
Stomatitis
Symptom
Vitamin deficiency
Wernicke–Korsakoff syndrome
White muscle disease
Xerophthalmia
Xerosis

I. The Concept of Vitamin Deficiency

What Is Meant by the Term *Vitamin Deficiency?*

Because the gross functional and morphological changes caused by deprivation of the vitamins were the source of their discovery as important nutrients, these signs have become the focus of attention for many with interests in human and/or veterinary health. Indeed, freedom from clinical diseases caused by insufficient vitamin nutriture has generally been used as the main criterion by which vitamin requirements have been defined. The expression **vitamin deficiency**, therefore, simply refers to the basic condition of **hypovitaminosis**. Vitamin deficiency is distinct from but underlies the various biochemical changes, physiological and/or functional impairments, or other overt disease signs by which the need for a vitamin is defined.

A vitamin deficiency is …
… the shortage of supply of a vitamin relative to its needs by a particular organism.

Vitamin Deficiencies Involve Cascades of Progressive Changes

The diseases associated with low intakes of particular vitamins typically represent clinical manifestations of a progressive sequence of lesions that result from biochemical perturbations (e.g., diminished enzyme activity due to lack of a coenzyme or cosubstrate; membrane dysfunction due to lack of a stabilizing factor) that lead first to cellular and subsequently to tissue and organ dysfunction. Thus, the clinical signs of a vitamin deficiency are actually the end result of a chain of events that starts with the diminution in cells and tissues of the metabolically active form of the vitamin (see Fig. 4-1).

Stages of vitamin deficiency

Marginal deficiency

Stage I	Depletion of vitamin stores, which leads to …
Stage II	Cellular metabolic changes, which lead to …

Observable deficiency

Stage III	Clinical defects, which ultimately produce …
Stage IV	Morphological changes

Marks[1] illustrated this point with the results of a study of thiamin depletion in human volunteers (Fig. 4-2). When the subjects were fed a thiamin-free diet, no changes of any type were detected for 5 to 10 days, after which the first signs of decreased saturation of erythrocyte transketolase with its essential cofactor, thiamin pyrophosphate (TPP), were noted. Not for nearly 200 days of depletion (i.e., long after tissue

---

[1] Marks, J. (1968). *The Vitamins in Health and Disease: A Modern Reappraisal.* Churchill, London.

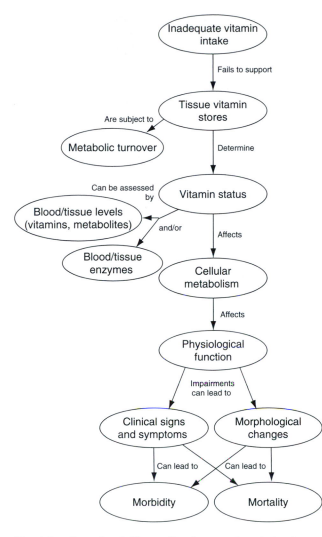

Fig. 4-1 Cascade of effects of inadequate vitamin intake.

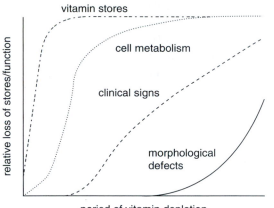

Fig. 4-2 Overtime, thiamin-deprived human subjects experience the four stages of vitamin deficiency, starting with tissue depletion, and ending with morphological changes. (*After* Marks [1968].)

stitutes good nutrition; this perspective ignores the importance of preventing the early functional impairments that can progress to overt clinical signs. Therefore, the modern view of nutritional adequacy must focus on maintenance of normal metabolism and, in several cases, body reserves as criteria of adequate vitamin status.[3]

thiamin levels and transketolase–TPP saturation had declined) were classic **clinical signs**[2] of thiamin deficiency (**anorexia**, weight loss, malaise, insomnia, hyperirritability) detected.

Marginal deficiencies of vitamins in which the impacts of poor vitamin status are not readily observed without chemical or biochemical testing are often referred to as *subclinical deficiencies* for that reason. They involve depleted reserves or localized abnormalities, but without the presence of overt functional or morphological defects. The traditional perspective has been that the absence of overt, clinical manifestations of deficiency con-

Intervention Is Most Effective in Early Stages of Vitamin Deficiency

That vitamin deficiencies[4] are not simply specific morphological events but, rather, cascades of biochemical, physiological, and anatomical changes is the key point in both the assessment of vitamin status and the effective treatment of hypovitaminoses. Because the early biochemical and metabolic effects of specific vitamin deficiencies are almost always readily reversed by therapy with the appropriate vitamin, in contrast to the later functional and anatomical changes, which may be permanent, intervention to correct hypovitaminoses is most effective when the condition is detected in its early and less severe stages. In this respect, the management of vitamin deficiencies is not different from that of other diseases—treatment

---

[2] A *symptom* is a change, whereas a *clinical sign* is a change detectable by a physician.

[3] By such criteria, marginal vitamin status in the United States appears to be quite prevalent, even though the prevalence of clinically significant vitamin deficiencies appears to be very low. Estimates of marginal status with respect to one or more vitamins have been as high as 15% of adolescents, 12% of persons 65 years of age and older, and 20% of dieters.

[4] This discussion, of course, is pertinent to *any* class of nutrients.

is generally most effective when given at the stage of cellular biochemical abnormality rather than waiting for the appearance of the ultimate clinical signs.[5] For this reason, the early detection of insufficient vitamin status using biochemical indicators has been and will continue to be a very important activity in the clinical assessment of vitamin status.

II. The Many Causes of Vitamin Deficiencies

Primary and Secondary Causes of Vitamin Deficiencies

The balance of vitamin supply and need for a particular individual at a given point in time is called *vitamin status*. Reductions in vitamin status can be produced either by reductions in effective vitamin supply or by increases in effective vitamin need. Vitamin deficiency occurs when vitamin status is reduced to the point of having metabolic impact (i.e., stage II); if not corrected, continued reductions in vitamin status lead inevitably to the observable stages of vitamin deficiency (stages II and IV), at which serious clinical and morphological changes can become manifest. When these changes occur as the result of the failure to ingest a vitamin in sufficient amounts to meet physiological needs, the condition is called a *primary deficiency*. When these changes come about as a result of the failure to absorb or otherwise utilize a vitamin owing to an environmental condition or physiological state and not to insufficient consumption of the vitamin, the condition is called a *secondary deficiency*.

Two fundamental ways in which vitamin deficiencies can be caused

> *Primary deficiencies* ... involve failures to ingest a vitamin in sufficient amounts to meet physiological needs.
> *Secondary deficiencies* ... involve failures to absorb or otherwise utilize a vitamin postabsorptively.

Causes of Vitamin Deficiencies in Humans

Many of the ways in which vitamin deficiencies can come about are interrelated. For example, poverty is often accompanied by gross ignorance of what constitutes a nutritionally adequate diet. People living alone, and especially the elderly and others with chronic disease, tend to consume foods that require little preparation but that may not provide good nutrition. Despite these potential causes of vitamin deficiency, in most of the technologically developed parts of the world the general level of nutrition is high. In those areas, relatively few persons can be expected to show signs of vitamin deficiency; those that do present such signs will most frequently be found to have a potentiating condition that affects either their consumption of food or their utilization of nutrients. In the developing parts of the world, however, famine is still the largest single cause of general malnutrition today. People affected by famine show signs of multiple nutrient deficiencies, including lack of energy, protein, vitamins, and minerals.

Potential causes of vitamin deficiencies in humans

Primary deficiencies have psychosocial and technological causes:

> Poor food habits
> Poverty (i.e., low food-purchasing power)
> Ignorance (i.e., lack of sound nutrition information)
> Lack of total food (e.g., crop failure)
> Lack of vitamin-rich foods (e.g., consumption of highly refined foods)
> Vitamin destruction (e.g., during storage, processing, and/or cooking)
> Anorexia (e.g., homebound elderly, infirm, dental problems)
> Food taboos and fads (e.g., fasting, avoidance of certain foods)
> Apathy (lack of incentive to prepare adequate meals)

---

[5] Marks (1968) makes this point clearly with the example of diabetes, which should be treated once hypoglycemia is detected, thus reducing the danger of diabetic arteriosclerosis and retinopathy.

Secondary deficiencies have biological causes:

Poor digestion (e.g., **achlorhydria**—absence of stomach acid)

Malabsorption (impaired intestinal absorption of nutrients; e.g., as a result of diarrhea, intestinal infection, parasites, pancreatitis)

Impaired metabolic utilization (e.g., certain drug therapies)

Increased metabolic need (e.g., pregnancy, lactation, rapid growth, infection, nutrient imbalance)

Increased vitamin excretion (e.g., diuresis, lactation, excessive sweating)

High-Risk Groups for Vitamin Deficiencies

Pregnant women
Infants and young children
Elderly people
Poor (food-insecure) people
People with intestinal parasites or infections
Dieters
Smokers

Causes of Vitamin Deficiencies in Animals

Many of the same primary and secondary causal factors that produce vitamin deficiencies in humans can also produce vitamin deficiencies in animals. In livestock, however, most of the very serious cases of vitamin deficiency in animals are due to human errors involving improper or careless animal husbandry.

Potential causes of vitamin deficiencies in livestock and other managed animal species

Primary deficiencies have physical causes:

Improperly formulated diet (i.e., error in vitamin premix formulation)

Feed mixing error (e.g., omission of vitamin from vitamin premix)

Vitamin losses (e.g., destruction during pelleting or extrusion, losses during storage)

Poor access to feed (e.g., competition for limited feeder space, improper feeder placement, breakdown of feed delivery system)

Secondary deficiencies have biological causes:

Poor feed intake (e.g., poor palatability, heat stress)

Poor digestion

Malabsorption (e.g., diarrhea, parasites, intestinal infection)

Impaired postabsorptive utilization (e.g., certain drug therapies)

Increased metabolic demand (e.g., infection, low environmental temperature, egg/milk production, rapid growth, pregnancy, lactation)

III. Clinical Manifestations of Vitamin Deficiencies

Many Organ Systems Can Be Affected by Vitamin Deficiencies

Every organ system of the body can be the target of a vitamin deficiency. Some vitamin deficiencies affect certain organs preferentially (e.g., vitamin D deficiency chiefly affects calcified tissues); others affect several or many organs in various ways. Because the diagnosis of a vitamin deficiency involves its differentiation from other potential causes of similar clinical signs, it is useful to consider the various morphologic lesions caused by vitamin deficiencies from an organ system perspective. After all, anatomical and/or functional changes in organs are the initial presentations of deficiencies of each of the vitamins. This is facilitated by presenting in Tables 4-1 through 4-10 the clinical signs of vitamin deficiencies, organized according to major organ system.

Summary of the Deficiency Diseases for Each Vitamin

It is also useful to consider the clinical signs of vitamin deficiencies according to the various vitamins. While this means of categorizing vitamin deficiency disorders has little relevance in the practical diagnosis of vitamin deficiencies, it is a most convenient (and certainly traditional) way to systematize this information for the purpose of learning about the vitamins. Tables 4.11A, 4.11B, and 4.11C present such a summary.

Table 4-1. Dermatologic disorders caused by vitamin deficiencies

Sign	Vitamins involved	Species affected	Specific diseases
Skin			
Subcutaneous hemorrhage	Vitamin K	Poultry	
Dermatitis[a]			
Scaly	Vitamin A	Cattle	
	Pantothenic acid	Rat	
	Biotin	Rat, mouse, hamster, mink, fox, cat	
	Riboflavin	Pig	
	Pyridoxine	Rat	**Acrodynia**[b]
Cracking	Niacin	Human, chick	**Pellagra**[c]
	Pantothenic acid	Chick (feet)	
	Biotin	Monkey (feet, hands), pig, poultry (feet)	
Desquamation[d]	Niacin	Human, chick	
	Biotin	Rat	
	Riboflavin	Rat, poultry, dog, monkey, human	
	Pyridoxine	Human	
Hyperkeratosis[e]	Niacin	Human, chick	Pellagra
	Biotin	Rat, mouse, hamster, mouse	
	Riboflavin	Rat	
Hyperpigmentation	Niacin	Human	Pellagra
Photosensitization	Niacin	Human	Pellagra
Stomatitis	Niacin	Human	Pellagra
	Pantothenic acid	Chick	
	Biotin	Chick	
	Riboflavin	Calf, human	
Edema[f]	Thiamin	Human	**Beriberi**[g]
Hair			
Rough	Vitamin A	Cattle	
Achromotrichia[h]	Pantothenic acid	Rat	
	Biotin	Rat, rabbit, mink, fox, cat, monkey	
Alopecia[i]	Pantothenic acid	Rat	
	Niacin	Pig, rat	
	Biotin	Rat, mouse, hamster, pig, rabbit, cat, mink, fox	Spectacle eye
	Riboflavin	Rat, pig, calf	
Blood-caked whiskers	Pantothenic acid	Rat	
Feathers			
Rough	Vitamin A	Poultry	
	Biotin	Poultry	
Impaired growth	Folic acid	Poultry	
	Biotin	Poultry	

[a]Inflammation of the skin.
[b]Swelling and **necrosis** (i.e., tissue and/or organ death) of the paws, tips of ears and nose, and lips.
[c]Pellagra, a disease characterized by lesions of the skin and mouth and by gastrointestinal and nervous symptoms, is caused by a deficiency of niacin.
[d]Shedding of skin.
[e]Thickening of the skin.
[f]Abnormal fluid retention.
[g]Beriberi, a disease characterized by polyneuritis, cardiac pathology, and edema, is caused by a deficiency of thiamin.
[h]Loss of normal pigment from hair or feathers.
[i]Baldness, or loss of hair or feathers.

Table 4-2. Muscular disorders caused by vitamin deficiencies

Sign/symptom	Vitamin involved	Species affected	Specific disease
General weakness	Vitamin A	Cat	
	Vitamin D	Human	Osteomalacia
	Pantothenic acid	Human	
	Ascorbic acid	Human	**Scurvy**[a]
	Thiamin	Rat, human	Beriberi
	Riboflavin	Dog, fox, pig	
	Pyridoxine	Rat, chick	
Skeletal **myopathy**[b]	Vitamin E	Monkey, pig, rat, rabbit, guinea pig, calf, chick, horse, goat, mink, duckling, salmon, catfish	**White muscle disease**[c]
		Lamb	Stiff lamb disease[d]
	Ascorbic acid	Guinea pig, human	Scurvy
	Thiamin	Rat, human	Beriberi
Hemorrhage of skeletal muscles	Vitamin K	Poultry	
	Pantothenic acid	Pig	
Cardiomyopathy[e]	Vitamin E	Pig	**Mulberry heart disease**[f]
	Vitamin E	Rat, dog, rabbit, guinea pig, calf, lamb, goat	
	Thiamin	Human, rat	Beriberi
Gizzard myopathy	Vitamin E	Turkey poults, ducklings	

[a]Scurvy, a disease characterized by weakness, anemia, and spongy gums, is caused by a deficiency of vitamin C.
[b]Any disease of muscle.
[c]Skeletal muscle degeneration in animals.
[d]Stiff lamb disease is a type of muscular dystrophy in lambs. The term **dystrophy** describes any disorder arising from poor nutrition.
[e]A general term indicating disease of the heart muscle.
[f]A form of congestive heart failure in swine.

Table 4-3. Reproductive disorders caused by vitamin deficiencies

Sign	Vitamin involved	Species affected	Specific disease
Female			
Vaginal **cornification**[a]	Vitamin A	Human, rat	
Ovarian degeneration	Vitamin A	Poultry	
Thin egg shell	Vitamin D	Poultry	
Low rate of egg production	Vitamin A	Poultry	
	Riboflavin	Poultry	
	Pyridoxine	Poultry	
Uterine **lipofuscinosis**[b]	Vitamin E	Rat	
Anestrus	Riboflavin	Rat	
Male			
Degeneration of germinal epithelium	Vitamin A	Rat, bull, cat	
	Vitamin E	Rat, rooster, dog, pig, monkey, rabbit, guinea pig, hamster	

(*Continued*)

Table 4-3. Reproductive disorders caused by vitamin deficiencies—Cont'd

Sign	Vitamin involved	Species affected	Specific disease
	Fetus		
Death	Vitamin A	Poultry	
	Vitamin E	Rat	
	Riboflavin	Chick	
	Folate	Chick	
	Vitamin B$_{12}$	Poultry	
Abnormalities	Riboflavin	Rat	
	Riboflavin	Chick	**Clubbed down**[c]
	Folate	Chick	Parrot beak

[a]Replacement of normal vaginal mucosa with a horny layer of cells.
[b]Accumulation of ceroid (**age pigments**), which are adducts of lipid breakdown products and proteins.
[c]Congenital deformation of embryonic feathers.

Table 4-4. Vascular disorders caused by vitamin deficiencies

Sign	Vitamin involved	Species affected	Specific disease
Blood vessels			
Increased capillary permeability	Vitamin E	Chick	**Exudative diathesis**[a]
		Pig	Visceral edema
Capillary fragility[b]	Vitamin C	Human	Scurvy
Hemorrhage		Guinea pig, monkey	Scurvy
Arteriosclerosis[c]	Pyridoxine	Monkey	
Blood cells			
Anemia[d]	Vitamin E	Human, monkey, pig	
	Vitamin K	Chick, rat	
	Niacin	Pig	
	Folate	Chick, rat, human	
	Riboflavin	Monkey, baboon	
	Pyridoxine	Human	
Erythrocyte fragility	Vitamin E	Human, rat, monkey, pig	
Leukopenia[e]	Folate	Guinea pig, rat	
Excess platelets	Vitamin E	Rat	
Increased platelet aggregation	Vitamin E	Rat	
Impaired clotting	Vitamin K	Chick, rat, pig, calf, human	

[a]Edema resulting from loss of plasma through abnormally permeable capillaries.
[b]A state in which capillaries become prone to disruption under conditions of stress.
[c]Thickening of the arterial walls.
[d]Subnormal amount of erythrocytes or hemoglobin in the blood.
[e]Subnormal number of leukocytes in the blood.

Table 4-5. Gastrointestinal disorders caused by vitamin deficiencies

Sign/symptom	Vitamin involved	Species affected	Specific disease
Intestine			
Lipofuscinosis	Vitamin E	Dog	**Brown bowel disease**[a]
Hemorrhage	Vitamin K	Poultry	
	Niacin	Dog	
	Thiamin	Rat	
Ulcer	Thiamin	Rat	
Diarrhea	Niacin	Dog, pig, poultry	
	Niacin	Human	Pellagra
	Riboflavin	Calf, dog, pig, chick	
	Vitamin B$_{12}$	Young pigs	
Constipation	Niacin	Human	Pellagra
Inflammation[b]	Niacin	Chick	
	Thiamin	Rat	
	Riboflavin	Dog, pig, chick	
Stomach			
Achlorhydria	Niacin	Human	Pellagra
Gastric distress	Thiamin	Human	Beriberi
Mouth			
Inflammation	Niacin	Poultry	
Glossitis[c]	Niacin	Human	Pellagra
Abnormal tongue papillae	Riboflavin	Rat, human	**Geographical tongue**[d]
	Niacin	Human	
Stomatitis[e]	Niacin	Human	Pellagra
	Riboflavin	Human	
Cheilosis[f]	Riboflavin	Human	

[a]Accumulation of lipofuscin pigments in the intestinal tissues.
[b]A response to injury characterized by pain, heat, redness, and swelling.
[c]Inflammation of the tongue.
[d]Abnormal textural appearance of the surface of the tongue.
[e]Inflammation of the oral mucosa (soft tissues of the mouth).
[f]Cracks and fissures at the corners of the mouth.

Table 4-6. Vital organ disorders caused by vitamin deficiencies

Sign	Vitamin involved	Species affected	Specific disease
Liver			
Necrosis	Vitamin E	Rat, mouse	Dietary liver necrosis
	Vitamin E	Pig	Hepatosis dietetica[a]
Steatitis[b]	Pantothenic acid	Chick, dog	
	Biotin	Chick	**Fatty liver and kidney syndrome**[c]
	Thiamin	Rat	
Cirrhosis[d]	Choline	Rat, dog, monkey	

(Continued)

Table 4-6. Vital organ disorders caused by vitamin deficiencies—Cont'd

Sign	Vitamin involved	Species affected	Specific disease
Kidney			
Nephritis[e]	Vitamin A	Human	
Steatosis	Biotin	Chick	Fatty liver and kidney syndrome
	Riboflavin	Pig	
Hemorrhagic necrosis	Choline	Rat, mouse, pig, rabbit, calf	
Calculi	Pyridoxine	Rat	
Thymus			
Lymphoid necrosis	Pantothenic acid	Chick, dog	
Adrenal glands			
Hypertrophy	Pantothenic acid	Pig	
Hemorrhage	Riboflavin	Pig	
Necrosis	Pantothenic acid	Rat	
	Riboflavin	Baboon	
Adipose			
Lipofuscinosis	Vitamin E	Rat, mouse, cat, hamster, mink, pig	**Brown fat disease**[f]
Pancreas			
Insulin insufficiency	Pyridoxine	Rat	

[a]Any disorder of the liver that can be traced to a deficiency in the diet.
[b]Fatty degeneration.
[c]This condition is generally referred to as FLKS by poultry pathologists and nutritionists.
[d]The degeneration of the parenchymal cells of an organ, accompanied by hypertrophy of interstitial connective tissue.
[e]Inflammation of the kidney.
[f]Accumulation of lipofuscin pigments in adipose tissues.

Table 4-7. Ocular disorders caused by vitamin deficiencies

Sign/symptom	Vitamin involved	Species affected	Specific disease
Retina			
Night blindness[a]	Vitamin A	Rat, pig, sheep, cat, human	**Nyctalopia**[a]
Retinal degeneration	Vitamin E	Rat, dog, cat, monkey, human	**Retrolental fibroplasia**[b]
Cornea			
Xerophthalmia[c]	Vitamin A	Human, calf, rat	
Keratomalacia[d]	Vitamin A	Human, calf, rat	
Lens			
Cataract[e]	Vitamin E	Turkey embryo, rabbit	
Photophobia[f]	Riboflavin	Human	

[a]Nyctalopia is commonly referred to as *night blindness*.
[b]There is considerable debate as to the role of vitamin E status in the etiology of retrolental fibroplasia, a condition involving the abnormal growth of fibrous tissue behind the crystalline lens. The condition, occurring in premature infants maintained in high-O_2 environments, has been reported to be reduced in severity or prevented by treatment with vitamin E, which is known to be at low levels in such infants.
[c]Xerophthalmia is characterized by extreme dryness (i.e., **xerosis**) of the conjunctiva.
[d]*Xerotic keratitis*, i.e., dryness with ulceration and perforation of the cornea, resulting in blindness.
[e]Lens opacity.
[f]Abnormal sensitivity to light.

Table 4-8. Nervous disorders caused by vitamin deficiencies

Sign/symptom	Vitamin involved	Species affected	Specific disease
Excessive CSF[a] pressure	Vitamin A	Calf, pig, chick	
Ataxia[b]	Vitamin A	Calf, pig, chick, sheep	
	Thiamin	Calf, pig, rat, chick, rabbit, mouse, monkey	**Wernicke–Korsakoff syndrome**[c]
	Thiamin	Human	
	Riboflavin	Pig, rat	
Tremors	Niacin	Human	Pellagra
Tetany	Vitamin D	Pig, chick, children	**Rickets**[d]
Encephalopathy[e]	Vitamin E	Chick	**Encephalomalacia**[e]
	Thiamin	Human	Wernicke–Korsakoff syndrome
Nerve degeneration	Riboflavin	Rat, pig	
	Riboflavin	Chick	**Curled-toe paralysis**[f]
	Vitamin E	Monkey, rat, dog, duck	
	Niacin	Pig, rat	
	Pyridoxine	Rat	
	Vitamin B$_{12}$	Human	
Peripheral neuropathy[g]	Thiamin	Human	Beriberi
	Thiamin	Chick	**Polyneuritis**[h]
	Riboflavin	Human	
	Pantothenic acid	Human	Burning feet[i]
	Vitamin B$_{12}$	Human	
Abnormal gait	Pantothenic acid	Pig, dog	Goose-stepping
Seizures	Pyridoxine	Rat, human infant	
Opisthotonos[j]	Thiamin	Chicken, pigeon	Star-gazing
Paralysis	Pantothenic acid	Chick	
	Pantothenic acid	Poult	**Cervical paralysis**[k]
	Riboflavin	Rat	
	Riboflavin	Chick	Curled-toe paralysis
	Pyridoxine	Chick	
Nystagmus[l]	Thiamin	Human	Wernicke–Korsakoff syndrome
Irritability	Niacin	Human	Pellagra
	Thiamin	Human	Beriberi
	Pyridoxine	Rat, human	
	Vitamin B$_{12}$	Pig	

[a]CSF, Cerebrospinal fluid.
[b]Poor coordination.
[c]Condition, most frequent among alcoholics, characterized by Wernicke's syndrome (presbyophrenia, i.e., loss of memory, disorientation, and confabulation but integrity of judgment) and Korsakoff's psychosis (polyneuritic psychosis, i.e., imaginary reminiscences and agitated hallucinations).
[d]Rickets, a disease of growing bones, manifests itself in children as deformations of the long bones (e.g., bowed legs, knock knees, curvatures of the upper and/or lower arms), swollen joints, and/or enlarged heads.
[e]*Encephalopathy* describes any degenerative brain disease. In chicks, *encephalomalacia* is a disease characterized by ataxis, lack of coordinated movement, paralysis, and softening of the brain.
[f]Curled toe paralysis describes the disorder of chickens characterized by inability to extend the toes, owing to disease of the sciatic nerve.
[g]The term **neuropathy** describes any functional disorder of the nerves of the peripheral nervous system.
[h]The term *polyneuritis* describes an inflammation of the peripheral nerves.
[i]Parethesia of the feet.
[j]Tetanic spasm with spine and extremities bent with convexity forward, i.e., severe head retraction.
[k]Cervical paralysis is a disorder of young turkeys, characterized by rigid paralysis of the neck.
[l]Rhythmical oscillation of the eyeballs, either horizontal, rotary, or vertical.

Table 4-9. Psychological and emotional disorders associated with vitamin deficiencies in humans

Sign/symptom	Vitamin involved	Specific disease
Depression	Niacin	Pellagra
	Thiamin	Beriberi
Anxiety	Thiamin	Beriberi
Dizziness	Niacin	Pellagra
Irritability	Niacin	Pellagra
	Thiamin	Beriberi
	Pyridoxine	
Dementia[a]	Niacin	Pellagra
Psychosis[b]	Thiamin	Wernicke–Korsakoff syndrome

[a]*Dementia* is characterized by loss of memory, judgment, and ability to think abstractly.
[b]*Psychosis* is characterized by behavior incongruent with reality.

IV. Vitamin Deficiency Diseases: Manifestations of Biochemical Lesions

Relationships between Biochemical Lesions and Clinical Diseases of Vitamin Deficiencies

The clinical signs and **symptoms** that characterize the vitamin deficiency diseases are manifestations of impairments (i.e., *lesions*) in biochemical function that result from insufficient vitamin supply. This is a fundamental concept in understanding the roles of the vitamins in nutrition and health.

Hypovitaminosis of sufficient magnitude and duration is causally related to the morphological and/or functional changes associated with the latter stages of vitamin deficiency. Although the validity of this concept is readily apparent in the abstract, documentary evidence for it in the case of each vitamin deficiency disease, that is, direct cause-effect linkages of specific biochemical lesions and clinical changes, is for many vitamins not complete.

Vitamin A offers a case in point. While the role of vitamin A in preventing nyctalopia (night blindness) is clear from presently available knowledge of the essentiality of retinal as the prosthetic group of rhodopsin and several other photosensitive visual receptors in the retina, the amount of vitamin A in the retina and thus available for visual function is only about 1% of the total amount of vitamin A in the body. Further more, it is clear from the clinical signs of vitamin A deficiency that the vitamin has other essential functions unrelated to vision, especially some relating to the integrity and differentiation of epithelial cells. However, although evidence indicates that vitamin A is involved in the metabolism of mucopolysaccharides and other essential intermediates, present knowledge cannot

Table 4-10. Skeletal disorders caused by vitamin deficiencies

Sign	Vitamin involved	Species affected	Specific disease
Excess periosteal growth	Vitamin A	Calf, pig, dog, horse, sheep	Blindness
Undermineralization (epiphyseal abnormality)	Vitamin D	Children, chick, dog, calf	Rickets
Demineralization (bone deformation)	Vitamin D	Human adult	**Osteomalacia**[a]
Increased fractures	Vitamin D	Human adult	**Osteoporosis**[b]
	Vitamin D	Laying hen	**Cage layer fatigue**[c]
Dental caries[d]	Vitamin D	Human child	Rickets
	Pyridoxine	Human	
Chondrodystrophy[e]	Niacin	Chick, poult	**Perosis**[f]
	Biotin	Chick, poult	Perosis
Congenital deformities	Riboflavin	Rat	
	Pyridoxine	Rat	

[a]Osteomalacia is a disease characterized by gradual softening and bending of bones, with more or less severe pain; bones are soft because they contain osteoid tissue that has failed to calcify.
[b]Osteoporosis involves a reduction in the quantity of bone, i.e., skeletal atrophy; usually, the remaining bone is normally mineralized.
[c]Osteomalacia in high-producing laying hens who can experience a net loss of 0.1–0.2 g of calcium/egg laid and often produce an egg per day for several weeks.
[d]Tooth decay.
[e]Abnormal development of the cartilage.
[f]Perosis is a condition of slippage of the Achilles tendon such that extension of the foot and, therefore, walking are impossible; it occurs as the result of twisting of the tibial and/or metatarsal bones owing to their improper development.

Table 4-11A.   Summary of vitamin deficiency signs: vitamins A, D, E, and K

Organ system	Vitamin A	Vitamin D	Vitamin E	Vitamin K
General				
Appetite	Decrease	Decrease	Decrease	
Growth	Decrease	Decrease	Decrease	Decrease
Immunity	Decrease		Decrease[a]	
Dermatologic	Scaly dermatitis			Hemorrhage[b]
	Rough hair			
Muscular	Weakness	Weakness	Myopathy	Hemorrhage[c]
Gastrointestinal			Lipofuscinosis	Hemorrhage
Adipose			Lipofuscinosis	
Skeletal	Periosteal over-growth	Rickets		
		Osteomalacia[d]		
Vital organs	Nephritis		Liver necrosis	
Vascular				
Vessels			Exudative diathesis	
Erythrocytes			Anemia	Anemia
Platelets		Aggregation	Decreased clotting	
Nervous	High CSF pressure	Tetany	Encephalopathy	
	Ataxia	Ataxia	Axonal dystrophy	
Reproductive				
Male	Low sperm motility	Low sperm motility		
Female	Vaginal cornification	Less shell	Uterine lipofuscinosis	
Fetal	Death		Death, resorption	
Ocular				
Retinal	Nyctalopia			
Cornea	Xerophthalmia			
	Keratomalacia			
Lens			Cataract	
			Retrolental fibroplasia	

[a]Some aspects of immune function can be impaired, especially if selenium is also deficient.
[b]Subcutaneous.
[c]Intramuscular.
[d]Loss of mineralization of mature bone.

adequately explain the mechanism(s) of action of vitamin A in supporting growth, in maintaining epithelia, and so on. It has been said that 99% of our information about the mode of action of vitamin A concerns only 1% of vitamin A in the body.

The ongoing search for a more complete understanding of the mechanisms of vitamin action is, therefore, largely based on the study of biochemi-cal correlates of changes in physiological function or morphology effected by changes in vitamin status. Most of this knowledge has come from direct experimentation, mostly with animal models. Also informative in this regard has been information acquired from observations of individuals with a variety of rare, naturally occurring, hereditary anomalies involving vitamin-dependent enzymes and transport proteins. Most of

Table 4-11B. Summary of vitamin deficiency signs: vitamin C, thiamin, riboflavin, and vitamin B_6

Organ system	Vitamin C	Thiamin	Riboflavin	Vitamin B_6
General				
Appetite	Decrease	Severe decrease	Decrease	Decrease
Growth	Decrease	Decrease	Decrease	Decrease
Immunity	Decrease[a]			
Heat tolerance	Decrease			
Dermatologic	Edema	Cheilosis	Acrodynia	
			Stomatitis	
Muscular	Skeletal muscle atropy	Cardiomyopathy	Weakness	Weakness
		Bradycardia[b]		
		Heart failure		
		Weakness		
Gastrointestinal		Inflammation	Inflammation	
		Ulcer		
Adipose				
Skeletal		Deformities	Dental caries	
Vital organs	Fatty liver[c]	Fatty liver		
Vascular				
Vessels	Capillary fragility			Arteriosclerosis
	Hemorrhage			
Erythrocytes		Anemia	Anemia	
Platelets				
Nervous	Tenderness	Peripheral neuropathy	Paralysis	Paralysis
		Opisthotonos	Ataxia	**Convulsions**[d]
Reproductive				
Male			Sterility	
Female			Few eggs	Few eggs
Fetal			Death, malformations	
Ocular				
Retinal			Photophobia	
Corneal			Decreased vascularization	
Lens			Retrolental fibroplasia	

[a]Some aspects of immunity may be affected by vitamin C status.
[b]Abnormally slow heartbeat.
[c]Hepatic steatosis.
[d]Violent, involuntary contractions; seizures.

Table 4-11C. Summary of vitamin deficiency signs: niacin, folate, pantothenic acid, biotin, and vitamin B_{12}

	Vitamin				
	Niacin	**Folate**	**Pantothenic acid**	**Biotin**	**Vitamin B_{12}**
General					
Appetite	Decrease			Decrease	
Growth	Decrease	Decrease	Decrease	Decrease	Decrease
Immunity					
Dermatologic	Dermatitis	Alopecia	Scaly dermatitis	Dermatitis	
	Photosensitization		Alopecia		
Muscular			Hemorrhage		
			Weakness		
Gastrointestinal	Diarrhea				Diarrhea
	Glossitis				
Adipose					
Skeletal	Perosis[a]			Perosis	
Vital organs			Fatty liver	FLKS[b]	
			Thymus degeneration		
Vascular					
Vessels					
Erythrocytes	Anemia	Anemia			Anemia
Platelets					
Nervous	Ataxia		Abnormal gait		Peripheral neuropathy
	Dementia		Paralysis		
Reproductive					
Male					
Female					
Fetal					Death
Ocular					
Retinal					
Cornea					
Lens					

[a]Slipped Achilles tendon, *hock disease* in birds, resulting in crippling.
[b]FLKS, Fatty liver and kidney syndrome, involving both hepatic and renal steatosis.

the documented inborn metabolic errors have involved specific mutations manifest as either a loss or an aberration in single factors in vitamin metabolism —a highly targeted situation not readily produced experimentally.[6]

Tables 4-12 and 4-13 summarize in general terms current information concerning the interrelationships of the biochemical functions of the vitamins and the clinical manifestations of their deficiencies or anomalous metabolism.

---

[6] However, it is theoretically possible to produce transgenic animal models with similar metabolic anomalies.

Table 4-12. The underlying biological functions of the vitamins

Vitamin	Active form(s)	Deficiency disorders	Important biological functions or reactions
Vitamin A	Retinol, retinal, retinoic acid	Night blindness, xerophthalmia, keratomalacia	Photosensitive retinal pigment, regulation of epithelial cell differentiation
		Impaired growth	Regulation of gene transcription
Vitamin D	1,25-$(OH)_2$-D	Rickets, osteomalacia	Promotion of intestinal calcium absorption, mobilization of calcium from bone, stimulation of renal calcium, resorption, regulation of PTH secretion, possible function in muscle
Vitamin E	α-Tocopherol	Nerve, muscle degeneration	Antioxidant protector for membranes
Vitamin K	K, MK	Impaired blood clotting	Cosubstrate for γ-carboxylation of glutamyl residues of several clotting factors and other calcium-binding proteins
Vitamin C	Ascorbic acid Dehydroascorbic acid	Scurvy	Cosubstrate for hydroxylations in collagen synthesis, drug and steroid metabolism
Thiamin	Thiamin pyrophosphate	Beriberi, polyneuritis, Wernicke–Korsakoff syndrome	Coenzyme for oxidative decarboxylation of 2-keto acids (e.g., pyruvate and 2-keto-glutarate); coenzyme for pyruvate decarboxylase and transketolase
Riboflavin	FMN, FAD	Dermatitis	Coenzymes for numerous flavoproteins that catalyze redox reactions in fatty acid synthesis/degradation, TCA cycle
Niacin	NAD(H), NADP(H)	Pellagra	Cosubstrates for hydrogen transfer catalyzed by many dehydrogenases, e.g., TCA cycle respiratory chain
Pyridoxine	Pyridoxal-5'-phosphate	Signs vary with species	Coenzyme for metabolism of amino acids, e.g., side chain, decarboxylation, transamination, racemization
Folate	Polyglutamyl tetrahydrofolates	Megaloblastic anemia	Coenzyme for transfer of single-carbon units, e.g., formyl and hydroxymethyl groups in purine synthesis
Biotin	1'-N-Carboxybiotin	Dermatitis	Coenzyme for carboxylations, e.g., acetyl-CoA/malonyl-CoA conversion
Pantothenic acid	Coenzyme A	Signs vary with species	Cosubstrate for activation/transfer of acyl groups to form esters, amides, citrate, triglycerides, etc.
	Acyl carrier protein		Coenzyme for fatty acid biosynthesis
Vitamin B_{12}	5'-Deoxyadenosyl-B_{12}	Megaloblastic anemia	Coenzyme for conversion of methylmalonyl-CoA to succinyl-CoA
	Methyl-B_{12}	Impaired growth	Methyl group transfer from 5-CH_3-FH_4 to homocysteine in methionine synthesis

Abbreviations: PTH, parathyroid hormone; TCA, tricarboxylic acid cycle; CoA, coenzyme A; 5-CH_3-FH_4, 5-methyltetrahydrofolic acid.

Table 4-13. Vitamin-responsive inborn metabolic lesions

Curative vitamin	Missing protein or metabolic step affected	Clinical condition
Vitamin A	Apolipoprotein B	Abetalipoproteinemia; low tissue levels of retinoids
Vitamin D	Vitamin D receptor	Unresponsive to $1,25(OH)_2$-D; osteomalacia
Vitamin E	Apolipoprotein B	Abetalipoproteinemia; low tissue levels of tocopherols
Thiamin	Branched-chain 2-oxoacid dehydrogenase	Maple syrup urine disease
	Pyruvate metabolism	Lactic acidemia; neurological anomalies
Riboflavin	Methemoglobin reductase	Methemoglobinemia
	Electron transfer flavoprotein	Multiple lack of acyl-CoA dehydrogenations, excretion of acyl-CoA metabolites, i.e., metabolic acidosis
Niacin	Abnormal neurotransmission	Psychiatric disorders, tryptophan malabsorption, abnormal tryptophan metabolism
Pyridoxine	Cystathionine β-synthase	Homocysteinuria
	Cystathionine γ-lyase	Cystathioninuria; neurological disorders
	Kynureninase	Xanthurenic aciduria
Folate	Enteric absorption	Megaloblastic anemia, mental disorder
	Methylene-FH_4-reductase	Homocysteinuria, neurological disorders
	Glutamate formiminotransferase	Urinary excretion of FIGLU[a]
	Homocysteine/methionine conversion	Schizophrenia
	Tetrahydrobiopterin-phenylalanine hydrolase	Mental retardation, PKU[b]
	Dihydrobiopteridine reductase	PKU, severe neurological disorders
	Tetrahydrobiopterin formation	PKU, severe neurological disorders
Biotin	Biotinidase	Alopecia, skin rash, cramps, acidemia, developmental disorders, excess urinary biotin, and biocytin
	Propionyl-CoA carboxylase	Propionic acidemia
	3-Methylcrotonyl-CoA carboxylase	3-Methylcrontonylglycinuria
	Pyruvate carboxylase	Leigh disease, accumulation of lactate and pyruvate
	Acetyl-CoA carboxylase	Severe brain damage
	Holocarboxylase synthase	Lack of multiple carboxylase activities, urinary excretion of metabolites
Vitamin B_{12}	Intrinsic factor	Juvenile pernicious anemia
	Transcobalamin	Megaloblastic anemia, growth impairment
	Methylmalonyl-CoA mutase	Methylmalonic acidemia

[a]FIGLU, Formiminoglutamic acid.
[b]PKU, Phenylketonuria.

Study Questions and Exercises

1. For one major organ system, discuss the means by which vitamin deficiencies may affect its function.

2. List the clinical signs that have special diagnostic value (i.e., are specifically associated with insufficient status with respect to certain vitamins) for specific vitamin deficiencies.

3. For one fat-soluble and one water-soluble vitamin, discuss the relationships between tissue distribution of the vitamin and organ site specificity of the clinical signs of its deficiency.

4. List the animal species and deficiency diseases that, because they show specificity for certain vitamins, might be particularly useful in vitamin metabolism research.

5. Develop a decision tree for determining whether lesions of a particular organ system may be due to insufficient intakes of one or more vitamins

Recommended Reading

Gaby, S. K., Bendich, A., Singh, V. N., and Machlin, L. J. (1991). *Vitamin Intake and Health: A Scientific Review*. Marcel Dekker, New York.

Friedovich, W. (1988). *Vitamins*. Walter de Gruyter, New York.

Marks, J. (1968). *The Vitamins in Health and Disease: A Modern Reappraisal*. Churchill, London.

Rucker, R. B., Suttie, J. W., McCormick, D. B., and Machlin, L. J., eds. (2001). *Handbook of Vitamins*, 3rd ed. Marcel Dekker, New York.

Sauberlich, H. E., and Machlin, L. J. (eds.). (1992). Beyond deficiency: New views on the function and health effects of vitamins. *Ann. N.Y. Acad. Med.* **669.**

CONSIDERING THE INDIVIDUAL VITAMINS

II

Vitamin A

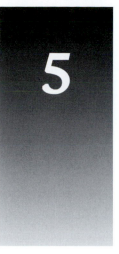

5

In … four [Southeast Asian] countries alone at least 500,000 preschool age children every year develop active xerophthalmia involving the cornea. About half of this number will be blind and a very high proportion, probably in excess of 60%, will die. The annual prevalence for these same countries of non-corneal xerophthalmia is many times higher, probably on the order of 5 million.… There can be no doubt about the claim that vitamin A deficiency is the most common cause of blindness in children and one of the most prevalent and serious of all nutritional deficiency diseases.

—D. S. McLaren

I.	Significance of Vitamin A	96
II.	Sources of Vitamin A	97
III.	Absorption of Vitamin A	99
IV.	Transport of Vitamin A	102
V.	Metabolism of Vitamin A	109
VI.	Excretion of Vitamin A	113
VII.	Metabolic Functions of Vitamin A	113
VIII.	Vitamin A Deficiency	130
IX.	Vitamin A Toxicity	135
X.	Case Studies	139
	Study Questions and Exercises	141
	Recommended Reading	141

Anchoring Concepts

1. Vitamin A is the generic descriptor for compounds with the qualitative biological activity of *retinol*, that is, retinoids and some (provitamin A) carotenoids.
2. Vitamin A-active substances are *hydrophobic* and thus are insoluble in aqueous environments (intestinal lumen, plasma, interstitial fluid, cytosol). *Accordingly, vitamin A-active substances are absorbed by micelle-dependent diffusion.*
3. Vitamin A was discovered by its ability to prevent *xerophthalmia*.

Learning Objectives

1. To understand the nature of the various sources of vitamin A in foods.
2. To understand the means of vitamin A absorption from the small intestine.
3. To become familiar with the various carriers involved in the extra- and intracellular transport of vitamin A.
4. To understand the metabolic conversions involved in the activation and degradation of vitamin A in its absorption, transport and storage, cellular function, and excretion.
5. To become familiar with current knowledge of the biochemical mechanisms of action of vitamin A and their relationships to vitamin A-deficiency diseases.
6. To understand the physiologic implications of high doses of vitamin A.

Vocabulary

Abetalipoproteinemia
Acyl-CoA:retinol acyltransferase (ARAT)
Alcohol dehydrogenase
all-*trans*-Retinal
all-*trans*-Retinoic acid
Apo-RBP
β-Carotene
β-Carotene 15,15′-dioxygenase
β-crypto xanthin
Bitot's spots
Bleaching
Canthoxanthin
Carotenodermia
Carotenoid
cGMP phosphodiesterase
Cholesteryl ester transfer protein
Chylomicron remnant

11-*cis*-Retinal
9-*cis*-Retinoic acid
11-*cis*-Retinoic acid
Conjunctival impression cytology
Corneal xerosis
CRABP (cellular retinoic acid-binding protein)
CRABP(II) (cellular retinoic acid-binding protein type II)
CRALBP (cellular retinal-binding protein)
CRBP (cellular retinol-binding protein)
CRBP(II) (cellular retinol-binding protein type II)
β-Cryptoxanthin
3,4-Didehydroretinol
Glycoproteins
High-density lipoproteins (HDLs)
Holo-RBP
Hyperkeratosis
Interphotoreceptor retinol-binding protein (IRBP)
Iodopsins
Keratomalacia
Low-density lipoproteins (LDLs)
Lecithin–retinol acyltransferase (LRAT)
Lycopene
Marasmus
Melanopsin
Meta-rhodopsin II
MRDR (modified relative dose–response) test
Night blindness
Nyctalopia
Pancreatic nonspecific lipase
Protein-energy malnutrition
Opsins
Otitis media
Relative dose–response (RDR) test
Retinal
Retinal isomerase
Retinal oxidase
Retinal reductase
Retinaldehyde reductase
Retinoic acid
Retinoic acid receptors (RARs)
Retinoic acid response elements (RAREs)
Retinoids
Retinoid X receptors (RXRs)
Retinol
Retinol dehydrogenases
Retinol equivalents (RE)
Retinol phosphorylase
Retinyl acetate
Retinyl-binding protein (RBP)
Retinyl ester hydrolase

Retinyl esters
Retinyl β-glucuronide
Retinyl palmitate
Retinyl phosphate
Retinyl stearate
Rhodopsin
Short-chain alcohol dehydrogenase/aldehyde reductase
Thyroid hormone (T_3)
Transducin
Transgenic
Transthyretin
Very low-density lipoproteins (VLDLs)
Xerophthalmia
Zeaxanthin

I. Significance of Vitamin A

Vitamin A is a nutrient of global importance. It is estimated to affect millions of children worldwide, some 90% of whom live in Southeast Asia and Africa. In recent years, substantial progress has been made in reducing the magnitude of this problem. In 1994, nearly 14 million preschool children (three-quarters from south Asia) were estimated to have clinical eye disease (**xerophthalmia**) due to vitamin A deficiency. Most recent estimates (2005) indicate that the prevalence of the clinical problem (corneal lesions and Bitot's spots) has declined (~0.5% per year) to affect at the present some 4.4 million children. However, at the same time the prevalence of subclinical deficiency (serum retinol levels < 0.7 μmol/L) has increased. Estimates range from 75 to 254 million preschool cases in at least two dozen countries. Almost 20 million pregnant women in developing countries are also vitamin A-deficient; a third have night blindness. It is possible that 40% of the world's children are growing up with insufficient vitamin A.

Vitamin A deficiency is now recognized as one of the most devastating of health problems, causing an estimated one million child deaths each year. It is the single most important cause of childhood blindness in developing countries, affecting 250,000 to 500,000 children each year (Table 5-1), two-thirds of whom die within months of going blind owing to their increased susceptibility to infections also caused by the deficiency. In addition, subclinical vitamin A deficiency also increases child mortality, having public health significance in at least 60 countries in Africa, southern and Southeast Asia, and some parts of Latin

Table 5-1. Prevalence of xerophthalmia among children[a] in the developing world

Region	Numbers affected (millions)	Prevalence (%)
Africa	1.3	1.4
Eastern Mediterranean	1.0	2.8
Latin America	0.1	0.2
Southern Asia	10.0	4.2
Western Pacific (including China)	1.4	1.3
Total	13.8	2.8

[a]From 0 to 5 years of age.
Source: United Nations Administrative Committee on Coordination—Subcommittee of Nutrition. (1993). *SCN News* **9**, 9.

America and the western Pacific. High rates of morbidity and mortality have long been associated with vitamin A deficiency; recent intervention trials have indicated that providing vitamin A can reduce child mortality by about 25% and birth-related, maternal mortality by 40%. Vitamin A deficiency in these areas does not necessarily imply insufficient national or regional supplies of food vitamin A, as vitamin A deficiency can also be caused by insufficient dietary intakes of fats and oils. Still, most studies show that children with histories of xerophthalmia consume fewer dark green leafy vegetables than their counterparts without such histories.

II. Sources of Vitamin A

Expressing the Vitamin A Activities in Foods

Vitamin A exists in natural products in many different forms. It exists as preformed **retinoids**, which are stored in animal tissues, and as provitamin A **carotenoids**, which are synthesized as pigments by many plants and are found in green, orange, and yellow plant tissues. In milk, meat, and eggs, vitamin A exists in several forms, mainly as long-chain fatty acid esters of **retinol**, the predominant one being *retinyl palmitate*. The carotenoids are present in both plant and animal food products; in animal products their occurrence results from dietary exposure. Carotenoid pigments are widespread among diverse animal species, with more than 500 different compounds estimated. About 60 of these have *provitamin A activity*, that is, those that can be cleaved by animals to yield at least one molecule of retinol. In practice, however, only five or six of these provitamins A are commonly encountered in foods. Therefore, the reporting of vitamin A activity from its various forms in foods requires some means of standardization. Two systems are used for this purpose: *international units* (*IU*) and **retinol equivalents (RE)**.[1]

Reporting food vitamin A activity

1 retinol equivalent (RE) = 1 μg all-*trans*-retinol

= 2 μg all-*trans*-β-carotene in dietary supplements

= 12 μg all-*trans*-β-carotene in foods

= 24 μg other provitamin A carotenoids in foods

for pharmaceutical applications:

1 USP[a] unit (or IU[b]) = 0.3 μg all-*trans*-retinol

= 0.344 μg all-*trans*-retinyl acetate

= 0.55 μg all-*trans*-retinyl palmitate

[a]United States Pharmacopecia.
[b]International Unit.

The retinol equivalency represents a 2001 revision by the Food and Nutrition Board of the Institute of Medicine from its previous values for provitamin A carotenoids. However, the estimated equivalency ratio for purified **β-carotene** in oils and nutritional supplements, 2:1, is weakly supported,[2] and other data suggest that a higher equivalency ratio (i.e., lower conversion efficiency) would be more appropriate.[3]

---

[1] USDA Handbook 8-9 lists both international units and retinol equivalents; the FAO tables list micrograms of retinol and β-carotene. The INCAP tables (Instituto de Nutrición de Centroamérica y Panamá) list vitamin A as micrograms of retinol; however, those values are not the same as RE values for the reason that a factor of one-half has been used to convert β-carotene to retinol, instead of the more common factor of one-sixth used to calculate RE values.

[2] The 2001 estimate was based on a single report (Sauberlich, H. E., Hodges, R. E., Wallace, D. L., Kolder, H., Canham, J. E., Hood, J., Raica, W., Jr., and Lowry, L. K. [1974]. Vitamin A metabolism and requirements in the human studied with the use of labeled retinol. *Vitamins Hormones* **32**, 251–275) of the efficacy of β-carotene in correcting impaired dark adaptation in two volunteers in a six-person study.

[3] The data of van Lieshout et al. (*Am. J. Clin. Nutr.* **77**, 12–28) suggest a ratio of 2.6 based on stable isotope (or circulating retinol) dilution studies in more than a hundred Indonesian children. Other recent iosotope dilution studies show the conversion of β-carotene to retinol by humans to be quite variable; for example, Wang et al. (*Br. J. Nutr.* **91**, 121–131) found individual equivalency ratios to vary from 2.0:1 to 12.2:1.

Dietary Sources of Vitamin A

Actual intake of vitamin A, therefore, depends on the patterns of consumption of vitamin A-bearing animal food products and provitamin A-bearing fruits and particularly in green leafy vegetables (Table 5-2). In American diets, it appears that each group contributes roughly comparably to vitamin A nutriture; however, these contributions are greatly influenced by personal food habits and food availability. For poor people in developing countries and vegetarians in industrialized countries, meat products comprise such low percentages of diets that the only real sources of

Table 5-2. Sources of vitamin A in foods

Food	Percentage distribution of vitamin A activity		
	Retinol	β-Carotene	Non-β-carotenoids
Animal foods			
Red meats	90	10	
Poultry meat	90	10	
Fish and shellfish	90	10	
Eggs	90	10	
Milk, milk products	70	30	
Fats and oils	90	10	
Plant foods			
Maize, yellow		40	60
Legumes and seeds		50	50
Green vegetables		75	25
Yellow vegetables[a]		85	15
Pale sweet potatoes		50	50
Yellow fruits[b]		85	15
Other fruits		75	25
Red palm oil		65	35
Other vegetable oils		50	50

[a]For example, carrots and deep-orange sweet potatoes.
[b]For example, apricots.
Source: Leung, W., and Flores, M. (1980). "Food Composition Table for Use in Latin America." Institute of Nutrition of Central America and Panama, Guatemala City, Guatemala; and Interdepartmental Committee on Nutrition for National Defense, Washington, DC.

vitamin A are plant foods. This fact makes it critical that the values used to estimate the bioavailabilities of provitamin A carotenoids in plant foods be accurate. In this regard, there has been reason to question previous RE equivalency estimates, as it is clear from isotope dilution studies that β-carotene from plant foods is utilized with much poorer efficiency than previously thought. In developing countries, several factors may reduce that bioconversion efficiency: low-fat intake, intestinal roundworms, recurrent diarrhea, tropical enteropathy, and other factors that affect the absorptive function of the intestinal epithelium and intestinal transit time. Solomons and Bulux (1993) have suggested that these factors may reduce by more than half the expected bioconversion of plant carotenoids. That the bioconversion of carotenoids to vitamin A does, indeed, vary considerably in practical circumstances is supported by findings that not all interventions with vegetables have produced improvements in vitamin A status (i.e., serum retinol concentrations) of deficient individuals. Such a negative finding came recently from a study of Indonesian women,[4] in which local green herbs consumed with adequate fat and cooked in the traditional manner were ineffective in raising serum retinol levels, whereas a food supplement fortified with purified β-carotene proved very effective.[5] Nevertheless, a number of studies from different parts of the world have shown positive impacts on vitamin A status of provitamin A-containing vegetables and fruits. These findings were considered by the Food and Nutrition Board in developing the 2001 estimates of RE values for β-carotene in foods (Table 5-2).

Foods Rich in Vitamin A

Several foods contain vitamin A activity (Table 5-3); however, relatively few are rich dietary sources, those being green and yellow vegetables,[6] liver, oily fishes, and vitamin A-fortified products such as margarine. It should be noted that, for vitamin A and other vitamins that are susceptible to breakdown during storage and cooking, values given in food composition tables are probably high estimates of amounts actually encountered in practical circumstances.

---

[4] de Pee, S., West, C. E., Muhilal, X., Karyadi, D., and Hautvast, J. G. A. J. (1995). Lack of improvement in vitamin A status with increased consumption of dark-green leafy vegetables. *Lancet* **346,** 75–81.

[5] If this phenomenon is found to be generally true, then there may be limits to the contributions of horticultural approaches (e.g., "home-gardening" programs) to solving problems of vitamin A deficiency.

[6] It is estimated that carotene from vegetables contributes two-thirds of dietary vitamin A worldwide and more than 80% in developing countries.

Table 5-3. Vitamin A activities of foods

Food	Vitamin A activity	
	IU/100 g	RE (µg)/100 g
Animal products		
Red meats	—	—
Beef liver	10,503	35,346
Poultry meat	41	140
Mackerel	130	434
Herring	28	94
Eggs	552	1,839
Swiss cheese	253	856
Butter	754	3,058
Plant products		
Corn	—	—
Peas	15	149
Beans	171	171
Chickpeas	7	67
Lentils	4	39
Soybeans	2	24
Green peppers	—	420
Red peppers	—	21,600
Carrots	—	11,000
Peach	—	1,330
Pumpkin	—	1,600
Yellow squash	—	—
Orange sweet potatoes	—	—
Margarine[a]	993	3,307

[a]Fortified with vitamin A.
Source: USDA (1978). USDA Science and Education Series, Handbook 8.

III. Absorption of Vitamin A

Absorption of Retinoids

Most of the preformed vitamin A in the diet is in the form of **retinyl esters**. Retinyl esters are hydrolyzed in the lumen of the small intestine to yield retinol; this step is catalyzed by hydrolases produced by the pancreas and situated on the mucosal brush border[7] or intrinsic to the brush border itself. The retinyl esters, as well as the carotenoids, are hydrophobic and thus depend on micellar solubilization for their dispersion in the aqueous environment of the small intestinal lumen. For this reason, vitamin A is poorly utilized from low-fat diets. The micellar solubilization of vitamin A facilitates access of soluble hydrolytic enzymes to their substrates (i.e., the retinyl esters), and provides a means for the subsequent presentation of retinol to the mucosal surface across which free retinol and intact β-carotene diffuse passively into the mucosal epithelial cells. The overall absorption of retinol from retinyl esters appears to be fairly high (e.g., about 75%); this process appears to be minimally affected by the level and type of dietary fat, although the absorption is appreciably less efficient at very high vitamin A doses.

Studies have shown that vitamin A can also be absorbed via nonlymphatic pathways. Rats with ligated thoracic ducts retain the ability to deposit retinyl esters in their livers. That such animals fed retinyl esters show greater concentrations of retinol in their portal blood than in their aortic blood suggests that, in mammals, the portal system may be an important alternative route of vitamin A absorption when the normal lymphatic pathway is blocked. This phenomenon corresponds to the route of vitamin A absorption in birds, fishes, and reptiles, which, lacking lymphatic drainage of the intestine, rely strictly on portal absorption. That retinyl esters can also be absorbed by other epithelial cells is evidenced by the fact that the use of vitamin A-containing toothpaste or inhalation of vitamin A-containing aerosols can increase plasma retinol levels.

Absorption of Carotenoids

The major sources of vitamin A activity for most populations are the provitamin A carotenoids. The carotenoids appear to be absorbed in the distal small intestine by micelle-dependent passive diffusion. A major factor limiting the utilization of carotenoids from food sources is their release from their original physical food matrix for solution in the bulk lipid phase of the ingesta. This process is affected by the distribution of carotenoids in food matrices. For example, carotenoids can occur in cytosolic crystalline complexes or in chromoplasts and chloroplasts, where they can be associated with proteins. Both types of complexes

---

[7] One of these activities appears to be the same enzyme that catalyzes the intralumenal hydrolysis of cholesteryl esters; it is a relatively nonspecific carboxylic ester hydrolase. It has been given various names in the literature, the most common being **pancreatic nonspecific lipase** and *cholesteryl esterase*.

are resistant to digestion without heat treatment. Carotenoid absorption can also vary according to the efficiencies of dispersion into and release from mixed micelles. Micellar incorporation, particularly of the less polar carotenoids, can be impaired by the presence of undigested lipids in the intestinal lumen; this has been demonstrated for sucrose polyesters. Micellar release is thought to involve the diffusion of carotenoids directly through the plasma membranes of the enterocytes. This process appears to be impaired by soluble dietary fiber and, likely, other factors that interfere with the contact of the micelle with the mucosal brush border. Limited evidence suggests that carotenoids may be mutually competitive during absorption. For example, high doses of **canthoxanthin** or **lycopene** have been shown to reduce the absorption of β-carotene. For these reasons, it has been technically very difficult to estimate quantitatively the efficiency of intact carotenoid absorption; available evidence indicates that for β-carotene it tends to be low (e.g., 11%) and highly variable. Recent evidence indicates that the enteric absorption of β-carotene may depend on the conditions of gastric acidity of the host, as human subjects with pharmaceutically obliterated gastric acid production showed reduced blood responses to test doses of β-carotene.[8]

Carotenoid Metabolism Linked to Absorption

Some carotenoids[9] can be provitamins A because they can be metabolized to yield **retinal** due to the action of retinal-forming carotene dioxygenases[10] (Fig. 5-1). Most of this bioconversion occurs via the central cleavage of the polyene moiety by a predominantly cytosolic enzyme, **β-carotene 15,15′-dioxygenase**, found in the intestinal mucosa, liver, and corpus luteum. The enzyme requires iron as a cofactor; studies have shown that its activity responds to dietary iron intake as well as to factors affecting iron utilization (e.g., copper, fructose). The retinal-forming carotenoid oxygenases contain ferrous iron (Fe^{++}) linked to a histidinyl residue at the axis of a seven-bladed, β-propeller-chain fold covered by a dome structure

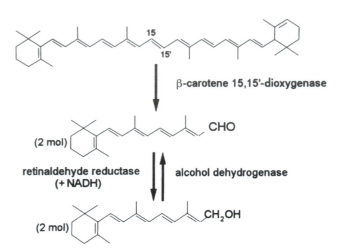

Fig. 5-1. Bioconversion of provitamins A to retinal.

formed by six large loops in the protein. Upon binding within that structure, the three consecutive *trans* double bonds of the carotenoid are isomerized to a *cis-trans-cis* conformation leading to the oxygen cleavage of the central *trans* bond.

Carotene dioxygenase activity is not highly specific for β-carotene, cleaving other carotenoids as well. In the case of β-carotene, the products of this cleavage are two molecules of retinal; other carotenoids have provitamin A activities to the extent that they yield retinal by the action of the dioxygenase (this is determined by both the chemical structure of the carotenoid and the efficiency of its enzymatic cleavage). Apo-carotenals yield retinal at higher rates than does β-carotene; epoxy-carotenoids are not metabolized. The reaction requires molecular oxygen, which reacts with the two central carbons (C-15 and C-15′), followed by cleavage of the C–C bond. It is inhibited by sulfhydryl group inhibitors and by chelators of ferrous iron (Fe^{++}). The enzyme, sometimes also called the *carotene cleavage enzyme*, has been found in a wide variety of animal species;[11] enzyme activities were found to be greatest in herbivores (e.g., guinea pig, rabbit), intermediate in omnivores (e.g., chicken, tortoise, fish), and absent in the only carnivore studied (cat). The activity of this enzyme is enhanced by the

---

[8] This finding has implications for millions of people, as atrophic gastritis and hypochlorhydria are common conditions, particularly among older people.

[9] Fewer than 10% of naturally occurring carotenoids are provitamins A.

[10] More than 100 enzymes in this group are known. Two occur in animals: β-carotene-15,15′-oxygenase and β-carotene-9′,10′-oxygenase.

[11] The β-carotene 15,15′-dioxygenase has also been identified in *Halobacterium halobium* and related halobacteria, which use retinal, coupled with an opsin-like protein, to form bacteriorhodopsin, an energy-generating light-dependent proton pump.

consumption of triglycerides,[12] suggesting that its regulation involves long-chain fatty acids. Low activities are associated with the absorption of intact carotenoids; this phenomenon is responsible for the yellow-colored adipose tissue, caused by the deposition of absorbed carotenoids, in cattle. Thus, at low doses β-carotene is essentially quantitatively converted to vitamin A by rodents, pigs, and chicks; cats, in contrast, cannot perform the conversion, and therefore β-carotene cannot support their vitamin A needs.

The turnover of carotenoids in the body occurs via first-order mechanisms that differ for individual carotenoids. For example, in humans the biological half-life of β-carotene has been determined to be 37 days, whereas those of other carotenoids vary from 26 days (lycopene) to 76 days (lutein).

The symmetric, central cleavage of β-carotene is highly variable between individuals. In the bovine corpus luteum, which also contains a high amount of β-carotene, it has been shown to vary with the estrous cycle, showing a maximum on the day of ovulation. Studies with the rat indicate that the activity is stimulated by vitamin A deprivation and reduced by dietary protein restriction.

Eccentric cleavage of carotenoids by apparently different enzymatic activities also occurs. This metabolism yields apo-carotenones and apo-carotenals, which can apparently be chain-shortened directly to yield retinal, or first oxidized to the corresponding apo-carotenoic acids and then chain-shortened to yield **retinoic acid**.[13] For example, the enzyme carotene-9′, 10′-oxygenase cleaves β-carotene asymmetrically to form apo-10′-β-carotenal. Intestinal enzymes can cleave 9-cis-β-carotene (which comprises 8 to 20% of the β-carotene in fruits and vegetables, but seems less well utilized than the all-trans isomer) to 9-cis-retinal which, in turn, appears to be oxidized to 9-cis-retinoic acid.

Retinoid Metabolism Linked to Absorption

Retinal produced by at least the central cleavage step is reduced in the intestinal mucosa to retinol. This step is catalyzed by another enzyme, **retinaldehyde reductase**, which is also found in the liver and eye. The reduction requires a reduced pyridine nucleotide (NADH/NADPH) as a cofactor and has an apparent K_m of 20 mM; this step can be catalyzed by a **short-chain alcohol dehydrogenase/aldehyde reductase**, and there is some debate concerning whether the two activities reside on the same enzyme.

Mucosal Metabolism of Retinol

Retinol, formed either from the hydrolysis of dietary retinyl esters or from the reduction of retinal cleaved from β-carotene,[14] is absorbed by facilitated diffusion via a specific transporter.[15] Then, retinol is quickly re-esterified with long-chain fatty acids in the intestinal mucosa. That 9-trans-retinol has been found in the plasma of human subjects given 9-cis-β-carotene indicates that cis-trans isomerization can occur in the enterocyte. That phenomenon would serve to limit the distribution of 9-cis-retinoids to tissues, thus rendering 9-cis-β-carotene an effective source of vitamin A.

Vitamin A is transported to the liver mainly (i.e., 80 to 90% of a retinol dose[16]) in the form of retinyl esters. The composition of lymph retinyl esters is remarkably independent of the fatty acid composition of the most recent meal. **Retinyl palmitate** typically comprises about half of the total esters, with **retinyl stearate** comprising about a quarter and retinyl oleate and retinyl linoleate being present in small amounts.

Two pathways for the enzymatic reesterification of retinol have been identified in the microsomal fraction of the intestinal muscosa. A low-affinity route (Fig. 5-2, top) involves uncomplexed retinol; it is catalyzed by **acyl-CoA:retinol acyltransferase (ARAT)**. A high-affinity route (Fig. 5-2, bottom) involves retinol complexed with a specific binding protein, **cellular retinol-binding protein type II [CRBP(II)[17]]**; it is catalyzed by **lecithin–retinol acyltransferase (LRAT)**. The expression of LRAT mRNA is induced by retinoic acid and downregulated by vitamin A depletion. It has been suggested that LRAT serves to esterify

---

[12] Triglycerides also increase CRBP(II) levels.

[13] Studies of these processes are complicated by the inherent instability of carotenoids under aerobic conditions; many of the products thought to be produced enzymatically are the same as those known to be produced by autoxidation.

[14] It has been estimated that humans convert 35 to 71% of absorbed β-carotene to retinyl esters.

[15] This transporter was discovered by Ong (1994), who found it to transport all-trans-retinol and 3-dehydroretinol. They found other retinoids to be taken up by enterocytes by passive diffusion.

[16] Humans fed radiolabeled β-carotene showed the ability to absorb some of the unchanged compound directly in the lymph, with only 60–70% of the label appearing in the retinyl ester fraction.

[17] CRBP(II) is a low-molecular-mass (15.6-kDa) protein that constitutes about 1% of the total soluble protein of the rat enterocyte.

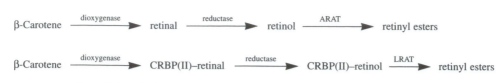

Fig. 5-2. Intestinal metabolism of vitamin A.

low doses of retinol, whereas ARAT serves to esterify excess retinol, when CRBP(II) becomes saturated. The identification of a retinoic acid-responsive element in the promoter region of the CRBP(II) gene suggests that the transcription of that gene may be positively regulated by retinoic acid, leading to increased CRBP(II) levels at high vitamin A doses. Experiments have shown that CRBP (II) expression is enhanced under conditions of stimulated absorption of fats, especially unsaturated fatty acids.

IV. Transport of Vitamin A

Retinyl Esters Conveyed by Chylomicra in Lymph

Retinyl esters are secreted from the intestinal mucosal cells in the hydrophobic cores of chylomicron particles, by which absorbed vitamin A is transported to the liver through the lymphatic circulation, ultimately entering the plasma[18] compartment through the thoracic duct. Carnivorous species in general, and the dog in particular, typically show high plasma levels. Retinyl esters are almost quantitatively retained in the extrahepatic processing of chylomicra to their remnants; therefore, chylomicron remnants are richer in vitamin A than are chylomicra. Retinyl and cholesteryl esters can undergo exchange reactions between lipoproteins, including chylomicra in rabbit and human plasma by virtue of a **cholesteryl ester transfer protein** peculiar to those species.[19] Although this kind of lipid transfer between lipoproteins is probably physiologically important in those species, the demonstrable transfer involving chylomicra is unlikely to be a normal physiological process.

Transport of Carotenoids

Carotenoids that are not metabolized at the intestinal mucosum are transported from that organ by chylomicra via the lymphatic circulation to the liver, where they are transferred to lipoproteins. It is thought that strongly nonpolar species such as β-carotene and lycopene are dissolved in the chylomicron core, whereas species with polar functional groups may exist at least partially at the surface of the particle. Such differences in spatial distribution would be expected to affect transfer to lipoproteins during circulation and tissue uptake. Indeed, the distribution of carotenoids among the lipoprotein classes reflects their various physical characteristics, with the hydrocarbon carotenoids being transported primarily in **low-density lipoproteins (LDLs)** and the more polar carotenoids being transported in a more evenly distributed manner among LDLs and **high-density lipoproteins (HDLs)** (Table 5-4). It is thought that small amounts of the nonpolar carotenoids are transferred from chylomicron cores to HDLs during the lipolysis of the

Table 5-4. Distribution of carotenoids in human lipoproteins

Carotenoid	VLDL	LDL	HDL
Zeaxanthin/lutein (%)	16	31	53
Cryptoxanthin (%)	19	42	39
Lycopene (%)	10	73	17
α-Carotene (%)	16	58	26
β-Carotene (%)	11	67	22

Source: Reddy, P. P., Clevidance, B. A., Berlin, E., Taylor, P. R., Bieri, J. G., and Smith, J. C. (1989). *FASEB J.* **3,** A955.

---

[18] On entering the plasma, chylomicra acquire apo-lipoproteins C and E from the plasma high-density lipoproteins (HDLs). Acquisition of one of these (apo C-II) activates lipoprotein lipase at the surface of extrahepatic capillary endothelia, which hydrolyses the core triglycerides, thus causing them to shrink and transfer surface components (e.g., apo A-I, apo A-II, some phospholipid) to HDLs and fatty acids to serum albumin, and lose apo A-IV and fatty acids to the plasma or other tissues. These processes leave a smaller particle called a **chylomicron remnant**, which is depleted of triglyceride but is relatively enriched in cholesteryl esters, phospholipids, and proteins (including apo B and apo E). Chylomicron remnants are almost entirely removed from the circulation by the liver, which takes them up by a rapid, high-affinity receptor-mediated process stimulated by apo E.

[19] This protein has not been found in several other mammalian species examined.

triglycerides carried by the former particles. However, because HDL transports only a small fraction of plasma β-carotene, the carrying capacity of the latter particles for hydrocarbon carotenoids would appear to be small. Therefore, it is thought that β-carotene is retained by the chylomicron remnants to be internalized by the liver for subsequent secretion in **very low-density lipoproteins (VLDLs)**.

Impact of Abetalipoproteinemia

The absorption of vitamin A (as well as the other fat-soluble vitamins) is a particular problem in patients with **abetalipoproteinemia**, a rare genetic disease characterized by general lipid malabsorption. These patients lack apo B and, consequently cannot synthesize any of the apo B-containing lipoproteins (i.e., LDLs, VLDLs, and chylomicra). Having no chylomicra, they show hypolipidemia and low plasma vitamin A levels; however, when given oral vitamin A supplementation, their plasma levels are normal. Although the basis of this response is not clear, it has been suggested that these patients can transport retinol from the absorptive cells via their remaining lipoprotein (HDLs), possibly by the portal circulation.

Vitamin A Is Stored in the Liver

Newly absorbed retinyl esters are taken up by the liver in association with chylomicron remnants by receptor-mediated[20] endocytosis on the part of liver parenchymal cells.[21] Within those cells, remnants are degraded by lysosomal enzymes. It appears that intact retinyl esters are taken up and are subsequently hydrolyzed to yield retinol. Retinol can be transferred from the parenchymal cells to *stellate cells*,[22] where it is re-esterified. It is likely that the re-esterification proceeds by a reaction similar to that of the

intestinal microsomal acyl-CoA:retinol acyltransferase (ARAT). The liver thus serves as the primary storage depot for vitamin A, normally containing more than 90% of the total amount of the vitamin in the body.[23] Most of this (about 90%) is stored in stellate cells (which account for only about 2% of total liver volume), with the balance stored in parenchymal cells (these two cell types are the only hepatocytes that contain retinyl ester hydrolase activities). Almost all (about 95%) of hepatic vitamin A occurs as long-chain retinyl esters, the predominant one being retinyl palmitate. Kinetic studies of vitamin A turnover indicate the presence, in both liver and extrahepatic tissues, of two effective pools (i.e., fast- and slow-turnover pools) of the vitamin. Of rat liver retinoids, 98% were in the slow-turnover pool (retinyl esters of stellate cells), with the balance corresponding to the retinyl esters of parenchymal cells. The storage or retinyl esters appears not to depend on the expression of **cellular retinol-binding protein** (**CRBP**), as **transgenic** mice that overexpressed CRBP in several organs have not shown elevated vitamin A stores in those organs. The metabolism of vitamin A by hepatic cytosolic retinal dehydrogenase increases with increasing hepatic retinyl ester stores.

Retinyl Ester Hydrolysis

Vitamin A is mobilized as retinol from the liver by hydrolysis of hepatic retinyl esters. This mobilization accounts for about 55% of the retinol discharged to the plasma (the balance comes from recycling from extrahepatic tissues). The **retinyl ester hydrolase** involved in this process shows extreme variation between individuals.[24] The activity of this enzyme is known to be low in protein-deficient animals and has been found to be inhibited, at least *in vitro*, by vitamins E and K.[25]

---

[20] Chylomicron remnants are recognized by high-affinity receptors for their apo E moiety.

[21] The parenchymal cell is the predominant cell type of the liver, comprising in the rat more than 90% of the volume of that organ.

[22] These are also known as *pericytes*, *fat-storing cells*, *interstitial cells*, *lipocytes*, *Ito cells*, or *vitamin A-storing cells*.

[23] Mean hepatic stores have been reported in the range of 171–723 μg/g in children and 0–320 μg/g in adults (Panel on Micronutrients, Food and Nutrition Board [2002]. Dietary Reference Intakes for Vitamin A, Vitamin K, Arsenic, Boron, Chromium, Copper, Iodine, Iron, Manganese, Molybdenum, Nickel, Silicon, Vanadium and Zinc. National Academy Press, Washington, DC: p. 95.)

[24] In the rat, hepatic retinyl ester hydrolase activities can vary by 50-fold among individual rats and by 60-fold among different sections of the same liver.

[25] Each vitamin has been shown to act as a competitive inhibitor of the hydrolase. This effect may explain the observation of impaired hepatic vitamin A mobilization (i.e., increased total hepatic vitamin A and hepatic retinyl esters with decreased hepatic retinol) of animals fed very high levels of vitamin E.

Retinol Is Transported Protein-Bound in the Plasma

Once mobilized from liver stores, retinol is transported to peripheral tissues by means of a specific carrier protein, plasma **retinol-binding protein (RBP)**. Human RBP consists of a single polypeptide chain of 182 amino acid residues, with a molecular mass of 21.2 kDa. Like several other of the retinoid binding proteins,[26] it is classified as a member of the lipocalin family of lipid-binding proteins. These are composed of an eight-stranded, antiparallel β-sheet that is folded inward to form a hydrogen-bonded, β-barrel that comprises the ligand-binding domain the entrance of which is flanked by a single-loop scaffold. Within this domain, a single molecule of all-*trans*-retinol is completely encapsulated, being stabilized by hydrophobic interactions of the β-ionnone ring and the isoprenoid chain with the amino acids lining the interior of the barrel structure. This structure protects the vitamin from oxidation during transport. RBP is synthesized as a 24-kDa *pre-RBP* by parenchymal cells, which also convert it to RBP by the cotranslational removal of a 3.5-kDa polypeptide.[27] This protein product (**apo-RBP**) is secreted in a 1:1 complex with all-*trans*-retinol (**holo-RBP**). Although it is not clear whether stellate cells also synthesize RBP, it is clear that they also contain the protein, albeit at much lower levels than parenchymal cells. It has been suggested that apo-RBP may be secreted from parenchymal cells to bind to stellate cells, thus mobilizing retinol to the circulation. According to this view, stellate cells may be important in the control of retinol storage and mobilization, a complex process that is thought to involve retinoid-regulated expression of cellular retinoid-binding proteins.

The secretion of RBP from the liver is regulated in part by estrogen levels[28] and by vitamin A status

Table 5-5. Percentage distribution of vitamin A in sera of fasted humans

Fraction	Retinol (%)	Retinyl palmitate (%)
VLDL	6	71
LDL	8	29
HDL	9	—
RBP	77	—
Total	100	100[a]

[a]This represents only about 5% of the total circulating vitamin A.

(i.e., liver vitamin A stores) protein, and zinc status; deficiencies of each markedly reduce RBP secretion and thus reduce circulating levels of retinol (Table 5-5). In cases of protein-energy malnutrition, RBP levels (and thus serum retinol levels) can be decreased by as much as 50%. Except in the postprandial state, virtually all plasma vitamin A is bound to RBP. In the plasma, almost all RBP forms a 1:1 complex with **transthyretin**[29] (a tetrameric, 55-kDa protein that strongly binds four thyroxine molecules). The formation of the RBP–*trans*thyretin complex appears to reduce the glomerular filtration of RBP and, thus, its renal catabolism.[30] The kidney appears to be the only site of catabolism of RBP, which turns over rapidly.[31,32] Under normal conditions, the turnover of holo-RBP is rapid—11 to 16 hours in humans.

Computer modeling studies indicate that more than half of hepatically released holo-RBP comes from apo-RBP recycled from RBP–*trans*thyretin complexes. Apo-RBP is not secreted from the liver. Vitamin A-deficient animals continue to synthesize apo-RBP, but the absence of retinol inhibits its secretion (a small amount of denatured apo-RBP is always found in the plasma). Owing to this hepatic

---

[26] The cellular retinal and retinoic acid binding proteins; see section on "Other Vitamin A-Binding Proteins Involved in Vitamin A Transport" and Table 5-6, both later in this chapter.

[27] Retinol-binding proteins isolated from several species, including rat, chick, dog, rabbit, cow, monkey, and human, have been found to have similar sizes and binding properties.

[28] Seasonally breeding animals show threefold higher plasma RBP levels in the estrous compared with the anestrous phase. Women using oral contraceptive steroids frequently show plasma RBP levels that are greater than normal.

[29] Previously called *prealbumin*.

[30] Studies have shown *holo*-RBP bound to transthyretin to have a half-life in human adult males of 11–16 hr; that of free RBP was only 3.5 hr. These half-lives increase (i.e., turnover decreases) under conditions of severe protein-calorie malnutrition.

[31] For this reason, patients with chronic renal disease show greatly elevated plasma levels of both RBP (which shows a half-life 10- to 15-fold that of normal) and retinol, while concentrations of transthyretin remain normal.

[32] Turnover studies of RBP and retinol in the liver and plasma suggest that some retinol does indeed recirculate to the liver; however the mechanism of such recycling, perhaps involving transfer to lipoproteins, is unknown.

accumulation of apo-RBP, vitamin A-deficient individuals may show a transient overshooting of normal plasma RBP levels on vitamin A realimentation.

Other factors can alter the synthesis of RBP to reduce the amount of the carrier available for binding retinol and secretion into the plasma. This occurs in response to dietary deficiencies of protein (e.g., **protein-energy malnutrition**) and/or zinc, which reduce the hepatic synthesis of apo-RBP. Because RBP is a negative acute-phase reactant, subclinical infections or inflammation can also decrease circulating retinol levels. Thus, low serum retinol levels in malnourished individuals may not be strictly indicative of a dietary vitamin A deficiency. Also, because vitamin A deprivation leads to reductions in plasma RBP only after the depletion of hepatic retinyl ester stores (i.e., reduced retinol availability), the use of plasma RBP/retinol as a parameter of nutritional vitamin A status can yield false-negative results in cases of vitamin A deprivation of short duration.

The retinol ligand of holo-RBP is taken into cells via specific receptor-mediated binding of RBP. Apparently, RBP binding facilitates the release of retinol to the target cell. This is accompanied by an increase in the negative charge of apo-RBP, which reduces its affinity for transthyretin, which is subsequently lost. The residual apo-RBP is filtered by the kidney, where it is degraded. Thus, plasma apo-RBP levels are elevated (by about 50%) under conditions of acute renal failure. Studies have shown that apo-RBP can be recycled to the holo form. Indeed, injections of apo-RBP into rats produced marked (70 to 164%) elevations in serum retinol levels. It is thought, therefore, that circulating apo-RBP may be a positive feedback signal from peripheral tissues for the hepatic release of retinol, the extent of which response is dependent on the size of hepatic vitamin A stores.

A two-point mutation in the human **RBP** gene has been shown to result in markedly impaired circulating retinol levels; surprisingly, this is associated with no signs other than night blindness.[33] This suggests that other pathways are also important in supplying cells with retinol, presumably via retinyl esters and/or β-carotene, and/or with retinoic acid. That the systemic functions of vitamin A can be discharged by retinoic acid, which is ineffective in supporting vision, indicates that the metabolic role of RBP is to deliver retinol to the pigment epithelium as a direct requirement of visual function and to other cells as a precursor to retinoic acid. Retinoic acid is not transported by RBP, but it is normally present in the plasma, albeit at very low concentrations (1 to 3 ng/ml), tightly bound to albumin. It is presumed that the cellular uptake of retinoic acid from serum albumin is very efficient.

Other Vitamin A-Binding Proteins Involved in Vitamin A Transport

The transport, storage, and metabolism of the retinoids involve their binding to several other binding proteins, four of which [**cellular retinol-binding protein types I and II, CRBPs(I) and (II), and cellular retinoic acid-binding protein types I and II, CRABPs(I) and (II)**; see Table 5-6] have the same general tertiary structure as the lipocalins, a class of low-molecular-weight proteins whose members bind hydrophobic ligands (e.g., fatty acids, cholesterol, biliverdin). Proteins of this family have multistranded β-sheets that are folded to yield a deep hydrophobic pocket suitable for binding appropriate hydrophobic ligands. Each of the retinoid-binding proteins has approximately 135 amino acid residues with pairwise sequence homologies of 40 to 74%. Each has been highly conserved (91 to 96% sequence homology among the human, rat, mouse, pig and chick proteins). Their genes also show similarities: each contains four exons and three introns, the latter being positioned identically. Therefore, it appears that these proteins share a common ancestral gene. The very close separation of the genes for CRBPs (I) and (II) (only 3 centimorgans) suggests that this pair resulted from the duplication of one of these two genes. They do, however, show very different tissue distributions: CRBP(I) is expressed in most fetal and adult tissues, particularly those of the liver, kidney, lung, choroids plexus, and pigment epithelium; CRNP(II) is expressed only in mature enterocytes in the villi of the mucosal epithelium (especially the jejunum) and in the fetal and neonatal liver.

Other retinoid-binding proteins, which are larger and not members of this family, have been characterized: **cellular retinal-binding protein (CRALBP)** and **interphotoreceptor retinol-binding protein**

---

[33] Biesalski, H. K., Frank, J., Beck, S. C., Heinrich, F., Ilek, B., Reifen, R., Gollnick, H., Seelinger, M. W., Wissinger, B., and Zrenner, E. (1999). *Am. J. Clin. Nutr.* **69**, 931–936.

Table 5-6. Vitamin A-binding proteins

| Binding protein | Abbreviation | Molecular weight | | K_d | |
		kDa	Ligand	nM	Location
Retinol-BP	RBP	21	all-*trans*-Retinol	20	Plasma
Cellular retinol-BP, type I	CRBP (I)	15.7	all-*trans*-Retinol	<10	Cytosol of most tissues
			all-*trans*-Retinal	50	except heart, adrenal, and ileum
Cellular retinol-BP, type II	CRBP(II)	15.6	all-*trans*-Retinol	–	Cytosol of enterocytes,
			all-*trans*-Retinal	90	fetal and neonatal liver
Cellular retinal-BP	CRALBP	36	11-*cis*-Retinol		Cytosol of retina
			11-*cis*-Retinal	15	
Cellular retinoic acid-BP, type I	CRABP (I)	15.5	all-*trans*-Retinoic acid	0.1	Cytosol of most tissues except liver, jejunum, ileum
Cellular retinoic acid-BP, type II	CRABP(II)	15	all-*trans*-Retinoic acid	0.1	Cytosol of embryonic limb bud
Epididymal retinoic acid-BP	–	18.5	all-*trans*-Retinoic acid		Lumen of epididymis
Uterine retinol-BP	–	22	all-*trans*-Retinol		Cytosol of uterus (sow)
Interphotoreceptor retinol-BP	IRBP	140	all-*trans*-Retinol and	50–100	Interphotoreceptor space
			11-*cis*-Retinol	50–100	
Retinol pigment epithelium protein	RPE65	65	all-*trans*-retinyl esters		Retinal pigment epithelium
Nuclear retinoic acid receptor-α	RARα	50	all-*trans*-Retinoic acid		Nuclei of most tissues except adult liver
Nuclear retinoic acid receptor-β	RARβ	50	all-*trans*-Retinoic acid		Nuclei of most tissues except adult liver
Nuclear retinoic acid receptor-γ	RARγ	50	all-*trans*-Retinoic acid		Nuclei of most tissues except adult liver
Nuclear retinoid X receptor-γ	RARγ	50	all-*trans*-Retinoic acid		Nuclei of most tissues except adult liver
Rhodopsin	–	41	11-*cis*-Retinal		Cytosol of retina
Melanopsin	–		11-*cis*-Retinal		Cytosol of retina, brain, skin[a]

[a]In *Xenopus* sp.

(IRBP). These are classified as in the group of intracellular lipid-binding proteins that included the fatty acid-binding proteins. Like the lipocalins, they also bind their lipophilic ligands with an antiparallel, β-barrel structure. Unlike those other proteins, however, they bind vitamin A in the reverse orientation: with its polar group buried internally and the β-ionone ring close to the surface. The IRBPs are unusual in that they can bind three retinol molcules (all other retinoid-binding proteins bind only a single-ligand molecule) as well as two long-chain fatty acid molecules.

Clearly, tissue levels of the CRBPs' mRNAs are influenced by nutritional vitamin A status. Both CRBP(I) protein and mRNA are reduced by deprivation of the vitamin; however, CRBP(II) protein and mRNA levels are increased by vitamin A deficiency. The CRBP gene appears to be inducible by retinoic acid, and a number of **retinoic acid response elements (RAREs)** have been identified in both the CRBP(I) and CRBP(II) promoters. Apparently, discrepant results have been obtained regarding the retinoic acid inducibility of the CRBP(II) gene. Whether other transcriptional factors also bind to those elements remains to be learned, yet it appears that these genes are responsive to other hormones, including glucocorticoids and 1,25-dihydroxyvitamin D_3, which have been shown to have negative effects on CRBP(I) and CRBP(II), respectively.

Cellular Uptake of Retinol

Due to their hydrophobic character, the plasma membranes do not present a barrier to retinol uptake, and thus, retinol can enter target cells by nonspecific partitioning into the plasma membrane from RBP. Nevertheless, most of the vitamin appears to enter cells through specific RBP–receptor-mediated mechanisms.[34] How this occurs for retinol and other retinoids is an intriguing question in view of their hydrophobic character and lability when dissolved in water; it is generally believed that this is a protein-mediated process. On entry into the target cell, holo-RBP interacts with a cell surface receptor. Retinol then combines with CRBP. Because CRBP(I) is present at high levels in cells that synthesize and secrete RBP, it has been suggested that it may interact at specific sites to effect the transfer of retinol to RBP for release to the general circulation. The synthesis and/or the retinol-binding affinity of CRBP(I) may be affected by thyroid and growth hormones; both hormones promote the cellular uptake of retinol.

Cells of many tissues also contain other retinoid-binding proteins that are thought to be involved in the transport of the hydrophobic retinoids within and between cells, and to effect presentation of their retinoid ligands to enzymes and to the nuclear receptors. These include CRABPs(I) and (II), and CRALBP,[35] which bind the dominant, hormonally active form retinoic acid, and several nuclear **retinoic acid receptors** (the **RAR** and **RXR** proteins).[36] Other vitamin A-binding proteins, with narrow tissue distributions, have been identified: IRBP in the retina, retinoic acid-binding proteins of the lumen of the epididymis, and a retinol-binding protein in the uterus.

Transport Roles of Vitamin A-Binding Proteins

The intracellular vitamin A-binding proteins appear to be important in the cellular uptake and the intra-cellular and transcellular transport of various vitamin A metabolites. Both CRBP and CRABP have been shown to serve as carriers of their ligands (retinol and retinoic acid, respectively) from the cytoplasm into the nucleus, where the latter are transferred to the chromatin such that the binding proteins are released, possibly to return to the cytoplasm.

CRBP also appears to have more specialized transport functions in certain tissues. In the liver, CRBP concentrations increase with increasing retinyl ester contents, suggesting that the binding protein may function in the transport of retinol from parenchymal cells into the stellate cells, which store retinyl esters. Specific and rich localization of CRBP has been identified in endothelial cells of the brain microvasculature, in cuboidal cells of the choroid plexus, in the Sertoli cells of the testis, and in the pigment epithelium of the retina. Because these tight-junctioned cells also have surface receptors for the plasma holo-RBP–transthyretin complex, it is thought that their abundant CRBP(I) concentrations are involved in the transport of retinal across the blood–brain, blood–testis, and retinal blood–pigment epithelium barriers. Studies with mice have shown that CRBP(I) is necessary for the hepatic uptake of retinol: CRBP(I)-null individuals exhausted their hepatic retinyl ester stores even when they were fed vitamin A.

CRBP(II) appears to be restricted largely to the enterocytes of the small intestine (particularly, the jejunum). Its abundance in mature enterocytes, where it comprises 1% of the total soluble protein, as well as the absence of CRBP(I) in these cells, suggest that CRBP(II) is involved in enteric absorption of vitamin A, presumably by transporting it across the cell. Both CRBP(II), as well as a high-capacity esterase that esterifies CRBP(II)-bound retinol, have been identified in hepatic parenchymal cells of fetal and newborn rats. After birth, CRBP(II) appears to be replaced by CRBP(I), such that mature animals show none of the former binding protein in that organ. The presence of CRBP(II) in fetal liver

---

[34] The existence of a membrane-associated retinol transporter is still controversial; that retinol can move spontaneously between the two layers of artificial phospholipid bilayers would argue against the need for a specific transporter.

[35] CRABP is related to the hepatic tocopherol binding protein.

[36] See the section "Vitamin A Regulation of Gene Transcription" for a discussion of the retinoid receptors.

corresponds to the increased concentration of retinyl palmitate in that organ at birth.

Some retinoid-binding proteins found extracellularly are believed to serve similar transport functions. These include two low-molecular-weight retinoic acid-binding proteins, generally related to RBP, that are secreted into the lumen of the epididymis, where they are thought to participate in the delivery of all-*trans*-retinoic acid to sperm in that organ, which also contain a particularly abundant supply of CRBP (I).[37] Other retinol-binding proteins are synthesized in the uterine endometrium and secreted into the uterus; these show some sequence homology with RBP but are slightly larger. They are thought to be involved in the transport of retinol to the fetus.

The IRBP of the interphotoreceptor space is thought to function in the transport of retinol between the pigment epithelium and photoreceptor cells. It is synthesized by the latter, in which its mRNA has been detected. Unlike the other retinoid-binding proteins, the IRBP is a large (140-kDa) glycoprotein; it can bind six moles of long-chain fatty acid in addition to two moles of retinol. It has been suggested that its relatively low affinity for retinol, in comparison with the other retinol-binding proteins, facilitates rapid, high-volume transport of that ligand along a series of IRBPs. That IRBP is involved in the visual process, perhaps by delivering the chromophore, is indicated by the finding that its binding specificity shifts from mainly 11-*cis*-retinol to mostly all-*trans*-retinol as eyes become more completely light adapted.[38]

The two IRBP binding sites for retinoids have been shown, using fluorescence techniques, to be quite different: a strongly hydrophobic binding pocket and a surface site that interacts with retinol via its polar head group. The protein shows higher affinities for all-*trans*-retinol and 11-*cis*-retinal than for other retinoids. Studies have shown that docosahexanoic acid (DHA) induces a rapid and specific release of 11-*cis*-retinal from the IRBP hydrophobic site, whereas palmitic acid is without effect. This finding suggests that DHA may function in the targeting of 11-*cis*-retinal to photoreceptor cells, the DHA concentrations of which are much greater than those of pigment epithelial cells.

A carotenoid-binding protein has been characterized in rat liver.[39] This protein binds β-carotene and is distributed predominantly in the mitochondria and lysosomes. The partially purified *carotenoprotein* is very sensitive to bright light and temperatures above 4°C.

Retinol Recycling

The majority of retinol that leaves the plasma appears to be recycled, as plasma turnover rates have been found to exceed (by more than an order of magnitude) utilization rates. Thus, kinetic studies in rats have indicated that a retinol molecule recycles via RBP 7 to 13 times before its irreversible utilization. Such data indicate that, in the rat, newly released retinol circulates in the plasma for 1 to 3.5 hours before leaving that compartment, and that it may take a week or more to recycle to the plasma. It is estimated that some 50% of plasma turnover in the rat is to the kidneys, 20% to the liver, and 30% to other tissues. It has been suggested that retinol leaves the plasma bound to RBP. Although the source of RBP for retinol recycling is not established, mRNA for RBP has been identified in many extrahepatic tissues, including kidney.

Plasma Retinol Homeostasis

In healthy individuals, plasma retinol is maintained within a narrow range (40–50 mg/ml in adults; typically, about half that in newborn infants) in spite of widely varying intakes of vitamin/provitamin A.[40] This control appears to be effected by several factors: regulation of CRBP(II) expression in stellate cells, regulation of enzymes that esterify retinol and hydrolyze retinyl esters, and other factors that may affect retinol release to the plasma and/or removal from it. The liver and kidneys appear to play important roles in these various processes. Indeed, renal dysfunction has been shown to increase plasma retinol levels; this has been suggested to involve a regulatory signal to the liver that alters the secretion of RBP–retinol. Serum retinol levels can also be affected by nutrition sta-

---

[37] The initial segment of the epididymis contains the greatest concentration of CRBP found in any tissue.

[38] IRBP is also found in another photosensitive organ, the pineal gland.

[39] Others have been identified in crustaceans, cyanobacteria, and carrots.

tus with respect to zinc, which is required for the hepatic synthesis of RBP.

Plasma levels of carotenoids, in contrast, do not appear to be regulated; they reflect intake of carotenoid-rich foods. Careful studies have revealed, however, cyclic changes of up to nearly 30% in the plasma β-carotene concentrations during the menstrual cycles of women. Whether these fluctuations are physiologically meaningful[41] or whether they relate to fluctuations in plasma lipids is not clear.

Vitamin A in Adipose Tissue

Appreciable amounts of vitamin A are stored in adipocytes: 15–20% of total body store, more than half as retinyl esters. Unlike other tissues, which take up retinol from RBP, adipocytes take up retinyl esters from chylomicra. Studies with the rat have shown that the mobilization of vitamin A from adipocytes also differs from that process in other cells. A cAMP-sensitve, hormone-dependent lipase converts adipocyte retinyl esters to retinal in a manner analogous to the liberation of free fatty acids from adipocyte triglyceride depots.

Milk Retinol

Retinol is transferred from mother to infant through milk. The retinol A content of milk is a function of two factors: the stage of lactation and the vitamin A status of the mother. Human breast milk from well-nourished, vitamin A-adequate mothers typically drops from ca. 5–7 μmol/L in colostrum to ca. 3–5 μmol/L in transitional milk to 1.4–2.6 μmol/L in mature milk. These levels are enough to meet the infant's immediate metabolic needs while also supporting the development of adequate vitamin A stores.[42] Over the first six months of life, such an infant will consume nearly 60 times as much vitamin A from breast milk (ca. 300 μmoles) than it accumulated throughout gestation. Vitamin A-deficient mothers, however, produce breast milk that is low in the vitamin; in vitamin A-deficient areas of the world,

levels average ca. 1 μmol/L (levels <1.05 μmol/L are considered indicative of maternal vitamin A deficiency[43]). This level appears to be sufficient to meet an infant's immediate metabolic requirements, as breastfed infants of vitamin A-deficient mothers are largely protected from xerophthalmia. However, higher levels (at least 1.75 μmol/L) are required to support adequate vitamin A stores to protect against the development of xerophthalmia during weaning. For this reason, vitamin A supplementation of mothers in vitamin A-deficient areas is regarded as a prudent public health strategy. A meta-analysis of randomized controlled trials showed that such measures have reduced infant mortality by 23% in children under five years of age in populations at risk to vitamin A deficiency.[44] The success of postpartum maternal supplementation depends on the prevailing breastfeeding practices, with the simultaneous promotion of optimal practices (including the feeding of colostrum) being highly effective in improving infant vitamin A status. For example, the administration of 60,000 RE to a low-vitamin A mother can produce a 29% increase in the retinol contents of her breast milk over six months.

V. Metabolism of Vitamin A

Metabolic Fates of Retinol

The metabolism of vitamin A (Fig. 5-3) centers around the transport form, retinol, and the various routes of conversion available to it: *esterification, conjugation, oxidation,* and *isomerization.*

Esterification

As discussed above, retinol is esterified in the cells of the intestine and most other tissues via enzymes of the endoplasmic reticulum, which use acyl groups from either phosphatidylcholine (lecithin–retinol acyltransferase, LRAT) or acylated coenzyme A (acyl-CoA:retinol acyltransferase, ARAT). These systems show marked specificities for saturated fatty

---

[41] It has been suggested that the oxidative enzymatic reactions involved in the synthesis of progesterone from cholesterol by the corpus luteum at midcycle may constitute an oxidative stress calling for protection by lipid-soluble antioxidants including β-carotene.

[42] The normal weight (ca. 3.2 kg) infant of a well-nourished, vitamin A-adequate mother is born with hepatic vitamin A stores of ca. 5 μmoles.

[43] Stoltzfus, R. J., and Underwood, B. A. (1995). *Bull WHO* **73**, 703–711.

[44] Beaton, G. H., Mortorell, R., Aronson, K. J., Edmonston, B., McCabe, G., Ross, A. C., and Harvey, B. (1993). Nutrition Policy Discussion Paper No. 13, UN Administrative Committee of Coordination—Subcommittee on Nutrition, New York, 120 pp.

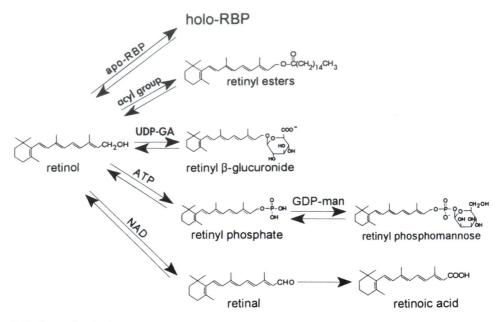

Fig. 5-3. Metabolic fates of retinol.

acids, in particular, palmitic acid; thus, the most abundant product is retinyl palmitate.

Conjugation

Retinol may also be conjugated in either of two ways. The first entails the reaction catalyzed by retinol-UDP-glucuronidase, present in the liver and probably other tissues, which yields **retinyl β-glucuronide**, a metabolite that is excreted in the bile.[45] The second path of conjugation involves ATP-dependent phosphorylation to yield **retinyl phosphate** catalyzed by **retinol phosphorylase**. That product, in the presence of guanosine diphosphomannose (GDP-man), can be converted to the glycoside retinyl phosphomannose, which can transfer its sugar moiety to glycoprotein receptors. However, because only a small amount of retinol appears to undergo phosphorylation *in vivo*, the physiological significance of this pathway is not clear.

Oxidation

Retinol can also be reversibly oxidized to retinal by NADH- or NADPH-dependent **retinol dehydro-genases**, which are also dependent on zinc. These cytosolic and microsomal activities are found in many tissues, the greatest being in the testis.[46] A short-chain **alcohol dehydrogenase** has been described that can oxidize 9-*cis*- and 11-*cis*-retinol to the corresponding aldehyde. This activity has been identified in several tissues, including the retinal pigment epithelium, liver, mammary gland, and kidney. That 9-*cis*-retinol can be converted to 9-*cis*-retinoic acid is evidenced by the finding of a 9-*cis*-retinol dehydrogenase. The enzyme in both humans and mice is inhibited by 13-*cis*-retinoic acid at levels similar to those found in human plasma, suggesting that 13-*cis*-retinoic acid may play a role in the regulation of retinoid metabolism. Retinal can be irreversibly oxidized by **retinal oxidase** to retinoic acid. Because retinoic acid is the active ligand for the nuclear retinoid receptors, it is very likely that this metabolism is tightly regulated.[47] The rate of that reaction is several fold greater than that of retinol dehydrogenase; that, plus the fact that the rate of reduction of retinal back to retinol is also relatively great, results in retinal being present at very low concentrations in tissues. The increasing

---

[45] About 30% of the retinyl β-glucuronide excreted in the bile is reabsorbed from the intestine and is recycled in an enterohepatic circulation back to the liver. For this reason, it was originally thought to be an excretory form of the vitamin. That view has changed with the findings that retinyl β-glucuronide is biologically active in supporting growth and tissue differentiation and that it is formed in many extrahepatic tissues.

[46] Male rats fed retinoic acid instead of retinol become aspermatogenic and experience testicular atrophy. It has been proposed that retinoic acid is required for spermatogenesis, but cannot cross the blood–testis barrier; this is supported by the fact that the rat testis is also rich in CRABP.

[47] Two microsomal proteins that catalyze this reaction have been isolated from rat liver; one has been shown to cross link with holo (but not apo)-CRBP in the presence of NADP.

analytical sensitivity afforded by developments in high-performance liquid–liquid partition chromatography, and mass spectrometry has resulted in the identification of an increasing number (approaching that of steroid hormones) of retinoic acid isomers in the plasma of various species;[48] the number of these with physiological significance is presently unclear.

Fates of Retinoic Acid

Once all-*trans*-retinoic acid is formed from all-*trans*-retinol, it is converted to forms that can be readily excreted (Fig. 5-4). It may be conjugated by glucuronidation in the intestine, liver, and possibly other tissues to retinyl β-glucuronide. Alternatively, it can be catabolized by further oxidization to several excretory end products, including several oxidative chain-cleavage metabolites that are conjugated with glucuronic acid, taurine,[49] or other polar molecules. The oxidation of retinoic acid to 4-oxo-retinoic acid is catalyzed by an enzyme CYP26, the mRNA of which is induced by retinoic acid and downregulated by vitamin A depletion. Both the production and

catabolism of all-*trans*-retinoic acid involve unidirectional processes; therefore, whereas the reduced forms of vitamin A (retinol, retinyl, esters, retinal) can be converted to retinoic acid, the latter cannot be converted to any of the reduced forms.

Isomerizations

Interconversion of the most common all-*trans* forms of vitamin A and various *cis* forms occurs in the eye and is a key aspect of the visual function of the vitamin, as the conformational change caused by the isomerization alters the binding affinity of retinal for the visual pigment protein *opsin*. In the eye, light induces the conversion of **11-*cis*-retinal** to **all-*trans*-retinal** (Fig. 5-5). The conversion back to the 11-*cis* form is catalyzed by the enzyme **retinal isomerase**, which also catalyzes the analogous isomerization (in both directions) of 11-*cis*- and all-*trans*-retinol. Some isomers (e.g., the 13-*cis* form) tend to be isomerized to the all-*trans* form more rapidly than others. The conversion of all-*trans*-retinoic acid to 9-*cis*-retinoic acid has also been demonstrated.

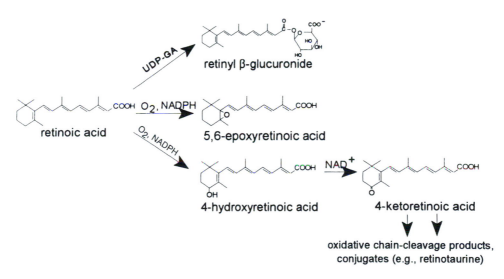

Fig. 5-4.   Catabolism of retinoic acid.

---

[48] In addition to all-*trans*-, 13-*cis*-, and 9-*cis*-retinoic acid, this number includes the 9,13-*dicis*-, 4-hydroxy-, 4-oxo-, 18-hydroxy-, 3,4-dihydroxy-, and 5,6-epoxy isomers, as well as such derivatives as retinotaurine.

[49] Significant amounts of retinotaurine are excreted in the bile.

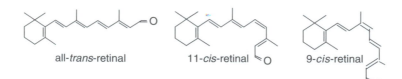

Fig. 5-5. Structures of the all-*trans,* 11-*cis,* and 9-*cis* isomers of retinal.

Role of Retinoid-Binding Proteins in Modulating Vitamin A Metabolism

In addition to serving as reserves of retinoids, the cellular retinoid-binding proteins also serve to modulate vitamin A metabolism, apparently both by holding the retinoids in ways that render them inaccessible to the oxidizing environment of the cell and by channeling the retinoids via protein–protein interactions among its enzymes (Fig. 5-6 and Table 5-7). Both CRBP and CRBP(II) function in directing the metabolism to their bound retinoid ligands by shielding them from some enzymes that would use the free retinoid substrate and by making them accessible to other enzymes important in metabolism. For example, the esterification of retinol by LRAT occurs while the substrate is bound to CRBP or CRBP(II). The abundance of CRBP in the liver and its high affinity for retinol suggest that its presence directs the esterification of the retinoid ligand to the reaction catalyzed by LRAT, rather than that catalyzed by ARAT, which can use only free retinol. This also appears to be the case for CRBP(II). Although it, unlike CRBP, can bind both retinol and retinal, only when retinal is bound to it can the reducing enzyme **retinal reductase** use the substrate. In addi-

tion, the binding of retinol to CRBP(II) greatly reduces the reverse reaction (oxidation to retinal). Thus, by facilitating retinal formation and inhibiting its loss, CRBP(II) seems to direct the retinoid to the appropriate enzymes, which sequentially convert retinal to the esterified form in which it is exported from the enterocytes. The preferential binding of 11-*cis*-retinal by CRALBP relative to CRBP appears to be another example of direction of the ligand to its appropriate enzyme, that is, a microsomal NAD-dependent retinal reductase in the pigment epithelium of the retina that uses only the carrier-bound substrate. In each of these cases, it is likely that the retinoid-binding protein–ligand complex interacts directly with the respective retinoid-metabolizing enzyme.

The nature of the role of CRABP in the transduction of endogenous retinoid signals is still unclear. That transgenic animals that overexpress CRABP show significant pathology[50] suggests an important function. On the other hand, mice in which expression of the gene is knocked out have been found to have normal phenotypes; importantly, they show normal susceptibility to the teratogenic effects of high doses of retinoic acid.

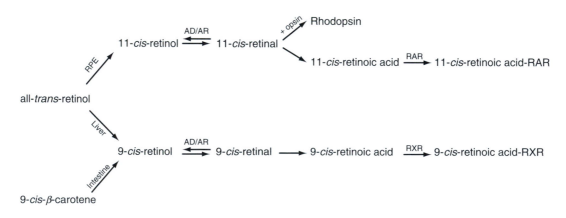

Fig. 5-6. Roles of binding proteins in vitamin A metabolism.

---

[50] For example, transgenic mice that expressed CRABP under the influence of lens-specific α-crystallin promoter developed cataracts and, later, pancreatic endocrine tumors.

Table 5-7. Apparent metabolic functions of the retinoid-binding proteins

Binding protein	Apparent function(s)
CRBP	Directs retinol to LRAT and oxidative enzymes; regulates retinyl ester hydrolase
CRBP(II)	Directs retinol to LRAT and oxidative enzymes
CRABP	Directs retinoic acid to catabolizing enzymes; and regulates free retinoic acid concentrations
CRABP(II)	Directs retinoic acid to catabolizing enzymes; and regulates free retinoic acid concentrations
CRALBP	Regulates enzymatic reactions of the visual cycle

VI. Excretion of Vitamin A

Vitamin A is excreted in various forms in both the urine and feces. Under normal physiological conditions, the efficiency of enteric absorption of vitamin A is high (80–95%), with 30–60% of the absorbed amount being deposited in esterified form in the liver. The balance of absorbed vitamin A is catabolized (mainly at C-4 of the ring and at C-15 at the end of the side chain[51]) and released in the bile or plasma, where it is removed by the kidney and excreted in the urine (i.e., short-chain, oxidized, conjugated products). About 30% of the biliary metabolites (i.e., retinoyl β-glucuronides) are reabsorbed from the intestine into the enterohepatic circulation back to the liver, but most are excreted in the feces with unabsorbed dietary vitamin A. In general, vitamin A metabolites with intact carbon chains are excreted in the feces, whereas the chain-shortened, acidic metabolites are excreted in the urine. Thus, the relative amounts of vitamin A metabolites in the urine and feces, vary with vitamin A intake (i.e., at high intakes fecal excretion may be twice that of the urine) and the hepatic vitamin A reserve (i.e., when reserves are above the low–normal level of 20 μg/g, both urinary and fecal excretion vary with the amount of vitamin A in the liver).

VII. Metabolic Functions of Vitamin A

Feeding provitamin A carotenoids, retinyl esters, retinol, and retinal can support the maintenance of healthy epithelial cell differentiation, normal reproductive performance, and visual function (Table 5-8). Each of these forms can be metabolized to retinol, retinal, or retinoic acid. But unlike retinol and retinal, retinoic acid cannot be reduced to retinal or retinol. Feeding retinoic acid can support only the *systemic* functions of vitamin A (e.g., epithelial cell differentiation). These observations and knowledge of retinoid metabolism led to the conclusion that whereas retinal discharges the visual functions, retinoic acid (and, specifically, **all-*trans*-retinoic acid**) must support the systemic functions of the vitamin.

Vitamin A in Vision

The best elucidated function of vitamin A is in the visual process where, as 11-*cis*-retinal, it serves as the photosensitive chromophoric group of the visual pigments of rod and cone cells of the retina. Rod cells contain the pigment **rhodopsin**; cone cells contain one of three possible **iodopsins**. In each case, 11-*cis*-retinal is bound (via formation of a Schiff base) to a specific lysyl residue of the respective apo-protein (collectively referred to as **opsins**) (see Fig. 5-7).

The visual functions of rhodopsin and the iodopsins differ only with respect to their properties of light absorbency,[52] which are conferred by the different opsins involved. In each, photoreception is effected by the rapid, light-induced isomerization of 11-*cis*-retinal to the all-*trans* form. That product, present as

Table 5-8. Known functional forms of vitamin A

Active form	Function
Retinol	Transport, reproduction (mammals)
Retinyl esters	Storage
Retinal	Vision
Retinoic acid	Epithelial differentiation, gene transcription, reproduction

---

[51] The chain terminal carbon atoms (C-14 and C-15) can be oxidized to CO_2; retinoic acid is oxidized to CO_2 to a somewhat greater extent than retinol.

[52] The absorbance maxima of the pigments from the human retina are as follows: rhodopsin (rods), 498 nm; iodopsin (blue cones), 420 nm; iodopsin (green cones), 534 nm; iodopsin (red cones), 563 nm.

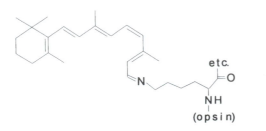

Fig. 5-7. 11-*cis*-Retinal binds to photopigment proteins via a lysyl linkage.

a protonated Schiff base of a specific lysyl residue of the protein, produces a highly strained conformation. This results in the dissociation of the retinoid from the opsin complex. This process (**bleaching**) is a complex series of reactions, involving progression of the pigment through a series of unstable intermediates of differing conformations[53] and, ultimately, to *N*-retinylidene opsin, which dissociates to all-*trans*-retinal and opsin (see Fig. 5-8).

The dissociation of all-*trans*-retinal and opsin is coupled to nervous stimulation of the vision centers of the brain. The bleaching of rhodopsin causes the closing of Na$^+$ channels in the rod outer segment, thus leading to hyperpolarization of the membrane.

This change in membrane potential is transmitted as a nervous impulse along the optic neurons. This response appears to be stimulated by the reaction of an unstable "activated" form of rhodopsin, **meta-rhodopsin II**, which reacts with **transducin**, a membrane-bound G protein of the rod outer segment disks. This results in the binding of the transducin α subunit with **cGMP phosphodiesterase**, which activates the latter to catalyze the hydrolysis of cGMP to GMP. Because cGMP maintains Na$^+$ channels of the rod plasma membrane in the open state, the resulting decrease in its concentration causes a marked reduction in Na$^+$ influx. This results in hyperpolarization of the membrane and the generation of a nerve impulse through the synaptic terminal of the rod cell.

The visual process is a cyclic one in that its constituents are regenerated. All-*trans*-retinal can be converted enzymatically in the dark back to the 11-*cis* form. After bleaching, all-*trans*-retinal is rapidly reduced to all-*trans*-retinol, in the rod outer segment. The latter is then transferred (presumably via IRBP) into the retinal pigment epithelial cells, where it is esterified (again, predominantly with palmitic acid) and stored in the bulk lipid of those cells. The regener-

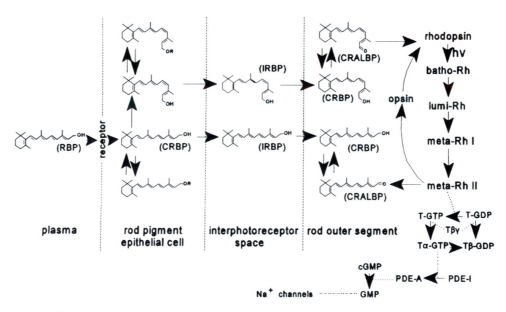

Fig. 5-8. Vitamin A in the visual cycle. Rh, rhodopsin; T, transducin; PDE-I, phosphodiesterase (inactive); PDE-A, phosphodiesterase (active).

---

[53] The conformation of rhodopsin is changed to yield a transient photopigment, *bathorhodopsin*, which, in turn, is converted sequentially to *lumirhodopsin*, *metarhodopsin I*, and (by deprotonation) *metarhodopsin II*.

ation of rhodopsin, which occurs in the dark-adapted eye, involves the simultaneous hydrolysis and isomerization of retinyl esters to yield 11-*cis*-retinol and then 11-*cis*-retinal which is transferred into the rod outer segment via IRBP. Studies have revealed that a protein, RPE65, has a key role in the *trans*-*cis* isomerization in the retinal pigment epithelium. That protein not only binds and stabilizes all-*trans*-retinyl esters, but also extracts from the retinal pigment epithelium endoplasmic reticular membrane for delivery to the isomerizing enzyme isomerohydrolase. Its activity appears to be regulated through the addition/release of palmitic acid: palmitoylation of the protein converts the protein from a form soluble in the cytosol to a membrane-bound form, thus controlling its capacity to present its retinoid ligand to cytosolic isomerohydrolase. Nervous recovery is effected by the GTPase activity of the transducin α subunit, which, by hydrolyzing GTP to GDP, causes the reassociation of transducin subunits and, hence, the loss of its activating effect on cGMP phosphodiesterase. Meta-rhodopsin II is also removed by phosphorylation to a form incapable of activating transducin, and by dissociation to yield opsin and all-*trans*-retinal.

The visual cycle of cones[54] differs from that of rods. Cones have much lower (100-fold) light sensitivity but faster (10-fold) recovery rates than rods. In cones the oxidation of 11-*cis*-retinol to 11-*cis*-retinal is NADP-dependent, and the isomerization of all-*trans* to 11-*cis*-retinal occurs in a two-step process apparently in Müller cells. In rods, the oxidation step is NAD-dependent, and the isomerization is a one-step process in the retinal pigment epithelium.

The vitamer 11-*cis*-retinal can also bind another rhodopsin-like proteins in the eye, **melanopsin**. The photosensitive pigment undergoes light-induced isomerization of 11-*cis*-retinal to 11-*trans*-retinal; but, unlike rhodopsin, it does not dissociate from the prosthetic group. That melanopsin is found in the inner retina but not in rods or cones, and in the site of the circadian clock of the brain[55] has led to the suggestion that the protein functions in photoperiod regulation.

Systemic Functions of Vitamin A

Although they are much less well understood, the extraretinal functions of vitamin A are clearly of greater physiological impact than the visual function. Whereas deprivation of vitamin A disrupts the visual cycle, resulting in impaired dark adaptation (**night blindness**, or **nyctalopia**), disruption of the vital functions of the vitamin is far more severe and often life-threatening (e.g., corneal destruction, infection, stunted growth). Vitamin A-deficient animals die, but not from lack of visual pigments. Collectively, the vital functions of vitamin A have been referred to as the *systemic functions* of the vitamin. More specifically, they include roles in the differentiation and growth of epithelial cells and in growth in general, in which the function of vitamin A resembles that of a hormone. Because the oxidation of retinal to retinoic acid is irreversible, retinoic acid can support only the systemic functions. Animals fed diets containing retinoic acid as the sole source of vitamin A grow normally and appear healthy in every way except that they go blind.

Chief among the systemic functions of vitamin A is its clear role in the differentiation of epithelial cells. It is well documented that vitamin A-deficient individuals (humans or animals) experience replacement of normal mucus-secreting cells by cells that produce keratin, particularly in the conjunctiva and cornea of the eye, the trachea, the skin, and other ectodermal tissues. Less severe effects are also produced in tissues of mesodermal or endodermal origin. It appears that retinoids affect cell differentiation through actions analogous to those of the steroid hormones; that is, they bind to the nuclear chromatin to signal transcriptional processes. In fact, studies have revealed that the differentiation of cultured cells can be stimulated by exposure to retinoids and that abnormal mRNA species are produced by cells cultured in vitamin A-deficient media.[56] Furthermore, retinoic acid has been found to stimulate, synergistically, with **thyroid hormone**, the production of growth hormone in cultured pituitary cells.

---

[54] Cones comprise only 5% of all photoreceptors in the human eye, although they are more numerous in other species. For example, cones comprise 60% of the photoreceptors in the chicken eye.

[55] The suprachiasmatic nucleus.

[56] Epidermal keratinocytes cultured in a vitamin A-deficient medium made keratins of higher molecular weight than those made by vitamin A-treated controls; this shift toward larger keratins was corrected by treatment with vitamin A. Different mRNA species were identified, which encoded the different proteins produced under each condition.

Vitamin A Regulation of Gene Transcription

Vitamin A discharges its systemic functions through the abilities of all-*trans*-retinoic acid and 9-*cis*-retinoic acid to regulate gene expression at specific target sites in the body. Retinoid regulation of transcription is receptor mediated. Retinoic acid binds to two members of a highly conserved superfamily of proteins that act as nuclear receptors for steroid hormones: 1,25-(OH)$_2$-vitamin D$_3$ and thyroid hormone (T$_3$).[57] These nuclear receptors have similar ligand-binding and DNA-binding domains and substantial sequence homology. Retinoic acid is thought to interact with them in a way similar to their other ligands: each receptor binds to regulatory elements upstream from the gene and acts as a ligand-activated transcription factor.

Two families of retinoic acid receptors have been identified: the retinoic acid receptors (**RARs**) and the retinoid "x" receptors (**RXRs**). All-*trans*-retinoic acid binds only the RARs, which it does with high affinity ($K_d = 1-5$ nmol/liter); three distinct subtypes of RAR have been identified (α, β, and γ). In contrast, **9-*cis*-retinoic acid**[58] binds both the RARs and RXRs with high affinity ($K_d = 10$ nmol/liter); three subtypes of the RXR have also been identified (α, β, and γ). For both the RAR and RXR subtypes, different variants have been identified.

The RARs resemble thyroid hormone receptors; the expression of RARs varies distinctly during development (Table 5-9). The ligand-binding domains of the RARs are highly conserved (showing 75% identity in terms of amino acid residues). That RARα1 and RARα2 share 7 of their 11 exons suggests that they have arisen from a common ancestral RAR gene. Different promoters, however, direct the expression of each in an unusual organization involving the 5′-untranslated region of genes divided among different axons. In the case of RARα1, the 5′ region is encoded in three axons: two contain most of the untranslated region; the third encodes the remainder of that region plus the first 61 amino acids that are peculiar to RARα1.

In contrast, the RXRs show only weak homology with the RARs, the highest degree of homology (61%) being in their DNA-binding domains. On the basis of homologies with an insect locus, it is thought that the RXRs may have evolved as the original retinoid-signaling system. Both receptors have been found in most tissues.[59] RXRα responds to some-

Table 5-9.   Nuclear retinoic acid receptors

Receptor	Isoforms[a]	Ligands	Tissue expression pattern	
			Embryo	Adult
RARα	RARα_1, RARα_2	all-*trans*-RA,[b] 9-*cis*-RA[b]	Widespread	Widespread
RARβ	RARβ_1, RARβ_2, RARβ_3	all-*trans*-RA, 9-*cis*-RA	Spatial, temporal	Specific (muscle, prostate)
RARγ	RARγ_1, RARγ_2[c]	all-*trans*-RA, 9-*cis*-RA	Spatial, temporal	Specific (skin, lung)
RXRα		9-*cis*-RA	Specific (intestine, skin, liver)	Specific (liver, skin, kidney)
RXRβ		9-*cis*-RA	Widespread	Widespread
RXRγ		9-*cis*-RA	Specific (brain, pituitary)	Specific (muscle, heart)

[a]Isoforms differ only in their N-terminal regions.
[b]Retinoic acid.
[c]Identified in *Xenopus laevis*.
[d]Identified in the newt.

[57] T$_3$, Triiodothyronine.

[58] Originally questioned as to whether it was a physiological metabolite, 9-*cis*-retinoic acid is now known to be produced from 9-*cis*-retinol (by 9-*cis*-retinol dehydrogenase with subsequent oxidation, by cleavage of 9-*cis*-β-carotene, and from the isomerization of all-*trans*-retinol in the lung.

[59] Greatest concentrations have been found in adrenals, hippocampus, cerebellum, hypothalamus, and testis.

what higher retinoic acid levels than other RXR isoforms.

These nuclear retinoic acid receptors comprise a two-component signaling system for the activation of the transcription of certain genes. It is thought that retinoic acid can act in either a paracrine or autocrine manner. Both all-*trans*-retinoic acid and 9-*cis*-retinoic acid can be synthesized within the target cell (from retinol *via* retinal) or be delivered to that cell from the circulation (see Fig. 5-9). On intracellular transport to the nucleus (presumably via CRABP), the ligand is thought to be transferred to the appropriate receptor (RAR, RXR), which then can bind to its respective, cognate, response element to regulate the transcription of target genes.

Two types of high-affinity retinoic acid response elements have been identified in the promoter regions of target genes near the transcription start: those that recognize the RXR homodimer and those that recognize the RXR–RAR heterodimer. The RXR–RAR heterodimer binds to retinoic acid response elements (RAREs), which consist of direct repeats of the consensus half-site sequence AGGTCA usually separated by five nucleosides. The RXR homodimer binds to retinoid X response elements (RXREs) most of which are direct repeats of AGGTCA with only one nucleoside spacing. Gene expression is effected by activating each response element present in the promoter regions of responsive genes.[60] The RXRs can also form homotetramers as well as dimers with other members of the steroid/thyroid/retinoic acid family; heterodimerization in this system has usually been found to increase the efficiency of interactions with DNA and, thus, transcriptional activation. Further regulation is effected in this signaling system as the RXR–RAR heterodimer appears to repress the transcription-activating function of RXR–RXR.

In the absence of retinoic acid, the apo-receptor pair (RXR–RAR/RXR) binds to the RAREs of target genes, and RAR recruits co-repressors that mediate negative transcriptional effects by recruiting histone deacetylase complexes, which modify histone proteins to induce changes in chromatin structure that reduce the accessibility of DNA to transcriptional factors. This process is reversed upon retinoic acid binding: a conformational change in the ligand-binding domain results in the release of the co-repressor and the recruitment of co-activators fo the AF-2 region of the receptor. Some cofactors interact directly to enhance transcriptional activation, whereas others can affect the acetylation histone proteins, causing the conformational opening of chromatin and the activation of transcription of the target gene. Impairments in the process can lead to carcinogenesis (see "Role of Vitamin A in Carcinogenesis," later in this chapter).

The general picture is one of RXRs forming heterodimers with RARs that are activated by retinoids, and with other receptors of the same superfamily

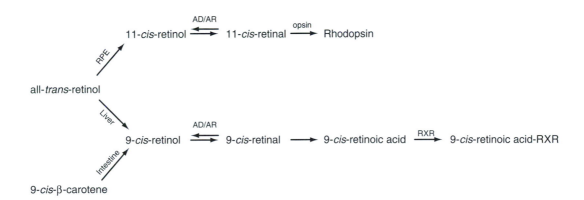

Fig. 5-9. Apparent roles of short-chain alcohol dehydrogenase/aldehyde reductase in the generation of retinoic acid isomers. (RPE = retinal pigment epithelium)

---

[60] The RXR–RAR response elements consist of polymorphic arrangements of the nucleotide sequence motif 5′-RG(G/T)TCA-3′. These gene elements are also responsive to thyroxine, suggesting that retinoic acid and thyroid hormone may control overlapping networks of genes.

(i.e., thyroid hormone receptors, the vitamin D_3 receptor, the peroxisome proliferator activating receptor, and, probably, others yet unidentified). The metabolite 9-*cis*-retinoic acid, which targets RXR, causes the formation of RXR homodimers that recognize certain RAREs. However, the same ligands inhibit the formation of heterodimers of RXR and the thyroid hormone receptor (TR), which reduce the expression of thyroid hormone-responsive genes.[61] In contrast, RXR-specific ligands do not appear to affect the formation of RAR-containing heterodimers. The retinoid binding protein CRABP(II) is directly involved in facilitating the interactions of RARα-RXRα heterodimers in the formation of a gene-bound receptor complex. In this role, CRABP(II) serves both to deliver retinoic acid to its nuclear receptors and to act as a co-activator of the expression of retinoic acid-responsive genes. Retinoid responses appear to be restricted to a subset of retinoid-responsive genes through the action of the orphan COUP (chicken ovalbumin upstream promoter) receptors, which have been found to form homodimers that avidly bind several retinoic acid response elements and repress both RAR–RXR and RXR homodimer activities. Retinoic acid receptors are abundant in the brain: RARα is distributed throughout, whereas RXRβ and RXRγ are found specifically in the striatal regions with dopaminergic neurons. These receptors in both the brain and pituitary gland function in the regulation of expression of the dopamine receptor.

Through this system, vitamin A and T_3 appear to play compensatory signaling roles. Studies with rats have shown that deprivation of either factor impairs thyroid signaling in the brain through reduced expression of RAR and TR as well as a neuronal protein neurogranin. This effect can be corrected by administering either vitamin A or T_3. Similarly, the regulation of the anterior pituitary hormone, thyroid-stimulating hormone (TSH), has been found to be dependent on the binding of both TR and RXR (which are activated by T_3 and 9-*cis*-retinoic acid, respectively) to the TSH gene.

The morphogenic role of retinoic acid in embryonic tissues appears to be affected by the establishment of concentration gradients of RARs/RXRs owing to the differential induction of the receptor by the retinoid.[62] Studies have found that CRABP mRNA is not transcribed in tissues expressing the RAR Minas, suggesting that CRABP is involved in regulating differentiation by controlling available free retinoic acid. Therefore, the retinoid-based transcription signaling system appears to involve the RXRs/RARs in a manner that is differentially controlled by the availability of both metabolically related ligands and intracellular binding proteins. The complexity of this signaling system is thought to be the basis of the pleiotropic effects of vitamin A.

Many proteins are known to appear during retinoic acid-induced cell differentiation. These include several that have been found to be induced by activation through RXR/RAR binding: growth hormone[63] (in cultured pituitary cells), the protein laminin (in mouse embryo cells), the respiratory chain-uncoupling protein of brown adipose tissue,[64] the vitamin K-dependent matrix Gla protein, and the RARs. The latter finding indicates autoregulation—that is, retinoic acid induces its own receptor. The induction of RARs appears to be differentially selective among various tissues; retinoic acid has been found to induce mainly RAR_α in hemopoietic cells, but RAR_β in other tissues.

A Coenzyme Role for Vitamin A?

A coenzyme-like role has been proposed for vitamin A. According to this hypothesis, vitamin A acts as a sugar carrier in the synthesis of **glycoproteins** (which function on the surfaces of cells to effect intercellular adhesion, aggregation, recognition, and other interac-

---

[61] This has been shown for the expression of uridine-5′-diphosphate-glucuronyl transferase, which is involved in the phase II metabolism of xenobiotic and endogenous substrates.

[62] Indeed, three RARs have been found to appear at different times in limb development in mouse embryos. The expression of one of these, RARs has been proposed to be associated with the programming of cell death, as in the developing mouse embryonic limb its mRNA has been found only in interdigital mesenchymal cells at the time of digit separation.

[63] That vitamin A may be required for the expression of growth hormone in humans is suggested by observations of a correlation of plasma retinol and nocturnal growth hormone concentrations in short children.

[64] This suggests that vitamin A may be involved in heat production and energy balance.

tions). Indeed, it has been observed that retinol can be phosphorylated to yield retinyl phosphate, which accepts mannose from its carrier GDP-mannose (to form retinyl phosphomannose) and donates it to a membrane-resident acceptor for the production of glycoproteins. Furthermore, vitamin A-deficient animals synthesize less glycoprotein in general (particularly in plasma, intestinal goblet cells, and corneal and trachea epithelial cells), relative to vitamin A-sufficient animals, and in addition produce abnormal glycoproteins.

Although changes in the glycan moieties of glycoproteins can certainly have great effects on cell functions, the actual physiologic significance of this sugar carrier role of vitamin A is not as clear. This is because the form that supports the systemic functions of vitamin A, retinoic acid, cannot serve as a sugar carrier because it cannot be reduced to form retinol. Furthermore, retinyl phosphate does not accept mannose. This problem has not been resolved; however, it has been proposed that retinoic acid may actually be hydroxylated *in vivo* to a derivative that is capable of being phosphorylated and, thus, serving as a sugar carrier.

Role of Vitamin A in Embryonic Development

Vitamin A is essential for growth, fetal development, and tissue maintenance. It has also become clear that retinoids play important fundamental roles as differentiating agents in morphogenesis. The discovery of the nuclear receptors for retinoic acid, the RARs and RXRs, has provided a means of understanding these effects at the gene level. The major organs affected in vitamin A deficiency are the heart and tissues of the ocular, circulatory, urogenital, and respiratory systems.

Vitamin A is required at various stages of embryonic development. Deprivation of vitamin A in the Japanese quail results in the loss of normal specification of heart left-right asymmetry. That this effect is associated with the decreased expression of RARβ_2 in the presumptive cardiogenic mesoderm suggests that retinoids may direct the differentiation of mesoderm into the heart lineage. Studies of the regenerating amphibian limb have revealed that retinoids

have profound effects, providing positional information enabling cells to differentiate into the pattern of structures relevant to their appropriate spatial locations. This morphogenic role may be discharged by retinoic acid or, as some data have suggested, one of its metabolites, all-*trans*-3,4-didehydroretinoic acid. That compound is produced by differentiating epithelial cells of the chick embryonic central nervous system,[65] which also responds to treatment with it. Vitamin A status has been found to modulate insulin-like growth factor I (IGF-1) as well as the gene expression of IGF-1, the IGF-1 receptor (IGF-1R), and the insulin receptor (IR) in differentiating tissues. Tissue IGF-1mRNA is downregulated in vitamin A deficiency, while the expression of IGF-1β and IR mRNA are generally upregulated under those conditions.

Role of Vitamin A in Reproduction

Vitamin A is necessary for reproduction, but the biochemical basis of this function is not known. It is apparent, however, that this role is different from the systemic one, as maintenance of reproduction is discharged by retinol and *not* retinoic acid, at least in mammals.[66] For example, rats maintained with retinoic acid grow well and appear healthy, but lose reproductive ability; that is, males show impaired spermatogenesis, and females abort and resorb their fetuses. Injection of retinol into the testis restores spermatogenesis, indicating that vitamin A has a direct role in that organ. It has been proposed that these effects are secondary to lesions in cellular differentiation and/or hormonal sensitivity. Several researchers have found that vitamin A-deficient dairy cows show reduced corpus luteal production of progesterone and increased intervals between luteinizing hormone peak and ovulation. There is some evidence indicating responses of these hormonal parameters to oral treatment with β-carotene but not preformed vitamin A.

Role of Vitamin A in Bone Metabolism

Vitamin A has an essential role in the normal metabolism of bone. This is indicated by the fact that both low and high vitamin A intakes lead to impaired bone

---

[65] *Floor plate* cells (i.e., epithelial cells at the ventral midline), derived from cells of *Hensen's node*.

[66] In the chicken, retinoic acid supports normal spermatogenesis, but in all mammalian species examined this function is supported only by retinol or retinal.

mineral density (in humans, bone mineral density is optimized with intakes of 0.6–0.9 mg RE/day). The mechanism of this role of vitamin A is not clear; it is presumed that retinoids are involved in regulating the phenotypic expression of bone-mobilizing cells. Osteoclasts are reduced in vitamin A deficiency, resulting in excessive deposition of periosteal bone by the apparently unchecked function of osteoblasts. This effect is associated with a reduction in the degradation of glycosaminoglycans.

Role of Vitamin A in Hematopoiesis

Because chronic deprivation of vitamin A leads to anemia, a role for the vitamin in hematopoiesis has been suggested. Cross-sectional studies have shown low hemoglobin levels to be associated with the prevalence of signs of xerophthalmia in children (Table 5-10), and children with mild-to-moderate vitamin A deficiency or mild xerophthalmia to have lower circulating hemoglobin levels than nondeficient children; serum retinol level has been shown to explain 4 to 10% of the variation in hemoglobin level among preadolescent children in developing countries. In such cases, the hematological response to vitamin A deficiency is biphasic: an initial fall in both hemoglobin and erythrocyte count due to an apparent interference in hemoglobin synthesis, followed by the rise in both factors late in deficiency due to hemoconcentration, apparently resulting from dehydration from reduced water intake and/or diarrhea.

Supplemental vitamin A has been shown to increase iron status in anemic, vitamin A-deficient humans and animals, and vitamin A can enhance the efficacy of iron supplements in reducing anemia (Table 5-11).

Retinoids are involved in the differentiation of myeloid cells into neutrophils, which occurs in the bone marrow; this function appears to involve all-*trans*-retinoic acid, as RARα is the predominant retinoid receptor type found in hematopoietic cells. Vitamin A-deficient animals have been found to sequester retinol in their bone marrow.[67] That vitamin A-deficient individuals do not necessarily show neutropenia suggests that local retinol sequestration is sufficient to meet the needs of myeloid cells for growth and differentiation into neutrophils, thus mitigating against the effects of low intakes of the vitamin.

The metabolic basis of the role of vitamin A in hematopoiesis appears to involve the mobilization and transport of iron from body stores as well as

Table 5-10. Prevalence of vitamin A deficiency related to hemoglobin status in Indonesian preschool children[a]

Hemoglobin g/dl	Prevalence of vitamin A deficiency[b] (%)
<11.0	54.2
11.0–11.9	43.3
≥12	34.3

[a]Lloyd-Puryear, M. A., Mahoney, J., Humphrey, F., Siren, N., Moorman, C., West, Jr., K. P. (1991). *Nutr. Res.* **11**, 1101–1110.
[b]Based on conjuctival impression cytological assessment.

Table 5-11. Efficacy of vitamin A supplementation on increasing hemoglobin levels in anemic subjects

Country	Subject age	Vitamin A dosage	Follow-up	n	Hemoglobin, g/dl Baseline	Follow-up
Indonesia[a]	<6 yrs.	0	5 mos.	240	11.4 ± 1.6	11.2 ± 1.5
		240 µg RE/d	5 mos.	205	11.3 ± 1.6	12.3 ± 1.6[*b]
Indonesia[c]	17–35 yrs.	0	2 mos.	62	10.4 ± 0.7	10.7 ± 0.6
		3 mg RE/d	2 mos.	63	10.3 ± 0.8	11.2 ± 0.8[*]
Guatemala[d]	1–8 yrs.	0	2 mos.	20	10.4 ± 0.7	10.7 ± 0.6
		2.4 mg RE/d	2 mos.	25	10.3 ± 0.8	11.2± 0.8[*]

[a]Mahilal, P. D., Idjradinata, Y. R., Muheerdiyantiningsih, K. D. (1988). *Am. J. Clin. Nutr.* **48**, 1271–1276.
[b]Significantly different from baseline level, $p < 0.05$.
[c]Suharno, D., West, C. E., Muhilal, K. D., Hautvast, J.G. (1993). *Lancet* **342**, 1325–1328.
[d]Mejia, L. A., Chew, F. (1988). *Am. J. Clin. Nutr.* **48**, 595–600.
[*]$p<0.05$

[67] Twinig et al. (*J. Nutr.* **126**, 1618, 1996) found bone marrow of vitamin A-deficient rats to contain about four times the retinol contained by that tissue from vitamin A-fed rats.

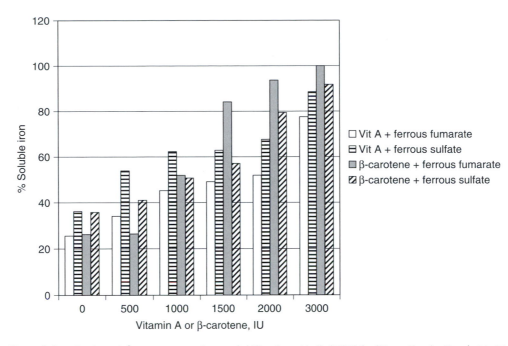

Fig. 5-10. Effect of vitamin A and β-carotene on iron solubility (at pH 6) (FGSN). (*From* Garcia-Casal, M. N., Layrisse, M., Solano, L., Baron, M. A., Arguella, F., Llovera, D., Ramirez, J., Leets, I., and Tropper, E. [1998]. *J. Nutr.* **128**, 646–650.)

the enhancement of nonheme-iron bioavailability. The results of cross-sectional studies in developing countries have found serum iron to be positively correlated with serum retinol levels, and animal studies have shown vitamin A deprivation to cause decreases in both hematocrit and hemoglobin levels, which precede other disturbances in iron storage and absorption. Vitamin A deficiency reduces the activity of ceruloplasmin, a copper-dependent protein with ferroxidase activity that is important in the enteric absorption of iron. This effect appears to occur as the result of a post-transcriptive disruption in the activity. In addition, the results of *in vitro* studies demonstrate that all-*trans*-retinol induces the differentiation and proliferation of pluripotent hemopoietic cells. These findings suggest that the anemia of vitamin A deficiency is initiated by impairments in erythropoiesis and accelerated by subsequent impairments in iron metabolism. The presence of vitamin A or β-carotene has been found to increase the enteric absorption of iron from both inorganic and plant sources. This has been explained on the basis of the formation of complexes with iron that are soluble in the intestinal lumen, thus blocking the inhibitory effects of

iron absorption of such antagonists as phytates and polyphenols (see Fig. 5-10; Table 5-12).

Role of Vitamin A in Immunity

Vitamin A is clearly important in supporting immunocompetence, in that deficiency affects immunity in several ways.[68] Vitamin A-deficient animals and humans are typically more susceptible to infection than are individuals of adequate vitamin A nutriture. Deficient animals show changes in lymphoid organ mass, cell distribution, histology, and lymphocyte characteristics. It is reasonable to suspect that the histopathological alterations caused by vitamin A deficiency provide environments conducive to bacterial growth and secondary infection in loci obstructed by keratinizing debris.[69] The latter hypothesis is supported by clinical findings: excess bacteriuria among xerophthalmic *versus* nonxerophthalmic, malnourished children in Bangladesh; negative correlation of plasma retinol level and bacteria adherent to nasopharyngeal cells of children in India. Vitamin A deficiency induces inflammation and exacerbates inflammatory states.

---

[68] In practice, it is difficult to ascribe such effects simply to the lack of vitamin A for the reason that individuals showing nutritional vitamin A deficiency generally also have protein-calorie malnutrition, which itself leads to impaired immune function.

[69] Such an example is Bitot's spots, which are patches of xerotic conjunctiva with keratin debris and bacillus growth.

Table 5-12. Effects of vitamin A and β-carotene on the bioavailability of nonheme plant iron for humans[a]

Iron source	Vit A μmol	β-Carotene μmol	Iron absorption (%)
Rice	0	0	2.1
	1.51	0	4.6[b]
	0	0.58	6.4[b]
	0	0.95	8.8[b]
Corn	0	0	3.0
	0.61	0	6.6[b]
	0	0.67	8.5[b]
	1	1.53	6.3[b]
Wheat	0	0	3.0
	.66	0	5.5[b]
	0	0.85	8.3[b]
	0	2.06	8.4[b]

[a]From Garcia-Casal, M. N., Layrisse, M., Solano, L., Baron, M. A., Arguella, F., Llovera, D., Ramirez, J., Leets, I., and Tropper, E. (1998). *J. Nutr.* **128**, 646–650.
[b]$p < 0.05$, n = 11–20 subjects.

Stimulation of immunity and resistance to infection are thought to underlie the observed effects of vitamin A supplements in reducing risks of mortality and morbidity from some forms of diarrhea, measles, HIV infection, and malaria in children. Nightblind women have a fivefold increased risk of dying from infections, and low doses of vitamin A have been found to reduce peri- and postpartum mortality in women (Table 5-13), presumably due to reduction in infections.

Evidence suggests that retinol may be a specific growth factor for B lymphocytes. That lymphocyte proliferation can be impaired by vitamin A deprivation suggests that cell-mediated immunity may be compromised by vitamin A deficiency. Decreased natural killer (NK) cell cytotoxic activity has been reported in vitamin A-deficient rats. Lower antibody titers have been reported for vitamin A-deficient children and experimental animals. It is well established that vitamin A deficiency increases the duration and severity of infection with the Newcastle disease virus in poultry, and vitamin A has been shown to enhance the immune responses of children vaccinated against measles. Studies have found apparently healthy older adults (with no signs of vitamin A deficiency) to show beneficial immunologic responses to vitamin A supplementation: increased numbers of T cells (CD3+, CD4+, but not CD8+), increased numbers and activities of NK cells, enhanced lymphocyte responses to phytohemagglutinin, increased production of interleukin-2 and expression of its receptor, and improved antibody responses to influenza vaccination. The enhancement by vitamin A of T cell-dependent antibody responses, and of the development of circulating CD4+ T cells, has suggested that the vitamin may contribute to maintaining immune functions in patients infected with the human immunodeficiency virus (HIV).

Because vitamin A deficiency impairs innate and adaptive immunity, it has been suggested that the deficiency may increase the risk of HIV transmission. Indeed, low serum retinol levels have been found to be more common among HIV-seroconverters than in HIV-negative individuals, and to be highly predictive of vaginal HIV-1 DNA shedding. Whether this is cause or effect is not clear, as serum retinol is known to decrease in the

Table 5-13. Efficacy of low-dose vitamin A supplements in reducing mortality related to pregnancy in Nepal

Parameter	Placebo	Vitamin A	β-carotene
Serum levels, midpregnancy,[a] μmol/L			
Retinol	1.02 ± 0.35	1.30 ± 0.33	1.14 ± 0.39
β-carotene	0.14 ± 0.12	0.15 ± 0.14	0.20 ± 0.17
Mortality, deaths/100,000 pregnancies (RR, 95% CL)			
During pregnancy	235 (1.0)	142 (0.60, 0.26–1.38)	111 (0.47, 0.18–1.20)
0–6 weeks postpartum	359 (1.0)	232 (0.65, 0.34–1.25)	222 (0.62, 0.31–1.23)
7–12 weeks postpartum	110 (1.0)	52 (0.47, 0.13–1.76)	28 (0.25, 0.04–1.42)

[a]The 3.5-year trial involved some 44,646 women who had more than 22,000 pregnancies, 7,200–7,700 in each treatment group. Vitamin A (retinol) or β-carotene were given in weekly dosages; post-hoc analyses revealed that only half of subjects took 80% of the intended doses (7000 IU), suggesting that the study underestimated the potential impact of vitamin A supplementation.
Source: West, K. P., Jr., Katz, J., Kharty, S. K., LeClerq, S. C., Pradham, E. K., Shrestha, S. R., Connor, P. B., Dali, S. M., Christian, P., Pokhrel, R. P., and Sommer, A. (1999). *Br. Med. J.* **318**, 570–574.

acute-phase response to infection. Three intervention studies have been conducted to test the hypothesis that maternal vitamin A supplementation can reduce the risk of perinatal HIV transmission. None found vitamin A supplements effective in reducing the prevalence of HIV infection in infants, despite the improvement in maternal vitamin A status (Table 5-14).

Retinoids and carotenoids may affect the immune system differently. Retinoids seem to act on the differentiation of immune cells, increasing mitogenesis of lymphocytes and phagocytosis of monocytes and macrophages. Carotenoids seem to affect immunosurveillance of activated NK cells and helper T cells by modifying the release of at least some cytokine-like products by activated lymphocytes and monocytes.

Active infection appears to alter the utilization or, at least, the distribution of vitamin A among tissues. Plasma retinol concentrations drop during malarial attacks, chickenpox, diarrhea,[70] measles, and respiratory disease. Ocular signs of xerophthalmia following measles outbreaks associated with declines in plasma retinol levels depend on the severity and duration of infection and can be as great as 50%. Episodes of acute infection have been found to be associated with substantive (e.g., eightfold) increases in the urinary excretion of retinol and RBP. That such insults to vitamin A status can be of clinical signifi-

cance is indicated by the fact that vitamin A treatment can greatly reduce the case morbidity and mortality rates in measles and respiratory diseases.[71]

Vitamin A deficiency is typically associated with malnutrition, particularly protein-energy malnutrition. This can be due to the common origins of each condition (i.e., in grossly unbalanced diets and poor hygiene), resulting in the fact that malnourished children are likely to be deficient in vitamin A and other essential nutrients. Protein deficiency also impairs the synthesis of apo-RBP, CRBP, and other retinol-binding proteins, impairing vitamin A transport and cellular untilization. Vitamin A deficiency is known to induce or exacerbate inflammation; DNA microarray technology has revealed inflammatory changes in the colon of the vitamin A-deficient rat that resemble those observed in colitis.

Epidemiologic studies have found that low vitamin A status is frequently associated with increased disease incidence and mortality rates. Indeed, many studies have found positive associations between mild xerophthalmia and risks of diarrhea, respiratory infection, and measles among children. A large longitudinal study of preschool children in Indonesia revealed that the overall mortality rate in children with xerophthalmia was four to five times that of children with no ocular lesions. Children with xerophthalmia were found to have low $CD4^+:CD8^+$ ratios as well as other immune abnormalities in T cell subsets (Table 5-15), each of which was reversible on supplementation with vitamin A. It appears that

Table 5-14. Vitamin A supplementation has failed to reduce mother-to-child HIV transmission

Trial	Intervention agent	RR[a] to being HIV+, by age			
		Birth	6 wks	12 wks	2 yrs
Malawi[b]	Retinol	—	0.96	—	0.84
Tanzania[c]	Retinol + β-carotene	1.60	1.22	—	1.38[d]
South Africa[d]	Retinol + β-carotene	0.85	—	0.91	—

[a]Ratio of % HIV+ children in treatment group to % HIV+ in control group.
[b]Kunwenda, N., Motti, P. G., Thaha, T. E., Broadhead, R., Biggar, R. J., Jackson, J. B., Melikian, G., Semba, R.D. (2002). *Clin. Infect. Dis.* **35**, 618–624.
[c]Fawzi, W. W., Msamanga, G. I., Hunter, D., Renjifo, B., Antelman, G., Bang, H., Manji, K., Kapiga, S., Mwakagile, D., Essex, M., Spiegelman, D. (2002). *AIDS* **16**, 1935–1944.
[d]$p < 0.05$.
[e]Coutsoudis, A., Pillay, K., Spooner, E., Kuhn, L., and Coovadia, L. H. M. (1999). *AIDS* **13**, 1517–1524.

Table 5-15. T cell abnormalities in children

Measure	Without xerophthalmia	With xerophthalmia
CD4/CD8	1.11 ± 0.04	0.99 ± 0.05
% CD4/CD45RA (naive)	34.9 ± 1.7	29.9 ± 2.1[a]
% CD4/CD45RO (memory)	18.0 ± 1.1	17.4 ± 1.2
% CD8/CD45RA	37.3 ± 1.7	41.6 ± 2.1
% CD8/CD45RO	7.6 ± 0.6	10.2 ± 0.9[a]
Plasma retinol (μM)	0.84 ± 0.06	0.57 ± 0.04[a]

[a]$p < 0.05$.
Source: Semba, R. D., Muhilal, X., Ward, B. J., Griffin, D. E., Scott, A. L., Natadisastra, G., West, K. P., Jr., and Sommer, A. (1993). *Lancet* **341**, 5–8.

---

[70] In Indonesia the presence of Bitot's spots is associated with intestinal worms, to the point that the spots are referred to as "worm feces."

[71] Of course, the first line of defense against such diseases as measles should be immunologic.

vitamin A deficiency can affect resistance to infection even before it is severe enough to cause xerophthalmia; but child mortality increases with increasing severity of the eye disease, and affected children die at nine times the rate of normal children.

Restoration of the adequate vitamin A status of deficient children can reduce morbidity rates, particularly for diarrhea and measles (Table 5-16). Meta-analyses of community-based, vitamin A intervention studies indicate an average 23% (range: 6–52%)[72] reduction in preschool mortality (Table 5-17). Vitamin A supplementation of children with active, severe, complicated measles has been shown to reduce in-hospital mortality by at least 50%. In other populations, vitamin A treatment has been shown to reduce the symptoms of diarrhea nearly as much (Table 5-18), as well as the symptoms of pneumonia and

other infections substantially. Although attendant reductions in morbidity would be expected, studies have shown those effects to be variable. That not all interventions with vitamin A have reduced mortality rates of vitamin A-deficient children is not surprising, as other factors (e.g., poverty, poor sanitation, inadequate diets) clearly contribute to the diminished survival of vitamin A-deficient children. It is likely that excess mortality occurs not only among xerophthalmic preschoolers but also among those who are mildly to marginally deficient in vitamin A but have not developed corneal lesions. In fact, a large portion of the deaths averted by vitamin A supplementation may be in this low-vitamin A group. Sommer and colleagues have estimated that the improvement of serum retinol levels in mildly deficient, asymptomatic children (with serum retinol levels of 18–20 µg/dl) to

Table 5-16. Effects of vitamin A on morbidity of children with measles in South Africa

Outcome	Hospital morbidity		Outcome	6-Month morbidity	
	Placebo	Vitamin A		Placebo	Vitamin A
Clinical pneumonia (days)	5.7 ± 0.8	3.8 ± 0.4[a]	Weight gain (kg)	2.37 ± 0.24	2.89 ± 0.23[a]
Diarrhea duration (days)	4.5 ± 0.4	3.2 ± 0.7	Diarrheal episodes	6	3
Fever duration (days)	4.2 ± 0.5	3.5 ± 0.3	Respiratory infections	8	3[a]
Clinical recovery (<8 days), %	65	96	Pneumonia episodes	3	0[a]
Integrated morbidity score[b]	1.37 ± 0.40	0.24 ± 0.15[a]	Integrated morbidity score	4.12 ± 1.13	0.60 ± 0.22

[a]$p < 0.05$.
Source: Coutsoudis, A., Broughton, M., and Coovadia, H. M. (1991). *Am. J. Clin. Nutr.* **54,** 890.

Table 5-17. Effects of vitamin A supplementation on child mortality

Trial	Observation (months)	Deaths/total control	Vitamin A	Odds ratio (95% CL)
Sarlahi, Nepal	12	210/14,143	152/14,487	0.70 (0.57–0.87)
Northern Sudan	18	117/14,294	123/14,446	1.04 (0.81–1.34)
Tamil Nadu, India	12	80/7,655	37/7,764	0.45 (0.31–0.67)
Aceh, Indonesia	12	130/12,209	101/12,991	0.73 (0.56–0.95)
Hyderabad, India	12	41/8,084	39/7,691	1.00 (0.64–1.55)
Jumia, Nepal	5	167/3,411	138/3,786	0.73 (0.58–0.93)
Java, Indonesia	12	250/5,445	186/5,775	0.69 (0.57–0.84)
Bombay, India	48	32/1,644	7/1,784	0.20 (0.09–0.45)

Source: Fawzi, W. W., Chalmers, T. C., Merrara, M. G., and Mosteller, F. (1993). *J. Am. Med. Assoc.* **269,** 898–903.

---

[72] Beaton, G. H., Martorell, R., L'Abbe, K. A., Edmonston, B., McCabe, G., Ross, A. C., and Harvey, B. (1992). Report to CIDA, University of Toronto; Sommer, A., West, K. P., Jr., Olson, J. A., and Ross, C. A. (1996). *Vitamin A Deficiency: Health, Survival, and Vision.* New York: Oxford University Press, p. 33.

Table 5-18. Effects of vitamin A supplementation on child cause-specific mortality

Study country	Relative risk[a] of death, by disease		
	Measles	Diarrhea	Respiratory disease
Indonesia[b]	0.58	0.48	0.67
Nepal[c]	0.24	0.61	1.00
Nepal[d]	0.67	0.65	0.95
Ghana[e]	0.82	0.66	1.00

[a]Ratio of deaths occurring in the vitamin A-treated group to those occurring in the untreated control group.
[b]Rahmathullah, L., Underwood, B. A., Thulasiraj, R. D., Milton, R. C., Ramaswamy, K., Rahmathullah, R., Babu, G. (1990). *N. Eng. J. Med.* **323**, 929–935.
[c]Reanalysis of data of West, Jr., K. P., Pokhrel, R. P., Katz, J., LeClarq, S. C., Khatry, S. K., Shrestha, S. R., Pradham, E. K., Tielsch, J. M., Pandey, M. R., Sommer, A. (1991). *Lancet* **338**, 67–71 cited in Sommer, A., West, Jr., K. P., Olson, J. A., and Ross, C. A. (1996). *Vitamin A Deficiency: Health, Survival, and Vision.* (New York: Oxford University Press), p. 41.
[d]Daulaire, N. M. P., Starbuck, E. S., Houston, R. M., Church, M. S., Stukel, T. A., and Pandey, M. R. (1992). *Br. Med. J.* **304**, 207–210.
[e]Ghana VAST Team (1993). *Lancet* **342**, 7–12.

serum levels of 30 µg/dl would be expected to reduce mortality by 30 to 50%.

Role of Vitamin A in Dermatology

Vitamin A appears to have a role in the normal health of the skin. Its vitamers, as well as carotenoids, are typically found in greater concentrations in the subcutis than in the plasma (significant amounts are also found in the dermis and epidermis), indicating the uptake of retinol from plasma RBP. Epithelial cell phenotypes are regulated by hormonal cycles and vitamin A intake; vitamin A deficiency impairs the terminal differentiation of human keratinocytes and causes the skin to be thick, dry, and scaly. It also results in obstruction and enlargement of the hair follicles.[73]

Owing to their similarities to changes observed in vitamin A-deficient animals, certain dermatologic disorders of keratinization (e.g., ichthyosis, Darier's disease, pityriasis rubra pilaris) have been treated with large doses of retinol. Clinical success of such treatments generally has been variable, and the high

doses of the vitamin needed for efficacy commonly produce unacceptable side effects. Therefore, the synthetic retinoids have commanded attention in the hope of finding therapeutically effective compounds of low toxicity. Of these, the most effective ones have been all-*trans*-retinoic acid,[74] 13-*cis*-retinoic acid,[75] and an ethyl ester of all-*trans*-retinoic acid.[76] The most successful of these compounds has been 13-*cis*-retinoic acid for the treatment of acne, in which it dramatically reduces sebum production. However, 13-*cis*-retinoic acid can also be teratogenic. Therefore, as acne patients will include women of child-bearing age, the compound must be used with strict medical supervision.

Clinical Applications of Retinoids in the Treatment of Dermatologic Diseases

Precancerous lesions: Actinic keratoses
Skin cancer: Nonmelanoma (squamous and basal) skin cancer
Photo-aging: Sun damage (roughness, drying, wrinkling, mottled pigmentation, laxity)
Acne vulgaris: Comedonal and cystic acne
Psoriasis and keratinization disorders: Erythrodermic, pustular, and calcitrant psoriasis

The mechanisms of the therapeutic activities of retinoids against dermatologic diseases are the subjects of current research. Because retinoids have been found to produce rapid reductions in the incidence of new nonmelanoma skin cancers in high-risk patients, it has been suggested that they function to produce regressions of prediagnostic malignant and/or premalignant lesions. Indeed, regressions of cutaneous metastases of malignant melanoma and cutaneous T cell lymphoma have been reported in response to retinoid therapy. Retinoids appear to affect photo aging by stimulating the production of the predominant collagen in the dermis.[77] The therapeutic efficacy of 13-*cis*-retinoic acid for acne vulgaris has been shown to involve its effects on all of the major pathogenic mechanisms involved in

---

[73] That is, follicular hyperkeratosis; this condition can also be caused by deficiencies of niacin and vitamin A.

[74] This compound, known generically as *tretinoin*, is effective in the treatment of acne vulgaris, photo aging, and actinic keratoses.

[75] 13-*cis*-Retinoic acid, known generically as *isotretinoin*, is effective in the treatment of cystic acne, rosacea, gram-negative folliculitis, pyoderma faciale, hidradenitis suppurativa, and cancers.

[76] This compound, known generically as *etretinate*, is effective in the treatment of psoriasis, ichthyosis, Darier's disease, palmoplantar keratodermas, and pityriasis rubra pilaris.

[77] Collagen I, which comprises some 85% of total dermal collagen.

the disease: It decreases sebum production, inhibits comedogenesis, reduces bacterial numbers in both the ducts and surface, and reduces inflammation by inhibiting the chemotactic responses of monocytes and neutrophils. The action of retinoids in psoriasis appears to involve thinning of the stratum corneum, reduced keratinocyte proliferation, and reduced inflammation.

Role of Vitamin A in Drug Metabolism

That the level of vitamin A intake has been found to affect negatively the genotoxic effect of several chemical carcinogens suggests that the vitamin may play a role in the cytochrome *P*-450-related enzyme system. Indeed, several studies have shown that vitamin A deficiency can reduce hepatic cytochrome *P*-450 contents and related enzyme activities, and vitamin A supplementation has been shown to increase the activities of cytochrome *P*-450 isozymes.[78]

Antioxidant Activities of Vitamin A and Carotenoids

It has been suggested that actions of vitamin A in supporting the health of the skin and immune systems may involve effects on systems that provide protection against the adverse effects of prooxidants.[79] Yet, it is unlikely that vitamin A itself is physiologically significant in this regard, as retinol and retinal cannot quench singlet oxygen ($^1O_2$) and have only weak capacities to scavenge free radicals. It can, however, affect tissue levels of other antioxidants. Animal studies have shown that deprivation of vitamin A leads to marked increases in the concentrations of

Table 5-19. Antioxidant abilities of carotenoid and other antioxidants

Compound	ROO· reduction[a]	$^1O_2$ quenching[a]
Lycopene	—	9×10^9
β-Carotene	1.5×10^9	5×10^9
α-Tocopherol	5×10^8	8×10^7
L-Ascorbate	2×10^8	1×10^7

[a]Bimolecular rate constants ($M^{-1} sec^{-1}$).
Source: Sies, H., and Stahl, W. (1995). *Am. J. Clin. Nutr.* **62**(Suppl.), 1315S–1321S.

α-tocopherol in the liver and plasma, whereas high intakes of retinyl esters can enhance the bioavailability of selenium, an essential constituent of several glutathione-dependent peroxidases.

Several carotenoids, on the other hand, have been shown to have direct antioxidant activities. These include β-carotene, lycopene, and some oxycarotenoids (**zeaxanthin**, lutein), which can quench $^1O_2$ or free radicals in the lipid membranes into which they partition (Table 5-19). These antioxidant activities are due to their extended systems of conjugated double bonds, which are thought to delocalize the unpaired electron of a free-radical reactant.[80] At low (physiologic) partial pressures of oxygen, carotenoids can also participate in the reduction of free radicals; xanthophyll carotenoids (lutein, lycopene, and **β-cryptoxanthin**) are more effective than β-carotene and more efficient than α-tocopherol *in vitro*. Despite these differences, the carotenoids tend to be less plentiful in tissues, for which reason their contributions to physiologic antioxidant protection are likely to be less important than those of the tocopherols except, perhaps, in cases of high carotenoid intake. Cooperative antioxidant interactions between

---

[78] These include CYP3A in rats, rabbits, and guinea pigs, and CYP2A in hamsters.

[79] Although aerobic systems rely on oxygen as the terminal electron acceptor for respiration, they must also protect themselves against the deleterious effects of highly reactive oxygen metabolites that can be formed either metabolically or through the action of such physical agents as ultraviolet light or ionizing radiation. These reactive oxygen species include singlet oxygen ($^1O_2$), superoxide ($O_2\cdot^-$), hydroxyl radical (OH·), and nitric oxide (NO·); they can react, either directly or indirectly, with polyunsaturated membrane phospholipids (to form scission products), protein thiol groups (to form disulfide bridges), nonprotein thiols (to form disulfides), and DNA (to cause base changes) to alter cellular function. They can also react with polyunsaturated fatty acid components of circulating lipoprotein complexes; such oxidative changes in low-density lipoproteins (LDLs) appear to be important in the development of atherosclerotic lesions. The systems that protect against these oxidative reactions include several reductants (e.g., tocopherols and carotenoids in membranes and lipoprotein complexes; glutathione, ascorbic acid, urate, and bilirubin in the soluble phases of cells) and antioxidant enzymes (e.g., superoxide dismutases, selenium-dependent glutathione peroxidases, catalase).

[80] This mechanism differs from that of the tocopherols, which donate a hydrogen atom to the lipid free radical to produce a semistable lipid peroxide; the tocopherols in turn become semiquinone radicals. (The antioxidant function of the tocopherols is discussed in detail in Chapter 7.)

α-tocopherol and β-carotene have been observed in model systems, and it is likely that *in vivo* carotenoids may serve to protect tocopherols.

The interactions of carotenoids with radicals result in the production of oxidation products of the carotenoids; this is manifested as bleaching of these pigments.[81] In ultraviolet (UV)-irradiated skin, lycopene is more susceptible to bleaching than is β-carotene, suggesting that it may be more important than β-carotene in antioxidant protection of dermal tissues. Supplementation with β-carotene has been found to improve antioxidant status *in vivo*. These results have included the following: reduced pentane[82] breath output in smokers; reduced plasma concentrations of malonyldialdehyde[83] in cystic fibrotics; reduced lipid peroxidation products (TBARS) in mice; reduced lethality to cultured cells of prooxidant drugs; and reduced acetaminophen toxicity[84] in mice. These and other non-provitamin A properties of carotenoids are discussed in greater detail in Chapter 18.

Role of Vitamin A in Reducing Heart Disease Risk

Epidemiologic investigations have repeatedly found inverse relationships between the level of consumption of provitamin A-containing fruits and vegetables and the risks of chronic diseases including cardiovascular disease, stroke, and cancer. Indeed, plasma retinol levels have been found to be related inversely to the risk of ischemic stroke, and low plasma β-carotene concentrations are associated with increased risk of myocardial infarction. Such findings have provided the bases for hypothetical actions of vitamin A or, more often, provitamin A carotenoids in chronic disease prevention. Unfortunately, many of these hypotheses have not withstood experimental challenge. Four well-designed, randomized, double-blind, clinical intervention trials have found supplements of β-carotene,[85,86] β-carotene and/or α-tocopherol,[87] or β-carotene and preformed vitamin A[88] to be ineffective in reducing the risk of either cardiovascular disease or angina pectoris. In fact, one of these found a slight increase in the incidence of angina associated with β-carotene use.

Role of Vitamin A in Carcinogenesis

Because vitamin A deficiency characteristically results in a failure of differentiation of epithelial cells without impairment of proliferation (i.e., the *keratinizing* of epithelia), it has been reasonable to question the possible role of vitamin A in the etiology of epithelial cell tumors (i.e., carcinomas). The squamous metaplastic changes seen in vitamin A deficiency are morphologically similar to precancerous lesions induced experimentally. Indeed, patients with oral leukoplakia, a precancerous condition of the buccal mucosa, have been found to have lower serum retinol levels than healthy controls, and treatment with retinol has been found to reduce the development of new lesions and to cause remissions in the lesions of some patients. It has been proposed that retinoic acid, which in high doses can inhibit the conversion of papillomas (benign lesions) to carcinomas, can upregulate its receptors (RARs),[89] which can, in turn, complex with protooncogenes such as c-fos to prevent malignant transformation.

---

[81] This is seen in the loss of pigmentation from the shanks of poultry, which sign has been used historically by poultry keepers to determine the reproductive status of their hens. Immature pullets deposit carotenoids in dermis, whereas those that are actively laying deposit the pigments in the lipids of the developing oocyte. The bleaching of the skin, therefore, is a positive sign of good laying condition.

[82] *n*-Pentane is a scission product of the peroxidative degradation of ω-6 fatty acids.

[83] Malonyldialdehyde is also a peroxidative scission product of polyunsaturated fatty acids. It can be detected by reaction with 3-thiobarbituric acid; it is the predominant, but not only, reactant in biological specimens. Because of the lack of absolute specificity, results are frequently expressed as total thiobarbituric-reactive substances (TBARS).

[84] The microsomal metabolism of acetaminophen, like that of other prooxidant drugs metabolized by cytochrome *P*-450-related enzymes, is known to produce $O_2 \cdot^-$. Antioxidant status has been shown to affect its acute toxicity in animal modes.

[85] The Physicians Health Study (22,071 male American physicians followed for 12 years).

[86] The Dartmouth Skin Cancer Study (1188 male and 532 female Americans followed for more than 4 years).

[87] The Alpha Tocopherol and Beta Carotene (ATBC) Cancer Prevention Trial (29,133 Finish male smokers followed for nearly 5 years).

[88] The Beta-Carotene and Retinol Efficacy Trial (CARET) (18,314 American male and female current and ex-smokers followed for 4 years of treatment).

[89] *In situ* hybridization studies have revealed RARα and RARγ in columnar and squamous epithelial cells of the skin.

From this theoretical basis, studies with animal tumor models have found vitamin A deficiency to enhance susceptibility to chemical carcinogenesis, and large doses of vitamin A (i.e., supranutritional but not toxic) to inhibit carcinogenesis in some models. On the basis of these findings, it was proposed that retinol can be anticarcinogenic by competing, at high levels in the cell, with carcinogens to prevent expression of malignant phenotypes and thus reinforce expression of the normal phenotype. However, the fact that high doses of vitamin A serve best to increase only the hepatic stores of retinyl esters rather than retinol concentrations in extrahepatic tissues led to retinoic acid and, subsequently, other retinoids being examined in animal tumor models.

Studies have demonstrated the efficacy of retinoic acid in inhibiting the growth of several types of cancer cells and tumors. Such effects appear to involve cells that do not express the RARβ gene even in the presence of physiological levels of vitamin A. The mechanism of silencing of RARβ gene expression is not clear, but it is thought not to involve alterations in the gene itself. Two other mechanisms have been proposed: (1) loss of heterozygosity of chromosome 3p24, the locus of RARβ; and (2) impaired expression of other factors[90] involved in RARβ expression.

Loss of RAR function under vitamin A-adequate conditions is associated with a variety of different cancers, the best studied of which is acute promyelocytic leukemia (APL[91]). This cancer has been found to result from a nonrandom, chromosomal translocation or deletion that leads to the production of a fusion of RARα gene on chromosome 17 to the promyelocytic (PML) gene on chromosome 15. When expressed, the fusion product represses translation and initiates leukemogenesis. This appears to occur through that action of the PML-RAR protein, which is a transcriptional activator of retinoic acid target genes. Studies with one specific target, the tumor suppressor gene RARβ2, have revealed that its promoter contains a high-affinity retinoic acid response element (RARE) near the transcription start site, but is inactivated by methylation.[92] It now appears that the PML-RAR fusion protein can form a complex with histone deacetylase, which, in turn, becomes oncogenic by recruiting DNA methyltransferases to the promoters of RARβ2 locking them in a stably silenced chromatin state by hypermethylation. Most (80%) APL patients, however, respond to treatment with very high doses of all-*trans*-retinoic acid, resulting in complete remission in more than half of cases. This effect appears to involve retinoic acid causing the dissociation of the PML-RAR protein-histone deacetylase complex, which converts the fusion protein into a transcriptional activator resulting in leukemia cell differentiation. Studies with breast cancer cells[93] suggest that retinoic acid can also cause histone acetylation (due to the release of histone deactylase) of the RARβ2 gene resulting in the inhibition of cell growth. Thus, in sensitive cells retinoic acid can reactivate RARβ2 gene expression through various epigenetic means.

While the use of retinoic acid, which is rapidly degraded and eliminated from the body, avoids the problem of chronic hypervitaminosis, its substantial toxicity makes it unsuitable for regular clinical use. Therefore, more than 1500 retinoids have been synthesized and tested for potential anticarcinogenicity.[94] A number of these[95] have been found to effectively inhibit experimentally induced tumors in several organs of animals[96] and have yielded hopeful results in clinical trials. The consensus, however, is that although retinoids currently available can delay

---

[90] Possibilities include the orphan receptors nurr77 and COUP-TF, both of which are overexpressed in retinoic acid-resistant cells.

[91] APL is characterized by a block in myeloid differentiation, resulting in the accumulation in the bone marrow of abnormal promyelocytes and in a coagulopathy involving disseminated intravascular coagulation and fibrinolysis.

[92] DiCroce, L., Raker V. A., Corsaro, M., Fazi, F., Fanelli, M., Faretta, M., Fuks, F., Lo, C. F., Kouzarides, T., Nervi, C., Minucci, S., and Pelicci, P. G. (2002). Methyltransferase recruitment and DNA hypermethylation of target promoters by an oncogenic transcription factor. *Science* **295**, 1079–1082.

[93] Sirchia, S. M., Ren, M., Pili, R., Sironi, E., Somenzi, G., Ghidoni, R., Toma, S., Nicolo, G., and Sacchi, N. (2002). Endogenous reactivation of the RARβ2 tumor suppressor gene epigenetically silenced in breast cancer. *Cancer Res.* **62**, 2455–2461.

[94] These compounds are formal derivatives of retinal differing by changes in the isoprenoid side chain (including modification of the polar end and cyclization of the polyene structure), or modifications of the cyclic head group (including replacement with other ring systems).

[95] For example, 13-*cis*-retinoic acid, *N*-ethylretinamide, *N*-(2-hydroxyethyl)-retinamide, *N*-(4-hydroxyphenyl)-retinamide, etretinate, *N*-(pivaloyloxyphenyl)-retinamide, *N*-(2,3-dihydroxypropyl)-retinamide.

[96] For example, several studies have shown that retinoids can inhibit the initiation and promotion of mammary tumorigenesis induced in rodents by dimethylbenz(α)anthracene or *N*-methyl-*N*-nitrosourea, as well as the induction of *ornithine decarboxylase*, an enzyme the induction of which appears to be essential in the development of neoplasia.

tumorigenesis, they cannot do so at doses that are not themselves toxic.

Epidemiological investigations of vitamin A intake and human cancer have produced results that support the plausibility of the hypothesis that low vitamin A status may increase cancer risk and that people who consume three or more servings of fruits and vegetables, particularly those rich in carotenoids, each day have lower risks of several types of cancers in comparison with those who eat less of such foods. Such results have come from both case control and cohort studies; these have shown notably consistent inverse associations of apparent pre-vitamin A (notably, β-carotene) intakes and risks of lung and stomach cancer. Modest protective effects of total dietary vitamin A intake have been indicated against cancers of the breast; however, such associations with prostate cancer have been inconsistent. Few studies have addressed relationships with colorectal cancer, although the available evidence suggests protective effects of preformed vitamin A rather than carotenoids. Among the problems that usually attend epidemiologic studies have been the variable and often imprecise ways of reporting the dietary intakes of vitamin A in free-living people, the difficulty in differentiating preformed vitamin A (retinol, retinyl esters) and carotenoids, and the difficulties in interpreting serum retinol concentrations. Nevertheless, the results of such surveys have fostered the hypothesis that β-carotene may have some beneficial effect unrelated to its role as a precursor of vitamin A (Table 5-20).

This hypothesis has been the subject of much debate. Supporting evidence comes from still-limited and somewhat varied findings of tumor inhibition by β-carotene in animal models (Table 5-21)[97]; from the demonstration that β-carotene can function as a membrane-resident antioxidant,[98] perhaps much like vitamin E; and from the finding that β-carotene-treated men showed increases in the production of a tumor cell recognition protein of monocytes (MHCII) and tumor necrosis factor α, indicative of enhanced

Table 5-20. Relationship of midpoint retinol and β-carotene status and human cancer outcome in a 12-year cohort study

Analyte	Plasma retinol concentration (μM)	
	Survivors[a]	Cancer cases[b]
Retinol	2.81 ± 0.01	2.81 ± 0.04
β-Carotene[c]	0.328 ± 0.005	0.342 ± 0.017[d]
Ascorbic acid	52.76 ± 0.44	47.61 ± 1.78[d]

[a] n = 2421.
[b] n = 204.
[c] Cholesterol corrected.
[d] $p < 0.01$.
Source: Stähelin, H. B., Grey, K. F., Eichholzer, M., and Lüdin, E. (1991). *Am. J. Clin. Nutr.* **53**(Suppl.), 265S–269S.

Table 5-21. Inhibition by β-carotene of chemical carcinogenesis in rats: reduced hepatic γ-glutamyltranspeptidase-positive foci

Treatment[a]	Foci (number/ cm²)	Focal area (percentage of total area)
Control	37.1 ± 9.7	1.267 ± 1.121
Retinyl acetate (10 mg/kg/2 days)	34.8 ± 9.6	0.911 ± 0.901
β-Carotene (70 mg/kg/2 days)	20.1 ± 12.5[b]	0.308 ± 0.208

[a] Rats were also treated with diethylnitrosamine/2-acetylaminofluorene.
[b] $p < 0.05$.
Source: Moreno, F. S., Wu, T. S., Penteado, M. V. C., Rizzi, M. B. S. L., Jordão, A. A., Jr., Almeida-Muradiau, L. B., and Dagli, M. L. E. (1995). *Int. J. Vit. Nutr. Res.* **65**, 87–94.

immune surveillance. Nevertheless, the correlations on which the hypothesis was based make it possible (perhaps probable) that β-carotene, as assessed in those epidemiological studies, may actually have been a proxy for some other factor(s) related to cancer causality.[99] Two facts further weaken the argument: β-carotene is much less abundant than vitamin E in tissues, and its antioxidant activity appears to be significant mainly at low oxygen tensions.[100] The antitumorigenic activities of retinoids have been cited as

---

[97] These include demonstrations of protection against tumors of the salivary gland, colon, stomach, pancreas, and skin.

[98] This is relevant to the view of one mechanism of carcinogenesis as apparently involving oxidant-induced DNA damage leading, if not repaired, to mutations in specific genes.

[99] For example, β-carotene may be a proxy for any of several other constituents of foods, including but not limited to the non-β-carotenoids; accordingly, many studies show the apparent inverse effect on cancer incidence to be greater for total fruits and vegetables than for β-carotene.

[100] At oxygen tensions characteristic of plasma, β-carotene has been shown to act as a prooxidant.

support for hypotheses that cancer-chemopreventive effects of β-carotene involve its conversion to vitamin A in target tissues; but that hypothesis is weakened by observations of the antitumorigenic efficacy of carotenoids (e.g., canthaxanthin) that are not metabolized to retinoids. Immunomodulatory effects of carotenoids have been reported.

The cancer-chemopreventive potential of supplemental β-carotene was tested in three large, well-designed, placebo-controlled, double-blind clinical intervention trials that yielded consistent results that jolted the nutrition and cancer research community. The first,[86] a 12-year study involving more than 22,000 American physicians, was stopped as planned; it found no health effects of β-carotene supplementation on the incidence of either cancer or heart disease. The second trial,[88] conducted in Finland with more than 29,000 men with histories of smoking, evaluated the health impacts of modest supplements of β-carotene (20 mg/day) and/or α-tocopherol (50 mg/day). Within 5 to 8 years of follow-up, results showed significantly greater total mortality (8%) and lung cancer incidence (18%) among men taking β-carotene in comparison with those not taking that supplement (Tables 5-22 and 5-23). The third trial,[89] which evaluated the health impact of a supplement containing both β-carotene (30 mg/day) and retinyl palmitate (25,000 IU/day) for American men and women at high risk for lung cancer,[101] also showed that, within only 4 years of follow-up, the treatment group developed, significantly greater lung cancer rates than the placebo controls.

Table 5-22. Lack of cancer protection by β-carotene among male smokers

Cancer site	Cancer incidence (per 10,000 person-years)	
	No β-carotene	β-carotene
Lung	47.5	56.3
Prostate	13.2	16.3
Bladder	9.0	9.3
Colon–rectum	8.6	9.0
Stomach	6.6	8.3
Other	44.9	42.3

Source: Alpha-Tocopherol, Beta-Carotene Cancer Prevention Study Group. (1994). *N. Engl. J. Med.* **330,** 1029–1035.

Table 5-23. Increased mortality among male smokers taking β-carotene

Causes of death	Mortality rate (per 10,000 person-years)	
	No β-carotene	β-Carotene
Lung cancer	30.8	35.6
Other cancers	32.0	33.1
Ischemic heart disease	68.9	77.1
Hemorrhagic stroke	6.0	7.0
Ischemic stroke	6.5	8.0
Other cardiovascular disease	14.8	14.8
Injuries and accidents	19.3	20.3
Other causes	23.5	22.5

Source: Alpha-Tocopherol, Beta-Carotene Cancer Prevention Study Group. (1994). *N. Engl. J. Med.* 330, 1029–1035.

The interpretation of these findings is not straightforward, as ample evidence also indicates that β-carotene at these levels is generally safe. It is possible, as some have suggested, that β-carotene may not be as safe for high-risk individuals (e.g., smokers) than for others, or that β-carotene in purified form may not be utilized in the way that it is from foods. It is also possible that β-carotene may stimulate cell growth in ways that enhance the latter stages of tumorigenesis.

VIII. Vitamin A Deficiency

The appreciable storage of vitamin A in the body tends to mitigate against the effects of low dietary intakes of the vitamin, as tissue stores are mobilized in response to low-vitamin A conditions. However, because there are two effective pools of vitamin A in the body, the rate of mobilization varies between tissues according to their respective proportions of fast-turnover and slow-turnover pools (Fig. 5-12). For this reason, rats showed faster losses of vitamin A from intestine than liver (71 vs. 53%) after being fed a vitamin A-deficient diet. It should be noted that, while hepatic stores are great enough to provide retinol, the plasma retinol level is only minimally affected by vitamin A deprivation (e.g., in the same experiment, it decreased by only 8%). Cellular functions of vitamin A can be expected to change only after transport of the vitamin is reduced, that is, after vitamin A stores have dropped to such levels as to reduce plasma retinol–RBP concentrations.

---

[101] These subjects were either smokers or asbestos workers.

Hepatic retinyl ester stores > 20 µg (>0.07 µmol) RE per gram indicate adequate vitamin A status.

Vitamin A deficiency can occur either because of a lack of both provitamins A and preformed vitamin A in diets (*primary vitamin A deficiency*) or because of failures in their physiologic utilization (*secondary vitamin A deficiency*). Primary vitamin A deficiency can occur among children and adults who consume diets composed of few servings of yellow and green vegetables and fruits and liver. For infants and young children, early weaning can increase the risk of primary deficiency. For livestock, it can occur with unsupplemented diets containing low amounts of yellow maize (corn) and corn gluten meal.

Secondary vitamin A deficiency can occur in several ways. One involves chronically impaired enteric absorption of lipids, such as in diseases affecting the exocrine pancreas (e.g., pancreatitis, cystic fibrosis, nutritional selenium deficiency) or bile production and release (e.g., biliary atresia, some mycotoxicoses in livestock), or due to the consumption of diets containing very low amounts of fat.[102] Chronic exposure to oxidants can also induce vitamin A depletion; an example is benzo(α)pyrene in cigarette smoke.[103] Nutritional deficiencies of zinc can also impair the absorption, transport, and metabolism of vitamin A, as zinc is essential for the hepatic synthesis of RBP and the oxidation of retinol to retinal, which is catalyzed by a zinc-dependent retinol dehydrogenase. Malnourished populations, which typically have low intakes of several essential nutrients including vitamin A and zinc, are at risk to vitamin A deficiency. A prevalence of 25% or more of individuals with plasma retinol levels < 0.70 µmol/L (<20/µg/dL) is indicative of populationwide inadequacy with respect to the vitamin.

Like most nutritional deficiencies in human populations, vitamin A deficiency is an outcome of a bio-eco-social system that fails to provide sources of the vitamin in ways that are at once accessible and utilizable. The complexity of this system has been captured in the WHO conceptual model (Fig. 5-11).

Vitamin A functions in many organs of the body. Therefore, insufficient intakes of the vitamin lead to a sequence of physiological events (Figs. 5-13 and 5-14) that ultimately are manifest in several clinical signs (Table 5-24). In fact, the only unequivocal signs of vitamin A deficiency are the ocular lesions nyctalopia and xerophthalmia. Nyctalopia, a disorder of dark adaptation of the retina, can take a year to develop after the initiation of a vitamin A-deficient diet,[104] but responds rapidly to vitamin A treatment. Xerophthalmia involves permanent morphological changes of the anterior segment of the eye that are not correctable without scarring. Early intervention is very important in cases of xerophthalmia (Table 5-25) in order to interrupt the progressive lesions in early stages before permanent blindness occurs.

Detection of Vitamin A Deficiency

Vitamin A deficiency can be detected by clinical diagnosis or by assessment of biochemical or histological indicators. Clinical signs include impaired dark adaptation, nyctalopia, and ocular lesions (Figs. 5-15–5-17, Table 5-26). Nyctalopia is the first functional sign of vitamin A deficiency that can be measured. It can be diagnosed by instrumental observation in the ophthalmology clinic, but in the field it is usually necessary to obtain this information about children from their caregivers. The condition can be detected by using the papillary response to a graduated light stimulus. Examination by slit lamp can reveal fundus specs and disrupted rod outer segments (with the possible involvement of similarly disrupted cones), signs suggestive of visual field alterations.

Ocular lesions including conjunctival xerosis with/without Bitot's spots, corneal xerosis, ulceration, and/or keratomalacia, and corneal scars can be diagnosed by direct examination of the eye. Morphological changes in epithelial cells blotted from the conjunctival surface can be detected by histologic examination, a procedure called **conjunctival impression cytology**.[105] The presence of enlarged, flattened

---

[102] There are few data on which to estimate the minimum amounts of dietary fat that are needed to support the absorption of vitamin A and the other fat-soluble vitamins; in the absence of empirical data, the estimate of 5 g/day is frequently used.

[103] That this effect can have practical significance was demonstrated by Christian et al. (*Eur. J. Clin. Nutr.* **58**, 204–211), who found that β-carotene supplementation of female Nepali smokers reduced the risk of pregnancy-related mortality.

[104] During this time, that is, prior to the development of clinically apparent night blindness, rod dysfunction can be detected by dark adaptation testing.

[105] This procedure involves blotting onto a piece of filter paper cells that are then fixed, stained, and examined microscopically. Normal conjunctival cells appear in sheets of small, uniform, nonkeratinized epithelial cells with abundant mucin-secreting goblet cells.

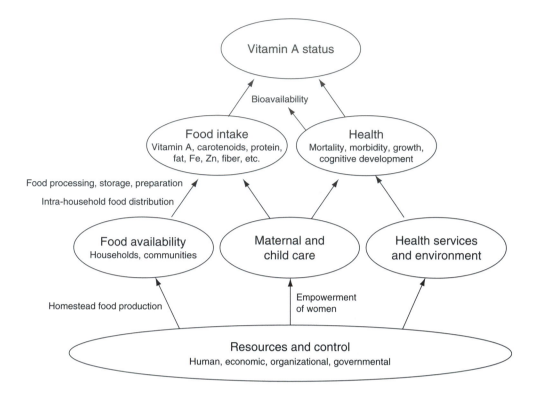

Fig. 5-11. WHO conceptual framework of causes of vitamin A deficiency in human populations. (From *UN Food Nutr. Bull.* **19,** 1998.)

epithelial cells and few or no goblet cells is indicative of vitamin A deficiency. With progressing vitamin A deficiency, the conjunctival surface takes on a dry, corrugated, irregular surface, ultimately developing an overlay of white, foamy, or "cheesy" material consisting of desquamated keratin and a heavy bacterial growth.[106] **Bitot's spots**, the *sine qua non* of conjunctival xerosis, are almost always bilateral oval or triangular structures first appearing temporal to the limbus and comprising a thickened, superficial layer of flattened cells usually with a keratinizing surface, a prominent granular cell layer, and acanthotic thickening with a disorganized basal cell layer, but with no goblet cells.

Conjunctival impression cytology has been shown to be capable of correctly identifying 82 to 93% of cases and 70 to 90% of normals; sensitivity declines and specificity increases when serum retinol or retinol relative dose–response cutoffs are also used in the definition of a case. The use of impression cytology yields estimates of vitamin A deficiency that are 5 to 10 times the rates of diagnosed xerophthal-

mia. Somer has suggested that vitamin A deficiency should be considered a public health problem when the prevalence of abnormal impression cytology reaches 20% in either women or children.

The earliest corneal signs of vitamin A deficiency are fine, fluorescein-positive, superficial punctuate keratopathy that usually begin in the inferior aspect of the cornea, particularly inferonasally. These lesions can be seen using the slit lamp microsope. Studies have revealed punctuate keratopathy in 60 to 75% of patients with nyctalopia or vitamin A-responsive conjunctival xerosis. With progressing vitamin A deficiency, the lesions become more numerous and concentrated, involving larger portions of the corneal surface. By the time most of the corneal surface is involved, the lesions are generally apparent by hand–light examination as a haziness and diminished wettability on the corneal surface. At that point the condition is called **corneal xerosis**. In addition to punctuate keratopathy, corneas affected at this level also show stromal edema, again mostly in the inferior aspect. If untreated, the condition progresses to the

---

[106] Most commonly the xerosis bacillus.

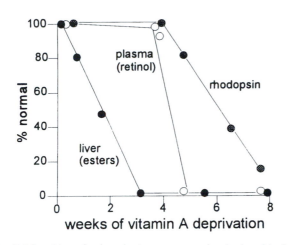

Fig. 5-12. Hepatic vitamin A stores must be depleted before changes in circulating retinol levels or photopigment concentrations occur.

point of corneal ulceration, frequently characterized by the presence of a single (in a minority of cases, by two to three) sharply defined ulcer varying in depth, usually one-fourth to one-half of corneal thickness, but sometimes deep enough to effect stromal loss. This can lead to deep stromal necrosis characterized by gray-yellow, edematous, and cystic lesions of varying size from 2 mm to most of the cornea.

The vitamers A can be accurately quantified in biological specimens using high-performance liquid–liquid partition chromatography (HPLC). Serum retinol is, therefore, a convenient parameter of vitamin A status. The homeostatic control of circulating retinol levels makes this parameter useful only in identifying subjects with chronically low vitamin A intakes sufficient to exhaust their hepatic stores that support the synthesis of RBP. With the caveats that vitamin A-deficient subjects with still-appreciable liver stores will have serum retinol levels in the normal range, and that deficiencies of protein and zinc, as well as hepatic illnesses, will depress serum RBP levels, RBP and retinol concentrations[107] less than 0.70 μM (20 $\mu g/dl$) are considered indicative of vitamin A deficiency. Still, almost 20% of nightblind children have serum retinol above this level (Table 5-27), children with greater serum retinol levels can show clinical xerophthalmia and or conjunctival metaplasia, and healthy adults depleted of vitamin A can show impaired dark adaptation at serum retinol levels of 20 to 30 $\mu g/dl$.

Because of the uncertainties associated with interpreting serum retinol values, additional tests have been devised to assess the mobilizable vitamin A

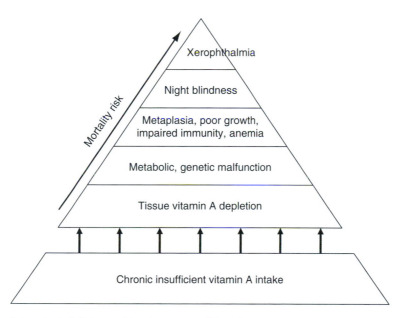

Fig. 5-13. Progression of vitamin A deficiency. (*From* West, K. P. [2002] *J. Nutr.* **132**, 2857S–2866S.)

---

[107] It should be remembered that RBP and retinol exist in the circulation in equimolar concentrations. Levels between 0.70 and 1.05 μM indicate marginal vitamin A status.

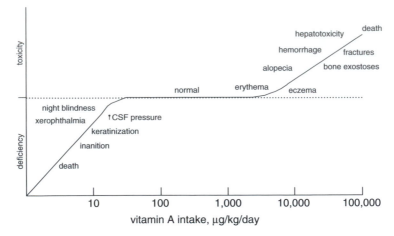

Fig. 5-14. Both low and high intakes of vitamin A can cause clinical signs.

Table 5-24. Signs of vitamin A deficiency

Organ system	Sign
General	Loss of appetite, retarded growth, drying and keratinization of membranes, infection, death
Dermatologic	Rough scaly skin, rough hair/feathers
Muscular	Weakness
Skeletal	Periosteal overgrowth, restriction of cranial cavity and spinal cord, narrowed foramina
Vital organs	Nephritis
Nervous system	Increased cerebrospinal fluid pressure, ataxia, constricted optic nerve at foramina
Reproductive	Aspermatogenesis, vaginal cornification, fetal death and resorption
Ocular	Nyctalopia, xerophthalmia, keratomalacia, constriction of optic nerve

Table 5-25. Stages of xerophthalmia

Stage	Signs
1. **Xerosis**	Dryness of conjunctiva
	Bitot's spots[a] (gray-white, foamy, greasy, "cheesy" deposits on the conjunctiva near the cornea; contain fatty degenerated epithelial cells and leukocytes)
	Ultimate extension to cornea
2. **Keratomalacia**	Softening of cornea
	Ultimate involvement of iris/lens
	Secondary infection

[a]There is some question about the relation of this sign, which can also occur in vitamin A-adequate individuals, to the deficiency.

capacity of the liver. These tests evaluate the serum responses to oral doses of either retinyl ester (acetate or palmitate) [in the **relative dose–response (RDR) test**] or the synthetic retinoid **3,4-didehydroretinol**[108] [in the modified relative dose–response (MRDR) test].[109] Such approaches have indicated that preterm infants generally have reduced hepatic vitamin A stores. The concentrations of vitamin A in breast milk (i.e., primarily retinyl palmitate in milk fat) drop in vitamin A deficiency and can, therefore, be used to detect the deficiency in mothers.[110]

---

[108] This compound has also been called dehydroretinol and vitamin A_2.

[109] The RDR test requires two samples of blood: a fasting sample drawn immediately before the administration of the test dose; another sample drawn 5 hr later. Retinol is determined in each sample, and the percentage response over baseline is calculated. For the MRDR, only a single blood sample is required; it is taken 4–6 hr after oral administration of 3,4-didehydroretinol. Both retinol and 3,4-didehydroretinol are determined in the sample, and the response is taken as the molar ratio of the two retinoids. Both tests assume that the appearance of retinoid in the plasma is a function of the amount also entering from endogenous hepatic stores. Therefore, an RDR value of ≥20% or an MRDR value of 20–30% is taken as indicative of inadequate hepatic storage (<0.07 μmol/g) of the vitamin; children with such low stores are almost certain to be vitamin A deficient.

[110] Breast milk retinyl palmitate concentrations typically fall in the range of 1.75–2.45 μM; levels ≤1.05 μM (i.e., ≤8 μg/g milk fat) are generally considered as indicative of vitamin A deficiency.

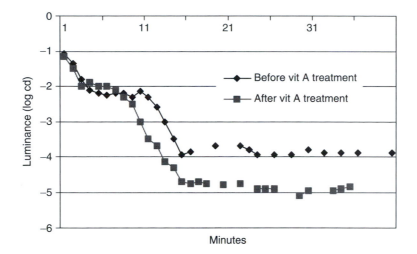

Fig. 5-15. Dark adaptation in a vitamin A-deficient individual before and after vitamin A treatment. (*After* Russell, R. M., Multack, R., Smith, V., Krill, A. and Rosenberg, I. H. [1973]. *Lancet* **2**, 1161–1164.)

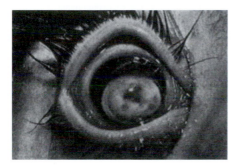

Fig. 5-16. Keratomalacia in a vitamin A-deficient child. (Courtesy of D. S. McLaren, American University of Beirut.)

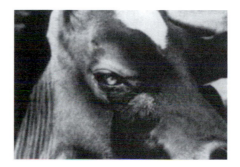

Fig. 5-17. Vitamin A-deficient calf: blind with copious lacrimation. (Courtesy of J. K. Loosli, University of Florida.)

Treatment of Vitamin A Deficiency

Because vitamin A is stored in appreciable amounts in the liver, it can be administered in relatively large, infrequent doses with efficacy. In cases of clear or suspected xerophthalmia, particularly in communities in which the deficiency is prevalent, vitamin A is administered orally in large doses, followed by an additional dose the next day and a third a few weeks later (Table 5-28). Oral administration of water miscible or oil solutions of the vitamin are as effective as water-miscible preparations administered parenterally. Water-miscible preparations are much more effective than oil solutions when administered parentally (i.e., by intramuscular injection). Topical administration on the skin is ineffective.

Night blindness due to vitamin A deficiency responds within hours to days upon the administration of vitamin A, although full recovery of visual function may take weeks and the fading of retinal lesions may take up to three months. Active Bitot's spots and the accompanying xerosis respond rapidly to vitamin A treatment with, in most cases, lesions regressing within days and disappearing within 2 to 3 weeks. Punctate keratopathy of the cornea also responds rapidly to vitamin A, improving within a week in response to a large oral dose.

IX. Vitamin A Toxicity

The hepatic storage of vitamin A tends to mitigate against the development of intoxication due to intakes in excess of physiological needs. However, persistent large overdoses (more than 1000 times the nutritionally required amount) can exceed the capacity of the liver to store and catabolize and will thus produce intoxication[111] (Fig. 5-14). This is marked by

---

[111] It has been suggested that the hepatic damage following hepatitis B infection may be due to the toxic effects of retinoids, which accumulate in the cholestatic liver.

Table 5-26. Clinical classification of eye lesions caused by vitamin A deficiency (from WHO)

Site affected	Clinical sign	Designation
Retina	Night blindness, *also* nyctalopia	XN
	Fundus specs	XF
Conjunctiva	Xerosis	X1A
	Bitot's spots	X1B
Cornea	Xerosis	X2
	Ulceration/keratomalacia < one-third of surface	X3A
	Ulceration/keratomalacia = one-third of surface	X3B
	Scar	XS

Table 5-27. Relationship of serum retinol level and clinical vitamin A deficiency in Indonesian preschool children[a]

Clinical status			Case frequency, by serum retinol level		
			Deficient	Low	Adequate
XN	X1B	n	<10 μg/dl	10–20 μg/dl	>20 μg/dl
+	–	174	27%	55%	18%
–	+	51	31%	57%	12%
+	+	79	38%	53%	9%
–	–	252	8%	37%	55%

[a]From Sommer, A., Hussaini, G., Muhilal, L., Tarwotjo, I., Susanto, D., Saroso, J. S. (1980). *Am. J. Clin. Nutr.* **33**, 887–891.

the appearance in the plasma of high levels of retinyl esters that, because they are associated with lipoproteins rather than RBP, are outside the normal strict control of vitamin A transport to extrahepatic tissues.

Four aspects of vitamin A metabolism tend to protect against hypervitaminosis:

1. Relatively inefficient conversion of the provitamins A in the gut
2. The unidirectional oxidation of the vitamin to a form (retinoic acid) that is rapidly catabolized and excreted

3. The relative excess capacity of CRBP(II) to bind retinol
4. Accelerated vitamin A catabolism

Hypervitaminosis A, therefore, requires high exposures. In humans it is manifest after single large doses (>660,000 IU for adults, >330,000 IU for children), or after doses exceeding 100,000 IU/day have been taken for several months. Children experiencing hypervitaminosis A develop transient (one to two days) signs: nausea, vomiting, signs due to increased cerebrospinal fluid pressure (headache, vertigo, blurred or double vision), and muscular incoordination. Most field studies have found that 3 to 9% of children given high single doses (>200,000 IU) for prophylaxis show transient nausea, vomiting, headache, and general irritability; a similar percentage of younger children may show bulging fontanelles[112] subsiding within 48 to 96 hours. Those reacting to extremely large doses of the vitamin show drowsiness, loss of appetite, and malaise, followed by skin exfoliation, itching (circumocular), and recurrent vomiting.

Chronic hypervitaminosis A occurs with recurrent exposures exceeding 12,500 IU (infants) to 33,000 IU (adult). It is manifest mainly as changes in the skin and mucous membranes. Dry lips (*cheilitis*) is a common early sign in humans, often followed by dryness and fragility of the nasal mucosa, leading to dry eyes and conjunctivitis. Skin lesions include dryness, pruritis, erythema, scaling, peeling of the palms and soles, hair loss (alopecia), and nail fragility. Headache, nausea, and vomiting (signs of increased intracranial pressure) have also been reported.

Hypervitaminosis A can affect bone; therefore, it has been suggested that high intakes of vitamin A may contribute to the pathogenesis of osteoporosis. Although most epidemiological studies have not revealed a relationship of vitamin A status and fracture risk, one study[113] found reduced bone mineral density with intakes greater than 0.6 mg RE (2000 IU)/day. According to the Third National Health and Nutrition Examination Survey (NHANES III), 50% of American adults consume more than that level. An analysis of results from more than 72,000 postmenopausal women in the Nurse's Health Study[114] found that individuals report-

---

[112] That is, the convex displacement of the infant's "soft spot" (the membranous covering of the cranial sutures) caused by fluid accumulation in the skull cavity or increased intracranial pressure.

[113] The Rancho Bernardo Study of 570 women and 388 men found a U-shaped relationship of bone mineral density and vitamin A intake, with optimal bone mineral density occurring at 2000–2800 IU (0.6–0.9 mg RE) per day (Promislow, J. H. E., Goodman-Gruen, D., Slymen, D. J. and Barret-Connor, E. [2002]. *J. Nutr.* **129**, 2246–2250).

[114] Feskanich, D., Singh, V., Willet, W. C., and Colditz, G. A. 2002. Vitamin A and hip fracture among postmenopausal women. *JAMA* **287**, 47–54.

Table 5-28. Treatment schedule for xerophthalmia[a]

		Vitamin A dose,[b] by age		
Case	Time	<6 mos.	6–12 mos.	>1 yr.
Xerophthalmia	Day 1	15,000 RE	30,000 RE	60,000 RE
	Next day	15,000 RE	30,000 RE	60,000 RE
	2–4 wks later	15,000 RE	30,000 RE	60,000 RE
Women of reproductive age without severe corneal lesions	Daily for 2 wks		3,000 RE	
Subjects with complicated measles	Day 1	15,000 RE	30,000 RE	60,000 RE
	Next day	15,000 RE	30,000 RE	60,000 RE
With severe protein-energy malnutrition	Day 1	15,000 RE	30,000 RE	60,000 RE
	Every 4–6 mos.[c]			60,000 RE
For prevention in high-risk populations	Once	15,000 RE	30,000 RE	60,000 RE[d]
	Every 4–6 mos.			60,000 RE

[a]From WHO (1997). *Vitamin A Supplementation: A Guide to Their Use in the Treatment and Prevention of Vitamin A Deficiency and Xerophthalmia*, 2nd ed., Geneva: WHO.
[b]Oil solution administered orally.
[c]Until signs of protein-energy malnutrition subside.
[d]Including postpartum mothers.

ing intakes of at least 2000 IU/d had twice the risk of hip fracture due to mild or moderate trauma than those reporting intakes less than 500 IU/d. Hypervitaminotic A animals frequently show bone abnormalities that apparently result from changes in impaired osteoclastic activities and enhanced osteoblastic activities resulting in overgrowth of periosteal bone in a non–vitamin D-dependent manner. This, in turn, can lead to impairments in visual function by restricting the optic foramina and pinching the optic nerve, and in motor function by increasing cerebrospinal fluid pressure. Because retinol has potent membranolytic activity, it has been proposed that disruption of cellular and subcellular membranes, with the consequent release of lysosomal enzymes, may be involved in these bone cell lesions. Signs of hypervitaminosis A (Table 5-29) are usually reversed upon cessation of exposure to the vitamin.

Table 5-29. Signs of hypervitaminosis A

Organ affected	Signs
General	Muscle and joint pains, headache
Skin	Erythema, desquamation, alopecia
Mucous membranes	Cheilitis, stomatitis, conjunctivitis
Liver	Dysfunction
Skeletal	Thinning and fracture of long bones

Signs of hypervitaminosis A are associated with plasma retinol levels >3 μmol/L and increases in serum retinyl ester levels without substantial increases in circulating holo-RBP. Dose-dependent elevations of plasma triglycerides and very low-density lipoprotein (VLDL) levels have been observed in patients on retinoid therapy. Several studies have found that about 30% of patients treated with 13-*cis*-retinoic acid (effective in treating globular acne) had increased LDL/HDL ratios; such an increase, if persistent, would increase the risk of ischemic heart disease. Some 15% of such patients report arthralgia and myalgia.

Embryotoxic Potential of High Levels of Vitamin A

Retinoids can be toxic to maternally exposed embryos, a fact that limits their therapeutic uses and raises concerns about the safety of high-level vitamin A supplementation for pregnant animals and humans. This is especially true for 13-*cis*-retinoic acid, which is very effective in the treatment of acne but can cause severe disruption of cephalic neural crest cell activity, which results in birth defects characterized by craniofacial, central nervous system, cardiovascular, and thymus malformations. Similar effects have been induced in animals by high doses of retinol, all-*trans*-retinoic acid, or 13-*cis*-retinoic acid. Animal model studies suggest that the teratogenic effects of excess vitamin A are due to the embryonic exposure to all-*trans*-retinoic acid (Table 5-30),[115] although those effects can be induced without substantially increasing maternal plasma concentrations of that metabolite. The mechanism of teratogenic action of retinoids is unclear, but it has been proposed that it involves the elevated production of mRNAs for specific isoforms of RARs,[116] leading to an imbalance in the heterodimers formed among the various RARs, RXRs, and other hormone receptors and consequently affecting the expression of a variety of genes.

The critical period for fetal exposure to maternally derived retinoids is the time when organogenesis is occurring—that is, before many women suspect they are pregnant. This is also before the development of fetal retinoid receptors as well as cellular and transport binding proteins, which serve to restrict maternal–fetal transfer of retinoids. Fetal malformations of cranial–neural crest origin have been reported in cases of oral use of all-*trans*-retinoic acid in treating acne vulgaris and of regular prenatal vitamin A supplements in humans. The latter have generally been linked to daily exposures at or above 20,000–25,000 IU. A retrospective epidemiologic study reported an increased risk of birth defects associated with an apparent threshold

exposure of about 10,000 IU of preformed vitamin A per day[117,118]; however, the elevated risk of birth defects was observed in a small group of women whose average intake of the vitamin exceeded 21,000 IU/day (Table 5-31).

Carotenoid Toxicity

The toxicities of carotenoids are considered low, and circumstantial evidence suggests that β-carotene intakes of as much as 30 mg/day are without side effects other than the accumulation of the carotenoid in the skin, with consequent yellowing of the skin (**carotenodermia**). Regular, high intakes of β-carotene can lead to accumulation in fatty tissues and thus to this condition. An intervention study with a small number of subjects showed that a daily intake of 30 mg of β-carotene from carotene-rich foods produced carotenodermia within 25 to 42 days of exposure;[119] the effect persisted for at least 14 days, and in some cases for more than 42 days, after cessation of carotene exposure. In addition to yielding retinal by symmetric cleavage, β-carotene can be cleaved asymmetrically to yield apo-carotenals and apo-carotenoic acids by a co-oxidative mechanism. Thus, it appears that under highly oxidative conditions β-carotene can yield oxidative breakdown products that can diminish retinoic acid signaling by interfering with the binding of retinoic acid

Table 5-30. Teratogenicity of vitamin A in rodent models

Species	Retinyl palmitate[a]		all-*trans*-Retinoic acid[a] (teratogenic)
	Highest nonteratogenic	Lowest teratogenic	
Rat[b]	30	90	6
Mouse[b]	15	50	3
Rabbit[c]	2	5	6
Hamster	—	—	7

[a]Dosage level (mg/kg/day).
[b]Exposed on gestational days 6–15.
[c]Exposed on gestational days 6–18.
Source: Kamm, J. J. (1982). *J. Am. Acad. Dermatol.* **64,** 552–559.

Table 5-31. Teratogenic risk of high prenatal exposures to preformed vitamin A

Retinol intake (IU/day)	Pregnancies	Cranial–neural crest defects	Total defects
0–5,000	6,410	33 (0.51%)	86 (1.3%)
5,001–10,000	12,688	59 (0.47%)	196 (1.5%)
10,001–15,000	3,150	20 (0.63%)	42 (1.3%)
>15,000	500	9 (1.80%)	15 (3.0%)

Source: Rothman, K. J., Moore, L. L., Singer, M. R., Nguyen, U. D. T., Mannino, S., and Milunsky, A. (1995). *N. Engl. J. Med.* **333,** 1369–1373.

---

[115] The embryo of dams exposed to high levels of vitamin A also show appreciable amounts of 4-oxo-retinoic acid and 5,6-epoxy-retinoic acid.

[116] That teratogenic doses of all-*trans*-retinoic acid produce prolonged increases in RARα2 mRNA levels supports this hypothesis.

[117] Rothman et al. (*N. Engl. J. Med.* **33,** 1995, p. 1369) estimated that apparent threshold, using regression techniques. That level of exposure to preformed vitamin A was associated with a birth defect risk of 1 in 57. This report has been criticized for suspected misclassification of malformations.

[118] This intake compares to the current RDA for pregnant women of 800 μg of RE (i.e., 2700 IU) per day.

[119] Carotenodermia was diagnosed only after plasma total carotenoid concentrations exceeded 4.0 mg/liter.

to RAR. This effect has been proposed as the basis for the finding that a regular daily dose of β-carotene increased lung cancer risk among smokers. (For further discussion, see "Role of Vitamin A in Carcinogenesis.")

X. Case Studies

Instructions

Review each of the following case reports, paying special attention to the diagnostic indicators on which the respective treatments were based. Then answer the questions that follow.

Case 1

The physical examination of a 5-month-old boy with severe **marasmus**[120] showed extreme wasting, apathy, and ocular changes: in the left eye, Bitot's spots and conjunctival and corneal xerosis; in the right eye, corneal liquefaction and keratomalacia with subsequent prolapse of the iris, extrusion of lens, and loss of vitreous humor. The child was 65 cm tall and weighed 4.5 kg. His malnutrition had begun at cessation of breast feeding at 4 months, after which he experienced weight loss and diarrhea.

Laboratory Results

Parameter	Patient	Normal range
Hb (hemoglobin)	10.7 g/dl	12–16 g/dl
HCT (hematocrit)	36 ml/dl	35–47 mg/dl
WBC (white blood cells)	15,000/μl	5000–9000/μl
Serum protein	5.6 g/dl	6–8 g/dl
Serum albumin	2.49 g/dl	3.5–5.5 g/dl
Plasma sodium	139 mEq/liter	136–145 mEq/liter
Plasma potassium	3.5 mEq/liter	3.5–5.0 mEq/liter
Blood glucose	70 mg/dl	60–100 mg/dl
Total bilirubin	1.1 mg/dl	<1 mg/dl
Serum retinol	5.5 μg/dl	30–60 μg/dl
Serum β-carotene	10.7 μg/dl	50–250 μg/dl
Serum vitamin E	220 μg/dl	500–1500 μg/dl

The child had an infection, showing **otitis media**[121] and *Salmonella* septicemia,[122] which responded to antibiotic treatment in the first week. The patient was given, by nasogastric tube, an aqueous dispersion of retinyl palmitate (with a nonionic detergent) at the rate of 3000 μg/kg per day for 4 days. This increased his plasma retinol concentration from 5 to 35 μg/dl by the second day, at which level it was maintained for the next 12 days. The child responded to general nutritional rehabilitation with a high-protein, high-energy formula that was followed by whole milk supplemented with solid foods. He recovered, but was permanently blind in the right eye and was left with a mild corneal opacity in the left eye. He returned to his family after 10 weeks of hospitalization.

Case 2

An obese 15-year-old girl, 152 cm tall and weighing 100 kg, was admitted to the hospital for partial jejunoileal bypass surgery for morbid obesity. She had a past history of obsessive eating that had not been correctable by diet. Except for massive obesity, her physical examination was negative.

Initial laboratory results

Parameter	Patient	Normal range
Hb	14 g/dl	12–15 g/dl
RBC	$4.5 \times 10^6/\mu l$	$4–5 \times 10^6/\mu l$
WBC	8000/μl	5000–9000/μl
Serum retinol	38 μg/dl	30–60 μg/dl
Serum β-carotene	12 μg/dl	50–300 μg/dl
Serum vitamin E	580 μg/dl	500–1500 μg/dl
Serum 25-OH-D$_3$	11 ng/dl	8–40 ng/dl

The following were within normal ranges: serum electrolytes, calcium, phosphorus, triglycerides, cholesterol, total protein, albumin, total bilirubin, iron, TBIC (total serum iron-binding capacity), copper, zinc, folic acid, thiamin, and vitamin B$_{12}$.

The patient encountered few postoperative complications except for mild bouts of diarrhea and some fatigue. Over the next year, she lost 45 kg of body

---

[120] Extreme emaciation or general atrophy, occurring especially in young children; it is caused by extreme undernutrition, owing primarily to lack of energy and protein.

[121] Inflammation of the middle ear.

[122] Presence in the blood of pathogenic, gram-negative, rod-shaped bacteria of the genus *Salmonella.*

weight while ingesting a liberal diet. She reported having three to four stools daily, but denied having any objectionable diarrhea or changes in stool appearance. Two years after surgery, she noted the onset of inflammatory horny lesions above her knees and elbows, and she experienced some difficulty in seeing at dusk. The skin lesions failed to respond to topical corticosteroids and oral antihistamine therapy. Because of intensification of these signs, she sought medical help; however, the cause was not determined.

She was readmitted to the hospital, complaining of her skin disorder and night blindness. At that time, she showed evidence of mild liver dysfunction, and her serum concentrations of retinol and β-carotene were 16 and 14 μg/dl, respectively. Her fecal fat was 70 g/day (normal, <7 g/day). Biopsies of the skin of her left thigh and right upper arm each showed **hyperkeratosis** and horny plugging of dilated follicles. She was treated with 15,000 μg of retinyl palmitate given orally three times daily for 6 months. By 1 month, the follicular hyperkeratosis had cleared and healed with residual pigmentation. By 2 months, the night blindness had subsided. At that time her serum retinol concentration was 54 μg/dl, β-carotene was 7 μg/dl, α-tocopherol was 1.6 μg/ml, and urinary [^{57}Co]B$_{12}$ was 6.7% (normal, 7–8%). She has been well on a daily oral supplement of 1500 μg of retinyl palmitate.

Case 3

A 41-year-old man was housed in a metabolic ward for 2 years during a clinical investigation of vitamin A deficiency. He weighed 77.3 kg and was healthy by standard criteria (history, physical examination, and laboratory studies). For 505 days, he was fed a casein-based formula diet that contained <10 μg of vitamin A per day. His initial plasma retinol concentration was 58 μg/dl, and his body vitamin A pool, determined by isotope dilution, was 766 mg (10 mg/kg). At the end of 1 year, his plasma retinol had declined to 25 μg/dl, and he began to show follicular hyperkeratosis (see Fig. 5-18). On day 300 his plasma retinol was 20 μg/dl, and he showed a mild anemia (Hb 12.6 mg/dl). Two months later, by which time his plasma retinol had dropped to 10 μg/dl, he developed night blindness as evidenced by changes in dark adaptation and electroretinogram. When his plasma retinol reached 3 μg/dl, his body vitamin A pool was 377 mg and repletion with vitamin A was begun with doses starting at 150 μg and increasing to 1200 μg of retinol per day over a 145-day period. After receiving 150 μg of retinol per day for 82 days, his night blindness was partially repaired, but his skin keratinization remained and his plasma retinol level was only 8 μg/dl. Then, after receiving 300 μg of retinol per day for 42 days, his follicular hyperkeratosis resolved and his plasma retinol level was 20 μg/dl.

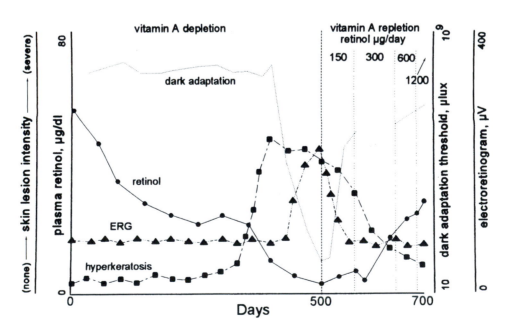

Fig. 5-18. Subject responses to vitamin deprivation and repletion. ERG, Electroretinogram.

At 600μg of retinol per day level, his plasma retinol was in the normal range, and all signs of vitamin A deficiency disappeared.

Case Questions

1. For each case, what signs/symptoms indicated vitamin A deficiency?

2. Propose hypotheses to explain why each patient in cases 1 and 2 responded to oral vitamin A treatment even though they had very different medical conditions. Outline tests of those hypotheses.

3. Comment on the value of serum retinol concentration for the diagnosis of nutritional vitamin A status.

Study Questions and Exercises

1. Discuss how the absorption, transport, tissue distribution, and intracellular activities of vitamin A relate to the concept of solubility.

2. Construct a flow diagram showing vitamin A, in its various forms, as it passes from ingested food, through the body where it functions in its various physiologic roles, and ultimately to its routes of elimination.

3. Construct a decision tree for the diagnosis of vitamin A deficiency in a human or animal.

4. Night blindness is particularly prevalent among alcoholics. Propose a hypothesis for the metabolic basis of this phenomenon and outline an experimental approach to test it.

5. Discuss the points of control, and intervention possibilities for each, in the WHO conceptual framework for vitamin A deficiency.

Recommended Reading

ACC/SCN Consultative Group. (1994). Controlling Vitamin A deficiency. Nutrition Policy Paper No. 14 (Gillespie, S., and Mason, J. B., eds.). United Nations Administrative Committee of Coordination—Subcommittee on Nutrition, New York, 81 pp.

Azais-Braesco, V., and Pascal, G. (2000). Vitamin A in pregnancy: Requirements and safety limits. *Am. J. Clin. Nutr.* **71**(Suppl.), 1325S–1333S.

Baurenfeind, J. C. (ed.) (1986). *Vitamin A Deficiency and Its Control.* Academic Press, New York.

Beaton, G. H., Mortorell, R., Aronson, K. J., Edmonston, B., McCabe, G., Ross, A. C., and Harvey, B. (1993). Effectiveness of Vitamin A Supplementation in the Control of Young Child Morbidity and Mortality in Developing Countries. Nutrition Policy Discussion Paper No. 13, United Nations Administrative Committee of Coordination—Subcommittee on Nutrition, New York, 120 pp.

Bendich, A., and Langseth, L. (1989). Safety of vitamin A. *Am. J. Clin. Nutr.* **49**, 358–371.

Bloem, M. W. (1995). Interdependence of vitamin A and iron: An important association for programmes of anemia control. *Proc. Nutr. Soc.* **54**, 501–508.

Blomhoff, R. (1994). Transport and metabolism of vitamin A. *Nutr. Rev.* **52**(Suppl.), S13–S23.

Blomhoff, R., Green, M. H., and Norum, K. R. (1992). Vitamin A: Physiological and biochemical processing. *Annu. Rev. Nutr.* **12**, 37–57.

Casetenmiller, J. J. M., and West, C. E. (1998). Bioavailability and bioconversion of carotenoids. *Ann. Rev. Nutr.* **18**, 19–38.

Chytil, F., and Ong, D. E. (1984). Cellular retinoid-binding proteins. In *The Retinoids* (J. C. Baurenfeind, ed.), pp. 89–123. Academic Press, New York.

Congdon, N. G., and West, K. P., Jr. (2002). Physiological indicators of vitamin A status. *J. Nutr.* **132**, 2889S–2894S.

Friedrich, W. (1988). Vitamin A and its provitamins. In *Vitamins*, pp. 65–140. Walter de Gruyter, New York.

Frolick, C. A. (1984). Metabolism of retinoids. In *The Retinoids* (J. C. Baurenfeind, ed.), pp. 177–208. Academic Press, New York.

Futoryan, T., and Gilchrest, B. A. (1994). Retinoids and the skin. *Nutr. Rev.* **52**, 299–310.

Gerster, H. (1993). Anticarcinogenic effect of common carotenoids. *Int. J. Vit. Nutr. Res.* **63**, 93–112.

Goodman, D. S. (1984). Plasma retinol-binding proteins. In *The Retinoids* (J. C. Baurenfeind, ed.), pp. 41–87. Academic Press, New York.

Harrison, E. H. (2005) Mechanisms of digestion and absorption of dietary vitamin A. *Ann. Rev. Nutr.* **25**, 87–103.

Hathcock, J. N., Hattin, D. G., Jenkins, M. Y., McDonald, J. T., Sundarsan, P. R., and Wilkening, V. L. (1990). Evaluation of vitamin A toxicity. *Am. J. Clin. Nutr.* **52**, 183–202.

Key, T. (1994). Micronutrients and cancer etiology: The epidemiological evidence. *Proc. Nutr. Soc.* **53**, 605–614.

Krinsky, N. I. (1994). Carotenoids and cancer: Basic research studies. In *Natural Antioxidants in Human Health and Disease* (B. Frei, ed.), pp. 239–261. Academic Press, New York.

Li, E., and Norris, A. W. (1996). Structure/function of cytosolic vitamin A-binding proteins. *Annu. Rev. Nutr.* **16**, 205–234.

Lippman, S. M., and Meyskens, F. L., Jr. (1989). Retinoids for the prevention of cancer. In *Nutrition and Cancer Prevention* (T. E. Moon and M. S. Miccozzi, eds.), pp. 243–272. Marcel Dekker, New York.

Maden, M. (1994). Vitamin A in embryonic development. *Nutr. Rev.* **52**(Suppl.), S3–S12.

Mangelsdorf, D. J. (1994). Vitamin A receptors. *Annu. Rev. Nutr.* **52**(Suppl.), S32–S44.

Mason, J. B., Lotfi, M., Dalmiya, N., Sethuraman, K., Deitchler, M., Geiber, S., Gillenwater, K., Gilman, A., Mason, K., and Mock, N. (2001). *The Micronutrient Report: Current Progress in the Control of Vitamin A, Iodine and Iron Deficiencies.* The Micronutrient Initiative, Ottawa, 116 pp.

McClaren, D. S., and Frigg, M. (1997). *Sight and Life Manual on Vitamin A Deficiency Disorders (VADD).* Task Force for Sight and Life, Basel, 138 pp.

Olson, J. A. (1996). Vitamin A. In *Present Knowledge in Nutrition* (E. E. Ziegler and L. J. Filer, Jr., eds.), 7th ed., pp. 109–119. ILSI Press, Washington, DC.

Ong, D. E. (1994). Cellular transport and metabolism of vitamin A: Roles of the cellular retinol-binding proteins. *Nutr. Rev.* **52**(Suppl.), S24–S31.

Packer, L. (ed.) (1993). *Methods in Enzymology*, Vol. 241: *Carotenoids, Part B: Metabolism, Genetics, and Biosynthesis.* Academic Press, San Diego, CA.

Parker, R. S. (1996). Absorption, metabolism and transport of carotenoids. *FASEB J.* **10**, 542–551.

Petkovich, M. (1992). Regulation of gene expression by vitamin A: The role of nuclear retinoic acid receptors. *Annu. Rev. Nutr.* **12**, 443–471.

Pfahl, M., and Chytil, F. (1996). Regulation of metabolism by retinoic acid and its nuclear receptors. *Annu. Rev. Nutr.* **16**, 257–283.

Prabhala, R. H., Garewal, H. S., Meyskens, F. L., Jr., and Watson, R. R. (1990). Immunomodulation in humans caused by beta-carotene and vitamin A. *Nutr. Res.* **10**, 1473–1486.

Reifen, R. (2002). Vitamin A as an anti-inflammatory agent. *Proc. Nutr. Soc.* **61**, 397–400.

Ross, C. (1992). Vitamin A status: Relationship to immunity and the antibody response. *Proc. Soc. Exp. Biol. Med.* **200**, 303–320.

Ross, J. S., and Harvey, P. W. J. (2003). Contribution of breastfeeding to vitamin A nutrition of infants: A simulation model. *Bull WHO* **81**, 80–86.

Russell, R. M. (2000). The vitamin A spectrum: from deficiency to toxicity. *Am. J. Clin. Nutr.* **71**, 878–884.

Solomons, N. W., and Bulux, J. (1993). Plant sources of provitamin A and human nutriture. *Nutr. Rev.* **51**, 199–204.

Sommer, A. (1994). Vitamin A: Its effect on childhood sight and life. *Nutr. Rev.* **52**(Suppl.), S60–S66.

Sommer, A. (1995). *Vitamin A Deficiency and Its Consequences: A Field Guide to Their Detection and Control*, 3rd ed. World Health Organization, Geneva.

Sommer, A., West, K. P., Jr., Olson, J. A., and Ross, C. A. (1996). *Vitamin A Deficiency: Health, Survival, and Vision.* Oxford University Press, New York, 452 pp.

Soprano, D. R., and Soprano, K. J. (1995). Retinoids as teratogens. *Annu. Rev. Nutr.* **15**, 111–132.

Soprano, D. R., Qin, P., and Soprano, K. J. (2004) Retinoic acid receptors and cancers. *Annu. Rev. Nutr.* **24**, 201–221.

Tompkins, A., and Hussey, G. (1989). Vitamin A, immunity and infection. *Nutr. Res. Rev.* **2**, 17–28.

Underwood, B. A. (1989). Teratogenicity of vitamin A. In *Elevated Dosages of Vitamins: Benefits and Hazards* (P. Walter, G. Brubacher, and H. Stähelin, eds.), pp. 42–55. Hans Huber, Berlin.

Underwood, B. A. (1990). Vitamin A prophylaxis programs in developing countries: Past experiences and future prospects. *Nutr. Rev.* **48**, 265–274.

Underwood, B. A. (1992). Was the "anti-infective" vitamin misnamed? *Nutr. Rev.* **52**, 140–143.

Underwood, B. A. (1994). Maternal vitamin A status and its importance in infancy and early childhood. *Am. J. Clin. Nutr.* **59**(Suppl.), 517S–524S.

Van den Berg, H. Carotenoid interactions. (1999). *Nutr. Rev.* **57**, 1–10.

Van Poppel, G., and Goldbohm, R. A. (1995). Epidemiologic evidence for β-carotene and cancer prevention. *Am. J. Clin. Nutr.* **62**(Suppl.), 1393S–1402S.

Wang, Z., Yin, S., Zhao, X., Russell, R. M., and Tang, G. (2004). β-Carotene-vitamin A equivalence in Chinese adults assessed by an isotope dilution technique. *Br. J. Nutr.* **91**, 121–131.

West, K. P., Jr. (2002). Extent of vitamin A deficiency among preschool children and women of reproductive age. *J. Nutr.* **132**, 2857S–2866S.

West, K. P., Jr., Howard, G. R., and Sommer, A. (1989). Vitamin A and infection: Public health implications. *Annu. Rev. Nutr.* **9**, 63–86.

Willett, W. C. (1990). Vitamin A and lung cancer. *Nutr. Rev.* **48**, 201–211.

Willett, W. C., and Hunter, D. J. (1994). Vitamin A and cancers of the breast, large bowel and prostate: Epidemiologic evidence. *Nutr. Rev.* **52**(Suppl.), S53–S59.

Wolf, G. (2004). The visual cycle of the cone photoreceptors of the retina. *Nutr. Rev.* **62**, 283–286.

Wolf, G. (2001). The enzymatic cleavage of β-carotene: End of a controversy. *Nutr. Rev.* **59,** 116–118.

Wolf, G. (1991). The intracellular vitamin A-binding proteins: An overview of their functions. *Nutr. Rev.* **49,** 1–12.

World Health Organization. (1995). Global prevalence of Vitamin A deficiency. MDIS Paper #2. World Health Organization, Geneva.

Yeum, K. J., and Russell, R. M. (2002). Carotenoid bioavailability and bioconversion. *Ann. Rev. Nutr.* **22,** 483–504.

Vitamin D

6

By following the reasoning that vitamin D is not required in the diet under conditions of adequate ultraviolet irradiation of skin and that it is the precursor of a hormone, it is likely that the vitamin is not truly a vitamin but must be regarded as a pro-hormone. These arguments, however, are only semantic; the fact remains that vitamin D is taken in the diet and is an extremely potent substance which prevents a deficiency disease.

—H. F. DeLuca

I.	Significance of Vitamin D	146
II.	Sources of Vitamin D	147
III.	Enteric Absorption of Vitamin D	150
IV.	Transport of Vitamin D	151
V.	Metabolism of Vitamin D	154
VI.	Metabolic Functions of Vitamin D	157
VII.	Vitamin D Deficiency	169
VIII.	Vitamin D Toxicity	175
IX.	Case Studies	176
	Study Questions and Exercises	177
	Recommended Reading	177

Anchoring Concepts

1. Vitamin D is the generic descriptor for *steroids*, exhibiting qualitatively the biological activity of cholecalciferol (i.e., vitamin D_3).
2. Most vitamers D are *hydrophobic* and thus are insoluble in aqueous environments (e.g., plasma, interstitial fluids, cytosol).
3. Vitamin D is not required in the diets of animals or humans adequately exposed to sources of *ultraviolet light* (e.g., sunlight).
4. Deficiencies of vitamin D lead to structural lesions of *bone*.

Learning Objectives

1. To understand the nature of the various sources of vitamin D.
2. To understand the means of endogenous production of vitamin D.
3. To understand the means of enteric absorption of vitamin D.
4. To understand the metabolism involved in the activation of vitamin D to its functional forms.
5. To understand the role of vitamin D and other endocrine factors in calcium homeostasis.
6. To understand the physiologic implications of high doses of vitamin D.

Vocabulary

Boron (B)
Cage layer fatigue
Calbindins
Calcidiol
Calcinosis
Calcipotriol
Calcitonin (CT)
Calcitriol
Calcitroic acid
Calcium (Ca)
Calcium-binding protein (CaBP)
Calmodulin
Cholecalciferol (vitamin D_3)
DBP (vitamin D-binding protein)
1,25-Dihydroxyvitamin D (1,25-[OH]$_2$-vitamin D)
7-Dehydrocholesterol
Diuresis
Epiphyseal plate
Ergocalciferol (vitamin D_2)
Ergosterol
Genu varum
25-hydroxyvitamin D (25-OH-vitamin D)
Hypercalcemia
Hyperphosphatemia
Hypersensitivity
Hypocalcemia
Hypoparathyroidism
Hypophosphatemia
Lead (Pb)
Milk fever
25-OH-Vitamin D 1-hydroxylase

Osteoblast
Osteocalcin
Osteochondrosis
Osteoclast
Osteomalacia
Osteon
Osteopenia
Osteoporosis
Parathyroid gland
Parathyroid hormone (PTH)
Prolactin
Provitamin D
Pseudofracture
Pseudohypoparathyroidism
Psoriasis
Rickets
Sarcopenia
Tibial dyschondroplasia
Transcaltachia
Transcalciferin
Varus deformity
Vitamin D-binding protein (DBP)
Vitamin D-dependent rickets type I, type II
Vitamin D receptors (VDRs)
Vitamin D$_2$
Vitamin D$_3$
Vitamin D 25-hydroxylase
Vitamin D-dependent rickets type I, type II
Vitamin D-responsive elements (VDREs)
Vitamin D-resistance

I. Significance of Vitamin D

Vitamin D,[1] the "sunshine vitamin," is actually a hormone produced from sterols in the body by the photolytic action of ultraviolet light on the skin; individuals who receive modest exposures to sunlight are able to produce their own vitamin D. However, this is not the case for many people, such as those who spend most of their days indoors, particularly those living in the northern latitudes, or animals reared in controlled environments. Such individuals must obtain the nutrient from their diets; for them it is, indeed, a vitamin in the traditional sense.[2]

Vitamin D plays an important role, along with the essential minerals **calcium**, phosphorus, and magnesium, in the maintenance of healthy bones and teeth; these are problems of major public health impact, particularly in industrialized countries. For example, each year Americans experience an estimated 13 million fractures,[3] including more than 350 hip fractures, and metabolic bone diseases are estimated to cost the United States some $13 billion in immediate medical care costs with as much as $8 billion lost annually from the U.S. economy in the form of extended treatment and lost productivity.[4] Metabolic bone diseases target women, who are more susceptible to **osteoporosis** (i.e., the loss of bone leading to increased bone fragility) than are men. Starting during the fourth or fifth decade of life, both men and women lose bone mass at similar annual rates;[5] but after the onset of menopause, the rate of bone loss in women can increase as much as tenfold[6] owing to diminished production of estrogen, which is required along with vitamin D to maintain bone mineralization. It has been estimated that among 50-year-old Americans half of all women and one-fifth of all men have signs of osteoporosis; accordingly, 75 to

---

[1] The use of the letter D without a subscript indicates either vitamin D$_2$ (ergocalciferol) or vitamin D$_3$ (cholecalciferol).

[2] Archeological studies have revealed low bone mass in a variety of past populations from various parts of the world. However, these were not necessarily associated with osteoporotic fractures. Nelson et al. (Nelson, D. A., Sauer, N. J., and Agarwal, S. C. [2004]. Evolutionary aspects of bone health, Chapter 1 in *Nutrition and Bone Health* [Holick, M. F., and Dawson-Hughes, B., eds.], Humana Press, Totowa, NJ, pp. 3–18.) have suggested that this apparent discrepancy may be explained on the basis of generally greater calcium intakes (e.g., at least 1500 mg/day) than are experienced by most people today. That phenomenon, they suggest, is a result of agricultural technologies that have emphasized the production of cereals containing less calcium than uncultivated plant foods used previously.

[3] Fractures of the vertebrae, hip, forearm, leg, and ankle, in that order, are the most common, although in many cases they may be asymptomatic. In 1999, hip fractures in the United States accounted for an estimated 338,000 physician office visits. Canadian health statistics show the risk of radial fractures for men and women to be about 25 per 100,000 until the fifth decade of life, after which it increases for women linearly to more than 200 per 100,000 by the seventh to eighth decades. Men, in contrast, do not show an appreciable age-related increase in risk.

[4] Only 25% of hip fracture patients can be expected to make full recoveries; 40% will require admission to nursing homes; half will be dependent on a cane or walker; and 20% will die within a year of various complications.

[5] Typical rates of bone loss of men and premenopausal women are in the range of 0.3–0.5%/year.

[6] Women can lose as much as 20% of their total bone mass within the first 5–7 years following menopause; by age 70–80, many women have lost 30–50% of their bone mass (in contrast with 20–30% losses for men).

80% of all hip fractures occur in women. As the U.S. population ages, these rates can be expected to increase; that of hip fractures is expected to triple by the year 2050.

II. Sources of Vitamin D

Distribution in Foods

Vitamin D, as either **ergocalciferol (vitamin D$_2$)** or **cholecalciferol (vitamin D$_3$)**, is rather sparsely represented in nature; however, its provitamins are common is both plants and animals. Ergocalciferol and its precursor **ergosterol** are found in plants, fungi,[7] molds, lichens, and some invertebrates (e.g., snails and worms). Some microorganisms are quite rich in ergosterol, in which it may comprise as much as 10% of the total dry matter.[8] Ergosterol does not occur naturally in higher vertebrates, but it can be present in low amounts in tissues of those species as the result of their consuming it. The actual distribution of ergocalciferol in nature is much more limited and variable than that of ergosterol (e.g., grass hays and alfalfa contain vitamin D only after they have been cut and left to dry in the sun). Whereas vitamin D$_2$ is probably present only in small amounts from natural sources, it has been a major synthetic form used in animal and human nutrition for four decades.

Cholecalciferol is widely distributed in animals, in which its provitamin D form, **7-dehydrocholesterol,** is a normal metabolite, but has an extremely limited distribution in plants. In animals, tissue cholecalciferol concentrations are dependent on the vitamin D content of the diet and/or the exposure to sunlight. Few foods, however, are rich in the vitamin. The richest natural sources are fish liver,

and oils[9] are particularly rich sources of vitamin D$_3$, which occurs in those materials in free form as well as esters of long-chain fatty acid esters. With a few notable exceptions, vitamin D$_3$ is not found in plants. Those exceptions include the species[10] *Solanum glaucophyllum, Solanum malacoxylon, Cestrum diurnum,* and *Trisetum flavescens* in which the vitamin occurs as water-soluble β-glycosides of **vitamin D$_3$**, **25-hydroxyvitamin D$_3$ (25-OH-D$_3$)**, and **1,25-dihydroxyvitamin D$_3$ (1,25-[OH]$_2$-D$_3$)**.[11]

Because most foods contain only very low amounts of vitamin D (see Table 6-1), it has become the practice in many countries to fortify certain common and frequently consumed foods (e.g., baked goods, grain products, milk[12] and milk products, infant foods) to prevent rickets. Both vitamers D$_2$ and D$_3$ are used in the fortification of foods. Some other foods may be enriched indirectly as the result of the supplementation of animal feeds with the vitamin. In general, therefore, the chief food sources of vitamin D in Western diets are fortified milk and cereals, and fatty fish.

Vitamin D can also be obtained from nutritional supplements. For example, multivitamin supplements typically contain 400 IU vitamin D, and pharmaceutical preparations can contain as much as 50,000 IU vitamin D$_2$ per capsule/tablet.

Biosynthesis of Vitamin D$_3$

Vitamin D is formed in animals by the action of ultraviolet (UV) light (295–300 nm) on 7-dehydrocholesterol in the skin (see Fig. 6-1). The activation reaction depends on the absorption of UV light by the 5,7-diene of the B ring of the sterol nucleus, causing it to open and isomerize to form the energetically more stable s-*trans,* s-*cis*-previtamin D$_3$. This physicochemical reaction appears to convert only 5 to 15% of the

---

[7] Ergosterol was named for the parasitic fungus, *ergot*, from which the sterol was first isolated.

[8] Provitamin D$_2$ accounts for virtually all of the sterols in *Aspergillus niger* and 80% of those in *Saccharomyces cerevisiae* (i.e., brewers' yeast).

[9] Fish oils typically have vitamin D$_3$ concentrations of about 50 µg/g, but cod, tuna and mackerel oils can contain 20 times that level. Marine mammals, which consume large amounts of such cold water fishes, accumulate vitamin D$_3$ from those sources in their livers. Therefore, peoples (e.g., Inuit, Faroe Islanders) who consume seals and whales obtain vitamin D$_3$ from those foods.

[10] Consumption of these plants has been associated with calcinosis in grazing ruminants; this observation was the basis of the discovery that they contained vitamin D.

[11] Both vitamin D$_3$-25-hydroxylase and 25-OH-vitamin D$_3$-1-hydroxylase activities have been found in *S. malacoxylon*, indicating that its ability to metabolize vitamin D is similar to that of higher animals.

[12] In the late 1950s, the American Medical Association recommended that milk be fortified with 400 IU (10 mcg) per quart; the U.S. Food and Drug Administration has specified that milk should contain 400–600 IU/qt. However, a survey by Tanner et al. (*J. Assoc. Off. Anal. Chem.* **71**, 607–610, 1988) showed that most fortified milk products failed to contain the specified amounts of vitamin D stated. Most European countries do not fortify milk with vitamin D.

Table 6-1. Vitamin D activities in foods

Food	Vitamin D (IU[a]/100 g)	Food	Vitamin D (IU[a]/100 g)
Animal products		Fish products (*Cont'd*)	
Milk		Sardines	1,500
Cow	0.3–54[b]	Shrimp	150
Human	0–10	Liver	
Dairy products		Beef	8–40
Butter	35	Chicken	50–65
Cheese	12	Pork	40
		Meats	
Cream	50	Beef	13
Eggs	28	Pork	84
Fish products		Poultry	80
Cod	85	Poultry skin	900
Cod liver oil	10,000	Plant products	
Herring	330	Cabbage	0.2
Herring liver oil	140,000	Corn oil	9
Mackerel	120	Spinach	0.2
Salmon	220–440		

[a]1 IU = 0.025 mg of vitamin D_2 or vitamin D_3.
[b]U.S. regulations specify that milk be fortified with 400 IU of vitamin D_3 per quart (about 37 IU/100 ml).

available 7-dehydrocholesterol to vitamin D_3.[13] That efficiency is affected by the physical properties of the skin and of the environment; thus, it differs between individuals and species, and it shows great variation according to time of day, season, and latitude.

The provitamin D sterol, 7-dehydrocholesterol, is both a precursor to and product of cholesterol (via different pathways). It is synthesized in the sebaceous glands of the skin, and it is secreted rather uniformly onto the surface, where it is reabsorbed into the various layers of the epidermis.[14] Thus, the skin contains very high concentrations of the sterol (e.g., 200 times that of liver). The distribution of 7-dehydrocholesterol in the epidermis varies according to its penetration from the surface. In humans, the greatest concentrations are found in the deeper *Malpighian layer*, whereas in the rat it is distributed more superficially in the *stratum*

corneum. In consequence of such a difference in **provitamin D_3** distribution, photoproduction in the rat can occur in the stratum corneum itself, whereas this reaction in humans occurs deeper and is therefore subject to the loss of UV owing to absorption by the stratum corneum layer. The thickness of that layer is a primary determinant of its transmission of UV light; the stratum corneum of black human skin tends to be thicker than that of white human skin and transmits much less UV light transmitted than the latter.[15]

Holick has estimated that exposure to the median erythemal dose[16] of sunlight can produce 10,000 to 25,000 IU of vitamin D; he recommends exposures of one-quarter of that amount of sunlight two to three times weekly to support the synthesis of physiologically relevant amounts, ca. 15,000 IU per week, of the vitamin.[17] The vitamin D biosynthetic response

---

[13] Excess irradiation does little to increase the efficiency of this activation step. Instead, it increases the photoproduction of biologically inactive forms (e.g., lumisterol-3, tachysterol-3, and 5,6-*trans*-vitamin D_3).

[14] In humans, the epidermis (particularly the stratum basale and stratum spinosum) contains twice as much 7-dehydrocholesterol as the dermis.

[15] While 20–30% of radiation at 295 nm is transmitted through the epidermis in Caucasians with skin type II, this transmission is only 2–5% in blacks with skin type V.

[16] 1 MED is that amount of sunlight that causes the skin to turn slightly pink and produce detectable erythema, the sign of mild sunburn.

[17] Holick, M. F., and Jenkins, M. (2003). *The UV Advantage*, ibooks, New York, p. 93.

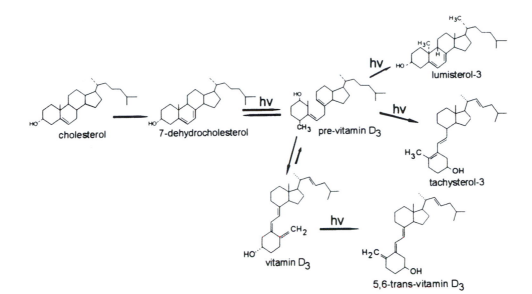

Fig. 6-1.   Biosynthesis of vitamin D_3 and its photolytic by-products.

to UV light is further diminished by the skin pigment *melanin*;[18] dark-skinned individuals appear to require longer UV doses than light-skinned individuals for comparable vitamin D biosynthesis. Both the thickness and 7-dehydrocholesterol content of skin decline with age, such that the vitamin D biogenic response to solar irradiation is diminished in older people (see Fig. 6-2). Accordingly, an age-related decline in plasma 25-OH-D_3 concentration is typically seen in individuals without significant dietary intakes of the vitamin.[19]

Physical factors that reduce the exposure of the skin to UV light also reduce the biosynthesis of vitamin D_3 (Figs. 6-2, 6-3, and 6-4). These include factors associated with the lifestyle of humans (e.g., clothing, indoor living, use of sunscreens) and practical management of livestock (e.g., confined indoor housing). Holick's group[20] has shown that the application of 5% p-aminobenzoic acid (PABA) with a sun protection factor of 8 completely prevented increases in serum vitamin D_3 in response to 1 MED of UV irradiation, indicating that a UV-blocking agent that prevents sun damage to

the skin will prevent the cutaneous production of vitamin D_3.

In addition, variations in environmental exposure to UV light result in corresponding variations in vitamin D biosynthesis (Table 6-2). Vitamin D-producing UV irradiation varies with the zenith angle of the sun, being greatest at noon (60% occurs between 10 A.M. and 2 P.M.), reaching an annual peak at midsummer and declining with the distance from the Earth's equator (e.g., in winter there is almost no UV light at latitudes north or south of 50°,[21] and above 40° N/S[22] there is virtually no vitamin D biosynthesis in the skin.

These factors lead to substantial variation in vitamin D_3 biosynthesis among people and animals. For many individuals, the aggregate effect is to render a need for exogenous (dietary) vitamin D. Indeed, that many people show seasonal changes in their serum 25-OH-D_3 levels (greatest concentrations occurring in the autumn) indicates that for most people sunlight is generally more important than diet as a source of the vitamin.

---

[18] Melanin, which absorbs solar radiation over the broad range of 290–700 nm, has been proposed as an evolutionary adaptation to protect against hypervitaminosis D due to excessive sunlight exposure in tropical latitudes, which was lost by populations migrating to areas distant from the equator.

[19] Need et al. (1993). *Am. J. Clin. Nutr.* **53**:882–885, found that the skinfold thickness of the back of the hand was significantly less for subjects in their 60s or 70s than for subjects in their 40s or 50s; this corresponded to lower serum concentrations of 25-OH-D_3 in the oldest group.

[20] Matsuoka et al. (1988). (*Arch. Dermatol.* **124**, 1802–1804.

[21] That is, that of Winnipeg, Frankfurt, Prague, and Kiev in the northern hemisphere, and Launceston (Tazmania) and the southern tips of Patagonia (Argentina) and Chile in the southern hemisphere. *Note:* The entire African and Australian contents lie north of 50°S.

[22] That is, that of Denver, Philadelphia, Toledo (Spain), Ankara, and Beijing in the northern hemisphere, and San Martin de los Andes (Argentina) in the southern hemisphere. *Note:* The entire African and Australian continents lie north of 40°S.

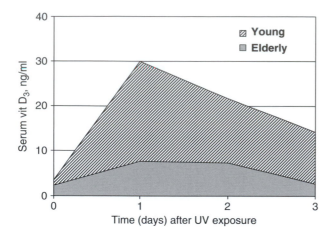

Fig. 6-2. Circulating vitamin D_3 responses of young and elderly human subjects. (*After* Holick et al. [1989]. *Lancet,* November 4, 1104–1105.)

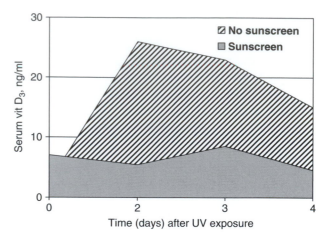

Fig. 6-4. Effects of sunscreen (SPF8) application on circulating vitamin D_3 responses of humans to 1 MED of UVB radiation. (*After* Matsuoka et al. [1987]. *J. Clin. Endocrinol. Med.* **64,** 1165–1168.)

III. Enteric Absorption of Vitamin D

Micelle-Dependent Passive Diffusion

Vitamin D is absorbed from the small intestine by nonsaturable passive diffusion that is dependent on micellar solubilization and, hence, the presence of bile salts. The fastest absorption appears to be in the upper portions of the small intestine (i.e., the duodenum and ileum), but, owing to the longer transit time of food in the distal portion of the small intestine, the greatest amount of vitamin D absorption probably occurs there. Like other hydrophobic substances absorbed by micelle-dependent passive diffusion in mammals, vitamin D enters the lymphatic circulation[23] predominantly (about 90% of the total amount absorbed) in association with chylomicra, with most of the balance being associated with the α-globulin fraction.[24] The efficiency of this absorption process for vitamin D appears to be about 50%.

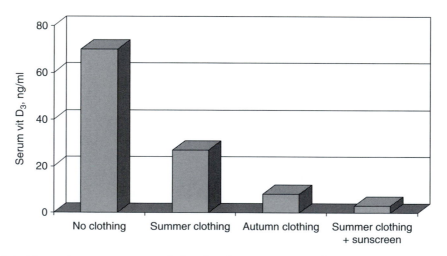

Fig. 6-3. Effects of clothing and sunscreen on circulating vitamin D_3 responses of humans to 1 MED of UVB radiation. (*After* Matsuoka et al. [1992]. *J. Clin. Endocrinol. Med.* **75,** 1099–1103.)

---

[23] In birds, reptiles, and fishes vitamin D, like other lipids, is absorbed into the portal circulation via portomicra.

[24] This is probably identical to the carrier, vitamin D-binding protein (DBP), in the plasma.

Table 6-2.   Effect of sun and dietary vitamin D on vitamin D status of women

Parameter	Low sunlight exposure		High sunlight exposure	
	Low vitamin D	High vitamin D	Low vitamin D	High vitamin D
Age (years)	84.9 ± 0.8	81.3 ± 1.6	83.6 ± 0.6	81.6 ± 1.5
		Summer		
Vitamin D intake (mg/day)	3.58 ± 0.53	16.05 ± 1.38^{a}	4.08 ± 0.65	14.53 ± 1.15^{a}
Plasma 25-OH-D_3 (nM)	44 ± 6	80 ± 8^{a}	57 ± 5	74 ± 6^{a}
		Winter		
Vitamin D intake (mg/day)	3.48 ± 0.45	16.33 ± 1.33^{a}	4.40 ± 0.78	14.63 ± 1.43^{a}
Plasma 25-OH-D_3 (nM)	35 ± 3	81 ± 7^{a}	42 ± 4	64 ± 4^{a}

$^{a}p < 0.05$.

Source: Salamone, L. M., Dallal, G. E., Zantos, D., Makrauer, F., and Dawson-Hughes, B. (1994). *Am. J. Clin. Nutr.* **59**, 80–86.

IV. Transport of Vitamin D

Transfer from Chylomicra to a Plasma

Almost all absorbed vitamin D is retained in nonesterified form, which is thought to be associated with the surface of *chylomicrons* (lipoprotein particles) because a portion of the vitamin D can be transferred from chylomicra to a binding protein in the plasma, either directly or during the process of chylomicron degradation. Vitamin D that is not transferred in the plasma is taken up with chylomicron remnants by the liver, where it is transferred to the same binding protein and released to the plasma.

Vtiamin D binding protein

Like other sterols, vitamin D is transported in the plasma largely in association with protein. Whereas some birds and mammals transport vitamin D in association with albumin, and fishes with cartilaginous skeletons (e.g., sharks and rays) transport it in association with plasma lipoproteins, most species[25] use a protein that has been called **transcalciferin** or, more commonly, **vitamin D-binding protein (DBP)** (Table 6-3). The DBP is a glycosylated, cysteine-rich, α-globulin of 55 kDa and 458 amino acids.[26]

Table 6-3.   Distribution of vitamin D_3 metabolites in human plasma

Metabolite	Percentage distribution			Normal concentration
	DBP	Lipoprotein	Albumin	
Vitamin D_3	60	40	0	2–4 ng/ml
25-OH-D_3	98	2	0	15–38 ng/ml
24,25-$(OH)_2$-D_3	98	2	0	—
1,25-$(OH)_2$-D_3	62	15	23	20–40 pg/ml

It binds vitamins D_2 or D_3 and their metabolites stoichiometrically,[27] with ligand-binding dependent on the *cis*-triene structure and C_3-hydroxyl grouping. Its binds 25-OH-D with an affinity an order of magnitude greater than those of 1,25-$(OH)_2$-D.[28] The concentration of DBP in the plasma, typically 4–8 μM, greatly exceeds that of 25-OH-D_3 (ca. 50 nM) and is remarkably constant, being unaffected by sex, age, or vitamin D status. In a survey of some 80,000 individuals, DBP was absent in none. Being synthesized by the liver, however, it is depressed in patients with hepatic disease; in addition, it is increased during estrogen therapy or pregnancy. It does not appear to cross the placenta;

---

[25] At least 140 different species in five classes have been examined.

[26] In contrast, the chicken has *two* distinct DBPs (54 and 60 kDa), each of which binds vitamin D_3 and its metabolites with greater affinities than vitamin D_2 and its metabolites.

[27] DBP also has a high affinity for actin, for reasons that are unclear. (The formation of this complex can interfere with the assay of 25-OH-D-1-hydroxylase in kidney homogenates.) It is likely, however, that the interaction of DBP with this widely distributed cellular protein may be the basis of reports of an intracellular 25-OH-D-binding protein

[28] K_A values: for 25-OH-D_3, 5×10^8 M^{-1}; for 1,25-$(OH)_2$-D_3, 4×10^7 M^{-1} (Haddad, J. G. [1999]. *Vitamin D: Physiology, Molecular Biology, and Clinical Applications* [M. F. Holick, ed.], Humana Press, Totowa, NJ, p. 102).

fetal DBP is immunologically distinct from the maternal protein. Human DBP shows genetic polymorphism[29] due to differences in both the primary structure of the protein and the carbohydrate moiety that is added post-translationally.

In addition to facilitating the peripheral distribution of vitamin D obtained from the diet, DBP functions to mobilize the vitamin produced endogenously in the skin. Indeed, vitamin D_3 found in the skin is bound to DBP.[30] It has been suggested that the efficiency of endogenously produced vitamin D_3 is greater than that given orally for the reason that the former enters the circulation strictly via DBP, whereas the latter enters as complexes of DBP as well as chylomicra. This would indicate that oral vitamin D remains longer in the liver and is thus more quickly catabolized to excretory forms. In support of this hypothesis, it has been noted that high oral doses of vitamin D can lead to very high levels of 25-OH-D_3 (>400 ng/ml) associated with intoxication, whereas intensive UV irradiation can rarely produce plasma 25-OH-D_3 concentrations greater than one-fifth that level, and hypervitaminosis D has never been reported from excessive irradiation. The DBP protein has also been found on the surfaces of lymphocytes and macrophages, although the functional significance of such binding is not clear.

Tissue Distribution

Unlike the other fat-soluble vitamins, vitamin D is *not* stored by the liver.[31] It reaches the liver within a few hours after being absorbed across the gut or synthesized in the skin, but from the liver it is distributed relatively evenly among the various tissues, where it resides in hydrophobic compartments. Therefore, fatty tissues such as adipose show slightly greater concentrations. However, in that tissue the vitamin is found in the bulk lipid phase, from which it is only slowly mobilized. About half of the total vitamin D in the tissues occurs as the parent vitamin D_3 species, with the next most abundant form, 25-OH-D_3, accounting for

about 20% of the total. In the plasma, however, the latter metabolite predominates by severalfold.[32,33] Tissues including those of the kidneys, liver, lungs, aorta, and heart also tend to accumulate 25-OH-D_3.[34] It is thought that the uneven tissue distribution of vitamin D, in its various forms, relates to differences in both tissue lipid content and tissue-associated vitamin D-binding proteins, the latter fraction being the smaller of the two intracellular pools of the vitamin.

The concentrations of both 25-OH-D_3 and 1,25-$(OH)_2$-D_3 are lower in the cord sera of fetuses and newborn infants than in the sera of their mothers. That fetal 25-OH-D_3 levels correlate with maternal levels (and show the same seasonal variations) suggests that the metabolite crosses the placenta. Such a correlation is not apparent for 1,25-$(OH)_2$-D_3. The extent of transplacental movement of the latter metabolite is not known; however, the placenta appears to be able to produce it from maternally derived 25-OH-D_3.

Vitamin D Receptor

Studies have revealed that both 1,25-$(OH)_2$-D_3 and its receptor are localized in the nuclei of certain tissues—the target tissues (bone, kidney, intestine) on which vitamin D exerts its classic actions, and also other tissues such as placenta, parathyroid, pancreatic islets, gastric endocrine cells, and certain cells of the brain (Table 6-4). Such findings indicate a breadth of vitamin D genomic functions. The gene in humans shows extensive polymorphism.

Vitamin D receptors (VDRs) have been identified in more than 30 different cell types; these include cells closely related to the maintenance of calcium homeostasis as well as immune, endocrine, hematopoietic, skin, and tumor cells. In intestinal cells, the VDR content is surprisingly low—fewer than 2000 binding sites per cell. In neonates, the intestinal receptor is absent until weaning, being induced on the feeding of solid foods, by a process that apparently involves cortisol. In at least some organs VDRs appear to be

---

[29] In humans, DBP is identical with group-specific component (G_c protein), a genetic marker of use in population studies and forensic medicine.

[30] DBP has practically no affinity for lumisterol$_3$ or tachysterol$_3$; therefore, these forms produced under conditions of excessive irradiation are not well mobilized from the skin.

[31] The high concentrations of vitamin D found in the livers of some fishes are important exceptions.

[32] The next most abundant form is 24,25-$(OH)_2$-vitamin D.

[33] The plasma concentrations of 25-OH-D_3 and 24,25-$(OH)_2$-D_3 of free-living persons vary seasonally, showing maxima in the summer months and minima in the winter. In contrast, plasma levels of 1,25-$(OH)_2$-D_3 are rather constant, indicating an effective regulatory mechanism for that metabolite.

[34] These organs are also prone to calcification in hypervitaminosis D.

Table 6-4.   Distribution of known nuclear vitamin D receptors

Organ system	Cell type
Bone	Osteoblasts
Alimentary tract	Epithelial cells, enterocytes, colonocytes, stomach
Liver	Hepatocytes
Kidney	Epithelial (proximal and distal) cells
Heart	Atrial myoendocrine cells, heart muscle cells
Skeletal, smooth muscle	Myocytes
Cartilage	Chondrocytes
Hematolymphopoietic	Activated T and B cells, macrophages, monocytes, spleen, thymus reticular cells and lymphocytes, lymph nodes, tonsillary dendritic cells
Reproductive	Amnion, chorioallantoic membrane, epididymus, mammary gland alveolar and ductal cells, ovary, oviduct, placenta, testis Sertoli and Leydig cells, uterus, yolk sac
Skin	Epidermis, fibroblasts, hair follicles, keratinocytes, melanocytes, sebaceous glands
Nervous	Brain (hippocampus, cerebellar Purkinje and granule cells, bed nucleus, stria terminalis, amygdala central nucleus), sensory ganglia, spinal cord
Other endocrine	Adrenal medulla and cortex, pancreatic β cells, pituitary, thyroid follicles and C cells, parathyroid gland
Other	Bladder, choroid plexus, lung, endothelial cells, parotid gland

inducible by estrogen treatment; in the guinea pig (and presumably in humans, who also require vitamin C) VDRs can be reduced in number by deprivation of ascorbic acid.[35] That VDRs plays key roles in mediating the physiological function of vitamin D is evidenced by the facts that: (i) low levels are associated with instestinal vitamin D resistance *in vitro*; (ii) defects are manifest as hereditary hypocalcemic, vitamin D-resistant rickets; and (iii) allelic variation is a predictor of bone mineral mass/density and risk of fracture.[36]

The VDR is classified in the family of steroid, thyroid hormone and retinoic acid receptor genes on the basis of its similar primary amino acid structure. The VDRs of different species vary in size (e.g., human, 48 kDa; avian, 60 kDa). Each is a sulfhydryl protein with an N-terminal recognition domain containing a cysteine-rich cluster comprising two "zinc finger" structures,[37] and a C-terminal region that binds 1,

$25\text{-}(OH)_2\text{-}D_3$ with high affinity utilizing the ligand's three hydroxyl groups ligand.

The liganded VDR is thought to be translocated from the cytosol into the nucleas via interactions with microtubules. While this mechanism is still unclear, it is thought to involve a sequence seen for other sterols: stimulation of protein kinase C (PKC), PKC-activation of guanylate cyclase, phosphorylation of microtubule-associated proteins, and association of VDR with importins. That the liganded VDR is less readily extractable from the nucleus than is the free receptor suggests that $1,25\text{-}(OH)_2\text{-}D_3$ binding causes a conformational change in the protein that increases its affinity for DNA.[38] After the manner of the other steroid hormone receptors, the VDR is an essential transactivator of the $1,25\text{-}(OH)_2\text{-}D_3$-dependent transcription of mRNAs for various proteins involved in calcium transport, the bone matrix, and cell cycle regulation. The VDR of intestinal epithelial cells can also bind bile acids, ultimately

---

[35] Guinea pig intestinal $1,25\text{-}(OH)_2\text{-}D_3$ receptors (occupied and unoccupied) were reduced by vitamin C deprivation. Whether this finding relates to the rickets-like bone changes observed in vitamin C-deficient guinea pigs and humans is not clear.

[36] In an 18-month study of elderly subjects typed by VDR allelic variant, Rizzoli et al. (1995). (*Lancet* **345**, 423–424, found 78% of *BB* homozygotes to lose bone mineral density at rates > 0.48%/year, whereas only 31% of *bb* homozygotes and only 41% of *Bb* heterozygotes experienced comparable losses.

[37] "Zinc fingers" are finger-like structures folded around a zinc atom tetrahedonally coordinated through the sulfhydryls of cysteine residues in the primary structure of the protein. This motif is similar to DNA-binding motifs found in other transcriptional regulating proteins.

[38] Two binding domains have been identified in nVDRs: a ligand-binding domain at the carboxyl-terminal end of the protein and a DNA-binding domain at the amino-terminal end.

leading to the detoxification of those inducers through the upregulation of a cytochrome P450 (CYP3A).

Evidence suggests that 1,25-(OH)$_2$-D$_3$ can exert certain rapid effects within cells that do not involve the nuclear receptor. Such effects are presumed to involve a membrane-bound receptor still to be characterized.

V. Metabolism of Vitamin D

Metabolic Activation

The metabolism of vitamin D (i.e., cholecalciferol/ergocalciferol) involves its conversions to a variety of hydroxylated products, each of which is more polar than the hydrophobic parent (Fig. 6-5).[39] The discovery of these metabolites, some of which are the actual metabolically active forms of the vitamin, explains the lag time that is commonly observed between the administration of vitamin D$_3$ and the earliest biological response. The metabolism of vitamin D, therefore, includes reactions that effect the metabolic activation of the ingested or endogenously produced vitamin.

25-Hydroxylation

Most of the vitamin D taken up by the liver from either DBP or lipoproteins is converted by hydroxy-lation of side-chain carbon C-25 to yield 25-OH-D$_3$, also called calcidiol, which is the major circulating form of the vitamin. This reaction is catalyzed by an enzyme limited to the liver in mammals but occurring in both liver and kidney in birds. That activity, **vitamin D 25-hydroxylase**, involves cytochrome P-450-dependent mixed-function oxygenases[40] of two types: a low-affinity, high-capacity enzyme associated with the endoplasmic reticulum;[41] and a high-affinity, low-capacity enzyme located in the mitochondria. The latter involves cytochrome P450c27 (also, CYP27), which also functions in side-chain hydroxylations in the synthesis of bile acids. That CYP27 also occurs in kidney and bone suggests extrahepatic 25-hydroxylation of vitamin D$_3$. The presence of two different mechanisms of 25-hydroxylation would appear to facilitate the maintenance of adequate vitamin D status under both deficient and excessive conditions of vitamin D intake/production. 25-Hydroxyvitamin D$_3$ is not retained within the cell, but is released to the plasma where it accumulates by binding with DBP. At normal plasma concentrations of this metabolite, only small amounts of 25-OH-D$_3$ are released from this pool to enter tissues. Therefore, the circulating level of 25-OH-D$_3$, normally 10–40 ng/ml (25–125 nM), is a good indicator of vitamin D status.

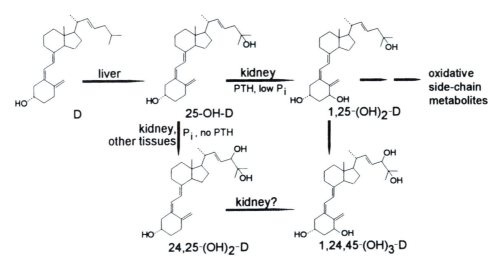

Fig. 6-5. Metabolism of vitamin D.

---

[39] In fact, it was the finding in the late 1960s of radioactive peaks migrating ahead of vitamin D (indicating greater polarity relative to vitamin D) in gel filtration of plasma from animals given radiolabeled cholecalciferol that first evidenced the conversion of vitamin D to other species, some of which have subsequently been found to be the metabolically active forms of the vitamin.

[40] A mixed-function oxygenase uses molecular oxygen (O$_2$) but incorporates only one oxygen atom into the substrate; a monooxygenase.

[41] In the rat, the microsomal hydroxylase is 5-fold more active in males than in females; in males it may involve cytochrome P4502C11, which does not occur in females.

1-Hydroxylation

The initial hydroxylation product of vitamin D (25-OH-D$_3$) is further hydroxylated at the C-1 position of the A ring to yield $1,25$-(OH)$_2$-D$_3$, which, being produced at a site distant from its target tissue to which it is transported in the blood, is properly classified as a hormone. This hydroxylation is catalyzed by **25-OH-vitamin D 1-hydroxylase**. This activity is located primarily in renal cortical mitochondria, but also in mitchondrial and microsmal fractions of at least some extrarenal tissues (e.g., bone cells, liver, placenta[42]) and has been detected in cultured cell lines (skin, bone, embryonic intestine, keratinocytes, dendritic cells, monocytes, calvarial cells). The 1-hydroxylase uses NADPH$_2$ as the electron donor and has three constituent proteins: ferridoxin reductase, ferridoxin, and cytochrome P-450.[43] The activity is widely distributed among animal species, being found in all but 2 of 28 species surveyed, with highest activities in rachitic chicks.

Despite its key role in discharging the actions of vitamin D, its tightly regulated production and relatively fast turnover[44] make $1,25$-(OH)$_2$-D$_3$ useless as a biomarker of vitamin D status. Circulating levels tend to be about 40 pg/ml (100 nM).

Catabolism

Vitamin D is catabolized in several different ways: oxidative cleavage of the side chain; hydroxylation of $1,25$-(OH)$_2$-D$_3$ to produce the trihydroxylated products $1,24,25$-(OH)$_3$-D$_3$ and $1,25,26$-(OH)$_3$-D$_3$; and formation of the $1,25$-(OH)$_2$-D$_3$-23,26-lactone. Other products, including glucuronides and sulfates, have also been identified. Most are excreted in the feces via the bile.

24-Hydroxylation

Hydroxylation at the C-24 of the side chain can occur to both 25-OH-D$_3$ or $1,25$-(OH)$_2$-D$_3$ to produce the di- and tri-hydroxy metabolites $24,25$-(OH)$_2$-**D$_3$** (also called **calcidiol**) and $1,24,25$-(OH)$_3$-D$_3$ (also called **calcitroic acid** or **calcitriol**), respectively. These reactions are catalyzed by the same activity, which may also catalyze further hydroxylations at the C-23 position. The 24-hydroxylase has a 10-fold greater affinity for $1,25$-(OH)$_2$-D$_3$ than for 25-OH-D$_3$, but the 1000-fold excess of the latter in the plasma suggests that the primary physiological significance of the hydroxylase is in the catabolism of excess 25-OH-D$_3$. The greatest activity of the 24-hydroxylase is found in renal mitochondria. Like the 1-hydroxylase, it is a cytochrome P-450-dependent enzyme requiring NADPH, but unlike the former activity, it is inhibited by **hypercalcemia** and **hyperphosphatemia.** The 24-hydroxylase activity is increased under these conditions but is very strongly induced by $1,25$-(OH)$_2$-D$_3$. Both calcitriol and $24,25$-(OH)$_2$-D$_3$ appear to be produced under conditions of vitamin D adequacy and normal calcium homeostasis. The latter metabolite has been show to inhibit the stimulatory effect of PTH on bone resorption by **osteoclasts,** suggesting that it may participate in local osteotropic control in bone. Calcitriol is a major biliary metabolite of the vitamin.

Other hydroxylations

More than three dozen other metabolites of vitamin D have been identified, most, if not all, of which appear to be physiologically inactive excretory forms.[45] The earliest of these to be identified is $25,26$-(OH)$_2$-D$_3$, which has a strong affinity for DBP and is detectable in the plasma of animals given large doses of vitamin D$_3$. Other 26-hydroxylated metabolites have been identified, the most abundant being the 26,23-lactone of 25-OH-D$_3$, which appears to be produced through sucessive extraheaptic CYP24-mediated 23- and 26-hydroxylations of 25-OH-D$_3$. 2-Hydroxyvitamin D$_3$ is also catabolized by an extrahepatic 24-hydroxylase that can also act on $1,25$-(OH)$_2$-D$_3$. These side-chain hydroxylations can produce 1-OH-24,25,26,27-*tetranor*-23-carboxycholecalciferol, which accounts for nearly one-fifth of the

---

[42] Maternal levels of 25-OH-vitamin D increase in the third trimester, presumably to assist the mother in providing Ca for the mineralization of the fetal skeleton.

[43] Cytochrome P450CYP1a, or CYP1a.

[44] Its half-life in the serum is 4–6 hr.

[45] It should be noted that about 95% of vitamin D excretion occurs via the bile; of that amount, only 2 to 3% of an oral or parenteral dose of vitamin D appears as vitamin D or the mono- or dihydroxy metabolites.

biliary excretion of the vitamin. Subsequent chain-shortening metabolism of hydroxylated metabolites with low affinities for DBP account for their clearance from the circulation and their subsequent conversion to fatty acid esters in tissues and to excretory forms including biliary glucuronides.

Regulation of Vitamin D Metabolism

Regulation of the vitamin D endocrine system is effected by tight control of the activity of the 1-hydroxylase by several factors: $1,25\text{-}(OH)_2\text{-}D_3$, PTH, **calcitonin** (CT), several other hormones,[46] as well as circulating levels of Ca^{2+} and phosphate. The 25-hydroxylase activity appears to be only poorly regulated, primarily by the hepatic concentration of vitamin D, with little or no inhibition by $25\text{-}OH\text{-}D_3$. It is increased by inducers of cytochrome $P\text{-}450$ (phenobarbital, diphenylhydantoin)[47] and is inhibited by isoniazid.[48]

The dominant renal synthesis of $1,25\text{-}(OH)_2\text{-}D_3$ is effected by the responses of PTH and CT to serum levels of Ca^{++} and phosphate. It is increased under three conditions:

- When serum Ca^{++} is low, the Ca receptor-mediated stimulation of the parathyroid to produce PTH, stimulates an increase in the renal 1-hydroxylase activity.
- When serum phosphate is low (in the presence of normal serum Ca^{++}), an unknown mechanism that appears to involve a pituitary gland hormone increases the 1-hydroxylase.
- When serum levels of both Ca^{++} and phosphate are low, both mechanisms result in the superstimulation of the 1-hydroxylase.

In all cases, the stimulation is lost upon the return of serum Ca^{++} to normal levels (as a result of $1,25\text{-}[OH]_2\text{-}D_3$-stimulated enteric absorption and bone mobilization of Ca^{++}). It has been suggested that some elderly people who cannot adapt to a low Ca diet by increasing enteric Ca absorption may suffer impaired PTH-dependent $1,25\text{-}[OH]_2\text{-}D_3$ upregulation.

The hormones PTH and CT both stimulate the renal 1-hydroxylase, the effect of PTH being rapid and mediated by cAMP, whereas the effect of CT is relatively slow, apparently acting at the level of transcription.[49] That ovariectomy reduces the synthesis of $1,25\text{-}(OH)_2\text{-}D_3$ in rat renal slices suggests that estrogen is also involved in the regulation of the 1-hydroxylase. That effect appears to be mediated via PTH, as parathyroidectomy has been found to block the stimulation of $1,25\text{-}(OH)_2\text{-}D_3$ production by estrogen treatment.

The regulation of the 1-hydroxylase in extrarenal tissues appears to be completely different. In macrophages, the production of $1,25\text{-}(OH)_2\text{-}D_3$ has been found to be insensitive to PTH but to be stimulated by such immune stimuli as interferon-gamma and lipopolysaccharide.

The catabolism of $1,25\text{-}(OH)_2\text{-}D_3$ is regulated by PTH, serum phosphate, and factors affecting the principal catabolizing enzyme, the hepatic 24-hydroxylase. Other enzymes also metabolize $1,25\text{-}(OH)_2\text{-}D_3$, as some 40 metabolites have been identified. The 1-hydroxylase is inhibited by strontium and is feedback-inhibited by $1,25\text{-}(OH)_2\text{-}D_3$.[50] Thus, when circulating levels of $1,25\text{-}(OH)_2\text{-}D_3$ are high, its renal synthesis is low. The tight regulation of the 1-hydroxylase activity results in the maintenance of nearly constant plasma concentrations of $1,25\text{-}(OH)_2\text{-}D_3$. 1,25-Dihydroxyvitamin D_3 activates its own breakdown by stimulating the transcription of the 24-hydroxylase gene; this stimulation is suppressed in conditions of low serum phosphate.

Role of protein binding

The DBP plays a critical role in the regulation of vitamin D metabolism by controlling the tissue distribution of vitamin D metabolites. Due to the excess of DBP over its ligands (4–8 μM vs. 50 nM for $25\text{-}OH\text{-}D_3$), nearly 90% of circulating vitamin D

---

[46] For example, prolactin, estradiol, testosterone, and growth hormone.

[47] Antiepileptic agents such as these reduce the half-life of vitamin D apparently by enhancing its conversion to 25-OH-D and other hydroxylated products.

[48] This appears to be the basis for the development of bone disease among patients on long-term isoniazid therapy.

[49] It has been suggested that the function of the CT-sensitive 1-hydroxylase, which is elevated in the fetus, may be to accommodate situations of increased need for $1,25\text{-}(OH)_2$-vitamin D.

[50] The hydroxylase is also inhibited by the $25\text{-}OH\text{-}D_3$-binding protein–actin complex. The effect of this inhibitor $in\ vitro$ can be overcome by using large amounts of $25\text{-}OH\text{-}D_3$ to saturate the binding protein; otherwise, it masks the 1-hydroxylase activity in kidney homogenates.

metabolites are bound to fewer than 5% of available DBP binding sites in vitamin D-adequate individuals. Furthermore, because of its avid binding of 25-OH-D$_3$, that metabolite accumulates in the plasma rather than other tissues, with concentrations of the free metabolite maintained at very low levels. Plasma DBP levels also correlate with those 1,25-(OH)$_2$-D$_3$; increasing plasma levels of the latter are accommodated by increased protein binding, maintaining very low circulating concentrations of the free form of the active metabolite.

Differential metabolism of vitamin D$_2$

Though a minor dietary form of the vitamin, vitamin D$_2$ is metabolized in many ways analogously to vitamin D$_3$. That is, the enzymes involved in the side-chain 1-, 24- and 25-hydroxylations do not descriminate between these vitamers. Vitamin D$_2$, however, appears to be metabolized to a number of mono- (24-), di- (1,24-; 24,26-) and tri- (1,25,28-) hydroxylated metabolites that are not produced from vitamin D$_3$. These, in turn, appear to be metabolized to a number of more polar tri- and tetra-hydroxylated forms some of which (e.g., 1,25,28-[OH]$_3$-D$_2$) are biologically active. That the net effect of this differential metabolism in most species is small is indicated by the fact that, for them, vitamins D$_2$ and D$_3$ have comparable biopotencies, for which reason vitamin D$_2$ is a useful dietary/supplemental form (see Table 6-5).

For birds and some mammals, however, vitamin D$_2$ is much less biopotent than vitamin D$_3$. This is because, in those species, the mono- and di-hydroxylated metabolites of vitamin D$_2$ are cleared faster

than those of vitamin D$_3$. For example, in the chick, the plasma turnover rates of vitamin D$_2$, 25-OH-D$_2$, and 1,25-(OH)$_2$-D$_2$ are 1.5-, 11- and 33-fold faster than those of the respective vitamin D$_3$ analogs. These differences in turnover rates are greater than those for the binding affinities to DBP (5-, 3.6-, and 3-fold, respectively) which (for each of the chicken's *two* DBPs) are greater for vitamin D$_3$ and its metabolites than for vitamin D$_2$ and its metabolites.

Bioactive Vitamin D Analogs

There are clear advantages of being able to provide vitamin D in effective forms to subjects, including those unable to produce the active metabolite efficiently, in ways that would not cause calcinosis. To this end, more than 2000 analogs of vitamin D have been developed for use as pro-drugs in treating disorders of vitamin D metabolism, such as vitamin D refractory rickets and hypocalcemia secondary to chronic renal disease, and cancer. Most contain structural deviations in the C and D rings of the steroid nucleas, or the side chain (Table 6-6).

VI. Metabolic Functions of Vitamin D

Vitamin D$_3$ as a Steroid Hormone

At least some, if not all, of the mechanisms of action of vitamin D fit the classic model of a steroid hormone. That is, it has specific cells in target organs with specific receptor proteins, and the receptor–ligand complex moves to the nucleus, where it binds to the chromatin at specific DNA sequences and stimulates

Table 6-5.   Effect of vitamin D$_2$ supplementation on plasma vitamin D metabolites in humans

Metabolite	Baseline	Control	Vitamin D$_2$ supplemented
D$_2$ (ng/ml)	0.3 ± 0.1	—	1.2 ± 0.2
D$_3$ (ng/ml)	1.1 ± 0.2	0.3 ± 0.2	1.0 ± 0.2
25-OH-D$_2$ (ng/ml)	1.7 ± 0.6	—	17.4 ± 1.6[a]
25-OH-D$_3$ (ng/ml)	16.9 ± 0.8	17.3 ± 2.0	19.0 ± 1.2
24,25-(OH)$_2$-D$_2$ (ng/ml)	—	—	0.5 ± 0.1[a]
24,25-(OH)$_2$-D$_3$ (ng/ml)	1.1 ± 0.4	1.0 ± 0.2	0.8 ± 0.3
1,25-(OH)$_2$-D$_2$ (pg/ml)	—	—	9.9 ± 0.2[a]
1,25-(OH)$_2$-D$_3$ (pg/ml)	47.2 ± 9.2	43.6 ± 5.2	35.4 ± 2.3

[a] $p < 0.05$.
Source: Takeuchi, A., Okano, T., Tsugawa, N., Tasaka, Y., Kabayashi, T., Kodama, S., and Matsuo, T. (1989). *J. Nutr.* **119,** 1639–1646.

Table 6-6. Bioactive vitamin D analogs

Dehydrotachysterol-2

1-OH-analogs (1-OH-D$_3$, 1-OH-D$_2$)

Cyclopropane ring-containing vitamin D analogs (e.g., calcipitriol)

Oxa-group containing analogs (e.g., 22-oxa-calcitriol)

Side-chain fluorinated analogs (e.g., F$_6$-1,25-(OH)2-D$_3$)

Unsaturated analogs (e.g., C$_{16}$=C$_{17}$ and C$_{22}$=C$_{23}$ analogs)

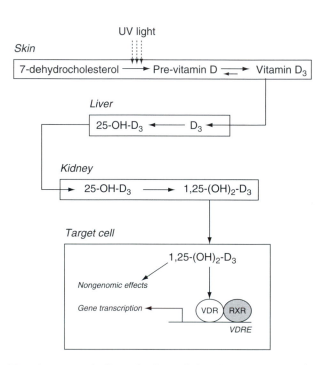

Fig. 6-6. Metabolic activation of vitamin D. (See text for abbreviations.)

the transcription of certain downstream genes to produce specific mRNAs that encode the synthesis of specific proteins (Fig. 6-6).

1,25-(OH)$_2$-D$_3$ as the Metabolically Active Form

The clearest physiological role of vitamin D is in the maintenance of calcium and phosphate homeostasis, impairment of which produces the lesions in bone called **rickets** and **osteomalacia**. In addition, other roles (e.g., induction of cell differentiation) have been proposed. In these roles, it is clear that vitamin D itself is not the functionally active form, but that it must be converted metabolically to a form(s) that exerts its biological activity. That form appears to be the dihydroxylated metabolite, 1,25-(OH)$_2$-D$_3$. The earliest evidence for this function was the shorter time to response and greater molar efficacy of 1,25-(OH)$_2$-D$_3$ than those of any other metabolite of the vitamin.

Genomic Pathways of Vitamin D Function

The target tissues for vitamin D contain a specific nuclear receptor to which the active metabolite binds. Autoradiographic studies have shown that 1,25-(OH)$_2$-D$_3$ is localized in the nuclei of many cell types that contain the nVDR. The VDR has been found in a wide variety of cell types inlcuding skin, lymphocytes, brain, and gonads. The VDR has been characterized, and the cDNA for it has been cloned; it has been found to have substantial sequence homology with receptors for other steroids, thyroid hormone, and retinoic acid. Specific, short, *cis*-acting, DNA base sequences, called **vitamin D-responsive elements (VDREs)**, have also been identified and sequenced; these are similar to those elements mediating the thyroid hormone or retinoic acid responses, consisting of imperfect direct repeats of six base-pair half-elements.[51] Binding of the 1,25-(OH)$_2$-D$_3$–VDR complex to VDREs involves one of the retinoid X receptors (RXRs); the preferred active species appears to be a VDR–RXR heterodimer,[52] although VDR homodimers are also thought to be formed. The VDRs and RXRs appear to occur in most cells; therefore, it may be the availability of 9-*cis*-retinoic acid that determines which set of genes is regulated by 1,25-(OH)$_2$-D$_3$. Involvement of other factors is also likely; for example, facilitation of the genomic action of 1,25-(OH)$_2$-D$_3$ by the thyroid hormone triiodothyronine (T$_3$) has been demonstrated. Transcriptional regulation by vitamin D is thought to involve a conformational change in VDR, effected by the phosphorylation of a specific serinyl residue upon the binding of 1,25-(OH)$_2$-D$_3$, that exposes domains of the protein capable of interacting with VDREs.

Some 50 genes have been identified as being regulated by vitamin D status (Table 6-7). These include genes associated with many aspects of metabolism, including cell differentiation and proliferation,

---

[51] Owing to their direct repeats, these lack the dyad symmetry of the classic steroid hormone-responsive elements.

[52] Interaction of these receptor proteins is thought to involve C-terminal dimerization interfaces in both.

Table 6-7.   Genes known to be regulated by vitamin D

Gene product	Tissue in which regulation has been demonstrated	Gene product	Tissue in which regulation has been demonstrated
Upregulated		**Upregulated (Cont'd)**	
Aldolase subunit B	Chick kidney	1,25-$(OH)_2$-D_3 receptor	Mouse fibroblasts
Alkaline phosphatase	Chick, rat intestine	Plasma membrane Ca^{2+} Pump	Chick intestine
ATP synthase	Chick intestine; rat intestine		
Calbindin-D_9 kDa	Chick kidney, skin, bone; rat intestine, skin, bone	Prolactin	Rat pituitary cells
		Protein kinase C	HL-60 cells
Calbindin-D_{28} kDa	Chick brain, kidney, uterus, intestine; mouse kidney; rat kidney, brain	Tumor necrosis factor α	U937, HL-60 cells
		Vitamin D receptor	Rat intestine, pituitary
Carbonic anhydrase	Marrow; myelomonocytes	**Downregulated**	
Cytochrome *c* oxidase		ATP synthase	Chick kidney
Subunit I	Chick intestine; rat intestine	Calcitonin	Rat thyroid gland
Subunit II	Chick intestine; rat intestine	CD23	PBMCs
Subunit III	Chick intestine; rat intestine	Collagen, type I	Rat fetal calvaria
Fibronectin	MG-63, TE-85, HL-60 cells	Cytochrome *b*	Chick kidney
c-Fms	HL-60 cells	Cytochrome *c* oxidase	
c-Fos	HL-60 cells	Subunit I	Chick kidney
Glyceraldehyde-3-phosphate dehydrogenase	BT-20 cells	Subunit II	Chick kidney
		Subunit III	Chick kidney
Heat shock protein 70	PBMCs	Fatty acid-binding protein	Chick intestine
Integrin$_{\alpha\gamma\beta3}$	Chick osteoclasts	Ferridoxin	Chick kidney
Interleukin 1	U937 cells	Granulocyte-macrophage colony-stimulating factor	Human T lymphocytes
Interleukin 6	U937 cells		
Interleukin 3 receptor	MC3T3 cells	Histone H_4	HL-60 cells
c-Ki-Ros	BALB-3T3 cells	Interferon γ	Human T lymphocytes
Matrix Gla protein	UMR106-01, ROS cells	Interleukin 2	Human T lymphocytes
Metallothionein	Rat keratinocytes	c-Myb	HL-60 cells
c-Myc	MG-63 cells	c-Myc	HL-60, U937 cells
NADH dehydrogenase		NADH dehydrogenase	
Subunit III	Chick intestine	Subunit I	kidney
Nerve growth factor	L-929 cells	Prepro-PTH	Rat, bovine parathyroid
Neutrophil-activating polypeptide	HL-60 cells		
		Protein kinase inhibitor	Chick kidney
Osteocalcin	ROS cells	PTH	Rat parathyroid
Osteopontin	ROS cells	PTH-related protein	T lymphocytes
1-OH-D3 24-hydroxylase	Rat kidney	Transferrin-receptor	PBMCs
		α-Tubulin	Chick intestine

Abbreviations: PTH, parathyroid hormone; BMCs, peripheral blood mononuclear cells.

energy metabolism, hormonal signaling, mineral homeostasis, oncogenes, and chromosomal proteins as well as vitamin D metabolism. For most of these genes, the regulation appears to involve 1,25-$(OH)_2$-D_3-dependent modulation of mRNA levels (i.e., regulation of transcription and/or message stability). To date, 1,25-$(OH)_2$-D_3-regulated transcription has been established for less than a dozen of these genes, and

VDREs have been reported for only four (calbindin$_{9k}$, integrin$_{\alpha\gamma\beta_3}$, osteocalcin and the plasma membrane Ca^{2+} pump). Evidence for posttranscriptional regulation of calbindin$_{9K}$ has been presented. From this emerging picture, it is clear that changes in vitamin D status have potential for pleiotropic actions.

The first gene product to be recognized as inducible by 1,25-(OH)$_2$-D$_3$ was for many years called **calcium-binding protein (CaBP)**. Different forms of CaBP have subsequently been described; these are now called **calbindins**.[53] Calbindins are widespread in animal tissues, with the greatest concentrations found in avian and mammalian duodenal mucosa, where they can comprise 1 to 3% of the total soluble protein of the cell. Two calbindins have been identified: calbindin-D$_{9k}$, occurring primarily in mammalian intestinal mucosa but also in kidney, uterus, and placenta; calbindin-D$_{28k}$, occurring in mammalian kidney (distal convoluted tubules), pancreas (β cells) and brain, and avian intestine and kindey. Calbindin-D$_{9k}$ can bind 2 Ca^{2+} atoms, while calbindin-D$_{28k}$ can bind 4 Ca^{2+} atoms. It is thought that calbindins function in the enteric absorption of calcium by facilitating the movement of calcium through the enterocytic cytosol while keeping the intracellular concentration of the free Ca^{2+} ion below hazardous levels. Calbindins are not expressed in vitamin D deficiency but are expressed in response to 1,25(OH)$_2$-D$_3$. That such treatment increases the expression of the protein without affecting its message suggests that vitamin D regulation of calbindin may occur at the translational level.

Nongenomic Pathways of Vitamin D Function

Some biological responses to vitamin D appear to be mediated by signal transduction mechanisms that are independent of transcription triggered by binding of the nuclear VDR. These nongenomic responses can be evoked within seconds by 1,25-(OH)$_2$-D$_3$. They include the stimulation of membrane phospholipid synthesis, cGMP levels, selenite (SeO_3^{-2}) uptake, and Ca^{2+} channel activation (which increases intracellular Ca^{2+} concentrations). The rapid Ca^{2+} transport response (sometimes referred to as **transcaltachia**) has been associated with a receptor for 1,25-(OH)$_2$-D$_3$ located in the plasmalemma. Substantial evidence

suggests that some aspects of intestinal calcium absorption are mediated by 1,25-(OH)$_2$-D$_3$ interacting with this cell surface receptor on the basal lateral membrane of the enterocyte to increase membrane Ca^{2+} permeability. Other studies, however have not found rapid transcaltachia to contribute significantly to the overall absorption of calcium across the gut.

Roles of Vitamin D in Calcium and Phosphorus Metabolism

The most clearly elucidated and, apparently, most physiologically important function of vitamin D is in the homeostasis of Ca^{2+} and phosphate. This is effected by a multihormonal system involving the controlled production of 1,25-(OH)$_2$-D$_3$, which functions in concert with PTH and calcitonin (CT). Regulation of this system occurs at the points of intestinal absorption, bone accretion and mobilization, and renal excretion.

Intestinal absorption of Ca^{2+}

Calcium is absorbed in the small intestine by both transcellular and paracellular mechanisms. The former is an active, saturable process, occurring in mammals primarily in the duodenum and upper jejunum and constitutes the most important means of absorbing calcium under conditions of low intake of the mineral; the latter is a nonsaturable process occurring throughout the intestine and is the most important means of absorbing calcium when calcium intake is high. The active metabolite, 1,25-(OH)$_2$-D$_3$, stimulates the enteric absorption of calcium through roles in both mechanisms, although its mechanism in the paracellular process is unclear. The availability of calcium for both processes is affected by both exogenous (e.g., inhibition by food phytates or phosphate) and endogenous (e.g., gastric acid secretion) factors.

When 1,25-(OH)$_2$-D$_3$ was found to induce called calbindins in the intestinal mucosa, it was logical to propose that those proteins must mediate the effect of vitamin D on the absorption of Ca^{2+} across the gut. Indeed, intestinal levels of 1,25-(OH)$_2$-D$_3$, calbindin mRNA, and Ca^{2+} uptake are highly correlated, but exposure to 1,25-(OH)$_2$-D$_3$ was found to cause measurable increases in Ca^{2+} absorption *before*

---

[53] Calbindins are members of a large family of Ca^{2+}-binding proteins having a distinctive helix-loop-helix sequence, the so-called EF hand.

increases in calbindin could be detected. Furthermore, the stimulatory effect of a single dose 1,25-$(OH)_2$-D_3 on Ca^{2+} absorption was found to decay long *before* intestinal calbindin levels started to fall.[54] Therefore, it is clear whether the effect of vitamin D on the enteric absorption of Ca^{2+} (particularly, rapid Ca^{2+} uptake) is mediated by calbindin or other processes. Subsequent research has revealed the process to be more complicated than envisioned.

The transcellular process of enteric calcium absorption is now seen as having three components, each of which is stimulated by 1,25-$(OH)_2$-D_3:

- *Uptake of Ca^{2+} from the intestinal lumen to the microvillus border.* This uptake of Ca2+ at the brush border involves a two-step mechanism involving a Ca^{2+} channel or integral membrane transporter (CaT1), followed by a channel-like flow gated by the intercellular concentration of Ca^{2+}, allowing the controlled movement of Ca^{2+} down a steep electrochemical gradient.[55] The latter is thought to involve the Ca^{2+}-binding protein **calmodulin**,[56] which can bind a number of target proteins, including myosin-I, a membrane ATPase that can tether F-actin filaments to the microvillar membrane perhaps affecting the permeability of the latter.
- *Translocation of Ca^{2+} across the cell to the basolateral membrane.* The movement of calcium across the enterocyte involves the vitamin-dependent Ca^{2+}-binding protein, calbindin, functioning as both a Ca^{2+} transporter and a cytosolic Ca^{2+} buffer. Calbindin appears to transport more than 90% of the transcellular calcium flux; its expression and thus calcium absorption, cease under conditions of vitamin D deficiency.
- *Active extrusion of Ca^{2+} into the circulation.* This occurs against a substantial thermodynamic

gradient involving a 50,000-fold differential in Ca^{2+} concentration and a positive electrical potential.[57] This action is facilitated by an Ca^{2+}-ATPase[58] residing in the basolateral membrane.

The paracellular process of calcium absorption is less well understood, although evidence suggests that it, too, is stimulated by 1,25-$(OH)_2$-D_3. Thus, it appears that vitamin D can affect the diffusional permeability of tight junction complexes to calcium, possibly by 1,25-$(OH)_2$-D_3-mediated second messengers.

Intestinal phosphate absorption

Vitamin D increases the mucosal uptake of phosphorus and enhances its absorption from the lumen of the gut. The active metabolite 1,25-$(OH)_2$-D_3 appears to modulate the number of carrier sites available at the mucosal membrane for a sodium-dependent phosphate entry.[59] At least in the duodenum, this process is independent of calcium absorption. The mechanism of vitamin D function in this process has not been elucidated.

Renal resorption of calcium and phosphate

Vitamin D, as 1,25-$(OH)_2$-D_3, stimulates the resorption of both phosphate and Ca^{2+} in the distal renal tubule.[60] The quantitative significance of this effect is greater for phosphate than it is for Ca^{2+}, as most (80%) of the latter is resorbed by passive, vitamin D-independent, paracellular routes in the proximal tubules and ascending loop of Henle. The transcellular process resembles that of the intestine in having a Ca^{2+} channel component, cytosolic Ca^{2+}-binding proteins (calbindin-D_{28k}) and a plasma membrane Ca^{2+} ATPase, all of which are expressed in 1,25-$(OH)_2$-D_3-responsive nephrons.

---

[54] This effect has been called **transcaltachia;** it is thought to involve the interaction of Ca^{2+} in the endocytic vesicles at the brush border, where they fuse with lysosomes to travel along the microtubules to the basolateral border where exocytosis occurs.

[55] Luminal concentrations of Ca^{2+} can be in the mM range, whereas intracellular concentrations of the free ion are in the of 50–100nM range.

[56] Calmodulin is a 17kD acidic protein (also of the "EF hand" family) that is expressed in many cell types and subcellular compartments. It can bind as many as 4 Ca^{2+} ions, which causes conformational changes and post-translational modifications that allow it also to bind to more than 100 target proteins. In this way, calmodulin serves as a major transducer of Ca^{2+}-signals in the control of cellular metabolism.

[57] It is estimated that the movement of 1 mole of Ca^{2+} against this gradient requires about 9.3kcal.

[58] The CaATPase spans the membrane, with a Ca2+-binding domain on the cytoplasmic side. It appears that phosphorylation-induced conformational changes in the protein allow it to form a channel-like opening through which Ca^{2+} is expelled, thus serving as a Ca "pump."

[59] Phosphate uptake by the brush border membrane takes place against an electrochemical gradient via a saturable Na^+–phosphate symport (common transport). The rate-limiting and regulated step for phosphate absorption appears to be at the brush border membrane entry.

[60] Each day a human filters some 8g calcium at the glomerulus, 98% of which is reabsorbed.

Bone mineral turnover

Bone is the largest target organ for vitamin D, accumulating more than one-quarter of a single dose of the vitamin within a few hours of its administration. That lesions in bone mineralization (rickets, osteomalacia) occur in vitamin D deficiency has long indicated its vital function in the metabolism of this organ.[61] The pattern of vitamin D metabolites in bone differs from that in intestine. Whereas the latter contains mainly $1,25\text{-}(OH)_2\text{-}D_3$, bone contains mainly $25\text{-}OH\text{-}D_3$, accounting for >50% of the vitamin D metabolites present, with $1,25\text{-}(OH)_2\text{-}D_3$ comprising less than 35%. As in plasma, the level of $24,25\text{-}(OH)_2\text{-}D_3$ in bone is fairly constant relative to that of $25\text{-}OH\text{-}D_3$.

Vitamin D plays roles in both the formation (*mineralization*) of bone and in the mobilization of bone mineral (*demineralization*). Some evidence suggests that bone mineralization may be mediated through $1,25\text{-}(OH)_2\text{-}D_3$, which is localized in the nuclei of the cells (*osteoblasts* and osteoprogenitor cells) that lay down bone mineral. These cells have been found to have $1,25\text{-}(OH)_2\text{-}D_3$ receptors that are stimulated by glucocorticoids. However, it is generally thought that $24,25\text{-}(OH)_2\text{-}D_3$ is also involved in this process; although the mechanism remains unclear, it appears to involve PTH. Interestingly, $1,25\text{-}(OH)_2\text{-}D_3$ has been found to stimulate bone growth *in vivo* but to inhibit bone accretion in tissue culture. The synthesis of the vitamin K-dependent Ca^{2+}-binding protein osteocalcin is increased by $1,25\text{-}(OH)_2\text{-}D_3$ both *in vivo* and in cultured cells. The relevance of this finding to bone mineralization is unclear, as osteocalcin is known to inhibit hydroxyapatite formation. It is possible that $1,25\text{-}(OH)_2\text{-}D_3$ may both stimulate *and* repress bone mineralization, according to such factors as its concentration, the presence of $24,25\text{-}(OH)_2\text{-}D_3$, and so on.

Vitamin D stimulates osteoclast-mediated bone resorption. This process appears to be mediated by $1,25\text{-}(OH)_2\text{-}D_3$, as it is the only form of vitamin D that is effective in anephric rats. It appears that, in this process, vitamin D has a role in the differentiation of macrophages to osteoclasts, as the number of these giant multinucleated bone-degrading cells is very low in bone from vitamin D-deficient animals. The demineralization of bone serves to mobilize Ca^{2+} and phosphate from that reserve, thus maintaining the homeostasis of those minerals in the plasma.[62] The process of bone resorption involves PTH, which appears to act via cAMP (i.e., PTH stimulates adenylcyclase activity) in a mechanism involving a $1,25\text{-}(OH)_2\text{-}D_3$-dependent factor. Because PTH is secreted in response to **hypophosphatemia**, nutritional deprivation of phosphate, too, can lead to bone demineralization.[63] The stimulation in bone cells of alkaline phosphatase activity, by a process inhibited by cycloheximide and actinomycin D and, therefore, involving *de novo* protein synthesis, has been demonstrated for $1,25\text{-}(OH)_2\text{-}D_3$.

Calcium and phosphate homeostasis

The normal concentration of Ca^{2+} in the serum of most species is about $10\,mg/dl$[64]; the vitamin D-dependent homeostatic system responds to perturbations of that level by modulating Ca^{2+} entry to and exit from the plasma via three portals: intestine, kidney, and bone (Fig. 6-7.) Diuresis For example, when the serum Ca^{2+} concentration falls below this target level (i.e., the development of **hypocalcemia**), PTH is secreted by the parathyroid glands, which function to detect hypocalcemia. The kidney responds to PTH in two ways: phosphate **diuresis** and stimulation of 25-OH-vitamin D 1-hydroxylase. The latter effect increases the production of $1,25\text{-}(OH)_2\text{-}D_3$, which acts (probably by inducing calbindin) in the intestine to increase the enteric absorption of both Ca^{2+} and phosphate. In addition, $1,25\text{-}(OH)_2\text{-}D_3$ acts jointly with PTH in bone to promote the mobilization of Ca^{2+} and phosphate. The aggregate result of these responses is to increase the concentrations of Ca^{2+} and phosphate in the plasma.

---

[61] Thus, the involvement of vitamin D in the metabolism of Ca and P was clear, as structural bone contains 99% of total body Ca and 85% of total body P, which in a 70-kg man are about 1200 and 770 g, respectively.

[62] The normal ranges of these parameters in human adults are as follows: calcium, 8.5–10.6 mg/dl; phosphorus, 2.5–4.5 mg/dl.

[63] Hypophosphatemia also increases the activity of 25-OH-vitamin D 1-hydroxylase and the accumulation of $1,25\text{-}(OH)_2\text{-}D_3$ in target tissues. These effects are associated with bone demineralization. In addition, hypophosphatemia can lead to bone resorption directly by a process that is independent of vitamin D.

[64] This level is 10,000 times greater than those within cells. Extracellular signals, such as hormones, stress, or pathogenesis, can disturb this ion gradient to produce transient increases intracellular Ca^{2+} concentrations. Such increases can signal a variety of cellular responses (e.g., transcriptional control, neurotransmitter release, muscular contraction) through the actions of binding proteins that serve as transducers of the Ca^{2+} signal.

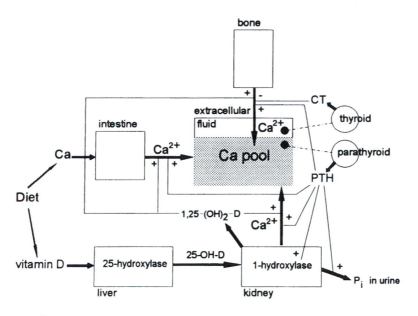

Fig. 6-7. Calcium homeostasis.

Under conditions of increased circulating concentrations of Ca^{2+} (**hypercalcemia**), calcitonin (CT) is secreted by the thyroid gland (i.e., C cells). That hormone suppresses bone mobilization and is also thought to increase the renal excretion of both Ca^{2+} and phosphate. In that situation, the 25-OH-vitamin D 1-hydroxylase may be feedback inhibited by 1,25-$(OH)_2$-D_3, and may actually be converted to the catalysis of the 24-hydroxylation of 25-OH-D_3. In the case of egg-laying birds, which show relatively high circulating concentrations of 1,25-$(OH)_2$-D_3, the 1-hydroxylase activity remains stimulated by the hormone **prolactin**.

Calcium deposition in the skeleton involves the intracellular synthesis of collagen and fibrils by the bone-forming osteoblasts, which extrude these fibrils to form the extracellular matrix of bone, portions of which can be mineralized.[65] Calcium mobilization from bone is directed by multinucleated osteoclasts that release proteins and lysosomal enzymes that dissolve bone mineral[66] and lyse its organic matrix. The accretion/mobilization of bone Ca^{2+}, therefore, involves the relative activities of osteoblasts and osteoclasts, with the bone surface serving, in effect, as a calcium buffer.

Roles of other minerals

Vitamin D function can be affected by several other mineral elements:

- *Zinc.* Deprivation of zinc has been found to diminish the 1,25-$(OH)_2$-D_3 response to low calcium intake,[67] and it has been suggested that zinc may indirectly affect renal 25-OH-D_3 1-hydroxylase activity.
- *Iron.* Iron deficiency has been shown to be associated with low serum concentrations of 24,25-$(OH)_2$-D_3 and reduced 25-OH-D_3 responses to supplementation with vitamin D_3. It has been suggested that iron deficiency, which is known to impair the enteric absorption of fat and vitamin A, may also impair the absorption of vitamin D.
- *Boron.* An interaction of vitamin D, magnesium and calcium has been demonstrated with **boron (B)**, an element known to be essential for plants. The feeding of low-boron diets has been shown to increase bone mobilization (indicated by increased serum alkaline phosphatase activities) in vitamin D-deficient chicks and rats if

---

[65] **Osteoblasts** synthesize bone matrix at the cartilaginous **epiphyseal plate** (growth plate) located at the ends of long bones in growing individuals. The epiphyseal plate disappears after puberty, an event referred to as *fusion of the epiphysis*. Osteoblasts are also active in the basic structural unit of bone, the tube-like **osteon**. Bone consists of arrayed osteons around which mineralization/demineralization occurs. The organic matrix produced by osteoblasts comprises a third of bone dry matter, some 90% of that fraction being collagen with the remaining portion composed of other proteins (osteonectin, **osteocalcin** [also called bone GLA-protein], bone sialoprotein, protein–chondroitin sulfate complexes).

[66] Bone mineral consists of submicroscopic (about 30 nm in diameter) crystalline particles similar in composition to hydroxyapatite $[Ca_{10}(PO_4)_6(OH)_2]$ but also containing carbonate and Na^+.

[67] This finding may have clinical significance, for in many parts of the world children are undernourished with respect to both zinc and calcium.

they were also fed deficient levels of magnesium and calcium. In addition, supplementation of chicks' diets with boron was found to correct several metabolic outcomes of vitamin D deficiency (e.g., elevated plasma levels of glucose, β-hydroxybutyrate, pyruvate, triglycerides, and triiodothyronine; depressed levels of Ca^{2+}) in the presence of calcium and magnesium deficiencies. The mechanisms of these effects are not clear.

- *Lead.* Exposure to **lead** also appears to impair the 1-hydroxylation of 25-OH-D_3. Ironically, that effect increases the amount of enterically absorbed lead that can be bound by the vitamin D-responsive protein, calbindin, implicated in enteric calcium absorption. In children, blood levels of 1,25-$(OH)_2$-D_3 and calcium have been found to be inversely related to blood lead concentrations,[68] suggesting that lead may inhibit the renal 1-hydroxylation of the vitamin, perhaps constituting an adaptation to protect against lead toxicity. This is consistent with 1,25-$(OH)_2$-D_3-mediated enhanced enteric lead absorption as a chief factor contributing to the elevated body lead burden generally observed in calcium deficiency (Table 6-8). Indeed, chronic ingestion of lead by calcium-deficient animals has been shown to reduce the metabolic production of 1,25-$(OH)_2$-D_3. This combination of effects allows the hormone system that is impaired by chronic lead ingestion to contribute to susceptibility to lead toxicity.[69]

Vitamin D and support of bone health

A recent meta-analysis of 12 randomized, controlled trials[70] revealed that vitamin D doses of 700 to 800 IU/day reduced the relative risk of hip fracture by 26% and of any nonvertebral fracture by 23%. Risk reductions were not oberved for trials that used a lower vitamin dose (400 IU/day).

Vitamin D Functions in Noncalcified Tissues

The finding of 1,25-$(OH)_2$-D_3 in tissues not involved in calcium homeostasis (e.g., β cells of the pancreas,[71] malpighian layer of the skin, specific cells of the brain, the pituitary, the mammary gland, endocrine cells of the stomach, the chorioallantoic membrane surrounding chick embryos)[72] suggests that this form of the vitamin may have a more general function in many cells (Table 6-9). The nature of such functions is still unclear, although it is reasonable to assume effects involving the regulation of the temporal/spatial distribution of intracellular calcium. Because such effects are observed at 1,25-$(OH)_2$-D_3 concentrations of 2 to 3 orders of magnitude greater than circulating levels, it is possible that they may normally be limited to specific sites of local production of the active metabolite such as during inflammation.

Role of vitamin D in immune function

That vitamin D functions in immunity is indicated by the identification of VDRs in most immune cells as

Table 6-8. Vitamin D-stimulated uptake and retention of lead[a]

		Kidney			Tibia	
Vitamin D treatment	Lead (%)	Calcium (ppm)	Lead (ppm)		Calcium (% ash)	Lead (ppm ash)
—	0	$69.0 \pm 8.8^*$	0^*		$33.2 \pm 0.4^*$	$23.4 \pm 14.3^*$
1,25-$(OH)_2$-D_3	0	$64.1 \pm 1.5^*$	0^*		$36.0 \pm 0.2^\dagger$	$10.9 \pm 6.7^*$
—	0.2	$56.6 \pm 3.8^*$	$4.8 \pm 0.5^\dagger$		$33.5 \pm 0.3^*$	$133.1 \pm 24.1^\dagger$
1,25-$(OH)_2$-D_3	0.2	$80.2 \pm 13.4^*$	$13.7 \pm 2.4\ddagger,\S$		$35.5 \pm 0.2^{\dagger,\ddagger}$	$335.1 \pm 15.8^\ddagger$
—	0.8	$62.4 \pm 2.4^*$	$9.2 \pm 0.9^\ddagger$		$32.8 \pm 0.2^*$	$299.8 \pm 4.8^\ddagger$
1,25-$(OH)_2$-D_3	0.8	$90.1 \pm 7.6^\dagger$	$32.4 \pm 7.6^\S$		$34.7 \pm 0.4^\ddagger$	$1008.8 \pm 71.2^\S$

[a]Entries with like superscripts are not significantly different ($p < 0.05$).
Source: Fullmer, C. S. (1990). *Proc. Soc. Exp. Biol. Med.* **194**, 258–264.

---

[68] The prevalence of lead toxicity among children is seasonal—for example, greatest in the summer months.

[69] Lead poisoning is a serious environmental health issue. In the United States alone, high blood lead levels are estimated in as many as 5 million school children and 400,000 pregnant women.

[70] Bischoff-Ferrari et al. (2005). *J. Am. Med. Assoc.* **293**, 2257–2264.

[71] Circulating insulin levels are reduced in vitamin D deficiency and respond quickly to treatment with 1,25-$(OH)_2$-D_3.

[72] Cytologic localization of 1,25-$(OH)_2$-D_3 has been achieved by the technique of frozen section autoradiography, made possible by the availability of radiolabeled 1,25-$(OH)_2$-D_3 of high specific activity.

Table 6-9. Experimental evidence for vitamin D functions in noncalcified tissues

Putative role	Observations
Cell differentiation	Promotion by 1,25-$(OH)_2$-D_3 of myeloid leukemic precursor cells to differentiate into cells resembling macrophages
Membrane structure	Alteration of the fatty acid composition of enterocytes, reducing their membrane fluidity
Mitochondrial metabolism	Decrease in isocitrate lyase and malate synthase (shown in rachitic chicks)
Muscular function	Stimulation of Ca^{2+} transport into the sarcoplasmic reticulum of cultured myeloblasts by 1,25-$(OH)_2$-D_3
	Easing, on treatment with vitamin D, of electrophysiological abnormalities in muscle contraction and relaxation in vitamin D-deficient humans
	Reduction, on treatment with vitamin D, of muscular weakness in humans
Pancreatic function	Stimulation of insulin production by pancreatic β cells in rats by 1,25-$(OH)_2$-D_3
	Impairment of insulin secretion, unrelated to the level of circulating calcium, shown in vitamin D-deficient humans
Immunity	Stimulation of immune cell functions by 1,25-$(OH)_2$-D_3
	Control of inflammation by 1,25-$(OH)_2$-D_3-dependent regulation of cytokine production
Neural function	Region-specific enhancement of choline acetyltransferase in rat brain by 1,25-$(OH)_2$-D_3
Skin	Inhibition of DNA synthesis in mouse epidermal cells by 1,25-$(OH)_2$-D_3
Parathyroid function	Inhibition of transcription of PTH gene via interaction of 1,25-$(OH)_2$-D_3 and DNA in parathyroid cells

well as the demonstration of effects of 1,25-$(OH)_2$-D_3 on the functional activities of those cells. This includes the inhibition of immunoglobulin secretion by B lymphocytes and the inhibition of production of interleukins 2 (IL-2) and 12 (IL-12), IL-2 receptor (IL-2R), granulocyte-macrophage colony-stimulating factor, and interferon-γ by T cells, and the inhibition of accessory cell and antigen-presenting cell activities. In addition, 1,25-$(OH)_2$-D_3 has been found to enhance macrophage and monocyte phagocytosis, bacterial killing, and heat shock protein production. The active metabolite 1,25-$(OH)_2$-D_3 has also been shown *in vitro* to suppress the antigen-presenting capacity of macrophages, apparently by reducing the expression of adhesion molecules necessary for full T-cell stimulation. Thus, 1,25-$(OH)_2$-D_3 has been found to suppress the development of various autoimmune diseases and to prolong the survival of allografts.

These effects appear to depend on VDRs, which mediate the 1,25-$(OH)_2$-D_3 signal to upregulate natural defense reactions by enhancing the functions of monocytes and macrophages. Vitamin D deficiency has been associated with inflammation; studies have shown the circulating marker of inflammation, C-reactive protein, to be inversely correlated with serum concentrations of 25-OH-D_3, and decreased in response to vitamin D treatment.[73] The active metabolite 1,25-$(OH)_2$-D_3 is also known to downregulate the production of pro-inflammatory cytokines by immune cells. However, that VDR-knockout mice show no immune abnormalities suggests that this function of the vitamin must be selective, depending on the nature of the immune challenge, or simply part of a higly reduntant system.

Vitamin D and noninsulin-dependent diabetes

For some years it has been known that vitamin D deficiency reduces the secretion of insulin but not other hormones produced by pancreatic beta cells, which have VDRs and express calbindin-D_{28k}. Furthermore, the insulin responses and glucose clearance rates of free-living humans has been found to vary according to VDR type. Subclinical, low-intensity, chronic inflammation has been associated with insulin resistance, which has been found to be inversely related to serum 25-OH-D_3 concentrations over a wide range.[74] Because insulin resistance is a major feature

[73] Timms et al. (2002). *Quarterly J. Med.* **95**, 787–796.
[74] Chiu et al. (2004). *Am. J. Clin. Nutr.* **79**, 820–825.

of non–insulin-dependent (type 2) diabetes mellitus (NIDDM), it is reasonable to ask whether low vitamin D status may play a role in the disease. To that point, results of the Third National Health and Nutrition Examination Survey (NHANES III) indicate an inverse association between quartiles of serum of 25-OH-D$_3$ levels and diabetes incidence in a multiethnic sample of over 6000 adults,[75] and Swedish researchers have found NIDDM incidence to be highest during the winter months when circulating 25-OH-D$_3$ levels are lowest.[76]

The relationship of vitamin D status and NIDDM risk appears to be greatest among overweight/obese individuals. Studies[77] have shown that serum 25-OH-D$_3$ levels are inversely correlated with body mass index[78] (Fig. 6-8) and body fat mass. One study[79] found that women with NIDDM and relatively high BMIs more frequently had low serum 25-OH-D$_3$ levels than did nondiabetic women with lower BMIs. These findings indicate low vitamin D status as a risk factor for NIDDM, an effect that can be exacerbated by adiposity ostensibly due to the removal of the vitamin from functional pools as a result of its partitioning into bulk lipid depots

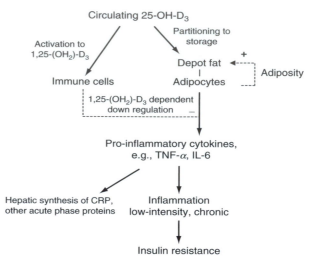

Fig. 6-9. Hypothetical relationships of vitamin D status and adiposity in affecting insulin resistance. *Abbreviations:* TNF-α, tumor necrosis factor α; IL-6, interleukin-6; CRP, C-reactive protein.

in adipose tissue. According to this hypothesis (Fig. 6-9), adipocytes would be involved in two opposing ways: responding to 1,25-(OH)$_2$-D$_3$ in the regulation of cytokine production; and sequestering 25-OH-D$_3$.

Vitamin D and autoimmune diseases

It has been suggested that vitamin D may play a role in insulin-dependent diabetes melitus (IDDM, type I diabetes), which results from the T-cell dependent destruction of insulin-producing pancreatic beta cells due to cytokines and perhaps free radicals from inflammatory infiltrates. Several epidemiological studies have indicated correlations between IDDM incidence and latitude (positive) and hours of sunlight (negative), and some prospective studies, including a large, multicenter case-control study,[80] have showed associations between vitamin D supplementation in infancy and reduced risk to IDDM later in life. Such protection may occur only with relatively large doses of the vitamin (50μg/day[81]).

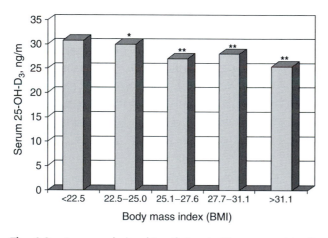

Fig. 6-8. Inverse relationship of vitamin D status and body mass index apparent in NHANES III subjects. Comparisons with lowest quintile: *$p < 0.05$, **$p < 0.01$. (*After* Black et al., [2005]. *Clin. Invest.* **128**, 3792–3798.)

[75] Scragg et al. (2004). *Diabetes Care* **27**, 2813–2818.

[76] Berger et al. (1999). *Diabetes Care* **22**, 773–777.

[77] Arunabh et al. (2003). *J. Clin. Endocrinol. Metab.* **88**, 157–161; Parikh et al. (2004). *J. Clin. Endocrinol. Metab.* **89**, 1196–1199.

[78] BMI = weight (kg)/height (m^2) or [weight (lb)/height (in^2)] × 705.

[79] Isaia et al. (2001). *Diabetes* **24**, 1496–1503.

[80] The EURODIAB Substudy 2 Study Group (1999). *Diabetologia* **42**, 51–54.

[81] Hyponen et al. (2001). *Lancet* **358**, 1500–1503.

Pancreatic beta cells express calbindin-D_{28k}, which has been found to protect them from cytokine-mediated cell death, and 1,25-$(OH)_2$-D_3 has been found to protect beta cells from cytokine-mediated dysfunction, known to be important in the pathogenesis of the disease. High doses of 1,25-$(OH)_2$-D_3 have been shown to reduce the incidence of diabetes in an animal model.[82] Two prospective trials have been conducted to evaluate the efficacy of vitamin D in preventing IDDM: One found positive effects of vitamin D doses of 50μg/day;[83] the other detected no effect using lower doses (<10μg/d).[84]

Studies have shown inverse associations of vitamin D intake, regardless of sun exposure, and the incidences of multiple sclerosis (MS) and rheumatoid arthritis (RA) which, like irritable bowel disease (IBD) and Crohn's disease are prevalent in northern lattitudes. Two studies have pointed to protective effects of vitamin D supplements against the clinical severity of MS and RA, but these trials have involved small numbers of patients and have not been placebo-controlled. Polymorphisms of VDR have been associated with increased risk of MS, RA, IBD, and IDDM. It appears that 1,25-$(OH)_2$-D_3 inhibits the symptoms of T-helper cell-driven autoimmune diseases, as VDR-knockout animal models do not show inflammatory signs attendant to experimentally induced asthma.

Vitamin D and periodontal disease

Circulating concentrations of 25-OH-D_3 have been found to be inversely correlated with the risk of periodontal disease in adults. This effect appears to be independent of those of bone mineral density. That it may involve the anti-inflammatory effects is supported by the finding that serum 25-OH-D_3 levels were inversely related to susceptibility to gingival inflammation and tooth loss in the NHANES III survey.

Vitamin D and cardiovascular disease

Epidemiological studies have shown that factors known to affect vitamin D status such as latitude,

altitude, and season are also associated with cardiovascular disease (CVD) mortality. For this reason, it has been suggested that low vitamin D status may be a risk factor for CVD. Although few intervention trials have been conducted to test this hypothesis, those that have indicate reductions in biomarkers of CVD risk, namely, CRP. Certainly, vitamin D is known to suppress several mechanisms of CVD pathogenesis: proliferation of vascular smooth muscle, vascular calcification, production of pro-inflammatory cytokines, and regulation of the renin-angiotensin system.

Vitamin D and proliferative skin diseases

The finding that 1,25-$(OH)_2$-D_3 can inhibit proliferation and induce terminal differentiation of cultured keratinocytes stimulated the study of its potential value in the treatment of proliferative skin disorders. Such studies have revealed that vitamin D has a paracrine function in skin keratinocytes: Those cells can produce vitamin D_3, metabolize it to 1,25-$(OH)_2$-D_3, and respond to the latter by changing from proliferating basal cells to terminally differentiated corneocytes. These effects appear to be among those mediated by VDRs, which are expressed throughout the epidermis as well as in skin immune cells,[85] and involve increases in intracellular free Ca^{2+} associated with increased phosphoinositide (inositol triphosphate and diacylglycerol) levels. Studies have shown that 1,25-$(OH)_2$-D_3 can decrease keratinocyte sensitivity to epidermal growth factor (EGF) receptor-mediated growth factors, can increase the transcription of transforming growth factor $β_1$ (TGF-$β_1$), and can regulate a cytokine cascade[86] involved in the accumulation of leukocytes during skin inflammation. Clinical studies have shown that both oral and topical applications of appropriate doses of either 1,25-$(OH)_2$-D_3 or the synthetic analog 1α,25-$(OH)_2$-D_3[87] can be safe and effective in the management of **psoriasis**.[88] Because the use of 1,25-$(OH)_2$-D_3 carries associated risks of hypercalcemia and hypercalciuria,

---

[82] Mathieu and colleagues have reported a 28% reduction in the autoimmune NOD mouse (Mathieu et al. [1994]. *Dabetologia* **37**, 552–558), but no effect in the BB rat model (Mathieu et al. [1997] in *Vitamin D and Diabetes* [Feldman, D., Glorieux, F., and J. Pike, eds.] pp. 1183–1196) Academic Press, San Diego.

[83] Hyponen et al. (2001). *Lancet* **358**, 1500–1503.

[84] Stene et al. (2003). *Am. J. Clin. Nutr.* **78**, 1128–1134.

[85] VDRs are expressed by the majority of Langerhans cells, macrophages, and T lymphocytes in skin.

[86] 1,25-$(OH)_2$-D_3 has been shown to inhibit the expression of mRNA for the neutrophil-activating peptide interleukin 8 (IL-8) in keratinocytes, dermal fibroblasts, and monocytes; these cells produce IL-8 in the skin of psoriatic but not nonpsoriatic patients.

[87] This analog is also called **calcipotriol**.

[88] Results of one clinical series showed that topical application of 1,25-$(OH)_2$-vitamin D_3 caused complete clearing of lesions in 60% of patients, with an additional 30% of patients showing significant decreases in scale, plaque thickness, and erythema.

there is interest in developing treatment regimens for such diseases involving the application of high doses of the vitamin in a safe and effective manner.

Vitamin D and muscular function

That vitamin D plays an important role in muscle is evidenced by the presence of VDR in myocytes and the lack of muscle development observed in VDR-knockout mice. Furthermore, myocytes treated with $1,25\text{-}(OH)_2\text{-}D_3$ respond by activating protein kinase C and transporting Ca^{2+} in the sarcoplasmic reticulum, an effect necessary for muscle contraction. Thus, it is not surprising that muscular weakness and hypotonia are seen in rickets, or that patients with osteomalacia frequently show myopathy. The latter affects primarily the type II muscle fibers that are the first to be recruited to avoid falling, resembling the **sarcopenia**[89] associated with aging. Therefore, it has been suggested that insufficient vitamin D status may increase the risk to bone fracture by affecting strength, balance, and gait. Although few intervention studies have addressed muscular function, those that have done so have shown that vitamin D supplementation (700–800 IU/day) of elderly subjects modestly improved muscle mass and function (as indicated by body sway, gait, balance) with as much as a halving in the frequency of falls.

Vitamin D and cancer

Epidemiologic studies have pointed to relationships of vitamin D status and cancer risk. Several studies in Europe and the United States have found positive associations between latitude and risk to cancers of the prostate, colon, and breast. Participants in the Nurses Health Study showed a significant inverse linear association between plasma 25-OH-D_3 and colon cancer risk.[90] Residents of the northern United States have nearly a twofold higher risk of total cancer mortality than those of the southern states. At least two studies have shown low serum $1,25\text{-}(OH)_2\text{-}D_3$ levels to be associated with increased risk of breast cancer (Fig. 6-10).

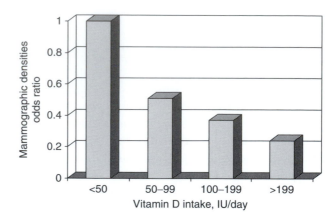

Fig. 6-10. Inverse relationship of frequency of mammographic breast density and vitamin D status in a cohort of 543 women aged 40–60 years undergoing screening mammographies. (*From* Berube et al. [2004]. *Cancer Epidemiol. Biomarkers Prev.* **13**, 1466–1472.)

That vitamin D may be protective against colon cancer is supported by the finding that cultured colonocytes have a high 1-hydroxylase capacity, converting 5 to 10% of 25-OH-D_3 to the active metabolite. Studies with a variety of cancer cell lines have shown that $1,25\text{-}(OH)_2\text{-}D_3$ can inhibit cell proliferation, induce cell differentiation, and induce apoptosis.[91] Physiological concentrations of 25-OH-D_3 inhibit mammary cells, which can also produce $1,25\text{-}(OH)_2\text{-}D_3$. Presumably, these effects result from the induction of gene expression[92] involved in the regulation of cell proliferation. In human leukemic cells,[93] $1,25\text{-}(OH)_2\text{-}D_3$ has been found to suppress cell division and induce differentiation by downregulating expression of the protooncogene c-*myc*. Thus, it has been proposed that this effect serves to bypass the cell cycle control (via synthesis or nuclear association) of c-*myc*. The antiproliferative effects of vitamin D may also involve its effects on cellular Ca^{2+} status and availability. Studies have shown that $1,25\text{-}(OH)_2\text{-}D_3$ can both attenuate the growth of rapidly dividing colonic tumor cells[94] and reverse colonocytes from a malignant to a normal phenotype. These effects depend on binding of the vitamer to VDRs and may involve opening of Ca^{2+} channels, leading to rapid

---

[89] Loss of muscle.

[90] Feskanich et al. (2004). *Cancer Epidemiol. Biomarkers* **13**, 1502–1508.

[91] Programmed cell death.

[92] Namely, such factors as cyclin D1, Kip1, WAF1, c-Fos, c-Myc, cyclin C, c-JUN and members of the TBF-beta family.

[93] HL-60 cells.

[94] Caco-2 cells.

reductions in the intracellular Ca^{2+} level, thus inducing apoptosis.[95] The mammary gland expresses VDR where the liganded receptor appears to function to oppose estrogen-driven proliferation and maintain differentiation. In that tissue 1,25-$(OH)_2$-D_3 has been shown to reduce the invasiveness of cancer cells and to inhibit angiogenesis. It has been suggested that polymorphisms in VDR may be associated with cancer risk; however, a recent meta-analysis indicated that such polymorphisms are unlikely to be major determinants of risk for at least prostate cancer.

Central Role of the Parathyroid Gland in Facilitating Vitamin D Function

The parathyroid gland has a central role in the physiological function of vitamin D. The gland senses serum calcium levels; when they drop, it increases secretion of PTH into the circulation (see Fig. 6-11). **Parathyroid hormone** is essential to vitamin D function. Increasing serum PTH levels stimulate the renal 25-OH-D_3 1-hydroxylase, thus increasing the production of 1,25-$(OH)_2$-D_3.[96] In addition, PTH facilitates the stimulation by 1,25-$(OH)_2$-D_3 of both osteoclastic activity and renal calcium resorption, both of which activities serve to restore the plasma Ca^{2+} concentration.

Secondary hyperparathyroidism, characterized by elevated serum PTH concentrations, is common among elderly people. The condition can reflect some degree of renal insufficiency, with associated reduction in renal 25-OH-vitamin D_3 1-hydroxylase activity. Serum concentrations of PTH can also increase owing to privational vitamin D deficiency, in which case it is manifested by low circulating levels of 25-OH-vitamin D_3. Accordingly, the PTH levels of people living in northern latitudes are highest during the winter for subjects not taking supplemental vitamin D.

Healthful Intakes of Vitamin D

Recognition of the roles of vitamin D beyond its long-established functions in bone mineralization has naturally led to questions about the levels required to support these aspect of health. Therefore, efforts have been made to ascertain the threshold intakes and biomarker levels for optimal bone mineral density, dental health, lower extremity function, and risks of falls, fractures, and cancer. A recent analysis concluded that, for these end points, the most advantageous serum 25-OH-D_3 concentration are 90 to 100 nmol/L (36–40 ng/ml) (Fig. 6-12). Such levels require regular daily vitamin D intakes of greater than 1000 IU (40 mcg).[97]

VII. Vitamin D Deficiency
Causes of Vitamin D Deficiency

Vitamin D deficiency can result from inadequate irradiation of the skin, insufficient intake from the diet, or impairments in the metabolic activation (hydroxylations) of the vitamin. Although sunlight can provide the means of biosynthesis of vitamin D_3, it is a well-documented fact that many people, particularly those in extreme latitudes during the winter months, do not receive sufficient solar irradiation to support adequate vitamin D status. Even people in sunnier climates may not produce adequate vitamin D if their lifestyles or health status keep them indoors, or if such factors as air pollution or clothing reduce their exposure to UV light. Most people, therefore, show strong seasonal fluctuations in plasma 25-OH-D_3 concentration; for some, this can be associated with considerable periods of suboptimal vitamin D status if not corrected by an adequate dietary source of the vitamin. Until the practice of vitamin D fortification

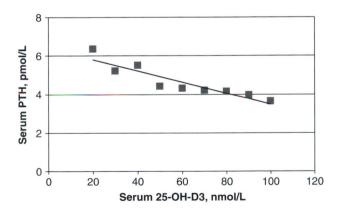

Fig. 6-11. Relationship of serum PTH and vitamin D status. (*From* Need et al. [2000]. *Am. J. Clin. Nutr.* **71**, 1577–1581.)

---

[95] The process of programmed cell death is called *apoptosis*.

[96] Parathyroidectomized animals cannot mount this 1-hydroxylase response unless they are treated with exogenous PTH.

[97] The analysis by Bischoff-Ferrari, H. A., et al. (2006). *Am. J. Clin. Nutr.* **84**, 18–28 indicated that vitamin D intakes of at least 1000 mcg/day are required to bring 50% of healthy American adults above the serum 25-OH-D_3 level of 75 nmol/L. Current recommended intakes for vitamin D are 200 and 600 IU/day in younger and older adults, respectively.

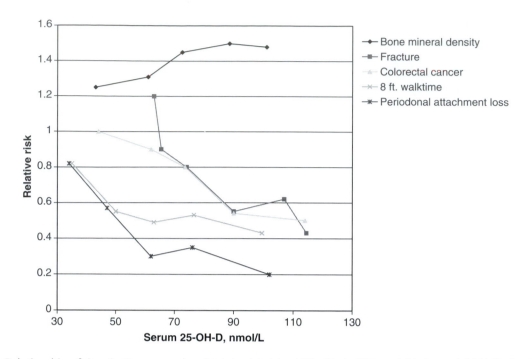

Fig. 6-12. Relationship of vitamin D status and multiple health risks. (*After* Bischoff-Ferrari, H. A., et al. [2006]. *Am. J. Clin. Nutr.* **84**, 18–28.)

of foods became widespread, at least in technologically developed countries, it was difficult to obtain adequate vitamin D from the diet, as most foods contain only minuscule amounts.[98] Therefore, vitamin D deficiency can have privational and/or nonprivational causes:

- *Privational causes* These involve inadequate vitamin D supply. They include:
  - ○ Inadequate exposure to sunlight
  - ○ Insufficient consumption of food sources of vitamin D
- *Nonprivational causes* These relate to impairments in the absorption, metabolism, or nuclear binding of the vitamin. They include:
  - ○ Diseases of the gastrointestinal tract (e.g., small bowel disease, gastrectomy, pancreatitis), involving malabsorption of the vitamin from the diet

  - ○ Diseases of the liver (biliary cirrhosis, hepatitis), involving reduced activities of the 25-hydroxylase
  - ○ Diseases of the kidney (e.g., nephritis, renal failure), involving reduced activities of the 1-hydroxylase, the major source of $1,25\text{-}(OH)_2\text{-}D_3$,[99] or of $25\text{-}OH\text{-}D_3$ as in individuals with nephrotic syndrome[100] who lose $25\text{-}OH\text{-}D_3$ along with its globulin-binding protein into the urine
  - ○ Exposure to certain drugs (e.g., the anticonvulsives phenobarbital, diphenylhydantoin), which induce the catabolism of 25-OH-D3 and 1,25-(OH)2-D3, reduce circulating levels of the former, and reduce elevated PTH levels[101]
  - ○ Impaired parathyroid function resulting in **hypoparathyroidism** (reduced production of PTH), which impairs the ability to respond to hypocalcemia[102] by increasing the conversion of $25\text{-}OH\text{-}D_3$ to $1,25\text{-}(OH)_2\text{-}D_3$

---

[98] Eggs are the notable exception. Even cows' milk and human milk contain only very small amounts of vitamin D.

[99] Chronic kidney disease leading to bone disease is called *renal osteodystrophy*. It is a frequent complication in renal dialysis patients, in which its severity varies directly with the reduction in the glomerular filtration rate. It is more common among children than adults, presumably owing to the greater sensitivity of growing bone to the deprivation of vitamin D, phosphate, and PTH that occurs in renal disease.

[100] A clinical condition, involving renal tubular degeneration, characterized by edema, albuminuria, hypoalbuminemia, and usually hypercholesterolemia.

[101] Vitamin D supplements (up to 4000 IU/day) are recommended to prevent rickets in children on long-term anticonvulsant therapy.

[102] Affected individuals show continued hypocalcemia leading to hyperphosphatemia. These conditions typically respond to treatment with $1,25\text{-}(OH)_2\text{-}D_3$ or high levels of vitamin D_3.

○ Genetic mutations resulting in impaired expression of the renal 25-(OH)-D3-1-hydroxylase in the condition referred to as **vitamin D-dependent rickets type I**, which can be managed using low doses of $1,25\text{-}(OH)_2\text{-}D_3$ or $1\alpha\text{-}OH\text{-}D_3$

○ Expression of a nonfunctional VDR and impairing the transcription of vitamin D-regulated genes involved in Ca and phosphorus homeostasis in the condition referred to as **vitamin D-dependent rickets type II**, the management of which requires relatively high doses of $1,25\text{-}(OH)_2\text{-}D_3$ or $1\alpha\text{-}OH\text{-}D_3$

○ Resistance of PTH target cells, resulting in **pseudohypoparathyroidism** and involving hypocalcemia without compensating renal retention or bone mobilization of Ca despite normal PTH secretion; the condition responds to low doses of $1,25\text{-}(OH)_2\text{-}D_3$ or $1\alpha\text{-}OH\text{-}D_3$[103]

○ **Vitamin D-resistance**[104] involving impaired phosphate transport in the intestine and reabsorption in the proximal renal tubules, hypersensitivity to PTH, and impaired 1-hydroxylation of 25-OH-D_3; the condition responds to phosphate plus either high-dose vitamin D_3 (25,000–50,000 IU/day) or low doses of $1,25\text{-}(OH)_2\text{-}D_3$ or $1\alpha\text{-}OH\text{-}D_3$.

Signs of Vitamin D Deficiency

General signs

Frank deficiency of vitamin D affects several sytems, most prominently skeletal and neuromuscular (Table 6-10).

Signs of Vitamin D Deficiency in Humans

Rickets

Rickets first appears in 6- to 24-month-old children, but can manifest at any time until the closure of the bones' epiphyseal growth plates. It is characterized by impaired mineralization of the growing bones with accompanying bone pain, muscular tenderness, and hypocalcemic tetany (Table 6-10). Tooth eruption may be delayed, the fontanelle may close late, and knees and wrists may appear swollen. Affected children develop deformations of their softened, weight-bearing bones, particularly those of the legs and arms—hence, the characteristic leg signs, *bowleg*,[105] *knock knee*,[106] and *sabre tibia*, which occur in nearly half of cases (Fig. 6-13). Radiography reveals enlarged epiphyseal growth plates resulting from their failure to mineralize and continue growth. Rickets is most frequently associated with low dietary intakes of calcium, as in the lack of access to or avoidance of milk products.[107]

Osteomalacia

Osteomalacia occurs in older children and adults with formed bones whose epiphyseal closure has rendered that region of the bone unaffected by vitamin D deficiency. The signs and symptoms of osteomalacia are more generalized than those of rickets, for example, muscular weakness and bone tenderness and pain, particularly in the spine, shoulder, ribs, or pelvis (Table 6-10). Lesions involve the failure to mineralize bone matrix, which continues to be synthesized by functional osteoblasts. Therefore, the condition is characterized by an increase in the ratio of nonmineralized bone to mineralized bone. Radiographic examination reveals abnormally low bone density (osteopenia) and the presence of pseudofractures, especially in the spine, femur, and humerus. Patients with osteomalacia are at increased risk of fractures of all types, but particularly those of the wrist and pelvis.

Osteoporosis

Although it is sometimes confused with osteomalacia, osteoporosis is a very different disease, being characterized by decreased bone mass with retention of normal histological appearance

---

[103] 0.25–3 mg/day.

[104] This is also called *hypophosphatemic rickets/osteomalacia* and *phosphate diabetes*.

[105] *Genu varum*.

[106] *Genu valgum*.

[107] Despite the notion that rickets has been eliminated (as a result of vitamin D fortification of dairy products), the facts show the disease to have reemerged. In the last decade, rickets has been reported in some 22 countries. Cases in Africa and South Asia appear to be caused primarily by deficiencies of calcium, which some have suggested may increase the catabolism of vitamin D. Other cases, however, appear to be due to insufficient vitamin D. These include most of the recent published cases in the United States, 83% of which were described as African American or black and 96% of which were breastfed with only 5% vitamin D supplementation during breast feeding.

Table 6-10. Signs of vitamin D deficiency

Organ system	Sign(s) of rickets	Sign(s) of osteomalacia
General	Loss of appetite, retarded growth	None
Dermatologic	None	None
Muscular	Weakness	Weakness
Skeletal	Failure of bone to mineralize: deformation, swollen joints, delayed tooth eruption, bone pain, and tenderness	Demineralization of formed bone: fractures, pseudofractures, bone pain, and tenderness
Vital organs	None	None
Nervous	Tetany, ataxia	None
Reproductive	None	Low sperm motility and number Birds: thin egg shells
Ocular	None	None

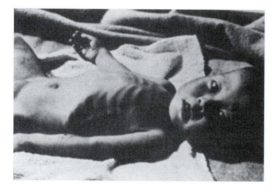

Fig. 6-13. Rachitic child (note beaded ribs).

(Table 6-10). Its etiology (loss of trabecular bone with retention of bone structure) is not fully understood; it is considered a multifactorial disease associated with aging and involving impaired vitamin D metabolism and/or function associated with low or decreasing estrogen levels. The disease is the most common bone disease of postmenopausal women and also occurs in older men[108] (e.g., nonambulatory geriatrics, postmenopausal women) and in people receiving chronic steroid therapy; these groups show high incidences of fractures, especially of the vertebrae, hip, distal radius, and proximal femur.[109]

In women, osteoporosis is characterized by rapid loss of bone (e.g., 0.5–1.5%/year) in the first 5 to 7 years after menopause.[110] The increased skeletal fragility observed in osteoporosis does not appear to be due solely to reductions in bone mass, but also involves changes in skeletal architecture and bone remodeling (e.g., losses of trabecular connectivity as well as inefficient and incomplete microdamage repair). Affected individuals show abnormally low circulating levels of 1,25-$(OH)_2$-D_3 (Table 6-11), suggesting that estrogen loss may impair the renal 1-hydroxylation step (i.e., that the disease may involve a bihormonal deficiency). Studies of the use of various vitamers D in the treatment of osteoporotic patients have produced inconsistent results; most of these studies have been fairly small (Table 6-12). Results of the Nurses' Health Study showed that adequate vitamin D intake ($\geq 12.5\,\mu g$/day) was associated with a 37% reduction in risk of osteoporotic hip fracture;[111] a meta-analysis of randomized intervention trials showed that 1,25-$(OH)_2$-D_3 treatment at doses of 0.5–1 μg/day decreased vertebral

---

[108] Osteoporosis is estimated to affect 25 million Americans, costing the U.S. economy some $13–18 billion per year. In women, bone loss generally begins in the third and fourth decades and accelerates after menopause; in men, bone loss begins about a decade later.

[109] Osteoporotic fractures appear to involve different syndromes. Type I osteoporosis is characterized by distal radial and vertebral fractures and occurs primarily in women ranging in age from 50 to 65 years; it is probably due to postmenopausal decreases in the amount of calcified bone at the fracture site. Type II osteoporosis occurs primarily among individuals over 70 years and is characterized by fractures of the hip, proximal humerus, and pelvis, where there has been loss of both cortical and trabecular bone.

[110] Therefore, the primary determinant of fracture risk from postmenopausal or senile osteoporosis in older people is the mass of bone each had accumulated during growth and early adulthood. This includes cortical bone, which continues to be accreted after closure of the epiphyses until about the middle of the fourth decade.

[111] Feskanich et al. (2003). *Am. J. Clin. Nutr.* **77**, 504–511.

Table 6-11. Abnormalities in vitamin D status of hip fracture patients

Parameter	Controls	Patients
Age (years)	75.6 ± 4.2	75.9 ± 11.0
Sunshine exposure (n)		
Low	9	51
Intermediate	26	38
High	39	31
Dietary intakes		
Calcium (mg/day)	696 ± 273	671 ± 406
Vitamin D (IU/day)	114 ± 44	116 ± 63
Serum analytes		
Calcium (mM)	2.35 ± 0.12	2.13 ± 0.16
Phosphate (mM)	1.09 ± 0.15	1.11 ± 0.26
Alkaline phosphatase (U/ml)	2.1 ± 0.5	2.0 ± 0.7
Albumin (g/liter)	41.9 ± 2.8	32.5 ± 4.8[a]
DBP (mg/liter)	371 ± 44	315 ± 60[a]
25-OH-D_3 (nM)	32.9 ± 13.6	18.5 ± 10.6[a]
24,25-$(OH)_2$-D_3 (nM)	1.8	0.5[a]
1,25-$(OH)_2$-D_3 (pM)	105 ± 31	79 ± 46[a]
PTH (µg Eq/liter)	0.12 ± 0.05	0.11 ± 0.05

[a]$p < 0.05$.
Source: Lips, P., van Ginkel, F. C., Jongen, M. H. M., Robertus, F., van der Vijh, W. J. F., and Netelenbos, J. C. (1987). *Am. J. Clin. Nutr.* **46,** 1005–1010.

Table 6-12. Reduction of fracture risk by 1,25-$(OH)_2$-vitamin D_3

Treatment	Year	Women in study	Women with new fractures	Number of new fractures
1,25-$(OH)_2$- vitamin D_3	1	262	14	23
	2	236	14	22
	3	213	12	21
Calcium	1	253	17	26
	2	240	30[a]	60[a]
	3	219	44[a]	69[a]

[a]$p < 0.01$.
Source: Tilyard, M. W., Spears, G. F. S., Thomson, J., and Dovey, S. (1992). *N. Engl. J. Med.* **326,** 357–362.

and at least some nonvertebral (e.g., forearm) fractures in postmenopausal women.[112]

---

[112] Papadimitropoulos et al. (2005). *Endocrine Rev.* **23,** 560–569.

Musculoskeletal pain

While deep pain is common among rickets patients, a recent study found persistent, nonspecific musculoskeletal pain among adults with low circulating levels of 25-OH-D_3 but not showing signs of osteomalacia or osteoporosis. Thus, it has been suggested that pain may be an early sign of severe hypovitaminosis D.

Signs of Vitamin D Deficiency in Animals

Rickets

Vitamin D-deficient, growing animals show rickets (Figs. 6-14 and 6-15). Species at greatest risk are those that experience rapid early growth, such as the chick. Rachitic signs are similar in all affected species: impaired mineralization of the growing bones with structural deformation in weight-bearing bones.

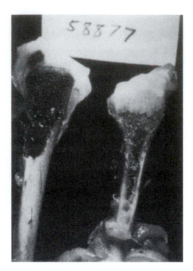

Fig. 6-14. Tibiae of normal (*left*) and rachitic (*right*) chicks.

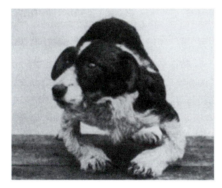

Fig. 6-15. Rachitic puppy.

Osteoporosis

Older vitamin D-deficient animals show the under-mineralization of bones that characterizes osteoporosis. This can be a practical problem in the high-producing laying hen,[113] in which it is called **cage layer fatigue.** The condiction is associated with reductions in egg production, feed intake, efficiency of feed utilzation, and survival.

Tibial dyschondroplasia

There appear to be other situations of impaired renal 1-hydroxylation of 25-OH-D$_3$, thus limiting the physiological function of the vitamin. One is the failure of bone mineralization seen in rapidly growing, heavy-bodied chickens and turkeys called **tibial dyschondroplasia**. The disorder is similar to the condition called **osteochondrosis** in rapidly growing pigs and horses; it is characterized by the failure of vascularization of the proximal metaphyses of the tibiotarsus and tarsalmetatarsus. It occurs spontaneously, but can be produced in animals made acidotic, a condition that reduces the conversion of 1-hydroxylation of 25-OH-D$_3$. Both the incidence and severity of tibial dyschondroplasia can be reduced by treatment with 1,25-(OH)$_2$-D$_3$ or 1α-OH-D$_3$ but not by higher levels of vitamin D$_3$ alone. That lesions in genetically susceptible poultry lines cannot be completely prevented by treatment with vitamin D metabolites suggests that tibial dyschondroplasia may involve a functional impairment in VDRs.

Milk fever

High-producing dairy cows can become hypocalcemic at the onset of lactation when they have been fed calcium-rich diets before calving. The condition, called **milk fever**, occurs when plasma calcium levels decrease to less than about 5.0 mg/dl; it is characterized by tetany and coma, which can be fatal. Milk fever results from the inability of the postparturant cow to withstand massive lactational calcium losses by absorbing dietary calcium and mobilizing bone at rates sufficient to support plasma calcium at normal levels. It can be prevented by preparing the pregnant cow for upregulated bone mobilization and enteric calcium absorption. In field practice, this is done by feeding her a relatively low-calcium diet (100 g/day); parenteral treatment with 1,25-(OH)$_2$-D$_3$ is also effective.

---

[113] In well-managed flocks, it is not uncommon for a hen to lay more than 300 eggs in a year, with 40 of these laid during the first 40 days after commencing egg laying. As each eggshell contains about 2 g of calcium and the hen is able to absorb only 1.8–1.9 g of calcium from the diet each day, she experiences a calcium debt of 0.1–0.2 g/day during that period. She accommodates this by mobilizing medullary bone; as her total skeleton contains only about 35 g of calcium, however, chronic demineralization at that rate without either decreasing the rate of egg production or increasing the efficiency of calcium absorption leads to osteoporosis characterized by fractures of the ribs and long bones.

VIII. Vitamin D Toxicity

Excessive intakes of vitamin D are associated with increases in circulating levels of 25-OH-D$_3$; this is especially true for vitamin D$_3$, exposure to high levels of which produces higher serum levels of the 25-OH metabolite than do comparable intakes of vitamin D$_2$.[114] The 25-OH metabolite is believed to be the critical metabolite in vitamin D intoxication. At high levels,[115] it appears to compete successfully for intracellular receptors for 1,25-(OH)$_2$-D$_3$, thus inducing the responses normally produced by the latter metabolite. Therefore, hypervitaminosis D involves increased enteric absorption and bone resorption of calcium, producing hypercalcemia, with attendant decreases in serum PTH and glomerular filtration rate and, ultimately, loss of calcium homeostasis. The mobilization of bone also results in increased serum concentrations of zinc from that reserve. Vitamin D-intoxicated individuals show a variety of signs (Table 6-13), including anorexia, vomiting, headache, drowsiness, diarrhea, and polyuria. With chronically elevated serum calcium and phosphorus levels, the ultimate result is **calcinosis**—the deposition of calcium and phosphate in soft tissues, especially heart and kidney, but also the vascular and respiratory systems and practically all other tissues.[116] It is not known whether calcinosis involves specific tissue lesions induced by high levels of vitamin D metabolites or whether it is simply a consequence of the induced hypercalcemia. Thus, the risk of hypervitaminosis D is dependent not only on exposure to vitamin D, but also on concomitant intakes of calcium and phosphorus.

Calcinosis in grazing livestock has been traced to the consumption of water-soluble glycosides of 1,25-(OH)$_2$-D$_3$ present in some plants. These appear to be deglycosylated to yield 1,25-(OH)$_2$-D$_3$, which is 100 times more toxic than the dominant circulating metabolite 25-OH-D$_3$.

There are no documented cases of hypervitaminosis D due to excessive sunlight exposure. A few cases of hypervitaminosis D, characterized by elevated serum concentrations of 25-OH-D$_3$ and vitamin D$_3$ and hypercalcemia, have been documented among consumers of milk that, through processing errors, was sporadically fortified with very high levels of the vitamin.[117]

Vitamin D **hypersensitivity** has been proposed as the basis for Williams-Beuren syndrome, a rare (1:47,000) condition of hypercalcemia and calcium hyperabsorption in humans. The syndrome is manifested in infancy; it is characterized by failure to thrive with mental handicap and long-term morbidity. Patients have been found to have normal circulating levels of 25-OH-D$_3$, but they appear to have exaggerated responses to oral doses of vitamin D$_3$. One report presented elevated serum levels of 1,25-(OH)$_2$-D$_3$ in patients.

The availability of synthetic 1α-OH-D$_3$ in recent years has meant that it can be used at very low doses to treat vitamin D-dependent or -resistant osteopathies.[118] This has reduced the risks of hypervitaminosis that attend the use of the massive doses of vitamin D$_3$ needed to provide effective therapy in such cases.

Table 6-13.   Signs of hypervitaminosis D

Anorexia
Gastrointestinal distress, nausea, vomiting
Headache
Weakness, lameness
Polyuria, polydypsia
Nervousness
Hypercalcemia
Calcinosis

---

[114] Vitamin D$_3$ is 10–20 times more toxic than vitamin D$_2$.

[115] That is, 100 times normal physiological requirements.

[116] The condition idiopathic infantile hypercalcemia, formerly thought to be due to hypervitaminosis D, appears to be a multifactorial disease with genetic as well as dietary components.

[117] Eight cases were described (Jacobus et al., *N. Engl. J. Med.* [1992], 326, 1173–1177); each consumed a local dairy's milk, samples of which were highly variable in vitamin D content (some samples contained as much as 245,840 IU of vitamin D$_3$ per liter). U.S. federal regulations stipulate that milk contain 400 IU/qt "within limits of good manufacturing practice"; however, a small survey concluded that milk and infant formula preparations rarely contain the amounts of vitamin D stated on the label, owing to both under- and overfortification.

[118] These diseases include hypoparathyroidism, genetic or acquired hypophosphatemic osteomalacias, renal osteodystrophy, vitamin D-dependent rickets, and osteomalacia associated with liver disease and enteric malabsorption.

IX. Case Studies

Instructions

Review each of the following case reports, paying special attention to the diagnostic indicators on which the respective treatments were based. Then answer the questions that follow.

Case 1

When the patient was first evaluated at the National Institutes of Health, he was a thin, short, bowlegged, 20-year-old male. His height at that time was 159 cm (below the 1st percentile), and he weighed 52 kg. In addition to his dwarfism, he showed a **varus deformity**[119] of both knees, and he walked with a waddling gait. Radiographs showed diffusely decreased bone density, subperiosteal resorption, and a **pseudofracture**[120] of the left ischiopubic ramus.[121]

Laboratory results at 20 years of age

Parameter	Patient	Normal range
Serum calcium	8.0 mg/dl	8.5–10.5 mg/dl
Serum phosphorus	2.2 mg/dl	3.5–4.5 mg/dl
Serum alkaline phosphatase	152 U/ml	<77 U/ml

Urine chromatography showed a generalized aminoaciduria.

The patient's history revealed that he had been a normal, full-term infant weighing 3.2 kg. He had been breastfed and had been given supplementary vitamin D. At 20 months, however, he failed to walk unsupported and was diagnosed as having active rickets, as revealed by **genu varum**, irregular cupped metaphyses, and widened growth plates,[122] with reductions of both calcium and phosphorus in his blood. The rickets did not respond to oral doses of ergocalciferol (normally effective in treating nutritional rickets), but healing was observed radiographically after intramuscular administration of 1,500,000 IU (37.5 mg) of vitamin D_2 weekly for 5 months. The patient continued to receive vitamin

D in the form of cod liver oil, approximately 5000–20,000 units/day. At 4 years of age, corrective surgery was performed for deformities of the tibias and femurs. At age 14, the patient's height was in the 15th percentile. Additional surgery was performed, after which vitamin D therapy was stopped, and, over the next 2 years, weakness and severe bone pain became evident. At age 19, bilateral femoral osteotomies[123] were performed again. As an outpatient at the NIH Clinical Center, the patient received oral ergocalciferol, 50,000 IU daily, for the next 6 years and experienced remission of pain and weakness and normalization of serum calcium and phosphorus levels. His height reached 161 cm (63.3 in.), which was still below the 1st percentile. At 27 years of age, his radiographs showed improved density of the skeletal cortices and healing of the pseudofractures, but the patient still showed the clinical stigmata[124] of rickets.

Laboratory results at 27 years of age

Parameter	Patient	Normal range
Serum PTH	0.31 ng/ml	<0.22 ng/ml
Urine cAMP	6 nmol/dl	2.3 ± 1.2 nmol/dl
^{47}Ca absorption	19%	33–43%
Plasma 25-OH-D_3	25 ng/ml	10–40 ng/ml
Plasma 1,25-$(OH)_2$-D_3	213 pg/ml	20–60 pg/ml
Plasma 24,25-$(OH)_2$-D_3	1.0 ng/ml	0.8–3 ng/ml

Two hundred micrograms of 25-OH-D_3 was then given orally daily for 2 weeks. Calcium retention improved, urinary cAMP fell, and plasma phosphorus and calcium rose, each to the normal level. Vitamin D_3 maintenance doses (about 40,000 IU, i.e., 1 mg/day) were given periodically to prevent recurrent osteomalacia.

Case 2

This patient was a sister of the patient described in Case 1. She was first evaluated at the NIH when she was 18 years old. She was a thin female dwarf (147 cm tall, below the 1st percentile) weighing 44.8 kg. She walked with a waddling gait and had mild bilateral varus deformities of the knees. *Chvostek's sign*[125] was

---

[119] That is, bowlegs.

[120] That is, new bone detected radiographically as thickening of the periosteum at the site of an injury to the bone.

[121] That is, a narrow process of the pelvis.

[122] Failure of mineralization of the growing ends of long bones.

[123] Surgical correction of bone shape.

[124] Abnormalities.

[125] That is, facial spasm (as in tetany), induced by a slight tap over the facial nerve.

present bilaterally. Analyses of her serum showed 7.0 mg of calcium and 3.0 mg of phosphorus per deciliter and alkaline phosphatase at 110 U/ml. Skeletal radiographs showed delayed ossification of several epiphyses and a pseudofracture in the left tibia. Her plasma 25-OH-D was 44 ng/ml, 1,25-$(OH)_2$-D_3 was 280 pg/ml, and 24,25-$(OH)_2$-D_3 was 2.5 ng/ml.

Her history showed that she had been a normal, full-term infant who weighed 3.8 kg at birth. At 5 months of age, she showed radiographic features of rickets. During infancy and childhood, she received vitamin D as cod liver oil, in doses of 2000–10,000 IU/day. She began to walk at 9 months and developed slight varus deformity of both legs. Her rate of growth was at the 5th percentile until the vitamin D was discontinued when she was 11 years old. Within 3 years, her height fell below the 1st percentile. From ages 15 to 16, the bowing of her legs progressed moderately. When she was 18 years old, at the time of her first admission to the NIH Clinical Center, she was treated with 200 μg of 25-OH-D_3 per day for 2 weeks. During this time, her calcium retention improved, and her serum calcium and phosphorus increased. Studies showed that 500 μg of vitamin D_3 per day was required to maintain her plasma calcium in the normal range. At this dose, her 25-OH-D_3 was 141 ng/ml, 1,25-$(OH)_2$-D_3

was 640 pg/ml, and 24,25-$(OH)_2$-D_3 was 3.6 ng/ml (above normal). When she was 24 years old (i.e., 6 years after her first admission to the center), she was readmitted for studies of the effectiveness of oral 1,25-$(OH)_2$-D_3 with a supplement of 800 mg of calcium per day. Serum calcium remained below normal on doses of 2–10 μg of 1,25-$(OH)_2$-D_3 per day. Only when the dose was increased to 14–17 μg of 1,25-$(OH)_2$-D_3 per day did her plasma calcium reach the normal range. Parthyroid hormone remained elevated at 0.40 ng/ml. At these high doses of 1,25-$(OH)_2$-D_3, her plasma 25-OH-D_3 was 26 ng/ml, and her 1,25-$(OH)_2$-D_3 was 400 pg/ml. While on 1,25-$(OH)_2$-D_3, her osteomalacia improved, and serum calcium and phosphorus entered normal ranges.

Case Questions

1. What are the common clinical features (physical and biochemical observations, response to treatment, etc.) of these two cases?

2. What can you infer about the nature of vitamin D metabolism in these siblings?

3. Propose a hypothesis to explain these cases of vitamin D-resistant rickets. How might you test this hypothesis?

Study Questions and Exercises

1. Construct a flow diagram showing the metabolism of vitamin D to its physiologically active and excretory forms.

2. Construct a "decision tree" for the diagnosis of vitamin D deficiency in a human or animal. How can deficiencies of vitamin D and calcium be distinguished?

3. How does the concept of solubility relate to vitamin D utilization? What features of the chemical structure of vitamin D relate to its utilization?

4. Relate the concept of organ function to the concept of vitamin D utilization/status.

5. Discuss the concept of homeostasis, using vitamin D as an example.

Recommended Reading

Angelo, G., and Wood, R. J. (2002). Novel intercellular proteins associated with cellular vitamin D action. *Nutr. Rev.* **60,** 209–214.

Bilke, D. D. (1995). 1,25$(OH)_2D_3$-Regulated human keratinocyte proliferation and differentiation: Basic studies and their clinical application. *J. Nutr.* **125**(Suppl.), 1709S–1714S.

Bischoff-Ferrari, H. A., Giovannucci, E., Willett, W. C., Dietrich, T., and Dawson-Huges, B. (2006). Estimation of optimal serum concentrations of 25-hydroxyvitamin D for multiple outcomes. *Am. J. Clin. Nutr.* **84,** 18–28.

Bonner, F. (2003). Mechanisms of intestinal calcium absorption. *J. Cell. Biochem.* **88,** 387–393.

Bouillon, R., Van Cromphaut, S., and Carmeliet, G. (2003). Intestinal calcium absorption: Molecular vitamin D mediate mechanisms. *J. Cell. Biochem.* **88,** 332–339.

Collins, E. D., and Norman, A. W. (2001). Vitamin D. In *Handbook of Vitamins* (R. B. Rucker, J. W. Suttie, D. B. McCormick, and L. J. Machlin, eds.), 3rd ed., pp. 51–113. Marcel Dekker, New York.

Christakos, S., Barletta, F., Huening, M., Dhawan, P., Liu, Y., Porta, A., and Peng, X. (2003). Vitamin D target proteins: Function and regulation. *J. Cell. Biochem.* **88**, 238–244.

Cross, H. S., Hulla, W., Tong, W. M., and Peterlik, M. (1995). Growth regulation of human colon adenocarcinoma-derived cells by calcium, vitamin D and epidermal growth factor. *J. Nutr.* **125**(Suppl.), 2004S–2008S.

Dawson-Hughes, B. (2004). Calcium and vitamin D for bone health in adults. Chapter 12 in *Nutrition and Bone Health* (M. F. Holick, and B. Dawson-Hughes, eds.), pp. 197–210. Humana Press, Totowa, NJ.

DeLuca, H. F. (2004). Overview of general physiologic features and functions of vitamin D. *J. Nutr.* **80**(Suppl.), 1689S–1696S.

DeLuca, H. F., and Zierold, C. (1998). Mechanisms and functions of vitamin D. *Nutr. Rev.* **56**, 4–10.

Fleet, J. C. (2004). Rapid, membrane-initiated actions of 1,25-dihydroxyvitamin D: What are they and what do they mean? *J. Nutr.* **134**, 3215–3218.

Flores, M. (2005). A role of vitamin D in low-intensity chronic inflammation and insulin resistance in type 2 diabetes? *Nutr. Res. Rev.* **18**, 175–182.

Grant, W. B., and Holick, M. F. (2005). Benefits and requirements of vitamin D for optimal health: A review. *Alt. Med. Rev.* **10**, 94–111.

Hannah, S. S., and Norman, A. W. (1994). 1α,25(OH)$_2$Vitamin D$_3$-regulated expression of the eukaryotic genome. *Nutr. Rev.* **52**, 376–382.

Harris, D. M., and Go, V. L. (2004). Vitamin D and colon carcinogenesis *J. Nutr.* **134**, 3463S–3471S.

Heaney, R. P. (1993). Nutritional factors in osteoporosis. *Annu. Rev. Nutr.* **13**, 287–316.

Heaney, R. P. (2003). Long-latency deficiency disease: Insights into calcium and vitamin D. *Am. J. Clin. Nutr.* **78**, 912–919.

Hoenderop, J. G. J., Nilius, B., and Bindels, R. J. M. (2002). Molecular mechanism of active Ca^{2+} reabsorption in the dital nephron. *Ann. Rev. Physiol.* **64**, 529–549.

Holick, M. F. (1999). *Vitamin D: Molecular Biology, Physiology and Clinical Applications*. Humana Press, Totowa, NJ, 458 pp.

Holick, M. F. (2003). Evolution and function of vitamin D. *Recent Results Cancer Res.* **164**, 3–28.

Holick, M. F. (2004). Vitamin D. Chapter 25 in *Nutrition and Bone Health* (M. F. Holick and B. Dawson-Hughes, eds.), pp. 403–440. Humana Press, Totowa, NJ.

Kragballe, K. (1992). Vitamin D analogues in the treatment of psoriasis. *J. Cell. Biochem.* **49**, 46–52.

Levine, A., and Li, Y. C. (2005). Vitamin D and its analogues: Do they protect against cardiovascular disease in patients with kidney disease? *Kidney Int.* **68**, 1973–1981.

Lou, Y. R., Qiao, S., Talonpoika, R., Syvälä, H., and Tuohimaa, P. (2004). The role of vitamin D3 metabolism in prostate cancer. *J. Steroid Biochem. Mol. Bol.* **92**, 317–325.

Mathieu, C., Gysemans, C., Giulietti, A., and Bouillon, R. (2005). Vitamin D and diabetes. *Diabetologia* **48**, 1247–1257.

Maxwell, J. D. (1994). Seasonal variation in vitamin D. *Proc. Nutr. Soc.* **53**, 533–543.

Montaro-Odasso, M., and Duque, G. (2005). Vitamin D in the aging musculoskeletal system: an authentic strength preserving hormone. *Mol. Aspects Med.* **26**, 203–219.

Nagpal, S., Na, S., and Rathnachalam, R. (2005). Noncalcemic actions of vitamin D receptor ligands. *Endocrinol. Rev.* **26**, 662–687.

Norman, A. W. (2001). Vitamin D. Chapter 13 in *Present Knowledge in Nutrition* (B. A. Bowman and R. M. Russell, eds.), 8th ed., pp. 146–155. ILSI Press, Washington, DC.

Omdahl, J. L., Morris, H. A., and May, B. K. (2002). Hydroxylase enzymes of the vitamin D pathway: Expression, function and regulation. *Ann. Rev. Nutr.* **22**, 139–166.

Pike, J. W. (1994). Vitamin D receptors and the mechanism of action of 1,25-dihydroxyvitamin D$_3$. Chapter 3 in *Vitamin Receptors: Vitamins as Ligands in Cell Communication* (K. Dakshinamurti, ed.), pp. 59–77. Cambridge University Press, Cambridge.

Posner, G. (2002). Low-calcemic vitamin D analogs (deltanoids) for human cancer prevention. *J. Nutr.* **132**(Suppl.), 3802S–3803S.

Schwartz, G. G. (2005). Vitamin D and the epidemiology of prostate cancer. *Semin. Dial.* **18**, 276–289.

Sergeev, I. N. (2005). Calcium signaling in cancer and vitamin D. *J. Steroid Biochem. Molec. Biol.* **97**, 145–151.

Shaffer, P. L., and Gewith, D. T. (2004). Vitamin D receptor-DNA interactions. *Vitamins Hormones* **68**, 257–273.

Standing Committee on the Scientific Evaluation of Dietary Reference Intakes. (1997). *Dietary Reference Intakes for Calcium, Phophorus, Magnesium, Vitamin D and Fluoride*. National Academy Press, Washington, DC., pp. 250–287.

Suda, T., Shinki, T., and Takahashi, N. (1990). The role of vitamin D in bone and intestinal cell differentiation. *Annu. Rev. Nutr.* **10**, 195–212.

Veith, R. (1999). Vitamin D supplementation, 25-hyroxyvitamin D concentrations, and safety. *Am. J. Clin. Nutr.* **69**, 842–856.

Wargovich, M. J. (1991). Calcium, vitamin D and the prevention of gastrointestinal cancer. In *Nutrition and Cancer Prevention* (T. E. Moon and M. S. Micozzi, eds.), pp. 291–304. Marcel Dekker, New York.

Wasserman, R. H. (2004). Vitamin D and the dual processes of intestinal calcium absorption. *J. Nutr.* **134**, 3137–3139.

Wharton, B., and Bishop, N. (2003). Rickets. *Lancet* **362,** 1389–1400.

Whitfield, G. K., Hsieh, J. C., Jurutka, P. W., Selznick, S. H., Haussler, C. A., MacDonald, P. N., and Haussler, M. R. (1995). Genomic actions of 1,25-dihydroxyvitamin D_3. *J. Nutr.* **125**(Suppl.), 1690S–1694S.

Willett, A. M. (2005). Vitamin E status and its relationship with parathyroid hormone and bone mineral status in older adults. *Proc. Nutr. Soc.* **64,** 193–203.

Ylikomi, T., Iaaksi, I., Lou, Y. R., Martinkainen, P., Miettinen, S., Pennanen, P., Purmonen, S., Syvälä, H., Vienonen, A., and Tuohimaa, P. (2002). Antiproliferative action of vitamin D. *Vitamins Hormones* **64,** 357–406.

Zittermann, A. (2003). Vitamin D in preventive medicine: are we ignoring the evidence? *Br. J. Nutr.* **89,** 552–572.

Zittermann, A., Schleithoff, S. S., and Koerfer, R. (2005). Putting cardiovascular diease and vitamin D insufficiency into perspective. *Br. J. Nutr.* **94,** 483–492.

Vitamin E

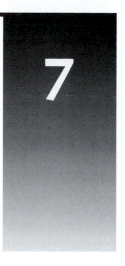

7

Vitamin E is a focal point for two broad topics, namely, biological antioxidants and lipid peroxidation damage. Vitamin E is related by its reactions to other biological antioxidants and reducing compounds (that) stabilize polyunsaturated lipids and minimize lipid peroxidation damage. In vivo lipid peroxidation has been identified as a basic deteriorative reaction in cellular mechanisms of aging processes, in some phases of atherosclerosis, in chlorinated hydrocarbon hepatotoxicity, in ethanol-induced liver injury and in oxygen toxicity. These processes may be a universal disease of which the chemical deteriorative effects might be slowed by use of increased amounts of antioxidants.

—A. L. Tappel

I.	Significance of Vitamin E	182
II.	Sources of Vitamin E	182
III.	Absorption of Vitamin E	184
IV.	Transport of Vitamin E	185
V.	Metabolism of Vitamin E	189
VI.	Metabolic Functions of Vitamin E	191
VII.	Vitamin E Deficiency	206
VIII.	Pharmacologic Uses of Vitamin E	207
IX.	Vitamin E Toxicity	208
X.	Case Studies	210
	Study Questions and Exercises	211
	Recommended Reading	212

Anchoring Concepts

1. Vitamin E is the generic descriptor for all tocopherol and tocotrienol derivatives exhibiting qualitatively the biological activity of α-tocopherol.
2. The vitamers E are hydrophobic and thus are insoluble in aqueous environments (e.g., plasma, interstitial fluids, cytosol).
3. By virtue of the phenolic hydrogen on the C-6 ring hydroxyl group, the vitamers E have antioxidant activities *in vitro*.
4. Deficiencies of vitamin E have a wide variety of clinical manifestations in different species.

Learning Objectives

1. To understand the various sources of vitamin E.
2. To understand the means of enteric absorption and transport of vitamin E.
3. To understand the metabolic interrelationships of vitamin E and other nutrients.
4. To understand the physiologic implications of high doses of vitamin E.

Vocabulary

Abetalipoproteinemia
All-*rac*-α-tocopheryl polyethyleneglycol-succinate
All-*rac*-α-tocopheryl succinate
Antioxidant
Apolipoprotein E (apoE)
Ataxia
α-Carboxyethylchromanol
Catalase
Chylomicra
Conjugated diene
Cysteine
Cytochrome P450
Encephalomalacia
Ethane
Exudative diathesis
Familial isolated vitamin E (FIVE) deficiency
Foam cells
Free radicals
Free-radical theory of aging
Glutathione (GSH)
Glutathione peroxidases
Glutathione reductase
Hemolysis
Hemolytic anemia
High-density lipoproteins (HDLs)
Hydroperoxide (ROOH)

Hydroxyl radical (HO•)
H_2O_2
Intraventricular hemorrhage
Ischemia-reperfusion injury
Lipid peroxidation
Lipofuscin
Lipoprotein lipase
Liver necrosis
Low-density lipoproteins (LDLs)
Malonyldialdehyde
Mulberry heart disease
Myopathy
5-Nitro-tocopherol
Oxidative stress
Oxidized glutathione (GSSG)
Oxidized LDLs
Pentane
Peroxide tone
Peroxyl radical (ROO•)
Phospholipid transfer protein
Polyunsaturated fatty acids (PUFAs)
Prooxidant
Reactive oxygen species
Resorption-gestation syndrome
Respiratory burst
Scavenger receptors
Selenium
Simon's metabolites
Steatorrhea
Superoxide dismutases
Superoxide radical, $O_2^{•-}$
α-Tocopherol
α-Tocopherol transfer protein (α–TTP)
β-Tocopherol
γ-Tocopherol
δ-Tocopherol
α-Tocopheronic acid
α-Tocopheronolactone
Tocopherol-associated proteins (TAPs)
Tocopherol radical tocopheryl quinone
α-Tocopheryl hydroquinone
α-Tocopheryl phosphate
Tocotrienols
Very low-density lipoprotein (VLDL)
White muscle disease

I. Significance of Vitamin E

Vitamin E has a fundamental role in the normal metabolism of all cells. Therefore, its deficiency can afffect several different organ systems. Its function is related to those of several other nutrients and endogenous factors that, collectively, comprise a multicomponent system that provides protection against the potentially damaging effects of reactive species of oxygen formed during metabolism or that are encountered in the environment. Therefore, both the need for vitamin E and the manifestations of its deficiency can be affected by such nutrients as **selenium** and vitamin C and by exposure to such **prooxidant** factors as **polyunsaturated fatty acids (PUFAs)**, air pollution, and ultraviolet (UV) light. Recent evidence indicates that vitamin E may also have non-antioxidant functions in regulating gene expression and cell signaling.

Unlike other vitamins, vitamin E is not only essentially nontoxic, but it also appears to be beneficial at dose levels appreciably greater than those required to prevent clinical signs of deficiency. Most notably, supranutritional levels of the vitamin have been useful in reducing the oxidation of **low-density lipoproteins (LDLs)** and thus reducing the risk of atherosclerosis. The ubiquitous and complex nature of its biological function, its demonstrated safety, and its apparent usefulness in combating a variety of **oxidative stress** disorders have generated enormous interest in this vitamin among the basic and clinical science communities as well as the lay public.

II. Sources of Vitamin E

Distribution in Foods

Vitamin E is synthesized only by plants and therefore is found primarily in plant products, the richest sources being plant oils. All higher plants appear to contain **α-tocopherol** in their leaves and other green parts. Because α-tocopherol is contained mainly in the chloroplasts of plant cells (whereas the β-, γ-, and δ-vitamers are usually found outside of these particles), green plants tend to contain more vitamin E than yellow plants. Wheat germ, sunflower, and safflower oils are rich sources of α-(RRR)-tocopherol, whereas corn and soybean oils contain mostly γ-(RRR)-tocopherol. Some plant tissues, notably bran and germ fractions,[1] can also contain tocotrienols, often in esterified form, unlike the tocopherols that exist only as free alcohols. Animal tissues tend to contain low amounts of α-tocopherol, the highest levels occurring in fatty tissues. These levels vary according to the dietary intake of the vitamin.[2] Because vitamin E occurs naturally in fats and oils, reductions in fat intake can be expected also to reduce vitamin E intake. A water-soluble metabolite, **α-tocopheryl phosphate**,[3] has also been idenfied at trace levels in animal tissues.

Synthetic Forms

Synthetic preparations of vitamin E are mixtures of all eight diastereoisomers, that is, 2RS,4′RS,8′RS-vitamers designated more commonly with the prefix all-rac- in both unesterified (all-rac-α-tocopherol) and esterified (all-rac-α-tocopheryl acetate) forms. Other forms used commercially include **all-rac-α-tocopheryl succinate** and **all-rac-α-tocopheryl polyethylene-glycol-succinate**.

Expressing Vitamin E Activity

Vitamin E activity is shown by several side-chain isomers and methylated analogs of tocopherol and tocotrienol (Table 7-1). These mono- (d-tocopherol), di- (ß- and γ-tocopherols) and tri-(α-tocopherol) methyl derivatives differ in vitamin E activity, the epimeric configuration at the 2-position being important in determining biological activity. Therefore, the use of an international standard facilitated the referencing of these various sources of vitamin E activity, which presumably relates to differences in their absorption, transport, retention, and/or metabolism. Although the original preparation d,l-α-tocopheryl acetate[4] that served as the international standard has not been extant for more than 30 years, R,R,R-α-tocopherol is now used as the international standardized[5] (see Chapter 3). This system distinguishes only the methylated analogs

and not the particular diastereoisomers possible for each.

Some of the vitamers E common in foods (β- and **γ-tocopherol**, the **tocotrienols**) have little biological activity. The most biopotent vitamer—the vitamer of greatest interest in nutrition is α-tocopherol, which occurs naturally as the RRR stereoisomer [(RRR)-α-tocopherol].

Dietary Sources of Vitamin E

The important sources of vitamin E in human diets and animal feeds are vegetable oils and, to lesser extents, seeds and cereal grains. The dominant dietary form (70% of tocopherols in American diets) is γ-tocopherol. Wheat germ oil is the richest natural source, containing 0.9 to 1.3 mg of α-tocopherol per gram, or, about 60% of its total tocopherols. The seeds and grains from which these oils are derived also contain appreciable amounts of vitamin E. Accordingly, cereals in general and wheat germ in particular are good sources of the vitamin. Foods that are formulated with vegetable oils (e.g., margarine, baked products) tend to vary greatly in vitamin E content owing to differences

Table 7-1. Relative biopotencies of tocopherols and tocotrienols by different bioassays

Compound	Fetal resorption (rat)	Hemolysis[a] (rat)	Myopathy prevention (chick)	Myopathy cure (rat)
α-Tocopherol	100	100	100	100
β-Tocopherol	25–40	15–27	12	—
γ-Tocopherol	1–11	3–20	5	11
δ-Tocopherol	1	0.3–2	—	—
α-Tocotrienol	28	17–25	—	28
β-Tocotrienol	5	1–5	—	—

[a]Describes the disruption of erythrocyte membranes causing cell lysis.

---

[1] Palm oil and rice bran have high concentrations of tocotrienols; other natural sources include coconut oil, cocoa butter, soybeans, barley, and wheat germ.

[2] Muscle from beef fed high levels of vitamin E (e.g., 1300 IU/day) before slaughter can yield vitamin E in excess of 16 nmol/g; this level is effective in reducing postmortem oxidation reactions, thus delaying the onset of meat discoloration due to hemoglobin oxidation and the development of oxidative rancidity.

[3] Water-soluble and resistant to both acid and alkaline hydrolysis, this metabolite has been missed by traditional methods of vitamin E analysis.

[4] At the time, the standard was called d,l-α-tocopheryl acetate; now it would be called (2RS)-α-tocopheryl acetate. Because of uncertainty about the proportions of the two diastereoisomers in that mixture, once the supply was exhausted it was impossible to replace it.

[5] 1 mg α-tocopherol equivalent = 1.49 IU.

in the types of oils used and to the thermal stabilities of the vitamers E present.[6]

The processing of foods and feedstuffs can remove substantial amounts of vitamin E. Vitamin E losses can occur as a result of exposure to peroxidizing lipids formed during the development of the oxidative rancidity of fats and to other oxidizing conditions such as drying in the presence of sunlight and air, the addition of organic acids,[7] irradiation, and canning. Milling and refining can reduce vitamin E content by removal of tocopherol-rich bran and germ fractions as well as through the use of bleaching agents (e.g., hypochlorous acid, ClO_2) to improve the baking characteristics of the flour. Some foods (e.g., milk and milk products) also show marked seasonal fluctuations in vitamin E content related to variations in vitamin E intake of the host (e.g., vitamin E intake is greatest when fresh forage is consumed). As a result of the many potential sources of vitamin E loss, the vitamin E contents of foods and feedstuffs vary considerably.[8]

The major form of vitamin E in most diets is not the most biopotent vitamer. γ-Tocopherol is the most prevalent form in foods (Tables 7-2 and 7-3)

and diets, and is also used in dietary supplements. Regardless of the form consumed, it is the main form found in tissues.

III. Absorption of Vitamin E

Micelle-Dependent Passive Diffusion

Vitamin E is absorbed from the upper small intestine by nonsaturable passive diffusion dependent on micellar solubilization and, hence, the presence of bile salts and pancreatic juice. The primary site of absorption appears to be the medial small intestine. Esterified forms of the vitamin E are hydrolyzed, probably by a duodenal mucosal *esterase*; the predominant forms absorbed are free alcohols. Most studies have shown no appreciable differences either in the efficiency of absorption of the acetate ester and free alcohol forms, or in the absorption of the various tocopherol and tocotrienol vitamers. It is clear, however, that regardless of the form absorbed, higher intakes lead to higher rates of absolute absorption but lower absorption efficiencies (that is, fractional

Table 7-2. Vitamin E in fats and oils

Item	Total vitamin E (mg/100 g)	Tocopherols (%) α	γ	δ	Tocopherols (%) α	β	γ	δ
Animal fats								
Lard	0.6–1.3	>90	<5		<5			
Butter	1–5	>90	<10					
Tallow	1.2–2.4	>90	<10					
Plant oils								
Soybean	56–160	4–18	58–69					
Cotton	30–81	51–67	33–49					
Maize	53–162	11–24	76–89					
Coconut	1–4	14–67		<17	<14	<3	<53	<17
Peanut	20–32	48–61	39–52					
Palm	33–73	28–50		<9	16–19	4	34–39	<9
Safflower	25–49	80–94	6–20					
Olive	5–15	65–85				15–35		

Source: Chow, C. K. (1985). *World Rev. Nutr. Diet.* **45,** 133–166.

---

[6] Tocotrienols tend to be less stable to high temperatures than tocopherols; therefore, baking tends to destroy them selectively.

[7] The addition of 1% propionic acid (as an antifungal agent) to fresh grain can destroy up to 90% of its vitamin E.

[8] For example, refining losses in edible plant oils are typically 10–40% but can sometimes be much greater.

Table 7-3. Vitamin E in grains and oil seeds

Item	Tocopherols (%)				Tocotrienols (%)	
	α	β	γ	δ	α	γ
Grains						
Maize	6–15		29–55		5–10	34–77
Oats	4–8	<1			10–22	
Milo	4–7		14–17		<1	
Barley	8–10	1–2	3–4		23–28	3
Wheat	8–12	4–6			2–3	
Oil seeds						
Soybean	1–3		3–33	2–6		Trace
Cotton seed	1–18		5–18			1–2

Source: Cort, W. M., Vincente, T. S., Waysek, E. H., and Williams, B. D. (1983). *J. Agric. Food Chem.* **31**, 1330–1333.

absorption). At nutritionally important intakes, variable (generally, 20 to 70%[9]) absorption efficiencies have been reported, with a large portion of ingested vitamin E appearing in the feces.

The enteric absorption of vitamin E is dependent on the adequate absorption of lipids. The process requires the presence of fat in the lumen of the gut, as well as the secretion of pancreatic esterases for the release of free fatty acids from dietary triglycerides and of bile acids for the formation of mixed micelles and ester-ases for the hydrolytic cleavage of tocopheryl esters when those forms are consumed. Individuals unable to produce pancreatic juice or bile (e.g., patients with biliary obstruction, cholestatic liver disease, pancreatitis, cystic fibrosis) can be expected to show impaired absorption of vitamin E, as well as other fat-soluble nutrients that are dependent on micelle-facilitated diffusion for their uptake. The micelle-dependent absorption of vitamin E would imply a need for dietary fat to facilitate the process. But the interaction of tocopher-ols with PUFAs in the intestinal lumen can result in absorption being stimulated by intragastric *medium-chain triglycerides* and inhibited by linoleic acid. The need for lipid would explain reports of vitamin E in dietary supplements not being well absorbed unless taken with a meal.[10] However, this need for lipid may be fairly low, as the absorption of all-*rac*-α-tocopheryl acetate by the rat was not impaired by feeding a diet containing only 7 grams of fat per kilogram (i.e., 1.6% of total calories). It has been suggested

that children can adequately absorb the fat-soluble vitamins with fat intake as low as 5 grams per day.

Other food components can interfere with the utilization of dietary vitamin E. For example, polyunsaturated fatty acids, particularly fish oils, can impair vitamin E retention; green tea catechins can interfere with the enteric absorption of tocopherols.

Absorbed vitamin E, like other hydrophobic substances, enters the lymphatic circulation[11] in association with the triglyceride-rich **chylomicra**. Studies measuring labeled compounds have shown the preferential lymphatic uptake of α-tocotrienol compared with γ- and δ-tocotrienols and α-tocopherol. The kinetics of vitamin E absorption are biphasic, reflecting the initial uptake of the vitamin by existing chylomicra followed by a lag phase due to the assembly of new chylomicra and intestinal VLDLs. Within the enterocytes vitamin E combines with other lipids and apolipoproteins to form chylomicra and very low-density lipoproteins (VLDLs). Chylomicron are released into the lymphatics in mammals or into the portal circulation in birds and reptiles.

IV. Transport of Vitamin E

Absorbed Vitamin E Transferred to Lipoproteins, Erythrocytes

Absorbed tocopherols can be transferred to tissues in several ways. The metabolism of ciculating chylomicra

---

[9] The enteric absorption of γ-tocopherol appears to be only 85% of that of α-tocopherol.

[10] Leonard, S. W., et al. (2004). *Am. J. Clin. Nutr.* **79,** 86–92.

[11] That is, the portal circulation in birds, fishes, and reptiles.

can result in tocopherols being transferred directly to tissues by partitioning into their plasma membranes, or indirectly by transfer to and between ciculating lipoproteins (Fig. 7-1). Unlike vitamins A and D, vitamin E does not appear to have a specific carrier protein in the plasma. Instead, it is rapidly transferred from chylomicra to plasma lipoproteins to which it binds nonspecifically, whereupon it is taken up by the liver and is incorporated into nascent VLDLs (with selectivity in favor of α-tocopherol over the γ-vitamer) secreted by the liver. Although the majority of the triglyceride-rich VLDL remnants are returned to the liver, some are converted by **lipoprotein lipase** to LDLs. It appears that, during this process, vitamin E also transfers spontaneously to apolipoprotein B-containing lipoproteins, including the **very low-density lipoproteins (VLDLs), low-density lipoproteins (LDLs)**, and **high-density lipoproteins (HDLs)**. Therefore, plasma tocopherols are distributed among these three lipoprotein classes, with the more abundant LDL and HDL classes comprising the major carriers of vitamin E. Nevertheless, as each class of lipoproteins derives its tocopherols ultimately from chylomicra, α-tocopherol transport by the latter is the major source of interindividual variation in response to ingested vitamin E.

These transport processes can be disrupted under hyperlipidemic conditions, as patients with hypercholesterolemia and/or hypertriglyceridemia show reduced plasma uptake of newly absorbed vitamin E.[12] Transport can also be disrupted by impairments in the expression of apolipoprotein B; patients with apobetalipoproteinemia become vitamin E-deficient due to very low rates of uptake regardless of dietary vitamin E status. The co-transport of vitamin E with other polyunsaturated lipids ensures protection of the latter from free-radical attack, and circulating tocopherol levels tend to correlate with those of total lipids and cholesterol.[13] That postprandial levels of tocopherols exceed those of tocotrienols reflects the more rapid metaabolic degradation of the latter.

Tocopherol exchanges rapidly between the lipoproteins[14] and erythrocytes (about one-fourth of total erythrocyte vitamin E turns over every hour); thus,

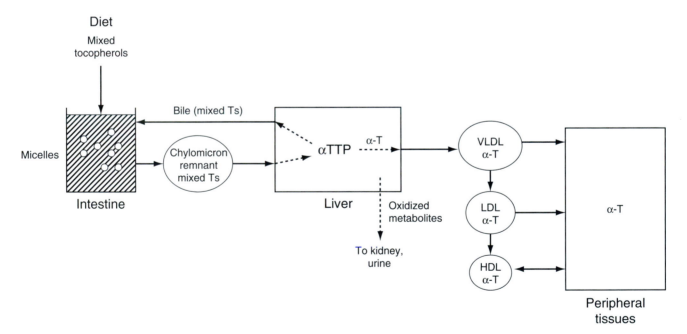

Fig. 7-1.   Absorption and transport of vitamin E. α-T, α-tocopherol; mixed Ts, mixed tocopherols; α-TTP, α-tocopherol transfer protein.

---

[12] Hall, W. L. Jeanes, Y. M., and Lodge, J. K. (2005). *J. Nutr.* **135**, 58–63.

[13] Therefore, high plasma vitamin E levels occur in hyperlipidemic conditions (hypothyroidism, diabetes, hypercholesterolemia), whereas low plasma vitamin E levels occur in conditions involving low plasma lipids (abetalipoproteinemia, protein malnutrition, cystic fibrosis).

[14] Rats, horses, and chicks transport 70–80% of plasma α-tocopherol with HDLs, 18–22% with LDLs, and < 8% with VLDLs. Human females, too, transport α-tocopherol preferentially with HDLs; but males transfer most (65%) with LDLs, only 24% with HDLs, and 8% with VLDLs.

the concentrations of vitamin E and of erythrocytes in plasma are highly correlated[15] (the latter containing 15 to 25% of total vitamin E in the plasma). Because vitamin E is membrane protective, plasma tocopherol levels are inversely related to susceptibility to oxidative **hemolysis**. This relationship makes the plasma α-tocopherol level useful as a parameter of vitamin E status; in healthy people, values ≥ 0.5 mg/dl are associated with protection against hemolysis and are taken to indicate nutritional adequacy (Table 7-4). Maternal tocopherol levels increase during pregnancy, but fetal levels remain low,[16] suggesting a barrier to transplacental movement of the vitamin. Because **apolipoprotein E (apoE)** affects the hepatic binding and catabolism of several classes of lipoproteins, it has been suggested that it can also affect the metabolism of tocopherols (Table 7-5).

Cellular Uptake

The cellular uptake of vitamin E differs according to cell type and appears to occur by established mechanisms of lipid transfer between lipoproteins and cells:

- *Uptake mediated by lipid transfer proteins and lipases.* Uptake of α-tocopherol from the amphipathic lipoprotein outer layer is mediated in a directional way by phospholipid transfer

protein[17] and by way of lipoprotein lipase-mediated exchange of α-tocopherol from chylomicra and lipoprotein remodeling. This lipase is thought to be involved in the transport of α-tocopherol across the blood–brain barrier and into the central nervous system.[18]

- *Receptor-mediated endocytosis of vitamin E-carrying lipoproteins.* Evidence has been presented that the binding of lipoproteins to specific cell surface receptors must occur to allow vitamin E to enter cells either by diffusion

Table 7-5. Relationship of apo E genotype to plasma tocopherol levels in free-living children

ApoE genotype	n	Plasma α-tocopherol (µmol/L)	Plasma γ-tocopherol (µmol/L)
E2/2	6	26.5[a] (23.8–29.2)	3.10[a] (2.27–4.22)
E3/2	89	20.8[b] (20.1–21.5)	1.90[b] (1.75–2.07)
E3/3	660	21.3[b] (21.1–21.6)	2.06[a,b] (2.00–2.12)
E4/3	150	21.4[b] (20.9–21.9)	2.05[a,b] (1.92–2.18)
E4/2	8	21.7[a,b] (19.4–23.9)	1.81[a,b] (1.39–2.36)
E4/4	13	19.0[b] (17.2–20.8)	1.84[a,b] (1.49–2.27)

[a,b] means sharing a common superscript are not significantly different ($p > 0.05$).

Source: Ortega, H., et al. (2005). *Am. J. Clin. Nutr.* **81**, 624–63.

Table 7-4. Serum α-tocopherol concentrations in humans

Group	α-Tocopherol (mg/dl)	Group	α-Tocopherol (mg/dl)
Healthy adults	0.85 ± 0.03	Infants	
Postpartum mothers	1.33 ± 0.40	Full term	0.22 ± 0.10
Children, 2–12 years old	0.72 ± 0.02	Premature	0.23 ± 0.10
Patients with cystic fibrosis, 1–19 years old	0.15 ± 0.15	Premature at 1 month	0.13 ± 0.05
		2 months, bottle-fed	0.33 ± 0.15
Patients with biliary atresia, 3–15 months old	0.10 ± 0.10	2 months, breastfed	0.71 ± 0.25
		5 months	0.42 ± 0.20
		2 years	0.58 ± 0.20

Source: Gordon et al. (1958). *Pediatrics* **21**, 673.

---

[15] Patients with abetalipoproteinemia are notable exceptions. They may show normal erythrocyte tocopherol concentrations, even though their serum tocopherols levels are undetectable.

[16] Serum tocopherol concentrations in infants are about 25% of those of their mothers. They increase to adequate levels within a few weeks after birth, except in infants with impaired abilities to utilize lipids (e.g., premature infants, biliary atresiacs); they show very low circulating levels of vitamin E.

[17] Mice lacking phospholipid transfer protein show high plasma levels of α-tocopherol in apo-B-containing lipoproteins (Jiang, X. C., et al. [2002]. *J. Biol. Chem.* **277**, 31850–31856).

[18] Mice lacking lipoprotein lipase show low brain α-tocopherol levels (although no associated pathologies have been reported, see Goti, B., et al. [2002]. *J. Biol. Chem.* **277**, 28537–28544).

and/or bulk entrance of lipoprotein-bound lipids.[19] That deficiencies in this pathway do not necessarily reduce tissue tocopherol levels suggests the similar function of other lipoprotein receptors.

- *Selective lipid uptake.* Evidence has been presented for the receptor-mediated uptake of lipoprotein-bound α-tocopherol without uptake of the apolipoprotein, in the manner described for the cellular uptake of cholesterol from HDLs. The process appears to involve the scavenger receptor class B type I (SR-BI).[20]

α-Tocopherol Transfer Protein

The intracellular transport of the α-vitamer appears to involve specific tocopherol-binding proteins. Originally discovered in the rat liver, 30-34-kDa cytoplasmic protein capable of high-affinity binding of α-tocopherol has been identified in liver, brain, spleen, lung, kidney, uterus, and placenta. Because it was shown to facilitate the transfer of α-tocopherol between microsomes and mitochondria, it has been called the **α-tocopherol transfer protein (α-TTP).** The α-TTP appears to be highly conserved: The rat and human liver proteins show 94% sequence homology as well as some homology to the interphotoreceptor retinol-binding protein (IRBP), cellular retinal-binding protein (CRALBP), and a phospholipid transfer protein. α-TTP recognizes the fully methylated chromanol ring of vitamers with a phytyl side chain in the *R* stereochemical configuration at the 2-position. It binds *RRR*-α-tocopherol more avidly than it does the *SRR* stereoisomer,[21] and the α-vitamer more avidly than the γ-vitamer. This selectivity appears to be the basis for the differences in the tissue retention and biopotency of these stereoisomers.[22] This would explain the fact that while γ-tocopherol is the dominant dietary form of vitamin E, α-tocopherol constitutes 90% of body vitamin E burden.

The human α-TTP gene has been localized on chromosome 8, and cases of genetic defects in the α-TTP gene have been described. This includes a group of American patients with sporadic or familial vitamin E deficiency;[23] they show poor incorporation of (*RRR*)-α-tocopherol into their VLDLs and an inability to discriminate between the *RRR* and *SRR* vitamers. These patients show exceedingly low circulating tocopherol concentrations unless maintained on high-level vitamin E supplements (e.g., 1 g/day); if untreated, they experience progressive peripheral neuropathy (characterized by pathology of the large-caliber axons of sensory neurons) and **ataxia**. Chromosome 8 defects have also been identified among the members of a number of inbred Tunisian families.[24] These patients also show low serum tocopherol levels and ataxia responsive to high-level vitamin E supplements. In this case, the defect has been shown to involve the deletion of the terminal 10% of the α-TTP peptide chain. A third group of subjects with isolated vitamin E deficiency has been identified in Japan. They have a point mutation[25] that results in their α-TTP having only 11% of the transfer activity of the wild-type protein. Individuals heterozygous for this trait show no clinical signs but have circulating tocopherol levels 25% lower than those of normal subjects. Deletion of the α-TTP gene in the mouse resulted in the accumulation of dietary α-tocopherol in the liver at the expense of α-tocopherol in peripheral tissues.[26]

The expresson of α-TTP occurs predominantly in the liver, apparently in response to vitamin E. Studies with the rat have shown that the α-TTP messenger RNA is increased in response to treatment with either α- or γ-tocopherol.[27] As α-TTP binds only the d-vitamer, this finding suggests the roles of these vitamers in regulating gene expression.

---

[19] Fibroblasts from an individual with a hereditary deficiency of LDL receptors were found to be unable to take up LDL-bound vitamin E at normal rates.

[20] Mice lacking SR-BI show marked reductions in the amounts of α-tocopherol in plasma (particularly, in the HDL fraction) and tissues (Mardones, P., et al. [2002]. *J. Nutr.* 132, 443–449).

[21] The preferential incorporation of the *RRR*-α-isomer into milk by the lactating sow (Lauridson, C., et al. [2002]. *J. Nutr.* **132**,1258–1264) suggests the presence of α-TTP in the mammary gland.

[22] Neither LDL receptor nor lipoprotein lipase mechanisms of vitamin E uptake by cells discriminate between these stereoisomers; yet α-tocopherol predominates in plasma owing to its preferential incorporation into nascent VLDLs, while the form often predominating in foods, γ-tocopherol, is left behind only to be more rapidly excreted.

[23] That is, **familial isolated vitamin E (*FIVE*) deficiency**, also referred to as *FIVE deficiency.*

[24] Previously called *Friedreich's ataxia*, this condition is now called *ataxia with vitamin E deficiency (AVED)*.

[25] This is a missense mutation that inserts histidine in place of glutamine at position 101.

[26] Leonard, S. W., et al. (2002). *Am. J. Clin. Nutr.* **75**, 555–560.

[27] Fechner, H. (1998). *Biochem. J.* **331**, 577–581.

Other Tocopherol-Binding Proteins

Other proteins with vitamin E-binding capacities have been identified. Because they do appear to participate in the intracellular transport of tocopherol, they are generally referred to as **tocopherol-associated proteins (TAPs)**. These have been found in several tissues (liver, heart, brain, intestinal mucosa, erythrocytes), with the greatest concentrations in liver, brain, and prostate. Tocopherol can also bind the IRBP, apparently at the same site as retinol, as the latter readily displaces it. This raises the possibility that some of the retinoid-binding proteins may also function in the intracellular transport of vitamin E.

Vitamin E Storage: Two Pools

In most nonadipose cells, vitamin E is localized almost exclusively in membranes. Kinetic studies indicate that such tissues have two pools of the vitamin: a *labile*, rapidly turning over pool; and a *fixed*, slowly turning over pool. Apparently, the labile pools predominate in such tissues as plasma and liver, as the tocopherol contents of those tissues are depleted rapidly under conditions of vitamin E deprivation. In contrast, in adipose tissue vitamin E resides predominantly in the bulk lipid phase, which appears to be a fixed pool of the vitamin. Thus, it is only slowly mobilized from that tissue (Fig. 7-2) and exhibits long-term physiological significance: Kinetic studies in humans have shown that, after a change in α-tocopherol intake, adipose tissue tocopherols may not reach a new steady state for two or more years. Neural tissues also exhibit very efficient retention (i.e., very low apparent turnover rates) of vitamin E.[28]

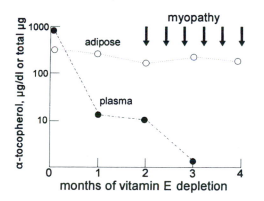

Fig. 7-2. Retention of α-tocopherol in guinea pig adipose tissue during vitamin E depletion. (*From* Machlin, L. J., et al. [1979]. *J. Nutr.* **109**, 105–109.)

Owing to the very slow rates of turnover of such fixed pools, the amounts of vitamin E in adipose tissue can be nearly normal even in animals showing clinical signs of vitamin E deficiency. Similarly, people on a weight-loss program were found to lose triglycerides but not vitamin E from their adipose tissues. However, circulating tocopherol levels have been found to rise significantly (10–20%) during intensive exercise, and it has been suggested that vitamin E may be mobilized from its fixed pools by way of the lipolysis induced under such conditions. Tissue tocopherol contents tend to be related exponentially to vitamin E intake; unlike most other vitamins, they show no deposition or saturation thresholds. Thus, the tocopherol contents of tissues vary considerably (Table 7-6), and are not consistently related to the amounts or types of lipids present.

V. Metabolism of Vitamin E

Limited Metabolism

The metabolism of vitamin E is limited; most tocopherols that are absorbed and retained are transported without transformation to the tissues. That a large fraction of α-tocopherol can be found in the skin after injection suggests that dermal elimination of the unchanged vitamin may also be significant. Excretion of the nonmetabolized α-tocopherol occurs only at high doses (e.g.,

Table 7-6. Concentrations of α-tocopherol in human tissues

Tissue	α-Tocopherol μ/g tissue	α-Tocopherol μ/g lipid
Plasma	9.5	1.4
Erythrocytes	2.3	0.5
Platelets	30	1.3
Adipose	150	0.2
Kidney	7	0.3
Liver	13	0.3
Muscle	19	0.4
Ovary	11	0.6
Uterus	9	0.7
Testis	40	1.0
Heart	20	0.7
Adrenal	132	0.7
Hypophysis	40	1.2

Source: Machlin, L. J. (1984). *Handbook of Vitamins*, p. 99. Marcel Dekker, New York.

---

[28] For example, weanling rats from vitamin E-adequate dams do not show neurologic signs of vitamin E deficiency for as long as 7 weeks when fed a vitamin E-free diet.

>50mg), which apparently exceed the binding capacity of α-TTP. The actual metabolism of tocopherols involves head-group and side-chain oxidation.

- *Oxidation of the chromanol ring.* Oxidation of the chromanol ring is the basis of the in *vivo* **antioxidant** function of the vitamin. It involves oxidation primarily to **tocopherylquinone**, which proceeds through the semis table tocopheroxyl radical intermediate (Fig. 7-3). It is important to note that, whereas the monovalent oxidation of tocopherol to the tocopheroxyl radical is a reversible reaction (at least *in vitro*), further oxidation of the radical intermediate is unidirectional. Because tocopherylquinone has no vitamin E activity, its production represents catabolism and loss of the vitamin from the system. Tocopherylquinone can be partially reduced to α-**tocopherylhydroquinone**, which can be conjugated with glucuronic acid and secreted in the bile, thus making excretion with the feces the major route of elimination of the vitamin. Under conditions of intakes of nutritional levels of vitamin E, less than 1% of the absorbed vitamin is excreted with the urine.
- *Oxidation of the phytyl side chain.* Vitamin E is catabolized to water-soluble metabolites by a **cytochrome P450**-mediated process initiated by a β-hydroxylation of a terminal methyl group of the phytyl side chain.[29] This hydroxylation step, which appears to be catalyzed by a cytochrome

P540 isoform (CYP3A) that is also involved in leucotriene β-hydroxylation, is followed by dehydrogenation to the 13´-chromanol, and subsequent truncation of the phytyl side chain through the removal of two- and three-carbon fragments. The resulting metolites include **tocopheronic acid** and **tocopheronolactone**[30] excreted in the urine often as glucuronyl conjugates. This pathway catabolizes γ-tocopherol much more extensively than it does α-tocopherol, apparently contributing to the much faster turnover of the former vitamer. However, it also appears to be upregulated by high doses of α-tocopherol, suggesting that it is also important in clearing that vitamer via conversion to the readily excreted α-**carboxyethylchromanol**.

- *Other reactions.* The detection of small amounts of α-tocopheryl phosphate in tissues of vitamin E-fed animals suggests that the vitamin can be phosphorylated. The metabolic significance of this metabolite is unclear, and a kinase has not been identified. Vitamin E can also be nitrated *in vivo*. In fact, **5-nitro-γ-tocopherol** has been identified in the plasma of cigarette smokers (Table 7-7), presumably due to the high amounts of reactive nitrogen species and the stimulatory effect of cigarette smoke on inflammatory responses. This reaction may be the basis for the enhanced turnover of tocopherols and reduced production of carboxyethylchromanol metabolites in smokers.

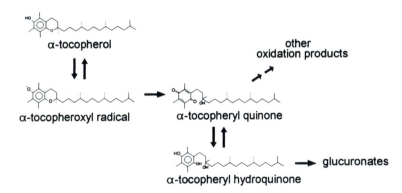

Fig. 7-3. Vitamin E metabolism.

---

[29] Sontag, T. J., and Parker, R. S. (2002). *J. Biol. Chem.* **277**, 25290–25296.

[30] These are collectively referred to as **Simon's metabolites**, after E. J. Simon, who described them in the urine of rabbits and humans. It is doubtful that these actually result from metabolism of the vitamin *in vivo* (e.g., by β oxidation in the kidney); they appear to be artifacts resulting from oxidation during their isolation.

α-tocopheronic acid   α-tocopheronolactone

Table 7-7.   Plasma tocopherols in smokers and nonsmokers

Metabolite	Nonsmokers (n = 19)	Smokers (n = 15)
α-tocopherol, μM	16.0 ± 4.0	15.9 ± 5.0
γ-tocopherol, μM	1.76 ± 0.98	1.70 ± 0.69
5-nitro-γ-tocopherol, nM	4.03* ± 3.10	8.02 ± 8.33

*$p < 0.05$.
Source: Leonard, S. W., et al. (2003). *Free Radical Biol. Med.* **12**, 1560–1567.

Vitamin E Recycling

A significant portion of vitamin E may be recycled *in vivo* by reduction of tocopheroxyl radical back to toco-pherol (Fig. 7-4). Several findings have been cited in support of this hypothesis: the very low turnover of α-tocopherol, the slow rate of its depletion in vitamin E-deprived animals, and the relatively low molar ratio of vitamin E to PUFA (about 1:850) in most biological membranes. Several mechanisms have been proposed for the *in vivo* reduction of to-copheroxyl by various intracellular reductants. *In vitro* studies have demonstrated that this can occur in liposomes by ascorbic acid, in microsomal suspensions by NAD(P)H, and in mitochondrial suspensions by NADH and succinate, with the latter two systems showing synergism with reduced glutathione (GSH) or ubiquinones. Indeed, a membrane-bound *tocoph-eroxyl reductase activity* has been suggested. To constitute a physiologically significant pathway *in vivo*, such a multicomponent system may be expected to link the major reactants, which are compartmentalized within the cell (e.g., ascorbic acid in the cytosol and

tocopheroxyl in the membrane). Thus, it is possible that the recycling of tocopherol may be coupled to the shuttle of electrons between one or more donors in the soluble phase of the cell and the radical intermediate in the membrane, resulting in the reduction of the latter.

According to this model, vitamin E[31] would be expected to be retained through recycling until the reducing systems in both aqueous and membrane domains become rate limiting. At this point the vitamin would be lost by the irreversible conversion of tocopheroxyl radical to tocopherylquinone, and **lipid peroxidation** and protein oxidation would increase.

Attractive though a model of vitamin E recycling may be, there is little direct evidence of this phenomenon *in vivo*. Although a few studies with experimental animals have found greater concentrations of vitamin E in tissues of ascorbic acid-fed animals, several others have not detected such evidence of nutritional *sparing* of vitamin E. A direct test of this hypothesis using deuterium-labeled α-tocopherol found no differences in α-tocopherol concentrations of plasma, platelets, buccal cells, or adipose in humans treated for 6 weeks with either deficient (5 mg/day) or excess (500 mg/day) levels of vitamin C.[32]

VI. Metabolic Functions of Vitamin E

Vitamin E as a Biological Antioxidant

The chief nutritional role of vitamin E is clearly that of a biological antioxidant.[33] In this regard, vitamin E

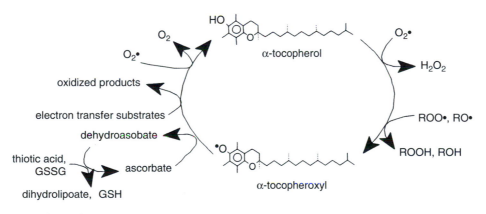

Fig. 7-4.   Vitamin E redox cycle.

---

[31] The analogous reactions would be expected for the tocotrienols.

[32] Jacob, R. A. et al. (1996). *J. Nutr.* **126**, 2268–2277.

[33] An **antioxidant** is an agent that inhibits oxidation and thus prevents such oxidation reactions as the conversion of polyunsaturated fatty acids to fatty hydroperoxides, the conversion of free or protein-bound sulfhydryls to disulfides, and so on.

is thought to have basic functional importance in the maintenance of membrane integrity in virtually all cells of the body. Its antioxidant function involves the reduction of **free radicals**, thus protecting against the potentially deleterious reactions of such highly reactive oxidizing species.

Production of free radicals and reactive oxygen species

Free radicals ($X^\bullet$) are produced in cells under normal conditions either by homolytic cleavage of a covalent bond, as in the formation of a C-centered free radical of a polyunsaturated fatty acid, or by a univalent electron transfer reaction. It has been estimated that as much as 5% of inhaled molecular oxygen (O_2) is metabolized to yield the so-called **reactive oxygen species**, that is, the one- and two-electron reduction products **superoxide radical $O_2^{\bullet-}$** and **H_2O_2**, respectively. There appear to be three sources of reactive oxygen species:

- *Normal oxidative metabolism* The mitochondrial electron transport chain, which involves a flow of electrons from NADH and succinate through a series of electron carriers to cytochrome oxidase, which reduces oxygen to water, has been found to leak a small fraction of its electrons, which reduce oxygen to $O_2^{\bullet-}$.
- *Microsomal cytochrome P-450 activity* Several xenobiotic agents are metabolized by the microsomal electron transport chain to radical species (e.g., the herbicide paraquat is converted to an N-centered radical anion) that can react with oxygen to produce $O_2^{\bullet-}$.
- *Respiratory burst of stimulated phagocytes* Macrophages produce $O_2^{\bullet-}$ and H_2O_2 during phagocytosis.

The half-life of $O_2^{\bullet-}$ appears to be only about 1 sec, and neither $O_2^{\bullet-}$ nor H_2O_2 is highly reactive. However, when exposed to transition metal ions (particularly Fe^{2+} and Cu^+), these two species can react to yield a very highly reactive free-radical species, the **hydroxyl radical HO**.

$$O_2^{\bullet-} + H_2O_2 + Fe^{2+} \rightarrow O_2 + HO^\bullet + HO^- + Fe^{3+}$$

These divalent metals can also catalyze the decomposition of H_2O_2 or fatty acyl **hydroperoxide (ROOH)** produced by lipid peroxidation to yield the oxygen-centered radical $RO^\bullet$ or $HO^\bullet$, respectively:

$$ROOH (HOOH) + Fe^{2+} \rightarrow RO^\bullet(HO^\bullet) + HO^- + Fe^{3+}$$

Targets of $HO^\bullet$ include:

- *DNA* Causing oxidative base damage[34]
- *Proteins* Causing the production of carbonyls and other amino acid oxidation products[35]
- *Lipids* Causing oxidation of PUFAs of membrane phospholipids, the formation of lipid peroxidation products (e.g., malonyldialdehyde, isoprostanes, pentane, ethane), and resulting in membrane dysfunction

Mechanism of lipid peroxidation

The PUFAs of biological membranes are particularly susceptible to attack by free radicals by virtue of their 1,4-pentadiene systems, which allow for the abstraction of a complete hydrogen atom (i.e., with its electron) from one of the $-CH_2-$ groups in the carbon chain, and the consequent generation of a *C-centered free radical* ($-C^\bullet-$) (Fig. 7-5). This initiation of lipid peroxidation can be accomplished by $HO^\bullet$ and possibly $HOO^\bullet$ (but *not* by H_2O_2 or $O_2^{\bullet-}$). The C-centered radical, being unstable, undergoes molecular rearrangement to form a **conjugated diene**, which is susceptible to attack by molecular oxygen (O_2) to yield a **peroxyl radical (ROO$^\bullet$)**. Peroxyl radicals are capable of abstracting a hydrogen atom from other PUFAs and thus propagating a chain reaction that can continue until the membrane PUFAs are completely oxidized to hydroperoxides (ROOH).

Fatty acyl hydroperoxides so formed are degraded in the presence of transition metals (Cu^{2+}, Fe^{2+}) and heme and heme proteins (cytochromes, hemoglobin, myoglobin) to release radicals that can continue the chain reaction of lipid peroxidation,[36] as well as

---

[34] Base damage products such as 8-hydroxydeoxyguanosine (8OHdG), presumably resulting from DNA repair processes, are excreted in the urine. Smokers typically show elevated 8OHdG excretion.

[35] For example, methionine sulfoxide, 2-ketohistidine, hydroxylation of tyrosine to DOPA, formylkynurenine, *o*-tyrosine, and protein peroxides

[36] Therefore, a single radical can initiate a chain reaction that may propagate over and over again.

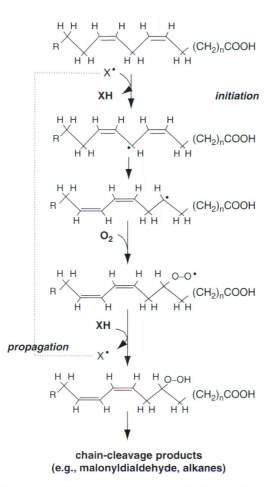

Fig. 7-5. The self-propagating nature of lipid peroxidation.

can also occur without significant lipid peroxidation, by oxidative damage to critical macromolecules (DNA, proteins), and by decompartmentalization of Ca^{2+}.[40]

Vitamin E as a scavenger of free radicals

Because of the reactivity of the phenolic hydrogen on its C-6 hydroxyl group and the ability of the chromanol ring system to stabilize an unpaired electron, vitamin E has antioxidant activity capable of terminating chain reactions among PUFAs in the membranes wherein it resides. This action, termed *free-radical scavenging*, involves the donation of the phenolic hydrogen to a fatty acyl free radical (or $O_2^{\bullet-}$) to prevent the attack of that species on other PUFAs. The antioxidant activities of the vitamers E thus relate to the leaving ability of their phenolic hydrogen. The tocopherols have greatest reactivities toward peroxyl and phenoxyl radicals but can also quench such mutagenic electrophiles as reactive nitrogen oxide species (NO_x). When assessed *in vitro* in chemically defined systems, activities are greatest for α-tocopherol,[41] with the β- and γ-vitamers roughly comparable and greater than the δ-vitamer. In contrast, reactive nitrogen species, NO_x, are trapped more effectively by γ-tocopherol than by the α-vitamer. The biological activities of the vitamers E are affected by both their intrinsic chemical antioxidant activities and their efficiencies of absorption and retention. Thus, γ-tocopherol has only 6 to 16% of the biological activity of the α-vitamer. An exception to this relationship has been identified in the case of sesame seed, lignans which act to potentiate the biopotency of γ-tocopherol such

other chain-cleavage products, **malonyldialdehyde**,[37] **pentane**, and **ethane**.[38] This oxidative degradation of membrane phospholipid PUFAs is believed to produce physicochemical changes, resulting in membrane dysfunction within the cell.[39] Cellular oxidant injury

---

[37] Although malonyldialdehyde (MDA) is a relatively minor product of lipid peroxidation, it has received a great deal of attention in part because of the ease of measuring it colorimetrically using 3-thiobarbituric acid (TBA). In fact, the TBA test has been widely used to assess MDA concentrations as measures of lipid peroxidation. It is important to note that the TBA test is subject to several limitations. Specifically, much of the MDA it detects may not have been present in the original sample, as lipid peroxides are known to decompose to MDA during the heating stage of the test, that reaction being affected by the concentration of iron salts.

[38] The volatile alkanes, pentane and ethane, are excreted across the lungs and can be detected in the breath of vitamin E-deficient subjects. Pentane is produced from the oxidative breakdown of ω-6 fatty acids (linoleic acid family), whereas ethane is produced from the ω-3 fatty acids (linolenic acid family).

[39] Whether lipid peroxidation does, indeed, occur *in vivo* has been surprisingly difficult to determine. Tissues of animals contain little or no evidence of lipid peroxides or their decomposition products. Although expired breath contains volatile alkanes that might have originated from the decomposition of fatty acyl hydroperoxides, it is difficult to exclude the possibility of their production by bacteria of the gut or skin. Perhaps the greatest presumptive evidence for *in vivo* lipid peroxidation is that biological systems have evolved redundant mechanisms of antioxidant protection, specifically involving the powerful chain-breaking antioxidant α-tocopherol in the membrane and several other antioxidants (glutathione, cysteine, ascorbate, uric acid, glutathione peroxidase, ceruloplasmin) in the soluble phase. Indeed, it is clear that deficiencies of this antioxidant defense system can greatly impair physiological function.

[40] For example, pulmonary injury by the bipyridilium herbicide paraquat involves lipid peroxidation only as a late-stage event, rather than as a cause of it.

[41] The antioxidant activity of α-tocopherol is about 200-fold that of the commonly used food antioxidant butylated hydroxytoluene (BHT).

that the vitamin in sesame oil, which consists exclusively of the γ-vitamer, has a biopotency equivalent to that of α-tocopherol. The identity of the potentiating antioxidant factor is believed to be a lignan phenol, sesamolin, to which antiaging properties have been attributed. In view of this finding, it has been suggested that γ-tocopherol, the predominant form of the vitamin in diets, may be important *in vivo* as a trap for electrophilic nitrogen oxides and other electrophilic mutagens. The tocotrienols are also active in scavenging the chain-propagating peroxyl radical.

In serving its antioxidant function, tocopherols and tocotrienols are converted from their respective alcohol forms to semistable radical intermediates, the *tocopheroxyl* (or *chromanoxyl*) *radical* (Fig. 7-6). Unlike the free radicals formed from PUFAs, the tocopheroxyl radical is relatively unreactive, thus stopping the destructive propagative cycle of lipid peroxidation. In fact, tocopheroxyl is sufficiently stable to react with a second peroxyl radical to form inactive, nonradical products including *tocopherylquinone*.[42] Because α-tocopherol can compete for peroxyl radicals much faster than PUFAs, small amounts of the vitamin are able to effect the antioxidant protection of relatively large amounts of the latter.

Although α-tocopherol is clearly the most abundant lipid-soluble, chain-breaking antioxidant, the fact that it is typically present in such low amounts relative to the membrane PUFAs it protects suggests that it is both recycled and highly mobile within the membrane. Evidence suggests the presence of two membrane pools of α-tocopherol: a highly mobile one and a relatively fixed one. A model that would appear to fit the latter was presented some years ago; it proposed that the vitamin may actually reside in intimate contact with PUFAs by virtue of their complementary three-dimensional structures (Fig. 7-7).

Interrelationships of Vitamin E and Other Factors in Antioxidant Defense

Factors that increase the production of reactive oxygen (e.g., xenobiotic metabolism, ionizing radiation, exposure to such prooxidants as ozone and NO_2) can be expected to increase the metabolic demand for antioxidant protection, including the need for vitamin E and the other nutrients involved in this system. Because it is hydrophobic and, therefore, distributed in membranes, vitamin E serves as a lipid-soluble biological antioxidant with high specificity for loci of potential lipid peroxidation. However, vitamin E is but one of several factors in an *antioxidant defense system* that protects the cell from the damaging effects of oxidative stress. This system (Fig. 7-8) includes:

- *Membrane antioxidants* The most important membrane antioxidants are the tocopherols, but the ubiquinones and carotenoids also participate in this function.
- *Soluble antioxidants* Soluble antioxidants include NADPH and NADH, ascorbic acid, reduced glutathione and other thiols, uric acid,

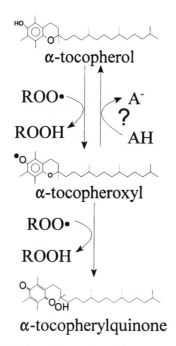

Fig. 7-6. Oxidation of tocopherols by reaction with peroxyl radicals.

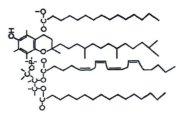

Fig. 7-7. Proposed interdigitation of tocopherols and polyunsaturated fatty acids in biological membranes.

---

[42] Evidence indicates that tocopherylquinones can induce apoptosis in cancer cells.

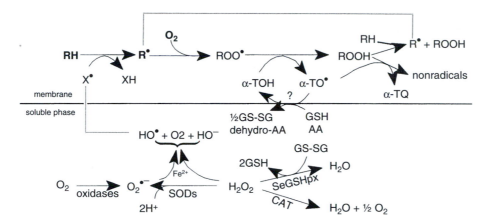

Fig. 7-8. The cellular antioxidant defense system. CAT, catalase; GSH, reduced glutathione; GSSG, oxidized glutathione; α-TQ, α-tocopherylquinone; α-TO·, α-tocopheryl radical; α-TOH, α-tocopherol; SeGSHpx, selenium-dependent glutathione peroxidase; SOD, superoxide dismutase.

thioredoxin, bilirubin, polyphenols, and several metal-binding proteins (copper: ceruloplasmin, metallothionine, albumin; iron: transferrin, ferritin, myoglobin).

- *Antioxidant enzymes*   Antioxidant enzymes include the superoxide dismutases,[43] the glutathione peroxidases,[44] thioredoxin reductase,[45] and catalase.[46]

In this multicomponent system, vitamin E scavenges radicals within the membrane, where it blocks the initiation and interrupts the propagation of lipid peroxidation. The group of metalloenzymes collectively blocks the initiation of peroxidation from within the soluble phase of the cell: the **superoxide dismutases** convert $O_2^{\bullet-}$ to $H_2O_2^{\bullet}$; **catalase** and the **glutathione peroxidases** each further reduce H_2O_2. The aggregate effect of this enzymatic system is to clear $O_2^{\bullet-}$ by reducing it fully to H_2O, thus preventing the generation of other, more highly reactive oxygen species [e.g., $HO^{\bullet}$ and singlet oxygen ($^1O_2$)]. Glutathione peroxidases can also reduce fatty acyl hydroperoxides to the corresponding fatty alcohols, thus serving to interrupt the propagation of lipid peroxidation.

Some components of this system are endogenous (e.g., NADPH, NADH, and, for most species, ascorbic acid), whereas other components must be obtained, at least in part, from the external chemical environment. That they are mutually affected by changes in status is indicated by the finding of increased plasma ascorbic acid concentrations in response to vitamin E supplementation (Table 7-8). The diversity of this system implies the ability to benefit from various antioxidants and other key factors obtained from dietary sources in variable amounts. That the various components of the defense system function cooperatively is evidenced by the nutritional sparing observed particularly for vitamin E and selenium in the etiologies of several deficiency diseases (e.g., **exudative diathesis** in chicks, **liver necrosis** in rats, **white muscle disease** in lambs and calves). In those species, nutritional deprivation of either vitamin E or selenium alone is usually asymptomatic, whereas deficiencies of both nutrients are required to produce disease.

---

[43] The superoxide dismutases (SODs) are metalloenzymes. The mitochondrial SOD contains manganese at its active center, whereas the cytosolic SOD contains both copper and zinc as essential cofactors. Although not found in animals, an iron-centered SOD has been identified in blue-green algae.

[44] The glutathione peroxidases contain selenium at their active centers and are dependent on adequate supplies of that element for their synthesis. There are at least four isoforms; each uses reducing equivalents from reduced glutathione (GSH) to reduce H_2O_2 to water or fatty acyl hydroperoxides to the corresponding fatty alcohols. One isoform is found in membranes and has specificity for esterified hydroperoxides; the others are soluble and have specificities for nonesterified hydroperoxide substrates including H_2O_2. The activities of these enzymes depend on a functioning glutathione cycle (i.e., the flavoenzyme **glutathione reductase**) to regenerate GSH from its oxidized form (GSSG).

[45] Thioredoxin reductase has been found to contain selenium at its active center and depends on adequate selenium nutriture for its synthesis.

[46] Catalase has an iron redox center. Because its distribution is almost exclusively limited to the peroxisomes/lysosomes, it is probably not important in antioxidant protection in the cytosol.

Table 7-8. Effects of vitamin E supplementation on circulating antioxidants in humans

Antioxidant	Baseline	Postsupplementation[a]
Plasma		
α-tocopherol, μmol/l	26.8 ± 1.03	32.3 ± 0.92[b]
Ascorbate, μmol/l	64.4 ± 3.18	76.3 ± 4.20[b]
Urate, μmol/l	262 ± 13.9	246 ± 12.6[b]
Whole blood		
GPX,[c] U/gHb	48.8 ± 2.39	53.5 ± 2.90[b]

[a]73.5 mg RRR-α-tocopheryl acetate per day for 6 weeks.
[b]$p < 0.05$.
[c]Selenium-dependent glutathione peroxidase activity.
Source: Hamilton, I. M. J., et al. (2000). Br. J. Nutr. **84**, 261–267.

The activities of various components of this system, as well as the cellular redox state, have been found to change markedly during cellular differentiation, corresponding to increased oxidant production under those conditions. That gradients of reactive oxygen species and/or the redox state may be important in influencing genetic expression is indicated by several lines of evidence; oxidizing conditions have been found to affect cellular ion distribution; chromatin-controlling proteins; the cytoskeleton and nuclear matrix, which in turn affect chromatic configuration and pre-mRNA processing. Thus, it appears that the antioxidant defense system actually serves to control **peroxide tone**, such that the beneficial effects of prooxidizing conditions are realized and their deleterious effects are minimized.

Prooxidant Capabilities of Vitamin E

That α-tocopherol can promote lipid peroxidation in LDLs in the absence of ascorbic acid or coenzyme Q_{10} to reduce the α-tocopheroxyl radical suggests that the vitamin can be prooxidative under some conditions.

Non-Antioxidant Functions of Vitamin E

The recognition in the early 1990s that vitamin E could inhibit cell proliferation and protein kinase C activity suggested that vitamin E may function *in vivo* in ways that are unrelated to its function as a bio-

logical antioxidant. Since then, research has revealed such actions of α-tocopherol in two general areas:

- *Transcriptional regulation* The possibility of regulation at the transcriptional level by vitamin E has been suggested by findings of vitamin E-induced regulation of several genes involved in tocopherol uptake/metabolism (TTP, CYP3A), lipid uptake (scavenger receptors CD36, SR-BI, and SR-AI/II), extracellar proteins (α-tropomyosin, collagen-α1, matrix metalloproteinases-1 and -19, and connective tissue growth factor), inflammation and cell adhesion (E-selectin, ICAM-1, integrins, glycoproteins IIb, interleukins-2, -4 and -ß), and cell signaling and cell cycle regulation (PPAR-γ, cyclins D1 and E, Bcl12-L1, p27 and CD95).[47] The underlying mechanisms for these effects may involve the antioxidant response element (ARE) or the transforming growth factor beta response element (TGF-ß-RE). A tocopherol-dependent transcription factor, tocopherol-associated protein, has been identified.
- *Signal transduction* At physiologically relevant concentrations, α-tocopherol has been shown to inhibit PKC, 5-lipoxygenase, and phospholipase A2, and to activate protein phospatase 2A and diacylglycerol kinase through post-translational mechanisms. These effects signal antiproliferative effects on a variety of cells, resulting in inhibition of inflammation, cell adhesion, platelet aggregation, and smooth muscle cell proliferation.

Vitamin E in Health and Disease

Vitamin E has been proposed as playing an important role in general health with specific implications regarding protection from conditions thought to involve reactive oxygen species (Table 7-9).

Aging

Experimental data suggest a causative role for reactive oxygen species in aging processes. An array of oxidative lesions, many likely to be caused by reactive oxygen species, has been found to accumulate with age. Mitochondria, which process 99% of the oxygen utilized by the cell, are thought to be the main

---

[47] Azzi, A., et al. (2004). *J. Biol. Chem.* **385**, 585–591.

Table 7-9 .   Conditions associated with oxidative damage

Aging

Cancer

Cardiovascular disease

Cataracts

Diabetes

Exercise

Hemodialysis

Immunity and infection

Inflammatory disease

Ischemia-reperfusion injury

Lung disease

Neurodegenerative diseases

Preeclampsia

Skin disorders

Smoking

source of reactive oxygen species. Oxidative damage to mitochondrial DNA, proteins, and lipids increases with age. The accumulation of lipid-soluble, brown to yellow, autofluorescent pigments,[48] collectively called **lipofuscin**, has been demonstrated in several tissues (e.g., retinal pigment epithelium, heart muscle, brain) of aging individuals. Vitamin E deficiency has been shown to increase the accumulation of these so-called *age pigments* in experimental animals; but there is no evidence that supranutritional levels of vitamin E are any more effective than nutritionally adequate levels in reducing their buildup.

That these changes are related causally to aging is suggested by interspecies observations that mammalian life span potentials tend to correlate inversely with metabolic rate and directly with tissue concentrations of tocopherols and other antioxidants (e.g., carotenoids, urate, ascorbic acid, superoxide dismutase activity).[49,50] According to the **free-radical theory of aging**, it is proposed that cumulative damage by reactive oxygen species, accompanied by grad-

ual decreases in repair capacity, contribute to aging. Mechanistic hypotheses have included adverse effects on gene expression, diminished immune functions, and enhanced genetically programmed cell death (called *apoptosis*) due to increases in peroxide tone (i.e., the net amount of reactive oxygen species within the cell).

Cancer

Chemical carcinogenesis is thought to involve the electrophilic attack of free radicals with DNA. Reactive oxygen (ROS) and nitrogen (RNS) species are mutagenic by inducing DNA damage,[51] including the production of 8-OH-2-deoxyguanosine. If this base modification is replicated before it can be repaired, a G to T transversion mutation occurs. That mutation in the p53 gene results in a gene product with reduced tumor-suppressing activity; it occurs in more than half of human cancers. The generation of ROS and RNS has been found to correlate with the initiation, promotion, and progression of tumors in animal models, and a product of lipid peroxidation, malonyldialdehyde, has been found to increase tumor production in animals. Therefore, it would seem reasonable to expect that, as an antioxidant, vitamin E may have a role in cancer prevention.

Alternatively, because ROS is involved in the signal cascade that results in the activation of caspases and endonucleases that effect the apoptotic removal of damaged cells, it is possible that vitamin E deficiency may enhance apoptosis, thereby suppressing tumor growth.[52] In support of this hypothesis, two studies with transgenic animal models have found vitamin E-deficient animals to show lower rates of growth of brain and mammary tumors compared to vitamin E-adequate controls.

Treatment with α-tocopheryl succinate has been found to stimulate apoptosis in nonmalginant mesothelioma cells and human malignant prostate cells. That this effect may be due to the intact ester and not to the hydrolysis product α-tocopherol is indicated by *in vitro* studies in which α-tocopheryl succinate

---

[48] Lipofuscins are generally thought to be condensation products of proteins and lipid. There is some evidence that the pigments isolated from the retinal pigment epithelium contain, at least in part, derivatives of vitamin A (e.g., *N*-retinylidene-*N*-retinylethanolamine).

[49] See review by Cutler, R. G. (1991). *Am. J. Clin. Nutr.* **53**, 373S–379S.

[50] It is likely that caloric restriction, which has been shown to increase longevity in experimental animals, may have that effect by reducing the metabolic rate and, hence, the endogenous production of reactive oxygen species.

[51] See review by Cooke, M. S., et al. (2002). *Nutr. Res. Rev.* **15**, 19–41.

[52] The corollary to this hypothesis, that antioxidant supplementation could enhance tumorigenesis, has been proposed to explain the unexpected finding of increase lung cancer risk in smokers supplemented with β-carotene in the ATBC trial (Albanes, D., et al. [1996]. *Am. J. Clin. Nutr.* **62**, 1427S–1430S.

induced apoptosis, particularly in cancer cells lacking hydrolytic capacity.[53] A nonhydrolyzable analog, *RRR*-α-tocopherol ether-linked acetic acid, has been found to be a potent inducer of apoptosis in a variety of cancer cells and to be effective in inhibiting tumorigenesis in murine mammary and xenograft tumor models.[54]

Studies have found treatment with vitamin E to inhibit tumorigenesis in animal models of mammary, colon, oral, or skin tumors. For example, topically applied α-tocopheryl acetate was shown to reduce UV-induced skin cancers in mice by nearly 60%, and oral α-tocopheryl succinate reduced pre-neoplastic lesions of the rat colon. Other studies have not shown protection. It is possible that nutritional status with respect to selenium and/or other antioxidants may not have been adequately controlled in every case.

Epidemiological studies have shown the consumption of vitamin E-rich foods to be inversely associated with cancer risk, and the dozen longitudinal studies[55] that have compared circulating tocopherol levels and total cancer risk have found those levels to be only slightly lower (about 3%) in cancer patients than in healthy controls. A greater difference was observed between cancer patients and controls in a large study in Finland,[56] which also found individuals with relatively low serum α-tocopherol levels to have a 1.5-fold greater risk of cancer than those with higher serum vitamin E levels.

Nevertheless, the results of most studies to date are inconsistent with respect to relationships of vitamin E and incidence of site-specific cancers. Plasma α-tocopherol levels have been related inversely to risks of cancers of the lung, prostate, cervix, colon, head, and neck, and melanoma, although null associations have also been observed. A case-control study nested within the Physician's Health Study showed that individuals with high plasma α-tocopherol levels (>14.44 mg/ml) had significantly fewer aggressive prostate cancers than those with low levels of the vitamin (<8.56 mg/ml).[57] Men entering the SU.VI.MAX study with low concentrations of serum vitamins E and C showed greater risks of developing cancer than those with higher baseline levels.[58] The CPS-II Nutrition Cohort showed long-term use of vitamin E supplement intake to be associated with reduced risk of bladder cancer but not prostate cancer.[59] Studies have pointed to some protection against breast cancer risk by vitamin E in foods, but there is no evidence of protection by vitamin E supplements.

Only a few randomized clinical trials have been conducted to evaluate the cancer-chemo-preventive potential of supplemental vitamin E. The SU.VI.MAX trial found that a vitamin E-containing antioxidant supplement reduced the risk of cancer in men (but not women), particularly those with low baseline serum levels of α-tocopherol, ascorbic acid, and β-carotene.[58] Of three studies of lung cancer risk that have employed vitamin E, one found the combination of vitamin E, selenium, and β-carotene to reduce lung cancer risk by an apparent 45%.[60] Vitamin E treatment resulted in a 34% reduction in risk of prostate cancer with trends toward risk reductions for colorectal and stomach cancers in the ATBC trial.[61] The SELECT trial will evalutate the efficacy of vitamin E, both alone and in combination with selenium, for reducing prostate cancer risk.[62]

Cardiovascular disease

Cardiovascular disease (CVD) is multifactorial, involving high concentrations of ciculating lipids and inflammation of the arterial intima with associated oxidative stress. This leads to the accumulation of lipids and the formation of arterial lesions with endothelial activation and adhesion by immune cells ultimately producing endothelial dysfunction. Chemotactic factors are released upon the rupture of atherosclerotic lesions, producing platelet aggregation, arterial thrombosis, and heart attack. Evidence suggests that oxidative stress caused by oxidation of LDL contributes to the inflammation leading to the

[53] See review, Basu, A., and Imrhan, V. (2005). *Nutr. Rev.* **63**, 247–501.

[54] Kline, K., et al. (2004) *J. Nutr.* **134**, 3458S–3462S.

[55] See review by Kneckt, P. (1994). *Natural Antioxidants in Human Health and Disease* (B. Frei, ed.), pp. 199–238. Academic Press, New York.

[56] The Finnish Mobile Clinic Health Survey, which involved more than 36,000 subjects; Kneckt, P., et al. (1991). *J. Clin. Nutr.* **53**, 283S–286S.

[57] Gann, P. H., et al. (1999). *Cancer Res.* **59**, 1225–1230.

[58] The SUpplementation en Vitamines et Minereaux AtioXidants study. Galan, P., et al. (2005). *Br. J. Nutr.* **94**, 125–132.

[59] Cancer Prevention Study II (CPS-II). Rodriguez, C. (2004). *Cancer Epidemiol. Biomarkers Prev.* **13**, 378–382.

[60] Blot et al. (1994). *J. Natl. Cancer Inst.* **85**, 1483–1490.

[61] Albanes, D. (1996). *Am. J. Clin. Nutr.* **62**, 1427S–1430S.

[62] The Selenium and Vitamin E Cancer Prevention Trial (SELECT) is a 12-year trial started in 2001 involving 32,400 men in the United States and Canada (Klein, E. A. [2003]. *World J. Urol.* **21**, 21–27).

formation of atherosclerotic lesions, although there is some question as to whether this is the cause or result of inflammation of the arterial wall.

At least 15 studies have shown the beneficial effects of dietary vitamin E or high circulating α-tocopherol levels on CVD risk.[63] One study found the plasma vitamin E level to account for 63% of observed differences in mortality from ischemic heart disease[64] in 16 different European populations; the plasma vitamin E concentration was also found to be inversely associated with risk of angina.[65] A pair of large, cohort studies (one of women; one of men) provides strong evidence that vitamin E protects against coronary heart disease (Table 7-10).[66] Each cohort showed vitamin E intake to be inversely related to coronary heart disease risk; but significant effects were detected only for high vitamin E intake achieved through the use of dietary supplements and for high-level intake for at least 2 years' duration. For women, apparently protective effects were also observed for total cardiovascular mortality, ischemic stroke, coronary artery surgery, and overall mortality, although these were less pronounced than the effect on major coronary heart disease incidence.

Clinical trials have produced inconsistent results. The ATBC trial found no effects of a nutritional dose (20 IU/day) of the vitamin on either ischemic heart disease mortality or total cardiovascular disease mortality, and a marginally significant *increase* in mortality from hemorrhagic stroke.[67] The CHAOS trial, which used high doses (400 or 800 IU/day), showed that patients with symptomatic coronary atherosclerosis and treated with the vitamin had a significantly lower risk of myocardial infarction (relative risk = 23%) in comparison with patients given a placebo, and that benefits were apparent after a year of

Table 7-10. High vitamin E intakes associated with reduced coronary heart disease risks in two cohorts of Americans

Parameter	Quintile group for vitamin E intake[a]					p Value for trend
	1	2	3	4	5	
Women[b]						
Median vitamin E intake (IU/day)	2.8	4.2	5.9	17	208	
Relative risk[c,e]	1.0	1.00	1.15	0.74	0.66	<0.001
Men[d]						
Total vitamin E intake (IU/day)						
Median	6.4	8.5	11.2	25.2	419	
Relative risk[c,e]	1.0	0.88	0.77	0.74	0.59	0.001
Dietary vitamin E intake (IU/day)						
Range	1.6–6.9	7.0–9.8	8.2–9.3	9.4–11.0	11.1	
Relative risk[c,e]	1.0	1.10	1.17	0.97	0.79	0.11
Supplemental vitamin E intake (IU/day)						
Range	0	<25	25–99	100–249	≥250	
Relative risk[c,e]	1.0	0.85	0.78	0.54	0.70	0.22

[a]Includes vitamin E from both foods and supplements.
[b]A total of 87,245 nurses (679,485 person-years of follow-up); data from Stampfer, M. J., Hennekens, C. H., Manson, J. E., Colditz, G. A., Rosner, B., and Willett, W. C. (1993). *N. Engl. J. Med.* **328,** 1444–1449.
[c]Adjusted for age and smoking.
[d]A total of 39,910 health professionals (139,883 person-years of follow-up); data from Rimm, E. B., Stampfer, M. J., Ascherio, A., Giovannucci, E., Colditz, G. A., and Willett, W. C. (1993). *N. Engl. J. Med.* **328,** 1450–1456.
[e]Ratio of events in each quintile to those in the lowest quintile.

---

[63] See review by Meydani, M. (2004). *Ann. N.Y. Acad. Sci.* **1031,** 271–279.

[64] That is, disease due to local hypoxia caused by obstructed blood flow to the heart.

[65] That is, *angina pectoris*, severe chest pains radiating from the heart region to the left shoulder and down the arm to the fingers.

[66] Stampfer et al. (1993). *N. Engl. J. Med.* **328,** 1444–1449; Rimm et al. (1993). *N. Engl. J. Med.* **328,** 1450–1456.

[67] The Alpha-Tocopherol, Beta-Carotene (ATBC) Trial: Alpha-Tocopherol, Beta-Carotene Cancer Prevention Study Group. (1994). *N. Engl. J. Med.* **330,** 1029–1035.

treatment.[68] The SPACE study found vitamin E treatment to reduce primary cardiovascular end points.[69] In contrast, several large primary and secondary prevention studies have found no benefits of vitamin E supplementation. For example, the HOPE study of men and women at risk of cardiovascular disease found no significant effects on CVD outcomes.[70] The VEAPS study found no effects of vitamin E treatment on common carotid intimal medial thickness.[71] It has been suggested that, in consideration of their metabolic interactions in redox recycling, it may be necessary to combine vitamins E and C, and perhaps other antioxidants, in order to reduce CVD risk.

The protective effects of vitamin E against cardiovascular disease would appear to involve its function as a protective antioxidant in LDLs. A growing body of evidence indicates that oxidative damage to LDLs greatly increases the risk of atherosclerosis.[72] Being rich in both cholesterol and PUFA (Table 7-11), LDLs are susceptible to peroxidation by the oxidative attack of reactive oxygen species. Research has shown that **oxidized LDLs** stimulate the recruitment, in the subendothelial space of the vessel wall, of monocyte-macrophages that can take up the oxidized particles via **scavenger receptors**[73] to form the lipid-containing **foam cells** found in the early stages of atherogenesis. Studies *in vitro* have shown that the peroxidation of LDL PUFAs occurs only after a lag phase caused by the loss of LDL antioxidants. Enrichment of LDLs with vitamin E, the predominant antioxidant occurring naturally in those particles, increases the lag phase, thus indicating increased resistance to oxidation. This has been achieved with oral supplements of the vitamin (Table 7-12).

The protection of LDLs by vitamin E appears to be dependent on the presence of other antioxidants, as high tocopherol concentrations have been found *in vitro* to act as prooxidants in the absence

Table 7-11. Lipid and antioxidant contents of human low-density lipoproteins

Component	Moles per mole LDL
Total phospholipids	700 ± 122
Fatty acids	
Free	26
Total	2700
Troglycerides	170 ± 78
Cholesterol	
Free	600 ± 44
Esters	1600 ± 119
Total	2200
Antioxidants	
α-Tocopherol	6.52
γ-Tocopherol	1.43
Ubiquinonol-10	0.33
β-Carotene	0.27
Lycopene	0.21
Cryptoxanthin	0.13
α-Carotene	0.11

Source: Adapted from Keaney, J. F., Jr., and Frei, B. (1994). *Natural Antioxidants in Human Health and Disease* (B. Frei, ed.), pp. 306–307. Academic Press, San Diego, CA; with unpublished data from G. F. Combs, Jr. (1995).

of water-soluble antioxidants (e.g., ascorbate, urate). Under such conditions, the tocopheroxyl radical formed on the LDL surface moves into the particle's core, where it can abstract hydrogen from a cholesteryl-PUFA ester to yield a peroxyl radical. Under such circumstances, vitamin E serves as a chain-transfer agent to propagate lipid peroxidation in the lipid core rather than as a chain-breaking antioxidant to block that process. This implies that both vitamins E and C are needed to prevent LDL oxidation.

---

[68] The Cambridge Heart Antioxidant Study (CHAOS), Stephens, N. G., et al. (1996). *Lancet* **347**, 781–786.

[69] Secondary Prevention with Antioxidants of Cardiovascular Disease in End-stage Renal Disease, Boaz, M., et al. (2000). *Lancet* **356**, 1213–1218.

[70] The Heart Outcomes Prevention Evaluation, Usuf, S., et al. (2000). *N. Engl. J. Med.* **342**, 154–160.

[71] Vitamin E Atherosclerosis Prevention Study, Hodis, H., et al. *Ciculation* **106**, 1453–1459.

[72] Atherosclerosis is the focal accumulation of acellular, lipid-containing material as plaques in the intima of the arteries. The subsequent infiltration of the intima by fatty substances (arteriosclerosis) and calcific plaques, and the consequent reduction in the lumenal cross-sectional area of the vessels, result in a reduction in blood flow to the organs served by the affected vessels, causing such symptoms as angina, cerebrovascular insufficiency, and intermittent claudication.

[73] Monocyte-macrophages have very few LDL receptors, which are downregulated. Therefore, when incubated with nonoxidized LDLs they do not form foam cells, as the accumulation of cholesterol further reduces LDL receptor activity. However, these cells have specific "scavenger" receptors for modified LDLs. It is thought that LDL lipid peroxidation products may react with amino acid side chains of apo B to form epitopes with affinities for the scavenger receptor.

Table 7-12.   Reduced low-density lipoprotein susceptibility to lipid peroxidation by oral vitamin E in humans

Treatment	Time of sampling	LDL α-tocopherol (μmol/g protein)	LDL oxidation[a]	
			Lag phase (hr)	Rate (μmol/g protein/hr)
Placebo	Baseline	14.3 ± 5.0	2.1 ± 0.9	396 ± 116
	8 weeks	15.8 ± 6.1	2.0 ± 0.8	423 ± 93
Vitamin E[b]	Baseline	13.8 ± 4.1	1.9 ± 0.6	373 ± 96
	8 weeks	32.6 ± 11.5[c]	2.9 ± 0.8[c]	367 ± 105

[a]Lipid peroxide formation.
[b]A total of 1200 IU/day as *RRR*-α-tocopherol.
[c]Significantly different ($p < 0.05$) from corresponding placebo value.
Source: Fuller, C. J., Chandalia, M., Garg, A., Grundy, S. M., and Jialal, I. (1996). *Am. J. Clin. Nutr.* **63,** 753–759.

Evidence indicates that vitamin E can also affect the adherence and aggregation of platelets, reductions of which would prevent the progression of a fatty streak and cell proliferation to advanced lesions (Fig. 7-9). Studies have shown that vitamin E supplementation at levels of about 200 IU/day reduced the adhesion of human platelets to a variety of adhesive proteins.

Cataracts

Cataracts result from the accumulation in the lens of damaged proteins that aggregate and precipitate, resulting in opacification of the lens.[74] Much of this damage involves oxidations characterized by the loss of sulfhydryls, the formation of disulfide and nondisulfide covalent linkages, and the oxidation of tryptophan residues. Several epidemiological studies have found plasma or serum tocopherol levels or vitamin E intake to be significantly inversely associated with cataract risk. Vitamin E has been shown to reduce or delay cataracts induced by galactose or aminotriazol treatment and to reduce the photoperoxidation of lens lipids. These effects may involve its direct action as an antioxidant or its indirect effect in maintaining glutathione in the reduced state.

Diabetes

Subjects with high plasma glucose tend to have higher levels of peroxidation products and lower levels of reduced glutathione, indicative of oxidative stress. That patients respond to such oxidative stress is indicated by findings that the circulating vitamin E and coenzyme Q_{10} levels of poorly controlled diabetics (Hb A1c > 8%) tend to exceed those of well-controlled patients. That oxidative stress plays a role in the pathogenesis of complications of diabetes is indicated by the finding that, in comparison with controls, diabetic erythrocytes have significantly more lipid peroxidation[75] which, by altering membrane fluidity, is thought to render erythrocytes hypercoagulable and more ready to adhere to endothelial cells. Membrane lipid peroxidation correlates with erythrocyte contents of glycosylated hemoglobin, and supplementation of non–insulin-dependent diabetics with high levels of vitamin E has been found to reduce hemoglobin damage. Studies have found diabetics to have

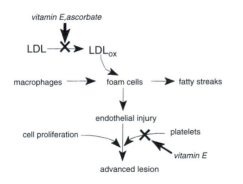

Fig. 7-9.   Model for prevention of atherogenesis by vitamin E.

---

[74] Cataracts constitute a significant public health problem in the United States, where a million cataract extractions are performed annually at a cost of some $5 billion. The prevalence of cataracts among Americans increases from about 5% at age 65 years to about 40% at age 75 years. These rates are considerably (up to fivefold) greater in less developed countries.

[75] That is, thiobarbituric acid-reactive substances.

low plasma tocopherols (Table 7-13) and high-level vitamin E supplements (e.g., 900 mg of *RRR*-α-tocopherol per day) to enhance the action of insulin by improving responsiveness to the hormone in both normal and diabetic individuals. Studies in rats have shown that the age-related decline in the major glucose transporter (Glut3) is exacerbated by vitamin E deprivation. One intervention trial failed to find vitamin E effective in delaying the development of diabetic vascular complications, but another showed significant protection by vitamin E against the development of diabetes among subjects with impaired glucose tolerance.[76] These results summarized above suggest the possibility that vitamin E may be useful in the management of this disease.

Exercise

Because exercise increases oxidative metabolism and the endogenous production of reactive oxygen species[77] and increases the turnover of vitamin E,[78] it has been proposed that exercise-induced injuries to muscle membranes may be due to the enhancement of oxidative reactions. Indeed, studies have shown that exercise increases the metabolism of vitamin E as well as other components of the cellular antioxidant defense system (e.g., ascorbic and uric acids), which appear to be increased in regularly exercised muscles. Because exercise increases mitochondrial number, it can be anticipated that trained muscles, which have more mitochondria, generate higher levels of free radicals than do nontrained ones. Accordingly, studies with rats have found lower vitamin E concentra-

tions in muscles of trained individuals than in those from sedentary ones. Studies with humans, though not extensive, have nevertheless shown that vitamin E supplementation can reduce the oxidative stress and lipid induced by exhaustive exercise. One study found that a daily supplement of 400 IU of vitamin E prevented decreases in anaerobic thresholds of high-altitude mountain climbers (Table 7-14); another[79] found that combined supplementation with vitamins E and C reduced decrements in muscular function after eccentric contraction. Collectively, these findings support the hypothesis that rigorous exercise increases the need for vitamin E.

Hemodialysis

Hemodialysis patients are exposed to oxidative stress. This is indicated by the enhanced susceptibility of their LDLs to oxidation *in vitro*. Beneficial effects of vitamin E supplementation have been reported for parameters of oxidation in hemodialysis patients.

Immunity and infection

Vitamin E is essential for normal immune function, which is also stimulated by supranutritional levels of intake. Its role appears to be that of a biological antioxidant protecting immune cells from reactive oxygen species produced during the inflammatory process. Those species are produced mostly by phagocytic cells attracted to the site of tissue injury. On encountering or ingesting a bacterium or other foreign particle, activated[80] neutrophils and macrophages produce large

Table 7-13. Effects of diabetes on tocopherol status

Patient group	Plasma vitamin E, mg/L	LDL vitamin E, mg/g
Nondiabetic	17.4 ± 3.7	6.4 ± 1.3
Diabetic	12.9[a] ± 2.9	5.5 ± 3.8

[a] $p < 0.05$

Source: Quilliot, D., et al. *Am. J. Clin. Nutr.* **81**, 1117–1125.

Table 7-14. Antioxidant protection by vitamin E in high-altitude climbers

Treatment group	Percentage change in pentane exhalation[a]		
	Median	Lower quartile	Upper quartile
Placebo	+104.0	+25.5	+121.5
Vitamin E[b]	−3.0	−7.4	+2.9

[a] Change observed after 4 weeks at high altitude.
[b] A total of 400 IU/day.

Source: Simon-Schnass, I., and Pabst, H. (1988). *J. Vitam. Nutr. Res.* **58**, 49–54.

---

[76] Mayer-Davis, E. J., et al. (2002). *Diabetes Care* **25**, 2172–2177.

[77] Oxygen utilization increases 10- to 15-fold during exercise.

[78] Mastaloudis, A., et al. (2001). *Free Radical Biol. Med.* **31**, 911–922.

[79] Shafat, A., et al. (2004). *Eur. J. Appl. Physiol.* **93**, 196–202.

[80] Various cytokines, such as tumor necrosis factor or interferon γ, can activate phagocytic cells to increase their $O_2^{\bullet}$ generation.

amounts of $O_2^{\bullet}$ and H_2O_2 in a process referred to as the respiratory burst. The sources of production of reactive oxygen species by those cells include myeloperoxidase, which catalyzes the H_2O_2-dependent oxidation of halide ions, yielding such powerful oxidizing agents as hypochlorous acid; and xanthine oxidase, which catalyzes the reaction of xanthine or hypoxanthine with molecular oxygen to generate uric acid. These reactions are important in killing pathogens, but they can also be deleterious to immune cells themselves. If not controlled, they can contribute to the pathogenesis of disease. Therefore, it appears that adequate antioxidant status is required to maintain appropriate *peroxide tone.*

Vitamin E deficiency has been shown in experimental animals and children to compromise both humoral and cell-mediated immunity. Deficient individuals have polymorphonucleocytes with impaired phagocytic abilities, suppressed oxidative burst and bactericidal activities, and decreased chemotactic responses. They also can show generally suppressed lymphocyte production, impaired T-cell functions. and decreased antibody production. Vitamin E deprivation has been found to increase susceptibility to viral infections and to enhance the virulence of certain viruses passed through vitamin E-deficient hosts. These effects are thought to involve loss of peroxide tone and appear to involve impaired cellular membrane fluidity and enhanced prostaglandin E_2 production.

Supranutritional intakes of vitamin E have been found to stimulate many immune functions, including antibody production. Experimental animal studies have shown these effects to result in increased resistance to infection. A controlled clinical study found a high level of vitamin E (800 IU/day) to increase T cell-mediated responses (delayed-type hypersensitivity, mitogenesis, and interleukin 2 production) and to decrease phytohemagglutinin-stimulated prostaglandin production. These responses typically decline with aging, and other studies found older subjects to show improvements in delayed-type hypersensitivity in response to vitamin E more frequently than younger subjects (Table 7-15), and vitamin E to reduce the age-related decline in T-cell signaling.[81] Animal studies have found optimization of certain immune parameters to call for intakes of at least an order of magnitude greater than the levels of the vitamin required to prevent clinical signs of deficiency. One trial found such levels of vitamin E supplementation to reduce the incidence of common colds in elderly subjects;[82] another, of acute respiratory infections, showed no protective effects.[83]

Inflammatory disease

Levels of oxidative DNA damage are elevated in several inflammatory dieases including chronic hepatitis, cystic fibrosis, atopic dermatitis, and rheumatoid arthritis. Indirect evidence suggests that in rheumatoid arthritis ROS produced during inflammation[84] causes oxidation of lipids in the synovial

Table 7-15. Enhancement of immune responses by vitamin E supplementation of healthy older adults

Treatment	Days of treatment	Vitamin E in PMNs[a] (nmol)	DTH[b] index (mm)	PMN proliferation[c] (× 10^3 cpm)	IL-2 production[d] (kU/liter)
Placebo	0	0.14 ± 0.04	16.5 ± 2.2	24.48 ± 2.73	31.8 ± 8.3
	30	0.19 ± 0.03	16.9 ± 2.1	21.95 ± 2.90	37.5 ± 12.5
Vitamin E[e]	0	0.12 ± 0.02	14.2 ± 2.9	20.55 ± 1.93	35.6 ± 9.1
	30	0.39 ± 0.05[f]	18.9 ± 3.5[f]	23.77 ± 2.99[f]	49.6 ± 12.6[f]

[a]Polymorphonucleocyte α-tocopherol content.
[b]Delayed-type hypersensitivity skin test.
[c]Concanavalin A-induced proliferation of polymorphonucleocytes.
[d]Concanavalin A-induced production of interleukin 2 by polymorphonucleocytes.
[e]A total of 800 IU of all-*rac*-α-tocopheryl acetate per day.
[f]$p < 0.05$.
Source: Maydani, S. N., Barkland, M. P., Liu, S., Meydani, M., Miller, R. A., Cannon, J. G., Morrow, F. D., Rocklin, R., and Blumberg, J. B. (1990). *Am. J. Clin. Nutr.* **52**, 557–563.

---

[81] That is, improve the percentage of CD4+ T cells capable of forming a functional immune synapse.
[82] Meydani, S. N., Han, S. N., and Hamer, D. H. (2004). *Ann. N.Y. Acad. Sci.* **1031**, 214–222.
[83] Great, J. M., Schouten, E. G., and Kok, E. J. (2002). *J. Am. Med. Assoc.* **288**, 715–721.
[84] This process is discussed in the section Vitamin E and Immunity and Infection.

fluid, increasing the viscosity of that fluid. Vitamin E supplementation can reduce joint swelling in animal models of the disease, and each of the seven double-blind, placebo-controlled, clinical intervention trials designed to evaluate vitamin E in the management of arthritis patients has shown high-level supplementation with the vitamin (100–600 IU/day) to relieve pain and to be anti-inflammatory.

Ischemia–reperfusion injury

Vitamin E and other free-radical scavengers have been found to affect the functions of mitochondria and sarcoplasmic reticula in animal models of myocardial injury induced by **ischemia–reperfusion**. That injury, which occurs in tissues reperfused after a brief period of ischemia, appears to be due to the oxidative stress of reoxygenation, involving the production of reactive oxygen species. The phenomenon has been demonstrated for several tissues (heart, brain, skin, intestine, and pancreas) and has relevance for the preservation of organs for transplantation. Reactive oxygen species are thought to contribute to milder forms of tissue injury at the time of reperfusion (e.g., myocardial stunning, reperfusion arrhythmias); however, it is not clear to what extent free radicals are responsible for the acute tissue damage seen under those circumstances. Intervention trials with antioxidants have yielded conflicting results, but it is possible that preoperative treatment with vitamin E may be useful in reducing at least some of this type of injury.

A disorder that appears to involve natural ischemia–reperfusion injury is **intraventricular hemorrhage**[85] of the premature infant. The results of a randomized clinical trial clearly demonstrate that vitamin E supplements (given by intramuscular injection) can be very effective in protecting premature infants against intraventricular hemorrhage. In disorders of this type, it is thought that vitamin E may act as a radical scavenger to protect against the oxidative stress associated with ischemia–reperfusion.

Lung disease

The lungs are continuously exposed to relatively high concentrations of O_2 as well as a variety of environmental oxidants and irritants. The first line of defense of the respiratory epithelium, respiratory tract lining fluid, contains antioxidants, including vitamin E as well as relatively high concentrations of vitamin C, urate, reduced glutathione, extracellular superoxide dismutase, catalase, and glutathione peroxidase. Vitamin E deficiency has been found to increase the susceptibility of experimental animals to the pathological effects of ozone and nitrogen dioxide,[86] air pollutants that are known to react with PUFAs to form free radicals. Thus, it has been suggested that supplements of the vitamin may protect humans against harmful effects of chronic exposure to ozone in smog. Good vitamin E status has been associated with positive effects on lung function and symptoms in cross-sectional studies as well as in studies of asthmatics. However, a randomized controlled trial found vitamin E supplementation not to affect the incidence or duration of lower respiratory tract infections in elderly patients.

Neurodegenerative disorders

Several facts make it reasonable to expect neuronal tissue to be susceptible to oxidative stress: neurons contain large amounts of both PUFAs and iron, but do not have extensive antioxidant defense systems, making them vulnerable to free-radical-mediated damage; neurons are terminally differentiated and do not replicate when damaged; Parkinson-like neuronal damage can be caused by a redox cycling drug[87] that generates reactive oxygen species; the metabolism of dopamine by monoamine oxidase B in dopaminergic neurons generates H_2O_2; exposure to hyperbaric oxygen can cause seizures in animals and humans; and vitamin E deficiency is characterized by neurological signs.[88]

---

[85] Hemorrhage in and around the lateral ventricles of the brain occurs in about 40% of infants born before 33 weeks of gestation.

[86] Ozone (O_3) is produced in photochemical smog from nitrogen dioxide (NO_2), oxygen, and uncombusted gasoline vapors; NO_2 is produced in internal combustion engines. Both can generate unstable free radicals that damage lungs through oxidative attack on polyunsaturated membrane phospholipids.

[87] 1-Methyl-4-phenyl-1,2,3,6-tetrahydropyridine.

[88] Chronic, severe vitamin E deficiency results in encephalopathy in most species. A neurodegenerative disorder resembling amyotrophic lateral sclerosis has been described in vitamin E-fed horses: equine motor neuron disease. Affected animals show little, if any, vitamin E in their plasma. Although the metabolic basis of the disease is not clear, it may involve an abnormal tocopherol-binding protein that renders affected animals unable to retain the vitamin.

Parkinson's disease is thought to involve mitochondrial oxidative stress and damage to cells in the substantia nigra. A large, randomized, controlled trial with patients with early Parkinson's disease found no beneficial effects of 2000 IU of α-tocopherol per day, but another using 3200 IU α-tocopherol plus 3000 mg vitamin C per day showed a 2.5-year delay in the need for the use of levodopa due to the supplement.

Age-related increase in vulnerability to reactive oxygen species is thought to contribute to Alzheimer's disease, characterized by regional neuronal degeneration, synaptic loss, and the presence of neurofibrillary tangles and senile plaques. The etiology of the disease appears to involve the neuronal secretion of the Aß peptide, which activates inflammatory pathways by inceasing the release of pro-inflammatory cytokines. Vitamin E has been shown to inhibit this inflammatory response by influencing the phosphorylation of PKC, a key player in the signaling of cytokines. Whether this is due to antioxidant or non-antioxidant effects of the vitamin is not clear; but there is ample evidence for an association of Alzheimer's disease risk reduction with dietary intake of either vitamin E or vitamin C, which suggests an antioxidant effect at least. The Chicago Health and Aging Study (CHAP) found that a high intake of α- and γ-tocopherols from foods has been associated with reduced risk to Alzheimer's disease (Table 7-16). That this relationship did not obtain for vitamin E from dietary supplements may indicate the functions of non–α-vitamers present in foods, particularly γ-tocopherol, which has been shown to be an efficient scavenger of reactive nitrogen species.

Modest protection has been reported for vitamins E and C in producing mild positive effects on symptoms of amyotrophic lateral sclerosis. However, a meta-analysis of 19 randomized, controlled trials found insufficient evidence of effects in treating this disease.

Preeclampsia

The condition of preeclampsia—pregnancy-induced hypertension and proteinuria—is a major cause of maternal and fetal morbidity and mortality. Increasing evidence suggests that the condition involves the oxidative stress associated with the threefold increase in intraplacental oxygen levels resulting from the establishment of the maternal intervillous circulation after embryogenesis. It is

Table 7-16. Adjusted differences in the rate of change in cognitive performance (β) per designated increase in food tocopherols

Vitamer	Median intake	Increase in[a] intake, mg/dβ	
Total vitamin E	24.9	5	0.0049 ± 0.0016^b
α-Tocopherol	7.1	5	0.0082 ± 0.0030^b
γ-Tocopherol	12.0	5	0.0065 ± 0.0030^b
d-Tocopherol	3.5	1	0.0029 ± 0.0018
ß-Tocopherol	0.8	1	0.0071 ± 0.0091

Source: Morris, C. M., et al. (2005). Am. J. Clin. Nutr. **81**, 508–514.
[a] Change in cognitive score per unit increase in tocopherol.
[b] $p < .05$

thought that this shift from the low-oxygen environment of the first trimester can produce oxidative damage to trophoblasts, the impairment of which can lead to the premature unplugging of vessels resulting in overwhelming oxidative stress and pregnancy failure. One intervention study has showed that mid-pregnancy supplementation with vitamins E and C can reduce the risk of preeclampsia.

Radiation protection

Radiation damages cells by direct ionization of DNA and other cellular targets and by indirect effects of reactive oxygen species that are also produced. Vitamin E has been shown to decrease radiation-induced chromosome damage in animal models. This effect may be the basis of the links detected epidemiologically of antioxidant-rich foods and reduced cancer risk.

Skin disorders

The skin is subject to the oxidizing effects resulting from exposure to ultraviolet light, which is known to generate reactive oxygen species from the photolysis of intracellular water. Studies with animal models have shown that the tocopherol content of dermal tissues decreases with UV irradiation, presumably owing to that oxidative stress. Topical treatment with vitamin E has been found to confer protection against UV-induced skin damage, as measured by reduction in erythemal responses and delays in the onset of tumorigenesis. One study reported that regular topical application of vitamin E reduced wrinkle amplitude and skin roughness in about half of cases.

Smoking

Smoking constitutes an oxidative burden on the lungs and other tissues owing to the sustained exposure to free radicals from tar and gas phases of the cigarette smoke.[89] This effect is characterized by decreased circulating levels of ascorbic acid and vitamin E and increased levels of peroxidation products (e.g., malonyldialdehyde in plasma, ethane and pentane in breath) and nitated metabolites (e.g., 5-nitro-γ-tocopherol in plasma, Table 7-7), resulting in enhanced turnover of tocopherols and increased dietary needs.[90] One intervention trial found that modest supranutritional doses of vitamin E (up to 560 mg of α-tocopherol per day) reduced the peroxidation potential of erythrocyte lipids (Table 7-17). The ATBC trial[91] found intervention with α-tocopherol to reduce pneumonia risk for smokers who started at later ages, but not to benefit other smokers.

Table 7-17 Comparison of effect of vitamin E on erythrocyte lipid peroxidation in smokers and nonsmokers

Group	Weeks of vitamin E administration[b]	Vitamin E in erythrocytes (μmol/g Hb)	*In vitro* lipid peroxidation (nmol MDA[a]/g Hb)
Nonsmokers	0	20.0 ± 4.5	141 ± 54
	20	36.1 ± 8.2	86 ± 51
Smokers	0	18.0 ± 4.2	291 ± 102
	20	32.8 ± 8.2	108 ± 53

[a]MDA, Malonyldialdehyde.
[b]A total of 70 IU/day.
Source: Brown *et al.* (1977). *Am. J. Clin. Nutr.* **65**, 496–502.

Other disorders

Vitamin E has frequently proven effective as a therapeutic measure in several disorders of humans, even though it may not be directly involved in their etiologies. These include *hemolytic anemia of prematurity, intermittent claudication,*[92] and *chronic hemolysis* in patients with glucose-6-phosphate dehydrogenase deficiency. In veterinary practice, vitamin E (most frequently administered with selenium) has had reported efficacy in the treatment of several disorders, including *tying up* in horses and postpartum placental retention in cows. Formerly, vitamin E was thought to protect against retinopathy of prematurity.[93] However, a controlled clinical trial has shown that its use failed to reduce the prevalence of the syndrome. A study of adults with major depression found plasma α-tocopherol level to be inversely related to depression score.[94]

VII. Vitamin E Deficiency

Vitamin E deficiency can result from insufficient dietary intake or impaired absorption of the vitamin. Several other dietary factors affect the need for vitamin E. Two are most important in this regard: selenium and PUFAs. Selenium spares the need for vitamin E. Accordingly, animals fed low-selenium diets generally require more vitamin E than animals fed the same diets supplemented with an available source of selenium. In contrast, the dietary intake of PUFAs directly affects the need for vitamin E; animals fed high-PUFA diets require more vitamin E than those fed low-PUFA diets.[95] Other factors that can be expected to increase vitamin E needs are deficiencies of sulfur-containing amino acids;[96] deficiencies of copper, zinc,

---

[89] Cigarette smoke contains a number of compounds that produce free radicals. It also increases the number of free-radical-producing inflammatory cells in the lungs.

[90] Bruno, R. S., and Traber, M. G. (2005). *J. Nutr.* **135**, 671–674.

[91] Alpha-Tocopherol, Beta-Carotene Trial, Hemilä, H., et al. (2004). *Chest* **125**, 557–565.

[92] Nocturnal leg cramps.

[93] This disorder was formerly called *retrolental fibroplasia*. Its pathogenesis involves exposure to a hyperoxic environment during neonatal oxygen therapy. Retrolental fibroplasia can affect as many as 11% of infants with birth weights below 1500 g, resulting in blindness of about one-quarter of them.

[94] Estimated vitamin E intake generally met recommended levels and did not correlate with depression score. Owen, A. J., et al. (2005). *Eur. J. Clin. Nutr.* **59**, 304–306.

[95] Various researchers have suggested values for the incremental effects of dietary PUFA level on the nutritional requirement for vitamin E in the range of 0.18–0.60 mg of α-tocopherol per gram of PUFA. Although the upper end of that range is frequently cited as a guideline for estimating vitamin E needs, it is fair to state that there is no consensus among experts in the field as to the quantitation of this obviously important relationship.

[96] **Cysteine**, which can be synthesized via transsulfuration from methionine, is needed for the synthesis of glutathione (i.e., the substrate for the selenium-dependent glutathione peroxidase).

and/or manganese;[97] and deficiency of riboflavin.[98] Alternatively, vitamin E can be replaced by several lipid-soluble synthetic antioxidants[99] (e.g., BHT,[100] BHA,[101] DPPD[102]) and, possibly, by vitamin C.[103]

Conditions involving the malabsorption of lipids can also lead to vitamin E deficiency (Table 7-18). Such conditions include those resulting in loss of pancreatic exocrine function (e.g., pancreatitis, pancreatic tumor, nutritional pancreatic atrophy in severe selenium deficiency), those involving a lumenal deficiency of bile (e.g., biliary stasis due to mycotoxicosis, biliary atresia), and those due to defects in lipoprotein metabolism (e.g., **abetalipoproteinemia**[104]). Premature infants, who are typically impaired in their ability to utilize dietary fats, are also at risk of vitamin E deficiency.

Mutations in the α-TTP gene can produce tissue-level vitamin E deficiency due to impaired uptake and transport of α-tocopherol (see α-Tocopherol Transfer Protein earlier in this chapter). A number of such mutations have been observed, with the affected individuals showing exceedingly low circulating tocopherol levels unless maintained on gram-level vitamin E supplementation. Otherwise, patients show progressive peripheral neuropathy characterized by pathology of the large axons of sensory neurons and ataxia.

The clinical manifestations of vitamin E deficiency vary considerably between species. In general, however, the targets are the *neuromuscular*,[105] *vascular*, and *reproductive systems* (Figs. 7-10 and 7-11). The various signs of vitamin E deficiency are believed to be manifestations of membrane dysfunction resulting from the oxidative degradation of polyunsaturated membrane phospholipids and/or the disruption of other critical cellular processes.[106] Many deficiency syndromes (e.g., **encephalomalacia** in the chick, intraventricular hemorrhage in the premature human infant, and at least some myopathies) appear to involve local cellular anoxia resulting from primary lesions of the vascular system. Others appear to involve the lack of protection from oxidative stress. It has also been proposed that some effects (e.g., impaired immune cell functions) may involve loss of control of the oxidative metabolism of arachidonic acid in its conversion to leukotrienes; vitamin E is known to inhibit the 5′-lipoxygenase in that pathway.

VIII. Pharmacologic Uses of Vitamin E

The efficacy of vitamin E as a biological antioxidant appears to be dependent on the amount of the vitamin present at critical cellular loci and the ability of the organism to maintain its supply and/or recycle it. Therefore, in the presence of other components of the cellular antioxidant defense system (a deficiency of which might allow tocopheroxyl to assume peroxidation chain-transfer activity), antioxidant protection would be expected to increase with increasing intake of vitamin E. High levels of vitamin E may therefore be appropriate in cases of oxidative stress. High levels of vitamin E are appropriate for supporting adequacy with respect to the vitamin in cases of its impaired utilization. For example, daily doses of 100–150 IU/kg body weight prevent neurological abnormalities in cases of abetalipoproteinemia or chronic

---

[97] These are essential cofactors of the superoxide dismutases.

[98] Riboflavin is required for the synthesis of FAD, the coenzyme for glutathione reductase, which is required for regeneration of reduced glutathione via the so-called *glutathione cycle*.

[99] The fact that vitamin E can be replaced by a variety of antioxidants was a point of debate concerning the status of the nutrient as a vitamin. Although such replacement can occur, the effective levels of other antioxidants are considerably greater (e.g., two orders of magnitude) than those of α-tocopherol. Therefore, it is now generally agreed that, although the metabolic role of vitamin E is that of an antioxidant that can be fulfilled by other reductants, tocopherol performs this function with high biological specificity and is, therefore, appropriately considered a vitamin.

[100] Butylated hydroxytoluene.

[101] Butylated hydroxyanisole.

[102] *N,N*′-Diphenyl-*p*-phenylenediamine.

[103] The sparing effect of vitamin C may involve its function in the reductive recycling of tocopherol.

[104] Humans with this rare hereditary disorder are unable to produce apoprotein B, an essential component of chylomicra, VLDLs, and LDLs. The absence of these particles from the serum prevents the absorption of vitamin E owing to the inability to transport it into the lymphatics. These patients show generalized lipid malabsorption with **steatorrhea** (i.e., excess fat in feces) and have undetectable serum vitamin E levels.

[105] The skeletal myopathies of vitamin E-deficient animals entail lesions predominantly involving type I fibers.

[106] It is interesting to note a situation in which vitamin E deficiency would appear advantageous: The efficacy of the antimalarial drug derived from Chinese traditional medicine, *qinghaosu* (artemisinin), is enhanced by deprivation of vitamin E. The drug, an endoperoxide, is thought to act against the plasmodial parasite by generating free radicals *in vivo*. Thus, depriving the patient of vitamin E appears to limit the parasite's access to the protective antioxidant.

Table 7-18. Signs of vitamin E deficiency

Organ system	Sign	Responds to: Vitamin E	Responds to: Selenium	Responds to: Antioxidants
General	Loss of appetite	+	+	+
	Reduced growth	+	+	+
Dermatologic	None			
Muscular	Myopathies			
	Striated muscle[a]	+	+	
	Cardiac muscle[b]	+		
	Smooth muscle[c]	+	+	
Skeletal	None			
Vital organs	Liver necrosis[d]	+	+	
	Renal degeneration[d]	+		+
Nervous system	Encephalomalacia[e]	+		+
	Areflexia, ataxia[f]	+		
Reproduction	Fetal death[g]	+	+	+
	Testicular degeneration[h]	+	+	
Ocular	Cataract[i]	+		
	Retinopathy[j]	+?		
Vascular	Anemia[j,k]	+		
	RBC hemolysis[l]	+		
	Exudative diathesis[e]	+	+	
	Intraventricular hemorrhage[j]	+		

[a]Nutritional muscular dystrophies (white muscle diseases) of chicks, rats, guinea pigs, rabbits, dogs, monkeys, minks, sheep, goats, and calves.
[b]**Mulberry heart disease** (a kind of congestive heart failure) of pigs.
[c]Gizzard **myopathy** of turkeys and ducks.
[d]In rats, mice, and pigs.
[e]In chicks.
[f]In humans with abetalipoproteinemia.
[g]In rats, cattle, and sheep, characterized by resorption of the dead fetus (**resorption-gestation syndrome**).
[h]In chickens, rats, rabbits, hamsters, dogs, pigs, and monkeys.
[i]Reported only in rats.
[j]Low vitamin E status is suspected in this condition in premature human infants.
[k]In monkeys, pigs, and humans.
[l]In chicks, rats, rabbits, and humans.

cholestasis, and intakes of 400–1200 IU/day are needed by individuals with familial isolated vitamin E deficiency. Supplements of 400 IU/day have been shown to support normal plasma tocopherol concentrations in patients with cystic fibrosis.

The use of high-level vitamin E supplementation of animals has potential practical value relative to food production. Supranutritional vitamin E supplements (e.g., α-tocopheryl acetate fed at levels 10- to 50-fold standard practice) to the diets of poultry, swine, and beef have been found effective in increasing the α-tocopherol contents of many tissues, and the residues in muscle serve to inhibit postmortem oxidative pro-

duction of off-flavors (oxidative rancidity of lipids) and color (hemoglobin oxidation). This increases the effective shelf-life of the retail meats.

IX. Vitamin E Toxicity

Vitamin E is one of the *least toxic* of the vitamins. Both animals and humans appear to be able to tolerate rather high levels. For animals, doses at least two orders of magnitude above nutritional requirements (e.g., to 1000–2000 IU/kg) are without untoward effects. Massive doses (e.g., 30–300 times required levels) of vitamin E have also been reported to

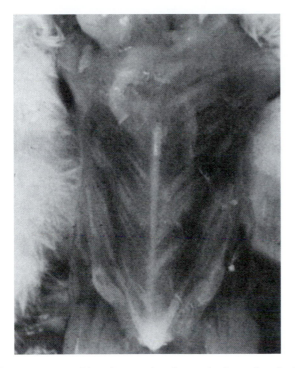

Fig. 7-10. Nutritional muscular dystrophy in a vitamin E-deficient chick; Zenker's degeneration of *M. pectorales* gives a striated appearance.

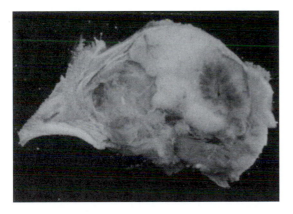

Fig. 7-11. Encephalomalacia in a vitamin E-deficient chick.

enhance atherogenesis in cholesterol-fed rabbits and DNA adduct formation in the rat. For humans, daily doses as high as 400 IU can be considered harmless, and large oral doses as great as 3200 IU have not been found to have consistent ill effects.

At very high doses, however, vitamin E can antagonize the functions of other fat-soluble vitamins. Thus, hypervitaminotic E animals have been found to show impaired bone mineralization, reduced hepatic storage of vitamin A, and coagulopathies. In each case, these signs could be corrected with increased dietary supplements of the appropriate vitamin (i.e., vitamins D, A, and K, respectively), and the antagonism seemed to be based at the level of absorption. Isolated reports of negative effects in human subjects consuming up to 1000 IU of vitamin E per day included headache, fatigue, nausea, double vision, muscular weakness, mild creatinuria, and gastrointestinal distress.

Potentially deleterious metabolic effects of high-level vitamin E status include inhibitions of retinyl ester hydrolase and vitamin K-dependent carboxylations. The former effect has been demonstrated in animals, where it results in impaired ability to mobilize vitamin A from hepatic stores. Evidence for the latter effect includes the findings that patients of normal coagulation status given high doses of vitamin E (at least 1000 IU/day) showed decreased γ-carboxylation and functionality of prothrombin.[107] This effect has implications for patients on anticoagulant therapy. Although the metabolic basis of the effect is not clear, it is thought to involve tocopherylquinone, which, bearing structural similarities to vitamin K, may act as an inhibitor of vitamin K metabolism.

A meta-analysis of 19 randomized trials suggested that vitamin E supplementation may increase all-cause mortality slightly in a dose-dependent way at surprisingly low doses (>150 IU/day).[108] This analysis has been widely criticized on a variety of methodological grounds, including the exclusion of trials with fewer than 10 deaths, heterogeneity of trial designs, confounding due to inclusion of mixed treatments including some with β-carotene, and overweighting of the vitamin E group for diseases and mortality risk factors.[109] From the dicussion precipitated by this report, as well as the supporting evidence presented, it appears that vitamin E is safe over a wide range of intakes; for humans that would extend to approximately 1600 IU/day for most healthy adults.

[107] Booth, S. L., et al. (2004). *Am. J. Clin. Nutr.* **80**, 143–148.

[108] Miller, E. R., et al. (2004). *Ann. Intern. Med.* **142**, 1–11.

[109] Hathcock, J. N., et al. (2005). *Am. J. Clin. Nutr.* **81**, 736–745; Blatt, D. H., and Pryor, W. A. (2005). *Ann. Int. Med.* **143**, 150–151; Krishman, K., et al. (2005). *Ann. Int. Med.* **143**, 151; Lim, W. S. et al. (2005). *Ann. Int. Med.* **143**, 152; Meydani, S. N., et al. (2005). *Ann. Int. Med.* **143**, 153; DeZee, K., et al. (2005). *Ann. Int. Med.* **143**, 153–154; Jialal, I., and Devaraj, S. (2005). *Ann. Int. Med.* **143**, 155; Carter, T. (2005). *Ann. Int. Med.* **143**, 155; Baggott, J. E. (2005). *Ann. Int. Med.* **143**, 155–156.

X. Case Studies

Instructions

Review the following case reports, paying special attention to the diagnostic indicators on which the treatments were based. Then answer the questions that follow.

Case 1

At birth, a male infant with *acidosis*[110] and **hemolytic anemia**[111] was diagnosed as having *glutathione (GSH) synthetase*[112] deficiency associated with *5-keto-prolinuria*;[113] he was treated symptomatically. During his second year, he experienced six episodes of bacterial *otitis media*.[114] His white cell counts fell to 3000–4000 cells/μl during two of these infections, with notable losses of polymorphonuclear leukocytes[115] (PMNs). Between infections, the child had normal white and differential cell counts, and PMNs were obtained for study.

Functional studies of PMNs showed the following results:

Laboratory results

Parameter	Finding
GSH synthetase activity	10% of normal
Phagocytosis of *Staphylococcus aureus*	Less than normal
Iodination of phagocytized zymosan particles	Much less than normal
H_2O_2 production during phagocytosis	Well above normal

The child was then treated daily with 30 IU of all-*rac*-α-tocopheryl acetate per kilogram body weight (about 400 IU/day). His plasma vitamin E concentration rose from 0.34 mg/dl (normal for infants) to 1.03 mg/dl. After 3 months of treatment, the same studies of his PMNs were performed. Although there were no changes in the activity of GSH peroxidase[116] or the concentration of GSH (which remained near 25% of normal during this study) in his plasma, the production of H_2O_2 by his PMNs had declined to normal levels, the iodination of proteins during phagocytosis had increased, and the bactericidal activity toward *S. aureus* had increased to the control level. Before his vitamin E therapy, electron microscopy of his neutrophils had revealed defective cytoskeletal structure, with more than the usual number of *microtubules*[117] seen at rest and a disappearance of microtubules seen during phagocytosis. This ultrastructural defect was corrected after vitamin E treatment.

Case 2

A 23-year-old woman with a 10-year history of neurologic disease was admitted complaining of severe ataxia,[118] titubation of the head,[119] and loss of proprioceptive sense in her extremities.[120] Her past history revealed that she had experienced difficulty in walking and was unsteady at age 10 years; there was no family history of ataxia, malabsorption, or neurologic disease. At 18 years of age, she had been hospitalized for her neurologic complaints; at that time, she had been below the 5th percentile for both height

---

[110] The condition of reduced alkali reserve.

[111] Reduced number of erythrocytes per unit blood volume, resulting from their destruction.

[112] This is the rate-limiting enzyme in the pathway of the biosynthesis of **glutathione (GSH)**, a tripeptide of glycine, cysteine, and glutamic acid, and the most abundant cellular thiol compound. **Oxidized glutathione (GSSG)** is a dimer joined by a disulfide bridge between the cysteinyl residues.

[113] This is the condition of abnormally high urinary concentrations of 5-ketoproline, the intermediate in the pathway of GSH biosynthesis (the γ-glutamyl cycle).

[114] Inflammation of the middle ear.

[115] The PMN is a type of white blood cell important in disease resistance, which functions by phagocytizing bacteria and other foreign particles.

[116] An enzyme that catalyzes the reduction of hydroperoxides (including H_2O_2) with the concomitant oxidation of glutathione (two GSH converted to GSSG).

[117] A subcellular organelle.

[118] Loss of muscular coordination.

[119] Unsteadiness.

[120] Senses of position, etc., originating from the arms and legs.

and weight. Her examination had revealed normal higher intellectual function, speech, and cranial nerve function; but her limbs had been found to be hypotonic[121] with preservation of strength and moderately severe ataxia. Her deep tendon reflexes were absent, plantar responses were abnormal, vibrational sense was absent below the wrists and iliac crests, and joint position sense was defective at the fingers and toes. Laboratory findings at that time had been negative; that is, she showed no indications of hepatic or renal dysfunction. No etiologic diagnosis was made. Two years later, when she was 20 years old, the patient was reevaluated. By that time, her gait had deteriorated, and her proprioceptive loss had become more severe.

Over the next 3 years, her symptoms worsened, and, by age 23 years, she had trouble walking unassisted. Still, she showed no sensory, visual, bladder, respiratory, or cardiac signs and ate a normal and nutritious diet. Her only gastrointestinal complaint was of constipation, with bowel movements only once per week. Nerve conduction tests revealed that the action potentials of both her sensory and motor nerves, recorded from the median and ulnar nerves, were normal. Electromyography of the biceps, vastus medialis, and tibialis anterior muscles was normal. However, her cervical and cortical somatosensory-evoked responses to median nerve stimulation were abnormal: there was no peripheral delay, and the nature of the response was abnormal. Furthermore, no consistent cortical responses could be recorded after stimulation of the tibial nerve at the ankle. These findings were interpreted as indicating spinocerebellar disease characterized by delayed sensory conduction in the posterior columns.

Routine screening tests failed to detect α-tocopherol in her plasma, although she showed elevated circulating levels of cholesterol (448 mg/dl versus normal: 150–240 mg/dl) and triglycerides (184 mg/dl versus normal: 50–150 mg/dl). Her plasma concentrations of 25-hydroxyvitamin D_3 [25-(OH)-D_3], retinol, and vitamin K-dependent clotting factors were in normal ranges. Tests of lipid malabsorption showed no abnormality. Her glucose tolerance and pancreatic function (assessed after injections of cholecystokinin and secretin) were also normal.

The patient was given 2 g of α-tocopheryl acetate with an ordinary meal; her plasma α-tocopherol level, which had been nondetectable before the dose, was in the subnormal range 2 hr later and she showed a relatively flat absorption[122] curve. She was given the same large dose of the vitamin daily for 2 weeks, at which time her plasma α-tocopherol concentration was 24 µg/ml. When her daily dose was reduced to 800 mg of α-tocopheryl acetate per day for 10 weeks, her plasma level was 1.2 mg/dl—in the normal range. During this time, she showed marked clinical improvement.

Case Questions

1. What inborn metabolic error(s) was (were) apparent in the first patient?
2. What sign/symptom indicated a vitamin E-related disorder in each case?
3. Why are PMNs useful for studying protection from oxidative stress, as in the first case?
4. What inborn metabolic error might you suspect led to vitamin E deficiency in the second patient?

Study Questions and Exercises

1. Construct a concept map illustrating the nutritional interrelationships of vitamin E and other nutrients.
2. Construct a decision tree for the diagnosis of vitamin E deficiency in a human or animal.
3. What features of the chemical structure of vitamin E relate to its nutritional activity?
4. How might vitamin E utilization be affected by a diet high in polyunsaturated fat? of a fat-free diet? of a selenium-deficient diet?
5. What kinds of prooxidants might you expect people or animals to encounter daily?
6. How can nutritional deficiencies of vitamin E and selenium be distinguished?

---

[121] Having abnormally low tension.

[122] That is, plasma α-tocopherol concentration versus time.

Recommended Reading

Allen, R. G. (1991). Oxygen-reactive species and antioxidant responses during development: The metabolic paradox of cellular differentiation. *Proc. Soc. Exp. Biol. Med.* **196,** 117–129.

Azzi, A. (2004). The role of α-tocopherol in preventing disease. *Eur. J. Nutr.* **43,** 1/18–1/25.

Azzi, A., Gysin, R., Kempná, P., Munteanu, A., Villacorta, L., Lisarius, T., and Zingg, J. M. (2004). Regulation of gene expression by alpha-tocopherol. *J. Biol. Chem.* **385,** 585–591.

Azzi, A., Gysin, R., Kempná, P., Ricciarelli, R., Villacorta, L., Visarius, T., and Zingg, J. M. (2003). The role of α-tocopherol in preventing disease: From epidemiology to molecular events. *Mol. Aspects Med.* **24,** 325–336.

Bendrich, A., and Machlin, L. J. (1988). Safety of oral intake of vitamin E. *Am. J. Clin. Nutr.* **48,** 612–619.

Bjrrneboe, A., Bjrrneboe, G. E., and Drevon, C. A. (1990). Absorption, transport and distribution of vitamin E. *J. Nutr.* **120,** 233–242.

Burton, G. W. (1994). Vitamin E: Molecular and biological function. *Proc. Nutr. Soc.* **53,** 251–262.

Brigelius-Flohé, R., Kelly, F. J., Salanen, J. T., Neuzil, J., Zingg, J. M., and Azzi, A. (2002). The European perspective on Vitamin E: Current knowledge and future research. *Am. J. Clin. Nutr.* **76,** 703–716.

Chow, C. K. (2001). Vitamin E. Chapter 4 in *Handbook of Vitamins* (R. B. Rucker, J. W. Suttie, D. B. McCormick, and L. J. Machlin, eds.), 3rd ed., pp. 165–197. Marcel Dekker, New York.

Cohn, W., Gross, P., Grun, H., Loechleiter, F., Muller, D. P. R., and Zulauf, M. (1992). Tocopherol transport and absorption. *Proc. Nutr. Soc.* **51,** 179–188.

Cooke, M. S., Evans, M. D., Mistry, N., and Lunec, J. (2002). Role of dietary antioxidants in the prevention of *in vivo* oxidative damage to DNA. *Nutr. Res. Rev.* **15,** 19–41.

Cutler, R. G. (2005). Oxidative stress profiling: Part I. Its potential importance in the optimization of human health. *Ann. N.Y. Acad. Sci.* **1055,** 93–135.

Cutler, R. G., Plummer, J., Chowdhury, K., and Heward, C. (2005). Oxidative stress profiling. Part I. Theory, technology and practice. *Ann. N.Y. Acad. Sci.* **1055,** 136–158.

Eitenmiller, R., and Lee, J. (2004). *Vitamin E: Food Chemistry, Composition, and Analysis.* Marcel Dekker, New York, 530 pp.

Frei, B. (2004). Efficacy of dietary antioxidants to prevent oxidative damage and inhibit chronic disease. *J. Nutr.* **134,** 3196S–3198S.

Jacob, R. A. (1995). The integrated antioxidant system. *Nutr. Res.* **15,** 755–766.

Jha, P., Flather, M., Lonn, E., Farouk, M., and Yusuf, S. (1995). The antioxidant vitamins and cardiovascular disease. A critical review of epidemiologic and clinical trial data. *Annu. Intern. Med.* **123,** 860–872.

Jiang, Q., Christen, S., Shigenaga, M. K., and Ames, B. N. (2001) γ-Tocopherol, the major form of vitamin E in the US diet, deserves more attention. *Am. J. Clin. Nutr.* **74,** 714–722.

Kappus, H., and Diplock, A. T. (1992). Tolerance and safety of vitamin E: A toxicological position report. *Free Rad. Biol. Med.* **13,** 55–74.

Kellym, F., Meydani, M., and Packer, L. (eds.) (2004). Vitamin E and Health. *Ann. N.Y. Acad. Sci.* **1031,** 463 pp.

Knekt, P. (1994). Vitamin E in cancer prevention. In *Natural Antioxidants in Human Health and Disease* (B. Frei, ed.), pp. 199–238. Academic Press, New York.

Maeda, H., and Akaike, T. (1991). Oxygen free radicals as pathogenic molecules in viral diseases. *Proc. Soc. Exp. Biol. Med.* **198,** 721–727.

Mardones, P., and Attilo, R. (2004). Cellular mechanisms of vitamin E uptake: Relevance in α-tocopherol metabolism and potential implications for disease. *J. Nutr. Biochem.* **15,** 252–260.

Martin, A., Youdim, K., Szprengiel, A., Shukitt-Hale, B., and Joseph, J. (2002). Roles of vitamins E and C on neurodegenerative diseases and cognitive performance. *Nutr. Rev.* **60,** 308–334.

Mergens, W. J., and Bhagavan, H. N. (1989). α-Tocopherols (Vitamin E). In *Nutrition and Cancer Prevention, Investigating the Role of Micronutrients* (T. E. Moon and M. S. Micozzi, eds.), pp. 305–340. Marcel Dekker, New York.

Meydani, M. (2004). Vitamin E modulation of cardiovascular disease. *Ann. N.Y. Acad. Sci.* **1031,** 271–279.

Packer, L. (1992). Interactions among antioxidants in health and disease: Vitamin E and its redox cycle. *Proc. Soc. Exp. Biol. Med.* **200,** 271–276.

Packer, L., and Fuchs, J. (eds.) (1993). *Vitamin E in Health and Disease.* Marcel Dekker, New York.

Pryor, W. A. (1991). Vitamin E. Chapter 14 in *Present Knowledge in Nutrition*, 8th ed. (B. A. Bowman and R. M. Russel, eds.), pp. 156–163. ILSI Press, Washington, DC.

Ricciarelli, R., Zingg, J. M., and Azzi, A. (2001). Vitamin E: Protective role of a Janus molecule. *FASEB J.* **15,** 2314–2325.

Rimbach, G., Minihane, A. M., Majewicz, J., Fischer, A., Pallauf, J., Virgli, F., and Wienberg, P. D. (2002). Regulation of cell signalling by vitamin E. *Proc. Nutr. Soc.* **61,** 415–425.

Schaffer, S., Müller, W. E., and Eckert, G. P. (2005). Tocotrienols: Constitutional effects in aging and disease. *J. Nutr.* **135,** 151–154.

Thurnham, D. I. (1990). Antioxidants and prooxidants in malnourished populations. *Proc. Nutr. Soc.* **49,** 247–259.

Traber, M. (2005). Vitamin E regulation. *Curr. Opin. Gastroenterol.* **21,** 223–227.

Traber, M. G., and Hiroyuki, A. (1999). Molecular mechanisms of vitamin E transport. *Ann. Rev. Nutr.* **19,** 343–355.

Traber, M. G., and Packer, L. (1995). Vitamin E: Beyond antioxidant function. *Am. J. Clin. Nutr.* **62,** 1501S–1509S.

Traber, M. G., and Sies, H. (1996). Vitamin E in humans: Demand and delivery. *Ann. Rev. Nutr.* **16,** 321–347.

Vitamin K

8

… Then Almquist showed
A substance, phthiocol, from dread T.B.,
Would cure the chicks …
And so the microbes of tuberculosis,
That killed the poet Keats by hemorrhage,
Has yielded forth the clue to save the lives
Of infants bleeding shortly after birth.
　　　　　　　　　—T. H. Jukes

I.	The Significance of Vitamin K	214
II.	Sources of Vitamin K	214
III.	Absorption of Vitamin K	216
IV.	Transport of Vitamin K	217
V.	Metabolism of Vitamin K	218
VI.	Metabolic Functions of Vitamin K	221
VII.	Vitamin K Deficiency	227
VIII.	Vitamin K Toxicity	229
IX.	Case Studies	230
	Study Questions and Exercises	232
	Recommended Reading	232

Anchoring Concepts

1. *Vitamin K* is the generic descriptor for 2-methyl-1,4-naphthoquinone and all its derivatives exhibiting qualitatively the antihemorrhagic activity of phylloquinone.
2. The vitamers K are side-chain homologs; each is hydrophobic and thus insoluble in such aqueous environments as plasma, interstitial fluids, and cytoplasm.
3. The 1,4-naphthoquinone ring system of vitamin K renders it susceptible to metabolic reduction.
4. Deficiencies of vitamin K have a narrow clinical spectrum: hemorrhagic disorders.

Learning Objectives

1. To understand the nature of the various sources of vitamin K.
2. To understand the means of absorption and transport of the vitamers K.
3. To understand the metabolic functions of vitamin K in the biosynthesis of plasma clotting factors and other calcium-binding proteins.
4. To understand the physiologic implications of impaired vitamin K function.

Vocabulary

Atherocalcin
γ-Carboxyglutamate (Gla)
Chloro-K
Coagulopathies
Collagen fibers
Coprophagy
Coumarin
Dicumarol
DT-diaphorase
Dysprothrombinemia
Extrinsic clotting system
Factor II
Factor VII
Factor IX
Factor X
Fibrin
Fibrinogen
Gas6
Gla
Hemorrhage
Hemorrhagic disease of the newborn
Heparin
Hydroxyvitamin K
Hypoprothrombinemia
Intrinsic clotting system
Matrix Gla protein
Menadione
Menadione sodium bisulfite complex
Menadione pyridinol bisulfite (MPB)
Menaquinones
Osteocalcin
Phylloquinones
Plasma thromboplastin
Proline-rich GLa proteins
Proconvertin

213

Protein C
Protein induced by vitamin K absence (PIVKA)
Protein M
Protein S
Protein Z
Renal Gla proteins
Serine protease
Stuart factor
Superoxide
Thrombin (factor IIa)
Tissue factor
Tissue thromboplastin under γ-carboxylated osteocalcin
Vitamin K deficiency bleeding (VKDB)
Vitamin K-dependent carboxylase
Vitamin K epoxidase
Vitamin K epoxide
Vitamin K epoxide reductase
Vitamin K quinine reductase
Vitamin K hydroquinone
Vitamin K oxide
Warfarin
Zymogens

I. The Significance of Vitamin K

Vitamin K is synthesized by plants and bacteria, which use it for electron transport and energy production. Animals, however, cannot synthesize the vitamin; still, they require it for blood clotting, bone formation, and other functions. These needs are critical to good health; yet the prevalent microbial synthesis of the menaquinones, including that occurring in the hindgut of humans and other animals (many of whom have *coprophagous* eating habits), results in frank deficiencies of this vitamin being rare. Nevertheless, vitamin K deficiency can occur in poultry and other monogastric animals when they are raised on wire or slatted floors and treated with certain antibiotics that reduce their hindgut microbial synthesis of the vitamin. Human neonates, particularly premature infants, can also be at risk of hemorrhagic disease by virtue of limited transplacental transfer of the vitamin.

The function of vitamin K in blood clotting is widely exploited to reduce risks to postsurgical thrombosis and cardiac patients. **Coumarin**-based drugs (e.g., **warfarin, dicumarol**) and other inhibitors of the vitamin K oxidation/carboxylation/reduction cycle are valuable in this purpose. In addition, vitamin K has clear but less well understood roles in

the metabolism of both calcified and noncalcified tissues. It may well prove that vitamin K functions with other vitamins in the regulation of intracellular Ca^{2+} metabolism, in signal transduction, and in cell proliferation—functions that have profound effects on health status.

II. Sources of Vitamin K

Vitamers K

There are two natural and one synthetic sources of vitamin K:

- *Phylloquinones* Green plants synthesize the phylloquinones (2-methyl-3-phytyl-1,4-naphthoquinones) as a normal component of chloroplasts.
- **Menaquinones** Bacteria (including those of the normal intestinal microflora) and some spore-forming *Actinomyces* spp. synthesize the menaquinones. The predominant vitamers of the menaquinone series contain 6 to 10 isoprenoid units; however, vitamers with as many as 13 isoprenoid groups have been identified.
- *Menadione* The formal parent compound of the menaquinone series does not occur naturally but is a common synthetic form called menadione (2-methyl-1,4-naphthoquinone). This compound forms a water-soluble sodium bisulfite addition product, **menadione sodium bisulfite**, whose practical utility is limited by its instability in complex matrices such as feeds. However, in the presence of excess sodium bisulfite, it crystallizes as a complex with an additional mole of sodium bisulfite (i.e., **menadione sodium bisulfite complex**), which has greater stability and, therefore, is used widely as a supplement to poultry feeds. A third water-soluble compound is **menadione pyridinol bisulfite** (**MPB**), a salt formed by the addition of dimethylpyridinol.

Biopotency of Vitamers K

The relative biopotencies of the various vitamers K differ according to the route of administration. Studies using restoration of normal clotting in the vitamin K-deficient chick have shown that, when administered orally, phylloquinone or menaquinone homologs with three to five isoprenoid groups had greater activities than those with longer side chains. The difference in biopotency appears to relate to the relatively poor absorption of the long-chain vitamers. In fact, studies with the vitamin K-deficient rat showed that the long-chain homologs (especially MK-9, i.e., menaquinone with nine iso-prenoid units) had the greatest activities when administered intracardially. Of the three synthetic forms, some studies indicate MPB to be somewhat more effective in chick diets; however, each is generally regarded to be comparable in terms of biopotency to phylloquinone.

Dietary Sources

Green leafy vegetables tend to be rich in vitamin K, whereas fruits and grains are poor sources. The vitamin K activities of meats and dairy products tend to be moderate. Unfortunately, data for the vitamin K contents of foods (Table 8-1) are limited by the lack of good analytical methods. Nevertheless, it is clear that, because dietary needs for vitamin K are low, most foods contribute significantly to those needs.[1] This is not true for breast milk (Table 8-2); most studies have shown this food to be of very low vitamin K

Table 8-1. Vitamin K contents of foods

Food	Vitamin K (μg/100 g)	Food	Vitamin K (μg/100 g)
Vegetables		Fruits	
Asparagus	39	Apples	4[a]
Beans		Bananas	0.5
Mung	33	Cranberries	1.4
Snap	28	Oranges	1.3
Beets	5	Peaches	3
Broccoli	154	Strawberries	14
Cabbage	149	Meats	
Carrots	13	Beef	0.6
Cauliflower	191	Chicken	0.01
Chick peas	48	Liver	
Corn	4	Beef	104
Cucumbers	5	Chicken	80
Kale	275	Pork	88
Tomatoes	48	Dairy products and eggs	
Lettuce	113	Milk, cow's	4
Peas	28	Eggs	50
Potatoes	0.5	Egg yolk	149
Spinach	266	Grains	
Sweet potatoes	4	Oats	63
Oils		Rice	0.05
Canola (rapeseed)	830	Wheat	20
Corn	5	Wheat bran	83
Olive	58	Wheat germ	39
Peanut	2		
Soybean	200		

[a]Almost 90% in the skin (peeling).
Source: United States Department of Agriculture. (1990). *National Nutrient Database.* U.S. Government Printing Office, Washington, DC.

[1] It is difficult to formulate an otherwise normal diet that does not provide about 100μg of the vitamin per day.

Table 8-2. Vitamin K contents of human milk

Sample	Vitamin K (nM)
Colostrum (30–81 hr)	7.52 ± 5.90
Mature milk	
1 month	6.98 ± 6.36
3 month	5.14 ± 4.52
6 month	5.76 ± 4.48

Source: Canfield, L. M., Hopkinson, J. M., Lima, A. F., Silva, B., and Garga, C. (1991). *Am. J. Clin. Nutr.* **53,** 730–735.

content and insufficient to meet the vitamin K needs of infants up to 6 months of age.[2]

Bioavailability

Little is known about the bioavailability of vitamin K in most foods. It appears, however, that only about 10% of the phylloquinone in boiled spinach is absorbed by humans.[3] This may relate to its association with the thylakoid membrane in chloroplasts, as the free vitamer was well absorbed (80%). This suggests that vitamin K may be poorly bioavailable from the most quantitatively important sources of it in most diets, green leafy vegetables.

Intestinal Microbial Synthesis

Microbial synthesis of vitamin K[4] in the intestine (Table 8-3) appears to have nutritional significance in most animal species. This is indicated by observations that germ-free animals have greater dietary requirements for the vitamin than do animals with normal intestinal microfloras (Table 8-4), and that prevention of coprophagy is necessary to produce vitamin K deficiency in some species (e.g., chicks, rats). The human gut contains substantial amounts of menaquinones of bacterial origin. The nutritional significance of this source of the vitamin is not clear, as the extent of absorption of those forms from the large intestine is not established. However, that menaquinones produced by the gut microflora are absorbed to some extent across the large intestine is indicated by the fact that the liver normally contains significant amounts of these vitamers.

III. Absorption of Vitamin K

Micellar Solubilization

The vitamers K are absorbed from the intestine into the lymphatic (in mammals) or portal (in birds, fishes, and reptiles) circulation by processes that first require that these hydrophobic substances be dispersed in the aqueous lumen of the gut via the formation of mixed micelles, in which they are dissolved.

Table 8-3. Menaquinones produced by several dominant species of enteric bacteria

Species	Major components	Minor components
Bacteroides fragilis	MK-10, MK-11, MK-12	MK-7, MK-8, MK-9
Bacteroides vulgatus	MK-10, MK-11, MK-12	MK-7, MK-8, MK-9
Veillonella sp.	MK-7	MK-6
Eubacterium lentum	MK-6[a]	
Enterobacter sp.	MK-8	MK-8[a]
Enterococcus sp.	MK-9	MK-6,[a] MK-7,[a] MK8[a]

[a]Includes demethylated derivatives.
Source: Mathers, J. C., Fernandez, F., Hill, M. H., McCarthy, P. T., Shearer, M. J., and Oxley, A. (1990). *Br. J. Nutr.* **63,** 639–652.

Table 8-4. Impaired clotting in germ-free rats

Treatment	Prothrombin time (sec)	Hepatic MK-4 (ng/g)
Germ free		
Vitamin K deficient	∞	8.3 ± 2.3
+ MK-4	5.8 ± 1.4[a]	66.5 ± 25.9
+ K$_3$	11.1 ± 2.5[a]	12.4 ± 2.0
Conventional		
Vitamin K deficient	12.7 ± 1.6	103.5 ± 44.9
+ MK-4	12.5 ± 2.0	207.6 ± 91.3
+ K$_3$	12.6 ± 0.9	216.2 ± 86.5

[a]$p < 0.05$.
Source: Komai, M., Shirakawa, H., and Kimura, S. (1987). *Int. J. Vitam. Nutr. Res.* **58,** 55–59.

---

[2] In consideration of the low vitamin K contents of breast milk and to prevent hemorrhagic disease, in the early 1960s the American Academy of Pediatrics recommended the intramuscular administration of vitamin K (1 mg) at the time of birth. This practice is now required by law in the United States and Canada. All commercial infant formulas are supplemented with vitamin K at levels in the range of 50–125 ng/ml.

[3] Gijsbers, B.L.M.G., et al. (1996). *Br. J. Nutr.* **76,** 223–229.

[4] Bacteria and plants synthesize the aromatic ring system of vitamin K from shikimic acid. The ultimate synthesis of the menaquinones in bacteria proceeds through 1,4-dihydroxy-2-naphthoic acid (*not* menadione), which is prenylated, decarboxylated, and then methylated.

Vitamin K absorption, therefore, depends on normal pancreatic and biliary function. Accordingly, conditions resulting in impaired lumenal micelle formation (e.g., dietary mineral oil, pancreatic exocrine dysfunction, bile stasis) impair the enteric absorption of vitamin K. It can be expected that any diet will contain a mixture of menaquinones and phylloquinones. In general, such mixtures appear to be absorbed with efficiencies in the range of 40–70%; however, these vitamers are absorbed via different mechanisms.

Active Transport of Phylloquinone

Studies of the uptake of vitamin K by everted gut sacs of the rat show that phylloquinone is absorbed by an energy-dependent process from the proximal small intestine. The process is not affected by menaquinones or menadione; it is inhibited by the addition of short- and medium-chain fatty acids to the micellar medium.

Other Vitamers Absorbed by Diffusion

In contrast, the menaquinones and menadione are absorbed strictly via non–carrier-mediated *passive diffusion*, the rates of which are affected by the micellar contents of lipids and bile salts. This kind of passive absorption has been found to occur in the distal part of the small intestine as well as in the colon. Thus, noncoprophagous[5] animals appear to profit from the bacterial synthesis of vitamin K in their lower guts by being able to absorb the vitamin from that location.[6]

IV. Transport of Vitamin K

Absorbed Vitamin K Transferred to Lipoproteins

On absorption, vitamin K is transported in the lymph in association with chylomicra, whereby it is transported to the liver. Vitamin K is rapidly taken up by the liver, but it has a relatively short half-life there (about 17 hr) before it is transferred to very low-density lipoproteins (VLDLs) and low-density lipoproteins (LDLs), which carry it in the plasma.

No specific carriers have been identified for any of the vitamers K. Plasma levels of phylloquinone are correlated with those of triglycerides and α-tocopherol; those of healthy humans are in the range of 0.1–0.7 ng/ml (Table 8-5).

Tissue Distribution

When administered as either phylloquinone or menaquinone, vitamin K is rapidly taken up by the liver (Table 8-6), which is the site of synthesis of the vitamin K-dependent coagulation proteins. In contrast, little menadione is taken up by that organ; instead, it is distributed widely to other tissues. Hepatic storage of vitamin K has little long-term significance, for the vitamin is rapidly removed from that organ and rapidly excreted. The vitamin is found at low levels in many organs; several tend to

Table 8-5. Vitamin K transport in humans

Fraction	Phylloquinones (% serum total)
Triglyceride-rich fraction	51.4 ± 17.0
LDLs	25.2 ± 7.6
HDLs	23.3 ± 10.9

Source: Kohlmeier, M., Solomon, A., Saupe, J., and Shearer, M. J. (1996). *J. Nutr.* **126,** 1192S–1196S.

Table 8-6. Vitamers K occurring in livers of several animal species

Vitamer	Species				
	Human	Cow	Horse	Dog	Pig
K_2	+++	+	+++		+
MK-4					+
MK-6				+	
MK-7	+++			+	
MK-8	+			+++	+++
MK-9	+			+++	+++
MK-10	+	+++		+++	+++
MK-11	+	+++		+	
MK-12		+++		+	
MK-13				+	

---

[5] The term **coprophagy** describes the ingestion of excrement. This behavior is common in many species and exposes them to nutrients such as vitamin K produced by the microbial flora of their lower guts. Coprophagy can be easily prevented in some species (e.g., chicks) by housing them on raised wire floors; it is very difficult to prevent it in others (e.g., rats) without the use of such devices as tail cups.

[6] Humans appear to be able to utilize menaquinones produced by their lower gut microflora. Indirect evidence for this is that hypoprothrombinemia is rare *except* among patients given antibiotics, even when vitamin K-free purified diets have been used.

concentrate it: adrenal glands, lungs, bone marrow, kidneys, lymph nodes. The transplacental movement of vitamin K is poor; the vitamin is frequently not detectable in the cord blood from mothers with normal plasma levels. For this reason, newborn infants are susceptible to hemorrhage.[7]

The tissues of most animals ingesting plant materials contain phylloquinones as well as menaquinones with 6–13 isoprenoid units in their side chains. That tissues show such mixtures of vitamers K, even when the sole dietary form is vitamin MK-4, indicates that much of the vitamin K in tissues normally has an intestinal bacterial origin. Animals fed phylloquinone show MK-4 widely distributed in their tissues. This fact was taken as evidence of microbial intercoversion of the phytyl side chain to a geranylgeranyl side chain; however, more recent evidence indicates such metabolic capability in rat tissues. Thus, it appears that the accumulation of MK-4 in extrahepatic tissues of phylloquinone-fed animals is due to local interconversion.

In each organ, vitamin K is found localized primarily in cellular membranes (endoplasmic reticulum, mitochondria). Under conditions of low vitamin K intake, the vitamin appears to be depleted from membranes more slowly than from cytosol.

V. Metabolism of Vitamin K

Side-Chain Modification

Dealkylation

That tissues contain menaquinones when the dietary source of vitamin K was phylloquinone was once taken as evidence for the metabolic dealkylation of the phylloquinone side chain (converting it to menadione), followed by its realkylation to the menaquinones. That the conversion appears to be greatest when phyolloquinone is taken orally[8] has suggested that this dealkylation is performed during intestinal absorption and/or by gut microbes. However, recent findings of MK-4 in tissues of germ-free animals given phylloquinone intraperitoneally (Fig. 8-1) make it clear that the conversion can be performed in several tissues.

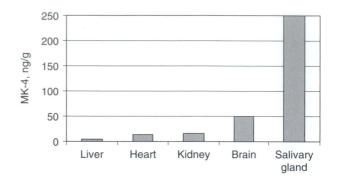

Fig. 8-1. Evidence of conversion of phylloquinone to menaquinone-4 in gnotobiotic animals: MK-4 levels in tissues of vitamin K-deficient rats treated with phylloquinone by intraperitoneal injection. (From Davidson, R.T., et al. (1998) *J. Nutr.* **128,** 220–223.)

Alkylation

The alkylation of menadione (either from a practical feed supplement or produced from microbial degradation of phylloquinone) does occur *in vivo*. This step has been demonstrated in chick liver homogenates, where it was found to use geranyl pyrophosphate, farnesyl pyrophosphate, or geranylgeranyl pyrophosphate as the alkyl donor in a reaction inhibitable by O_2 or **warfarin**. The main product of the alkylation of menadione is MK-4.

Redox Cycling

Vitamin K is subject to a cycle of oxidation and reduction that is coupled to the carboxylation of peptidyl glutamyl residues to produce various functional γ-carboxylated proteins. The redox cycling of vitamin K (Fig. 8-2) occurs in three steps:

1. *Oxidation of dihydroxyvitamin K to vitamin K 2,3-epoxide*   The production of the 2,3-epoxide, also called **vitamin K epoxide** or **vitamin K oxide,** is catalyzed by vitamin K γ-glutamyl carboxylase, a 94 kD protein located in the endoplasmic reticulum and Golgi apparatus. Vitamin K 2,3-epoxide comprises about 10% of the total vitamin K in the normal liver and can be the predominant form in the livers of rats treated with warfarin or other coumarin

---

[7] Furthermore, because human milk contains less vitamin K than cow's milk, infants who receive only their mother's milk are more susceptible to hemorrhage than are those who drink cow's milk.

[8] Thijssen, H.H.W., et al. (2006). *Br. J. Nutr.* **95**, 260–266.

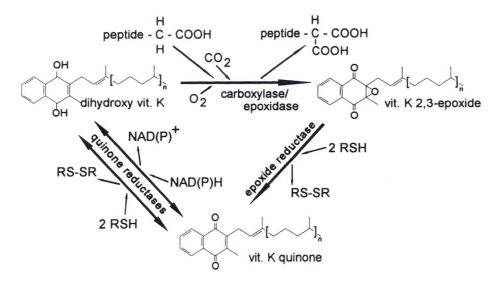

Fig. 8-2. The vitamin K cycle.

anticoagulants. Studies of the human, bovine, and rat carboxylase show high (88–94%) sequence homology. The carboxylase itself appears to be a protein, containing three **Gla** residues per mole of enzyme.[9]

2. *Reduction of the 2,3-epoxide to vitamin K quinone*   This step is catalyzed by **vitamin K epoxide reductase**, a dithiol-dependent, microsomal enzyme inhibited by the coumarin-type anticoagulants. Genetic variability in the vitamin K epoxide reductase is thought to account for the variability observed among patients in their responses to warfarin therapy. Studies have also demonstrated much greater hepatic concentrations of phylloquinone-2,3-epoxide in chicks compared with rats, corresponding (inversely) to a 10-fold marked difference in the hepatic activities of their hepatic vitamin K epoxide reductases (Table 8-7). These findings suggest that the inability to recycle the vitamin effectively is the basis for the relatively high dietary requirement of the chick.

3. *Reduction of the quinone to the active dihydroxyvitamin K*   This final reductive step can be catalyzed in two ways:
   a. By **vitamin K quinine reductase**, a dithiol-dependent microsomal enzyme that is inhibited by the coumarin-type anticoagulants; or
   b. By **DT-diaphorase**, a microsomal flavoprotein that uses NAD(P)H as a source of reducing equivalents. Unlike the dithiol-dependent enzyme, it is relatively insensitive to coumarin inhibition, such that reduction of vitamin K quinone persists in anticoagulant-treated individuals.

Catabolism

Menadione

Menaquinone is rapidly metabolized and excreted, leaving only a relatively minor portion to be converted to MK-4. It is excreted primarily in the urine (e.g., about 70% of a physiological dose may be lost within 24 hr) as the phosphate, sulfate, or glucuronide

Table 8-7.   Species differences in vitamin K metabolism

Enzyme	Substrate	V_{max}[a] Chick	V_{max}[a] Rat
Carboxylase	Phylloquinone	14 ± 2	26 ± 1
	MK-4	41 ± 3	40 ± 2
Epoxide reductase	Phylloquinone	26 ± 2	280 ± 2
	MK-4	55 ± 7	430 ± 10

[a]V_{max} is expressed as micromoles per minute per milligram.
Source: Will, B. H., Usui, Y., and Suttie, J. W. (1992). *J. Nutr.* **122,** 2354–2360.

---

[9] Berkner, K. L., and Pudota, B. N. (1998). *Proc. Natl. Acad. Sci. USA* **95,** 466.

of menadiol. It is also excreted in the bile as the glucuronide conjugate.

Menaquinone

Little is known about menaquinone metabolism, but it is likely that extensive side-chain conversion occurs. Its catabolism appears to be much slower than that of menadione.

Phylloquinone

The total body pool of phylloquinone, about 100 mg in an adult, appears to turnover in about 1.5 days. This involves the vitamer undergoing oxidative shortening of the side chain to 5- or 7-carbon carboxylic acids and a variety of other, more extensively degraded metabolites. A fifth of phylloquinone is ultimately excreted in the urine; however, the primary route of excretion of these metabolites is the feces, which contain glucuronic acid conjugates excreted via the bile.

Both vitamin K epoxide and hydroxyvitamin K are thought to be degraded metabolically before excretion. That these may have different routes of degradation is suggested by the finding that warfarin treatment greatly increases the excretion of phylloquinone metabolites in the urine while decreasing the amounts of metabolites in the feces. Another ring-altered metabolite has been identified:

3-hydroxy-2,3-dihydrophylloquinone, also called **hydroxyvitamin K**.

Vitamin K Antagonists

The coumarin-type anticoagulants block the thiol-dependent regeneration of the reduced forms of the vitamin, resulting in the accumulation of the 2,3-epoxide. The attendant loss of dihydroquinone results in a loss of protein γ-carboxylation and, consequently, the loss of active Gla-proteins.

These compounds were developed as a result of the identification of 3,3′methylbis-(4-hydroxycoumarin) as the active principle present in spoiled sweet clover and responsible for the hemorrhages and prolonged clotting times of animals consuming that as feed. Compounds in this family block the thiol-dependent, redox recycling of the vitamin by inhibiting the dithiol-dependent reductases. This results in diminished synthesis of the Gla proteins involved in the clotting pathway (see 'Blood Clotting' later in this chapter).[10] This has caused several substituted 4-hydroxycoumarins to be widely used in anticoagulant therapy in clinical medicine, as well as rodenticides. The most widely used for each purpose have been warfarin (3-[a-acetonylbenzyl]-4-hydroxycoumarin),[11] an analog of the naturally occurring hemorrhagic factor dicumarol, and its sodium salt.[12] Warfarin therapy is prescribed for a million patients each year in the

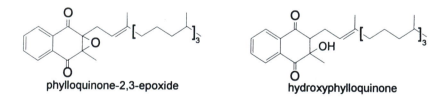

phylloquinone-2,3-epoxide   hydroxyphylloquinone

---

[10] This effect, by inhibition of vitamin K epoxide reductase, is very different from that of another anticoagulant, heparin, a polysaccharide that complexes with thrombin in the plasma to enhance its inactivation.

[11] This analog of the naturally occurring vitamin K antagonist, dicumarol, warfarin (4-hydroxy-3-[3-oxo-1-phenylbutyl]-2H-1-benzopyran-2-one), was synthesized by Link's group at the University of Wisconsin and named for the Wisconsin Alumni Research Foundation.

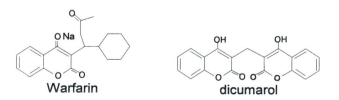

Warfarin   dicumarol

[12] Others include ethyl biscoumacetate (3,3′-carboxymethylenebis-[4-hydroxycoumarin) ethyl ester; and phenprocoumon (3-[1-phenylproyl]-4-hydroxycoumarin).

United States. While this therapy is regarded as important in preventing strokes, it is estimated that 12% of cases experience major bleeding episodes, which are fatal in some 2%.[13] For this reason there has been great interest in developing safer and effective anticoagulants.

Resistance to warfarin has been observed in rats and humans and is a significant problem in Europe and North America. It appears to involve a mutant form of the vitamin K epoxide reductase that is not sensitive to the coumarin. The vitamin K_1 analog, 2-chloro-3-phytyl-1,4-naphthoquinone (**chloro-K**), has proven to be very effective in warfarin-resistant rats, as it functions as a competitive inhibitor of the vitamin at the active site(s) in the vitamin K cycle. Other coumarins have also shown promise.[14]

VI. Metabolic Functions of Vitamin K

Vitamin K-Dependent γ-Carboxylations

Vitamin K is the cofactor of a specific microsomal carboxylase that uses the oxygenation of **vitamin K hydroquinone** to drive the γ-carboxylation of peptide-bound glutamic acid residues (Fig. 8-1). This **vitamin K-dependent carboxylase** is found predominantly in liver but also in several other organs.[15] In the reduced form, vitamin K provides reducing equivalents for the reaction, thus undergoing oxidation to vitamin K-2,3-epoxide. This is coupled to the cleavage of a C–H bond and formation of a carbanion at the γ-position of a peptide-bound glutamyl residue and followed by carboxylation.

The vitamin K-dependent γ-carboxylation of specific glutamyl residues on the zymogen precursors of each blood clotting factor occurs post-translationally at the N-terminus of the nascent polypeptide. In the case of prothrombin, all 10 glutamyl residues in positions 7–33 (but none of the remaining 33 glutamyl residues) are γ-carboxylated. Carboxylation confers

Ca^{2+}-binding capacities to these proteins. This facilitates the formation of Ca^{2+} bridges between the clotting factors and phospholipids on membrane surfaces of blood platelets and endothelial and vascular cells, as well as between Gla residues (i.e., glutamyl residues that have been carboxylated) to form internal Gla–Gla linkages.

The enzyme requires reduced vitamin K (vitamin K hydroquinone), CO_2 as the carboxyl precursor, and molecular oxygen (O_2).[16] It is frequently referred to as vitamin K carboxylase/epoxidase to indicate the coupling of the γ-carboxylation step with the conversion of vitamin K to the 2,3-epoxide. Normally, this coupling is tight; however, under conditions of low CO_2 levels or in the absence of peptidyl-Glu, the epoxidation of the vitamin, referred to as the **vitamin K epoxidase**, proceeds without concomitant carboxylation.

Vitamin K-Dependent Gla Proteins

Vitamin K functions in the post-translational modification of at least a dozen proteins via carboxylation of specific glutamate residues to γ-**carboxyglutamate** (**Gla**) residues. This unusual amino acid was discovered in investigations of the molecular basis of abnormal clotting in vitamin K deficiency. While it had been known that vitamin K deficiency and 4-hydroxycoumarin anticoagulant treatment each caused hypoprothrombinemia, studies in the early 1970s revealed the presence, in each condition, of a protein that was antigenically similar to prothrombin but that did not bind Ca^{2+} and therefore was not functional. Studies of the prothrombin Ca^{2+}-binding sites revealed them to have Gla residues, whereas these were replaced by glutamate (Glu) residues in the abnormal prothrombin. Subsequently, Gla residues were found in each of the other vitamin K-dependent clotting factors, as well as in several other Ca^{2+}-binding proteins in other tissues in at least a dozen proteins. These include several groupings of proteins in animals[17] (Table 8-8), each member of which is thought to function by binding negatively charged phospholipids

---

[13] Landefeld, C. S., et al. (1989). *Am. J. Med.* **87**, 144–152.

[14] For example, difenacoum (3-[3-p-diphenyl-1,2,3,4-tetrahydronaphth-1-yl]-4-hydroxycoumarin); bromodifenacoum (3-[3-{4′-bromodiphenyl-4-yl}-1,2,3,4-tetrahydronaphth-1-yl]-4-hydroxycoumarin).

[15] For example, lung, spleen, kidney, testes, bone, placenta, blood vessel wall, and skin.

[16] The *in vitro* activity of the carboxylase is stimulated almost fourfold by pyridoxal phosphate when the substrate is a pentapeptide. It is doubtful whether that cofactor is important *in vivo*, as no stimulation was observed in the carboxylation of endogenous microsomal proteins.

[17] The venomous cone snail has two small Gla-rich proteins that serve as paralyzing neurotoxins used to subdue prey.

Table 8-8. The vitamin K-dependent Gla proteins

Group	Member proteins
Clotting and regulatory proteins	Prothrombin (factor II)
	Factors VII, IX, and X
	Proteins C, M, S, and Z
Bone proteins	Osteocalcin
	Matrix Gla-protein
	Atherocalcin in atherosclerotic tissue
	A protein S-like protein in detine
	A Gla-protein in renal stones
Other proteins	Protein Z
	Gas6
	Proline-rich Gla proteins (PRGP1, PRGP2)

via Ca^{2+} held by their Gla residues. Each mammalian Gla-protein appears to contain a short, carboxylase-recognition sequence that binds covalently to glutamate-containing peptides to enhance catalysis and is cleaved after carboxylation.

Vitamin K-Dependent Proteins in Plasma

The eight vitamin K-dependent proteins in plasma (Table 8-9) have homologous amino acid sequences in the first 40 positions; all require Ca^{2+} for activity. Protein C inhibits coagulation, and, stimulated by protein S, it promotes fibrinolysis.

The four classic (long-known) clotting factors (II, VII, IX, and X) are components of a complex system of proteins that function to prevent **hemorrhage** and lead to thrombus formation. The protein components of this system circulate as **zymogens**—inactive precursors of the functional forms, each of which is a **serine protease** that participates in a cascade of proteolytic activation of a series of factors ultimately leading to the conversion of a soluble protein, **fibrinogen**, to insoluble **fibrin**, which cross links with platelets to form the blood clot. The conversions of vitamin K-dependent factors in this cascade each involve the Ca^{2+}-mediated association of the active protein, its substrate, and another protein factor with a phospholipid surface.

Blood Clotting

Blood clotting (Fig. 8-3) is initiated by injury to tissues through the release of **collagen fibers** and **tissue factor**, a cell surface protein, whereupon they interact with vitamin K-dependent Gla proteins in the circulation. These signals are amplified via the clotting pathway ultimately to form the clot. The key step in this system is the activation of **factor X** (also called **Stuart factor**), by the proteolytic removal of a short polypeptide from a zymogen. This can occur in two ways:

- By the actions of **factor IX** (also called Christmas factor, or plasma thromboplastin component), which is activated by **plasma thromboplastin** as the result of a contact with a foreign surface in what is referred to as the **intrinsic clotting system**
- By the action of **factor VII**,[18] which is activated by **tissue thromboplastin** released as the result of injury in what is called the **extrinsic clotting system**.

Once activated, factor X,[19] binding Ca^{2+} and phospholipid, catalyzes the activation of several coagulation factors:

Table 8-9. Characteristics of the vitamin K-dependent plasma proteins

Parameter	II[a]	VII	IX	X	C	M	S	Z
Level (μg/ml)	100	1	3	20	10	<1	1	<1
Molecular mass (kDa)	72	46	55	55	57	50	69	55
Percentage carbohydrate	8	13	26	13	8	+	+	+
Chains	1	1	1	2	2	1	1	1
Gla residues	10	10	12	12	11	+	10	13

[a]Prothrombin.

---

[18] Also called **proconvertin**, factor VII is also activated by a high-fat meal and has been associated with increased risk to ischemic heart disease in some studies (e.g., Junker, R., et al. [1997]. *Arterioscler. Thromb. Vasc. Biol.* **17**, 1539–1544).

[19] Polymorphisms of factor X have been identified; however, these do not appear to affect circulating factor X levels.

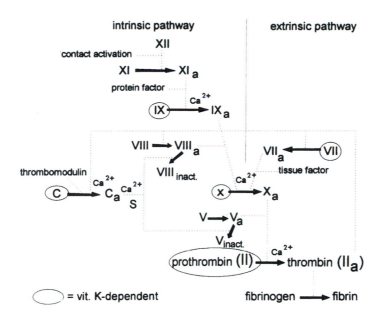

Fig. 8-3.   Roles of vitamin K-dependent factors in blood clotting.

- Prothrombin (**factor II**) to its active form, **thrombin (factor IIa)**, which catalyzes the proteolytic change in fibrinogen that renders it insoluble (as fibrin) for clot formation
- Factor V to its active form, factor Va
- Factor VIII to its active form factor VIIIa

This system also includes other vitamin K-dependent proteins.

- **Protein C**   This protein is activated by thrombin (factor IIa) in the presence of an endothelial cell protein, thrombomodulin, and acts in a complex with protein S by partially hydrolyzing the activated factors V and VIII, thus inactivating them. Activated protein C regulates the activities of coagulation factors (VIIIa and Va) that serve as cofactors for the activation of factor X and prothrombin, respectively, by mediating their cleavage. It also has anti-inflammatory and anti-apoptotic activities involving the binding to an endothelial receptor and the cleavage of a protease-activated receptor. These effects involve activation of a protease-activated receptor (PAR1) and the inhibition of the NF-κB pathway. That these functions are vital is evidenced by the fact that patients with inherited deficiency of factor C are at high risk of thromboses.

- **Protein S**   Unlike the other clotting factors, protein S is not a serine protease zymogen. It is found in the plasma both in free form and as a bimolecular complex with a regulatory component (C4b-binding protein) of the complement system. It has been suggested that protein S may thus have a role in regulation of that system. In support of this hypothesis are observations of cases of recurrent thrombosis in patients with inherited protein S deficiency.
- **Proteins M**   The physiological functions of this protein is presently unknown.
- **Protein Z**   Like Protein S, Protein Z is not a serine protease; instead, it is a 62 kD cofactor for the inhibition of factor Xa[20] by an inhibitor to which it is complexed in the plasma. Protein Z deficiency has been associated with a bleeding tendency in patients with factor V Lieden mutation.[21]

---

[20] The activated form of factor X.

[21] A point mutation in the gene encoding coagulation factor V results in the expression of a form of a factor Va that is resistant to activated protein C and a relatively hypercoagulable state. The mutation occurs in 4–6% of the U.S. population and is associated with increased risk to venous thromboembolism.

This system functions to contain coagulation to the site of injury and to curtail the process upon the formation of the clot. This regulation involves protein Z-dependent inhibition of factor Xa, and downregulation of thrombin production by thrombin bound to another protein, thrombomodulin, a complex that activates protein C[22] which, in turn, inactivates factors Va and VIIIa.[23]

Vitamin K-Dependent Proteins in Calcified Tissues

Osteocalcin

The best characterized vitamin K-dependent protein of calcified tissues is osteocalcin (also called bone GLA protein), a low-molecular-mass (about 5.7-kDa) protein found in rapidly growing regions of bones. Osteocalcin shows no apparent homology with the vitamin K-dependent plasma proteins; however, it is very homologous between various species. It contains three Gla residues in a 49-amino acid segment. It binds Ca^{2+} weakly, that binding serving both to maintain its secondary structure and to allow it to bind the mineralized bone matrix. It has been shown that osteocalcin is synthesized by osteoblasts. In fact, it is the second most abundant protein[24] in the bone matrix, comprising about 2% of total bone protein and 10–20% of noncollagen protein. Its synthesis is inhibited by warfarin treatment and is stimulated (at least in vitro) by 1,25-dihydroxyvitamin D_3 [1,25-$(OH)_2$-vitamin D_3]. An estimated 20% of osteocalcin is not bound to bone and is free to enter the plasma. Because it is synthesized only by osteoblasts that loses small amounts to the general circulation, osteocalcin can be used as a marker of bone formation. The greatest circulating levels of osteocalcin are found in young children and patients with Paget's disease[25] and other disorders involving increased bone resorption/mineralization (Table 8-10).

It has been suggested that osteocalcin may function in the regulation of calcification, perhaps by acting as an attractant for osteoclast progenitor cells. However, supporting evidence for this hypothesis is inconsistent. The 98% reduction of osteocalcin in vitamin K-deficient, nonhemorrhagic rats failed to affect bone growth, morphology, or mineralization[26] unless the treatment was continued for several months,[27] by which time other vitamin K-dependent bone proteins may also have been affected. On the other hand, osteocalcin-null transgenic mice show hyperostosos,[28] and undercarboxylated osetocalcin has been associated with risk to hip fracture (Table 8-11). Relatively high intakes of vitamin K appear to be required to support the maximal carboxylation of osteocalcin (Table 8-12).

Matrix Gla protein

This is a small (9.6kDa), insoluble polypeptide with a clear affinity for demineralized bone matrix and

Table 8-10. Plasma osteocalcin concentrations in humans

Group	Osteocalcin (ng/ml)
Children	10–40[a]
Adults	4–8
Women	
60–69 years of age	7
80–89 years of age	8
Patients with Paget's disease	39
Patients with secondary hyperparathyroidism	47
Patients with osteopenia	9

[a]Highest levels observed in patients 10–15 years of age.

---

[22] Activation is enhanced by endothelial cell protein C receptor.

[23] Inactivation is enhanced by protein S.

[24] Collagen is the most abundant protein in bone.

[25] Paget's disease, also called osteitis, is estimated to affect 3% of people over 40 years of age. It involves dysfunctional bone remodeling, with bone continually breaking down and rebuilding at rates faster than normal, resulting in bone being replaced with soft, porous, highly vascularized bone that can be weak and easily bend, leading to shortening of the affected part of the body, or with excess bone that can be painful and easily fractured. The disease most commonly affects the spine, pelvis, skull, femur, and tibia.

[26] Price, W. A., and Williamson, M. K. (1981). *J. Biol. Chem.* **256**, 12754–12759.

[27] Price, W. A., et al. (1982). *Proc. Natl. Acad. Sci. USA* **79**, 7734–7738.

[28] Iwamoto, J., et al. (2004). *Curr. Pharm. Des.* **10**, 2557–2576; Cockayne, S. (2006). *Arch. Intern. Med.* **166**, 1256–1261.

Table 8-11. Total and undercarboxylated osteocalcin in fracture and nonfracture patients

Parameter	Nonfracture	Fracture
N	153	30
Age, kg	82.5 ± 5.9	85.8 ± 6.5[a]
Body weight, kg	56.6 ± 11.5	49.4 ± 10.7[a]
Plasma osteocalcin, ng/ml		
Total	6.18 ± 3.34	7.90 ± 4.34[a]
Undercarboxylated	0.89 ± 0.89 (14)[b]	1.47 ± 1.65[a] (19)[b]
Carboxylyated	5.29 ± 2.69 (86)[b]	6.43 ± 2.94[a] (81)[b]
25-OH-D_3, ng/ml	17.4 ± 14.1	15.9 ± 10.8
PTH, pg/ml	47.0 ± 23.8	60.0 ± 40.9
Alkaline phosphatase IU/L	78 ± 37	92 ± 40[a]

[a] $p < 0.05$.
[b] n analyzed.
Source: Szulc, P., et al. (1996). Bone 18, 487–488.

Table 8-12. Signs of vitamin K deficiency

Organ system	Sign
General	
Growth	Decrease
Dermatologic	Hemorrhage
Muscular	Hemorrhage
Gastrointestinal	Hemorrhage
Vascular	
Erythrocytes	Anemia
Platelets	Decreased clotting

nonmineralized cartilage. It is structurally related to osteocalcin and is found predominantly in bone and cartilage, although its mRNA has been identified in several noncalcified tissues. Although its metabolic function remains unclear, it has been suggested that matrix Gla protein may serve in the clearance of extracellular Ca^{2+} to protect against calcification of soft tissues and to assist in calcification of bone matrix.

Protein S

The discovery that **protein S** is synthesized by osteoblasts suggests that it may have an activity in bone in addition to that apparent in the regulation of clotting. That protein S may have a role in bone metabolism was suggested by the finding of severe osteopenia, low bone mineral density, and vertebral compression fractures in two children with very low levels of the protein. The protein contains a thrombin-sensitive region, an epidermal growth factor-like domain, and a steroid hormone-binding domain. The nature of its role remains unclear.

Other calcification proteins

A Gla protein has been identified in rat dentine. It is thought to have a role in dental calcification.

Bone mineralization

Several studies have shown associations of serum vitamin K levels or vitamin K intake and bone mineral density or fracture risk.[29] The Nurses Health Study, a 10-year prospective study of more than 72,000 women, found the age-adjusted risk of hip fracture to be 30% less in women with vitamin K intakes >109 mcg/d than those consuming greater amounts.[30] A similar relationship was observed in the Framingham Heart Study: subjects in the highest quartile of vitamin K intake (median intake 254 mcg/day) had significant reductions in hip fracture risk compared to those in the lowest quartile (median intake 56 mcg/day).[31] At least a dozen intervention

---

[29] See review by Weber, P. (2001). *Nutr.* 17:880–887.
[30] Feskanich, D. et al. (1999). *Am. J. Clin. Nutr.* 69:74–81.
[31] Booth, S. L. et al. (2000). *Am. J. Clin. Nutr.* 71:1201–1208.

studies have shown vitamin K treatment to reduce the loss of bone mineral and/or reduce the incidence of fractures.

Other Vitamin K-Dependent Gla Proteins

The finding of other Gla proteins makes it is clear that vitamin K functions widely in physiological systems beyond those involved in blood clotting:

- **Atherocalcin** A Gla protein, atherocalcin, was discovered in calcified atherosclerotic tissue. With this finding, it was suggested that arterial vitamin K-dependent γ-glutamyl carboxylase, which is found in the walls of arteries but not veins, may be involved in the development of atherosclerosis.

- **Gas6**[32] Widely distributed in nervous tissue, Gas6 has 44% sequence homology with protein S and, like the latter, contains an epidermal growth factor-like domain. Unlike protein S, Gas6 lacks thrombin-sensitive motifs, thus its susceptibility to thrombin cleavage. Gas6 functions as a ligand for the reception tyrosine kinases Ax1 and Sky/Rse, and protects cells from apoptosis by activating Ark phosphorylation and inducing MAP kinase[33] activity. It has also been found to facilitate growth of smooth muscle cells, and it has been suggested that Gas6 may function as a ligand for Tyro 3 and thus serve as a neurotrophic factor.

- **Proline-rich Gla proteins** These small (*PRG1,* 23 kD; *PRG2,* 17 kD), single-pass, transmembrane proteins are expressed in a variety of extrahepatic proteins. Their functions are presently unknown.

- **Renal Gla protein** This protein is inhibited by parathyroid hormone (PTH), and vitamin D_3 has been described; it is thought to have some role in the transport/excretion of Ca^{2+} in the kidney.

- *Other Gla proteins* Other Gla proteins have been reported in sperm, urine, hepatic mitochondria, shark skeletal cartilage, and snake venom.

Vitamin K in Atherosclerosis

Vitamin K-dependent Gla proteins may play roles in atherogenesis, which involves thrombus-induced coagulation as well as intimal calcification. Gene deletion studies in mice suggest that matrix Gla protein may be a regulator of this process.[34] Undercarboxylation of matrix Gla protein results in arterial calcification in the warfarin-treated rat model. Osteocalcin, normally expressed only in bone, is upregulated in arterial calcification. It has been suggested that Gas6 and protein S may inhibit calcification through enhancing apoptosis, which is extensive in atherosclerotic lesions. Although the roles of vitamin K-dependent factors in atherogenesis remain unclear, it is possible that increased dietary intake of the vitamin may be useful in reducing atherosclerosis risk.

Vitamin K in Sulfatide Metabolism

Vitamin K is known to be required for the biosynthesis of sphingolipids by bacteria, by supporting the activity of serine palmitoyltransferase,[35] the initial enzyme in the sphingolipid pathway. A role of vitamin K in sphingolipid metabolism has not been reported in animals, although studies have shown that warfarin treatment reduces brain sulfatides and that vitamin K depletion treatment reduces the activity of brain glutathione *S*-transferase.

Vitamin K in the Nervous System

Vitamin K may also have a role in the nervous system. The vitamin is abundant in the rat brain, mostly as MK-4, which is highest in myelinated regions such as the pons medulla and midbrain. A function in brain sphingolipid metabolism could be important in nervous tissue, as sphingolipids are important components of membranes and also serve as a second messenger for intracellular signal transduction pathways. The chick embryo central nervous system has been found to demonstrate a vitamin K-dependent protein-tyrosine phosphorylation cascade, possibly involving the Gla protein Gas6 as a ligand for the reception tyrosine kinase Ax1. It is not clear whether

---

[32] Named for its gene, Growth Arrest Specific Gene 6.
[33] Mitogen-activated protein kinase.
[34] Luo, G., et al. (1997). *Nature* **386,** 78–81.
[35] That is, 3-keto-dihydrosphingosine synthase.

brain microsomes have γ-carboxylase activity, which would imply that the post-translational glutamation of Gas6 must occur in other tissues.

Vitamin K and Cancer

Vitamin K has been found to reduce carcinogenesis in animal models and to reduce cancer risk in human trials. The K_3 vitamer was found six decades ago to increase the survival of inoperable bronchial carcinoma patients. Vitamins K_2 has also been found effective in reducing cancer risk. In an eight-year randomized clinical trial, women receiving the vitamin (45 mg/day) showed a relative risk of hepatocellular carcinoma of 0.13 (95% confidence interval: 0.02–0.99, P = 0.05) compared to those in the placebo control group.[36]

These effects appear to involve two types of mechanisms:

- *Oxidative stress in malignant cells* The actions of vitamin K_3 have been attributed to the reactive oxygen species generated by the single-electron redox-cycling of the quinone, and to the depletion of glutathione due to its arylation by the vitamer.
- *Modulation of transcription factors* In cell culture, vitamers K_1, K_2, and K_3 have been shown to induce proto-oncogenes, increasing the levels of c-myc, c-jun, and c-fos, delaying the cell cycle, and enhancing apoptosis. Vitamin K_3 also appears to induce protein tyrosine kinase activation and to inhibit through direct interaction extracellular signal-regulated kinase (ERK) protein tyrosine phosphatases. These effects are associated with impaired proliferation.
- *Cell cycle arrest* Vitamin K_3 has been shown to inhibit cyclin-dependent kinases (CDKs) by binding to sulfhydryls at the active site of those enzymes. This effect is associated with inhibition of malignant cell proliferation at the G1/S and S/G2 phases of the cell cycle. Vitamin K_2 has been found to affect cyclin function, which is also manifest as cell cycle inhibition.

VII. Vitamin K Deficiency

Signs of Vitamin K Deficiency

Coagulopathy

The predominant clinical sign of vitamin K deficiency is hemorrhage (Table 8-12), which can lead to a fatal anemia. The blood shows prolonged clotting time and **hypoprothrombinemia**. Because a 50% loss of plasma prothrombin level is required to affect prothrombin time, prolongation of the latter is a useful biomarker for advanced subclinical vitamin D deficiency. Several congenital disorders of vitamin K-dependent proteins have been identified in human patients: at least a dozen forms of congenital **dysprothrombinemia**, at least three variants of **factor VII**, and a congenital deficiency of protein C. Patients with these disorders show **coagulopathies**; none respond to high doses of vitamin K.

Undercarboxylated proteins

A more sensitive indicator of low vitamin K status is the presence in plasma of under-γ-carboxylated vitamin K-dependent proteins. The first was originally thought to be a distinct protein produced only in vitamin K deficiency; it was referred to as the **protein induced by vitamin K absence** (**PIVKA**). Subsequently, it became clear that PIVKA was actually inactive prothrombin lacking Gla residues required for its Ca^{2+} binding. It is thus useful as a marker for subclinical vitamin K deficiency. Another marker is **under-γ-carboxylated osteocalcin** (Fig. 8-4), which is released from bone into the circulation. Studies have shown that increases in the serum concentrations of these factors are more sensitive to minidose warfarin therapy than are decreases in prothrombin or osteocalcin. Except for patients on anticoagulant therapy, undercarboxylation of bloodclotting factors is rare. The undercarboxylation of osteocalcin, however, is frequent among postmenopausal women.[37]

Importance of hindgut microbial biosynthesis

Vitamin K deficiency is rare among humans and most other animal species, the important exception being the rapidly growing chick raised in a wire-floored cage. This is due to the wide occurrence of vitamin K

---

[36] Habu, D. et al. (2004). *JAMA* **292**, 358–361.

[37] Clinical trials have found that members of this group respond to supplemental vitamin K with increases in bone formation and decreases in bone resorption.

in plant and animal foods and to the significant microbial synthesis of the vitamin that occurs in the intestines of most animals. In fact, for many species, including humans, the intestinal synthesis of vitamin K appears to meet normal needs. Species with short gastrointestinal tracts and very short intestinal transit times (e.g., about 8 hr in the chick), less than the generation times of many bacteria, do not have well-colonized guts. Being thus unable to harbor vitamin K-producing bacteria, they depend on their diet as the source of their vitamin K.

Risk factors for vitamin K deficiency

Thus, the most frequent causes of vitamin K deficiency are factors that interfere with the microfloral production or absorption of the vitamin:

- *Lipid malabsorption* Diseases of the gastrointestinal tract, biliary stasis, liver disease, cystic fibrosis, celiac disease, and *Ascaris* infection can interfere with the enteric absorption of vitamin K.
- *Anticoagulant therapy* Certain types of drugs can impair vitamin K function. These include warfarin and other 4-hydroxycoumarin anticoagulants, and large doses of salicylates, which inhibit the redox-cycling of the vitamin. In each case, high doses of vitamin K are generally effective in normalizing clotting mechanisms. In medical management of thrombotic disorders, over-anticoagulation with warfarin is common; this is reversed by warfarin dose reduction coupled with treatment with phylloquinone.[38]
- *Antibiotic therapy* Sulfonamides and broad-spectrum antibiotic drugs can virtually sterilize the lumen of the intestine, thus removing an important source of vitamin K for most animals. Therefore, it has been thought that patients on antibiotic therapy can be at risk of vitamin K deficiency.[39] Indeed, cases of hypoprothrominemia have been identified in association with the use of penicillin, semisynthetic penicillins,

and cephalosporins. The prevalence of such cases appeared to increase in the 1980s with the introduction of the β-lactam antibiotics.[40] Although these drugs are administered intravenously, it is possible that they may affect enteric bacterial metabolism via biliary release. Studies have shown that not all patients treated with β-lactam antibiotics show altered fecal menaquinones, although they show significant increases in circulating vitamin K-2,3-epoxide levels when treated with vitamin K. This observation led to the demonstration that the cephalosporin-type antibiotics can inhibit the vitamin K-dependent carboxylase to produce coumarin-like depressions of the activities of the vitamin K-dependent clotting factors. Unlike the coumarins, however, the β-lactam antibiotics are very weak anticoagulants, the effects of which are observed only in patients of low vitamin K status.

Neonates

Neonates are at special risk of vitamin K deficiency for several reasons:

- *Placental transport of the vitamin is poor.* Infants have very limited reserves of vitamin K; their serum levels are typically about half those of their mothers.
- *The neonatal intestine is sterile for the first few days of life.* The neonatal intestine thus does not provide an enteric microbial source of the vitamin.
- *Hepatic biosynthesis of the clotting factors is inadequate in the young infant.* The plasma prothrombin concentrations of fetuses and infants are typically one-quarter those of their mothers (Fig. 8-5).
- *Human milk is an inadequate source of vitamin K.* The frequency of vitamin K-responsive hemorrhagic disease in 1-month-old infants is 1/4000 overall, but 1/1700 among breastfed infants.

---

[38] Baker, P., et al. (2006). *Br. J. Haematol.* **133,** 331–336.

[39] This risk can be further increased by inanition. Because vitamin K is rapidly depleted from tissues, periods of reduced food intake, such as may occur postsurgically, can produce vitamin K deficiency in patients with reduced intestinal microbial synthesis of the vitamin.

[40] For example, cephalosporin, cefamandole, and the related oxa-β-lactam moxalactam.

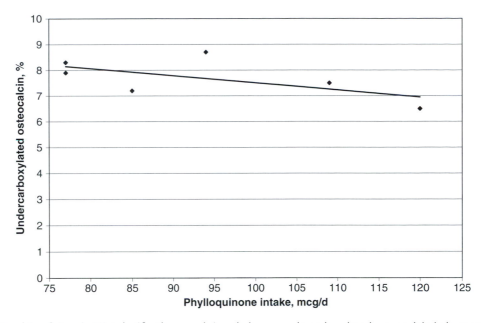

Fig. 8-4. Relationship of vitamin K intake (for three weeks) and plasma undercarboxylated osteocalcin in humans. (*From* Brinkley, N. C., et al. [2002]. *Am. J. Clin. Nutr.* **76**, 1055–1060.)

For these reasons, some infants[41] will develop hemorrhage if continuing intake of vitamin K is not provided. This condition of **vitamin K deficiency bleeding (VKDB)**, also called **hemorrhagic disease of the newborn**, can present in different ways, depending on the age of the infant:

- Newborns (first 24 hours)—cephalohematoma; intracranial, intrathoracic or intra-abdominal bleeding
- Newborns (first week)—generalized ecchymoses[42] of the skin; bleeding from the gastrointestinal tract, umbilical cord stump or circumcision site
- Infants (1–12 weeks)—intracranial, skin, or gastrointestinal bleeding

The major risk factors for VKDB are exclusive breast feeding, failure to give vitamin K prophylaxis, and certain maternal drug therapies. Exclusively breastfed infants who have not received vitamin K or who have gastrointestinal disorders involving lipid malabsorption (cystic fibrosis, biliary atresia, α_1-antitrypsin deficiency) can show signs within

several weeks as intracranial hemorrhage with liver disease, central nervous system damage, and high mortality due to bilirubinemia. Infants fed formula diets are at lower risk probably because of the greater amounts of vitamin K in infant formulas than in human milk. Hemorrhagic disease has also been reported for newborns of mothers on anticonvulsant therapy.

It has become a common practice in many countries to treat all infants at birth with parenterally administered vitamin K (1 mg phylloquinone). This practice has greatly reduced the incidence of hemorrhagic disease of the newborn, although much lower doses have been found to be effective.[43]

VIII. Vitamin K Toxicity

Phylloquinone exhibits no adverse effects when administered to animals in massive doses by any route. The menaquinones are similarly thought to have negligible toxicity. Menadione, however, can be toxic. At high doses, it can produce hemolytic anemia, hyperbilirubinemia, and severe jaundice. Accordingly, phylloquinone has replaced menadione for the

---

[41] Without vitamin K prophylaxis, the risk of hemorrhage for healthy, nontraumatized infants in the first two weeks of life has been estimated to be 1–2/1000, and for older infants a third of that level (Hey, E. www.archdischild.com, July 13, 2006).

[42] Sheet hemorrhages of the skin, *ecchymoses,* differ from the smaller *petechiae* only in size.

[43] Sutherland, J. M., et al. (1967). *Am. J. Dis. Child.* **113,** 524–533.

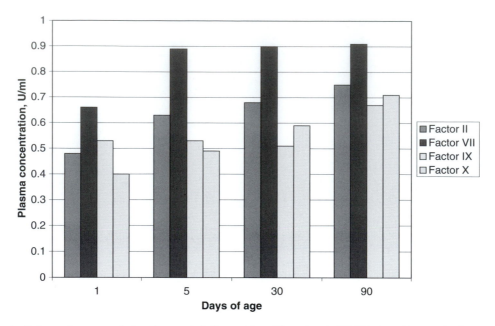

Fig. 8-5. Vitamin K-dependent coagulation factors in infants. (*From* Zipursky, A. [1999]. *Br. J. Haematol.* **104**, 430–437.)

vitamin K prophylaxis of neonates. The intoxicating doses of menadione appear to be at least three orders of magnitude above those levels required for normal physiological function. At such high levels, menadione appears to produce oxidative stress. This occurs as a result of the vitamer undergoing monovalent reduction to the semiquinone radical, which, in the presence of O_2, is reoxidized to the quinone, resulting in the formation of the **superoxide** radical anion. In addition, high levels of menadione are known to react with free sulfhydryl groups, thus depleting reduced glutathione (GSH) levels.

A review of the U.S. Food and Drug Adminstration database revealed 2236 adverse reactions reported for 1019 patients receiving intravenous vitamin K in 1968–1997.[44] Of those cases, 192 were anaphylactoid reactions and 24 were fatalities; those numbers were only 21 and 4, respectively, for patients given vitamin K doses < 5 mg. Persistent, localized eczematous plaque has been reported at the injection site for some patients given vitamin K_1 intramuscularly or subcutaneously.[45]

IX. Case Studies

Instructions

Review the following case report, paying special attention to the diagnostic indicators on which the treatments were based. Then answer the questions that follow.

Case 1

A 60-year-old woman involved in an automobile accident sustained injuries to the head and compound fractures of both legs. She was admitted to the hospital, where she was treated for acute trauma. Her recovery was slow, and for the next 4 months she was drowsy and reluctant to eat. Her diet consisted mainly of orange and glucose drinks with a multivitamin supplement that contained no vitamin K. Her compound fractures became infected, and she was treated with a combination of antibiotics (penicillin, gentamicin, tetracycline, and cotrimoxazole). She then developed intermittent diarrhea, which was treated with codeine phosphate. After a month, all antibiotics were stopped and 46 days later

---

[44] Fiore, L. D., et al. (2001). *J. Thromb. Thrombosis* **11,** 175–183.

[45] Wilkins, K., et al. (2000). *J. Cutan. Med. Surg.* **4,** 164–168.

(6 months after the injury) she experienced bleeding from her urethra. At that time other signs were also noted: bruising of the limbs, bleeding gums, and generalized *purpura*.[46] The clinical diagnosis was scurvy until it was learned that the patient was taking 25 mg of ascorbic acid per day via her daily vitamin supplement.

Laboratory results

Parameter	Patient	Normal range
Hb	9.0 g/dl	12–16 g/dl
Mean RBC volume	79 fl	80–100 fl
White cells	6.3×10^9/liter	5–10×10^9/liter
Platelets	320×10^9/liter	150–300×10^9/liter
Plasma iron	22 μg/dl	72–180 μg/dl
Total iron-binding capacity	123 μg/dl	246–375 μg/dl
Calcium	7.6 mg/dl	8.4–10.4 mg/dl
Inorganic phosphate	2.4 mg/dl	2.4–4.3 mg/dl
Folate	1.6 ng/ml	3–20 ng/ml
Vitamin B_{12}	110 ng/liter	150–1000 ng/liter
Prothrombin time	273 sec	13 sec (control)
Thrombin time	10 sec	10 sec (control)

When her abnormal prothrombin time was noted, specific coagulation assays were performed. These showed that the activity of each vitamin K-dependent factor (factors II, VII, IX, and X) was <1% of the normal level and that the activity of factor V was 76% of normal. A xylose tolerance test (to measure small bowel absorption), performed with a single oral dose of 5 g of xylose, showed tolerance within normal limits. A stool culture showed normal fecal flora. The patient was then given phylloquinone (10 mg daily, administered intravenously, for 3 days) and showed a complete recovery of all coagulation factor activities to normal. She was given a high-protein/high-energy diet supplemented with $FeSO_4$ and, for a week, daily oral doses of 10 mg of phylloquinone. Her diarrhea subsided, her wounds healed, and she returned to normal health.

Case 2

A 55-year-old man with arteriosclerotic heart disease and type IV hyperlipoproteinemia was admitted to the hospital with a hemorrhagic syndrome. Six months earlier, he had suffered a myocardial infarction[47] complicated by pulmonary embolism[48] for which he was treated with **heparin**[49] followed by warfarin. Two months earlier, he had been admitted for a cardiac arrhythmia, at which time his physical examination was normal and chest radiograph showed no abnormalities, but his electrocardiogram showed first-degree atrioventricular block[50] with frequent premature ventricular contractions. At that time, he was taking 5 mg of warfarin per day.

Laboratory findings 2 months before third admission[a]

Parameter	Patient	Normal
Prothrombin time	16.6 sec	12.7 sec
Plasma triglycerides	801 mg/dl	20–150 mg/dl
Serum cholesterol	324 mg/dl	150–250 mg/dl

[a]Blood count, blood urea nitrogen, blood bilirubin, and urinalysis were all normal.

He was treated with warfarin (5 mg/day), digoxin,[51] diphenylhydantoin,[52] furosemide,[53] potassium chloride,[54] and clofibrate.[55] Within a month, quinidine gluconate[56] was substituted for diphenylhydantoin because the patient showed persistent premature ventricular beats, but that drug was discontinued

[46] Subcutaneous hemorrhages.
[47] Dysfunction due to necrotic changes resulting from obstruction of a coronary artery.
[48] Obstruction or occlusion of a blood vessel by a transported clot.
[49] A highly sulfated mucopolysaccharide with specific anticoagulant properties.
[50] Impairment of normal conduction between the atria and ventricles.
[51] A cardiotonic.
[52] A cardiac depressant (and anticonvulsant).
[53] A diuretic.
[54] That is, to correct for the loss of K^+ induced by the diuretic.
[55] An antihyperlipoproteinemic.
[56] A cardiac depressant (antiarrhythmic).

because of diarrhea and so procainamide was used instead. At that time, his prothrombin time was 31.5 sec, and his warfarin dose was reduced first to half the original dose and then to one-quarter of that level.

At the time of the third admission, the patient appeared well nourished, but had ecchymoses on his arms, abdomen, and pubic area. He had been constipated with hematuria[57] for the preceding 2 days. His physical examination was unremarkable except for occasional premature beats, and his laboratory findings were similar to those observed on his previous admission, with the exception that his prothrombin time had increased to 36.6 sec. In questioning the patient, it was learned that he had been taking orally as much as 1200 mg of all-*rac*-α-tocopheryl acetate each day for the preceding 2 months.

Both his warfarin and vitamin E treatments were discontinued, and 2 days later his prothrombin time had dropped to 24.9 sec and his ecchymoses began to clear. The patient consented to participate in a clinical trial of vitamin E (800 mg of all-*rac*-α-tocopheryl acetate per day) in addition to the standard regimen of warfarin and clofibrate. The results were as follows:

Effect of vitamin E on the activities of the patient's coagulation factors

Activity	Initial value	+ Vitamin E (6 weeks)	− Vitamin E (1 week)	Normal range
Factor II (prothrombin)[a]	11	7	21	60–150
Factor VII[a]	27	16	20	50–150
Factor IX[a]	30	14	23	50–150
Factor X[a]	15	10	—	50–150
Prothrombin time (sec)	20.7	29.2	22.3	11.0–12.5

[a]Values represent a percentage of normal means.

Case Questions

1. What signs indicated vitamin K-related problems in each case?
2. What factors probably contributed to the vitamin K deficiency of the patient in case 1? Why was phylloquinone, rather than menadione, chosen for treatment of that patient?
3. What factors may have contributed to the coagulopathy of the patient in case 2? What might be the basis of the effect of high levels of vitamin E seen in that case?

Study Questions and Exercises

1. Construct a concept map to illustrate the ways in which vitamin K affects blood coagulation.
2. Construct a decision tree for the diagnosis of vitamin K deficiency in a human or an animal.
3. What features of the chemical structure of vitamin K relate to its metabolic function?
4. What relevance to their vitamin K nutrition would you expect of the rearing of experimental animals in a germ-free environment or fed a fat-free diet?
5. How does the concept of a coenzyme relate to vitamin K?

Recommended Reading

Berkner, K. L. (2005). The vitamin K-dependent carboxylase. *Ann. Rev. Nutr.* **25,** 127–149.

Berkner, K. L., and Runge, K. W. (2004). The physiology of vitamin K nutriture and vitamin K-dependent protein function in atherosclerosis. *J. Thrombosis Haematostasis* **2,** 2118–2132.

Booth, S. L., and Suttie, J. W. (1998). Dietary intake and adequacy of vitamin K. *J. Nutr.* **128,** 785–788.

Broze, Jr., G. J. (2001). Protein Z-dependent regulation of coagulation. *Thromb. Haemast.* **86,** 8–13.

---

[57] The presence of blood in the urine.

Bügel, S. (2003). Vitamin K and bone health. *Proc. Nutr. Soc.* **62,** 839–843.

Butenas, S., and Mann, K.G. (2002). Blood coagulation. *Biochem.* (Moscow) **67,** 3–12.

Dahlbäck, B., and Villoutreix, B. O. (2005). The anticoagulation protein C pathway. *FEBS Letts* **579,** 3310–3316.

Denisova, N. A., and Booth, S. A. (2005). Vitamin K and sphingolipid metabolism: Evidence to date. *Nutr. Rev.* **63,** 111–121.

Dowd, P., Ham, S. W., Naganathan, S., and Hershline, R. (1995). The mechanism of action of vitamin K. *Ann. Rev. Nutr.* **15,** 419–440.

Ferland, G. (2001). Vitamin K, Chapter 15 in *Present Knowledge in Nutrition*, 8th ed. (B. A. Bowman and R. M. Russell, eds.), pp. 164–172. ILSI Press, Washington, DC.

Furie, B., Bouchard, B. A., and Furie, B. C. (1999). Vitamin K-dependent biosynthesis of γ-carboxyglutamic acid. *Blood* **93,** 1798–1808.

Greer, F. R. (1995). The importance of vitamin K as a nutrient during the first year of life. *Nutr. Res.* **15,** 289–310.

Heaney, R. P. (1993). Nutritional factors in osteoporosis. *Annu. Rev. Nutr.* **13,** 287–316.

Kohlmeier, M., Salomon, A., Saupe, J., and Shearer, M. J. (1996). Transport of vitamin K to bone in humans. *J. Nutr.* **126,** 1192S–1196S.

Lamson, D. W., and Plaza, S. M. (2003). The anticancer effects of vitamin K. *Alt. Med. Rev.* **8,** 303–318.

Nelsestuen, G. L., Shah, A. M., and Harvey, S. B. (2000). Vitamin K-dependent proteins. *Vit. Hormones* **58,** 355–389.

Shearer, M. J. (1995). Vitamin K. *Lancet* **345,** 229–234.

Shearer, M. J., Bach, A., and Kohlmeier, M. (1996). Chemistry, nutritional sources, tissue distribution and metabolism of vitamin K with special references to bone health. *J. Nutr.* **126,** 1181S–1186S.

Stafford, D. W. (2005). The vitamin K cycle. *J. Thrombosis Haemostasis* **3,** 1873–1878.

Suttie, J. W. (2006). Vitamin K, Chapter 22, in Modern Nutrition in Health and Disease, 10th ed. (M. E. Shils, M. Shike, A. C. Ross, B. Caballero, and R. J. Cousins, eds.), pp. 412–425. Lippincott, New York.

Uprichard, J., and Perry, D. J. (2002). Factor X deficiency. *Blood Rev.* **16,** 97–110.

Vermeer, C., Shearer, M. J., Zitterman, A., Bolton-Smith, C., Szulc, P., Hodges, S., Walter, P., Rambeck W., Stöcllin, E., and Weber, P. (2004). Beyond deficiency: potential benefits of increased intakes of vitamin K for bone and vascular health. *Eur. J. Nutr.* **43,** 325–335.

Weber, P. (2001). Vitamin K and bone health. *Nutr.* **17,** 880–887.

Zipursky, A. (1999). Prevention of vitamin K deficiency bleeding in newborns. *Br. J. Haematol.* **104,** 430–437.

Vitamin C

I still had a gram or so of hexuronic acid. I gave it to [Svirbely] to test for vitaminic activity. I told him that I expected he would find it identical with vitamin C. I always had a strong hunch that this was so but never had tested it. I was not acquainted with animal tests in this field and the whole problem was, for me, too glamorous, and vitamins were, to my mind, theoretically uninteresting. "Vitamin" means that one has to eat it. What one has to eat is the first concern of the chef, not the scientist. Anyway, Svirbely tested hexuronic acid … after one month the result was evident: hexuronic acid was vitamin C.

—A. Szent-Györgyi

I.	The Significance of Vitamin C	236
II.	Sources of Vitamin C	236
III.	Absorption of Vitamin C	239
IV.	Transport of Vitamin C	240
V.	Metabolism of Vitamin C	241
VI.	Metabolic Functions of Vitamin C	243
VII.	Vitamin C Deficiency	254
VIII.	Pharmacological Uses of Vitamin C	257
IX.	Vitamin C Toxicity	258
X.	Case Studies	260
	Study Questions and Exercises	262
	Recommended Reading	263

Anchoring Concepts

1. Vitamin C is the generic descriptor for all compounds exhibiting qualitatively the biological activity of ascorbic acid.
2. Vitamin C-active compounds are hydrophilic and have an oxidizable/reducible 2,3-enediol grouping.
3. Deficiencies of vitamin C are manifest as connective tissue lesions (e.g., capillary fragility, hemorrhage, muscular weakness).

Learning Objectives

1. To understand the nature of the various sources of vitamin C.
2. To understand the means of vitamin C synthesis by most species.
3. To understand the means of enteric absorption and transport of vitamin C.
4. To understand the functions of vitamin C in connective tissue metabolism, in drug and steroid metabolism, and in mineral utilization.
5. To understand the physiologic implications of low and high intakes of vitamin C.

Vocabulary

Antioxidant
Ascorbate polyphosphate
Ascorbic acid
L-Ascorbic acid 2-sulfate
Ascorbyl free radical
Carnitine
Cholesterol 7α-hydroxylase
Collagens
Dehydroascorbic acid
Dehydroascorbic acid reductase
Dopamine β-monooxygenase
Elastin
Glucose transporters (GLUTs)
Glucuronic acid pathway
Guinea pig
L-Gulonolactone oxidase
Histamine
Homogentisate 1,2-dioxygenase
Hydroxylysine
4-Hydroxyphenylpyruvate
Hydroxyproline
Hypoascorbemia
Indian fruit bat
Insulin
Iron
Lysyl hydroxylase
Moeller–Barlow disease
Monodehydroascorbate
Monodehydroascorbate reductase
Oxalic acid
Peptidylglycine α-amidating monooxygenase
Petechiae
Prooxidant
Red-vented bulbul

L-Saccharoascorbic acid
Scurvy
Sodium-dependent vitamin C transporters (SVCTs)
Systemic conditioning
Tropoelastin
Tyrosine
Vitamin C

I. The Significance of Vitamin C

Vitamin C is required by only a few species, which, by virtue of a single enzyme deficiency, cannot synthesize it. For most species, *ascorbic acid* is a normal metabolite of glucose, but it is not an essential dietary constituent. Whether or not it is synthesized, ascorbic acid is important for several physiological functions. Many, if not all, of these functions involve redox characteristics that allow ascorbic acid to play an important role, along with α-tocopherol, reduced glutathione, and other factors, in the antioxidant protection of cells. Thus, ascorbic acid represents the major water-soluble antioxidant in plasma and tissues. As such, it is thought to support the redox recycling of α-tocopherol, the bioavailability of nonheme iron, and the maintenance of enzyme-bound metals in oxidation states appropriate for several enzymatic functions. It is fairly well established that compromises of these effects underlie the pathophysiology of vitamin C deficiency. Other beneficial health effects of ascorbic acid have been reported: reductions in hypertension, atherogenesis, diabetic complications, colds and other infections, and carcinogenesis. Although some of these claims have become widely accepted, the empirical evidence remains incomplete for many.

II. Sources of Vitamin C

Distribution in Foods

Vitamin C is widely distributed in both plants and animals, occurring mostly (80–90%) as **ascorbic acid** but also as **dehydroascorbic acid**. The proportions of both species tend to vary with food storage time, owing to the time-dependent oxidation of ascorbic acid. Fruits, vegetables,[1] and organ meats (e.g., liver and kidney) are generally the best sources; only small amounts are found in muscle meats (Table 9-1). Plants synthesize L-ascorbic acid from carbohydrates; most seeds do not contain ascorbic acid, but start to synthesize it upon sprouting. Some plants accumulate high levels of the vitamin (e.g., fresh tea leaves, some berries, guava, rose hips). For practical reasons, citrus and other fruits are good daily sources of vitamin C, as they are generally eaten raw and are, therefore, not subjected to cooking procedures that can destroy vitamin C. Processed foods, such as cured meats and some beverages, can also contain the analog, erythorbic acid,[2] which is used as a preservative. While that analog has no vitamin C activity *in vivo*, it can yield false positives in some analyses for plasma ascorbic acid.[3]

Stability in Foods

The vitamin C content of most foods decreases dramatically during storage owing to the aggregate effects of several processes by which the vitamin can be destroyed (Table 9-2). Ascorbic acid is susceptible to oxidation to dehydroascorbic acid, which itself can be irreversibly degraded by hydrolytic opening of the lactone ring to yield 2,3-diketogulonic acid, which is not biologically active. These reactions occur in the presence of O_2, even traces of metal ions, and are enhanced by heat and conditions of neutral to alkaline pH. The vitamin is also reduced by exposure to oxidases in plant tissues. Therefore, substantial losses of vitamin C can occur during storage and are enhanced greatly during cooking. For example, stored potatoes lose 50% of their vitamin C within 5 months, and 65% within 8 months of harvest. Apples and cabbage stored for winter can lose 50% and 40%, respectively, of their original vitamin C content. Losses in cooking are usually greater with such methods as boiling, because the stability of ascorbic acid is much less in aqueous solution. For example, potatoes can lose 40% of their vitamin C content by boiling. Alternatively, quick heating methods can protect food vitamin C by inactivating oxidases.

Vitamin C Bioavailability

Vitamin C in most foods appears to have biological activities comparable to those of purified L-ascorbic

---

[1] Historically, the potato was the best source of vitamin C in North America and Europe.

[2] Also referred to as D-isoascorbic acid or D-araboascorbic acid.

[3] This is not a problem for blood samples taken after an overnight fast, as erythorbic acid is cleared from the blood within 12 hr.

Table 9-1.   Vitamin C contents of some uncooked foods

Food	Vitamin C (mg/100 g)	Food	Vitamin C (mg/100 g)
Fruits		Vegetables	
Apple	10–30	Asparagus	15–30
Banana	10	Bean	10–30
Cherry	10	Broccoli	90–150
Grapefruit	40	Cabbage	30–60
Guava	300	Carrot	5–10
Hawthorn berries	160–800	Cauliflower	60–80
Melons	13–33	Celery	10
Orange, lemon	50	Collard greens	100–150
Peach	7–14	Corn	12
Raspberry	18–25	Kale	120–180
Rose hips	1000	Leek	15–30
Strawberry	40–90	Oat, wheat	0
Tangerine	30	Onion	10–30
Animal products		Pea	10–30
Meats	0–2	Parsley	170
Liver	10–40	Pepper	125–200
Kidney	10–40	Potato	10–30
Milk		Rhubarb	10
Cow	1–2	Rice	0
Human	3–6	Spinach	50–90

acid at doses in the nutritional range (15–200 mg). At higher doses bioavailability declines; doses greater than 1000 mg appear to be utilized with roughly 50% efficiency. Because dehydroascorbic acid can be reduced metabolically to yield ascorbic acid (after enteric absorption and subsequent cellular uptake), both forms present in foods have vitamin activity.

Table 9-2.   Two-day storage losses of vitamin C

Food	Percentage lost at:	
	4°C	20°C
Beans	33	53
Cauliflower	8	26
Lettuce	36	42
Parsley	13	70
Peas	10	36
Spinach	32	80
Spinach (winter)	7	22

Several synthetic ascorbic acid derivatives also have vitamin C activity and offer advantages of superior chemical stability. Forms, such as ascorbate 2-sulfate, ascorbate 2-monophosphate, ascorbate 2-diphosphate, and ascorbate 2-triphosphate (mixtures of the latter three are referred to as **ascorbate polyphosphate**), are useful as vitamin C supplements for fish diets where the intrinsic instability of ascorbic acid in aqueous environments is a problem. The more highly biopotent of these vitamers appear to be effectively hydrolyzed in the digestive tract and tissues to yield ascorbic acid (Table 9-3).

Biosynthesis of Ascorbic Acid

In addition to probably all green plants, most higher animal species can synthesize vitamin C (Table 9-4), which they make from glucose via the **glucuronic acid pathway**. The enzymes of this pathway are localized in the kidneys of amphibians, reptiles, and the more primitive orders of birds, but they occur in

Table 9-3. Vitamin C-active derivatives of ascorbic acid

Strong biopotency[a]	Weak biopotency[b]
Ascorbic acid 2-O-α-glucoside	L-Ascorbyl palmitate
6-Bromo-6-deoxy-L-ascorbic acid	L-Ascorbyl-2-sulfate
L-Ascorbate 2-phosphate	L-Ascorbate-O-methyl ether
L-Ascorbate 2-triphosphate	

[a]More than 50% of antiscorbutic activity of ascorbic acid.
[b]Less than 50% of antiscorbutic activity of ascorbic acid.

Table 9-4. Estimated rates of ascorbic acid biosynthesis in several species

Species	Synthetic rate (mg/kg body weight)	$T_{1/2}$[a] (days)	Turnover (%/day)
Mouse	125	1.4	50
Golden hamster	20	2.7	26
Rat	25	2.6	26
Rabbit	5	3.9	18
Guinea pig	0	3.8	18
Human	0	10–20	3

[a]Half-life in the body.

the livers of passerine birds and mammals. Egg-laying mammals synthesize ascorbic acid only in their kidneys, and many marsupials use both their liver and kidneys for this purpose. The transfer of ascorbic acid synthesis from the kidney to the larger liver has been interpreted as an evolutionary adaptation that provided increased synthetic capacity of the larger organ to meet the increased needs associated with homeothermy.

The biosynthesis of ascorbic acid may not occur early in fetal development and can be inhibited by deficiencies of vitamins A and E and biotin. It can be stimulated under conditions of glycogen breakdown, and by certain drugs (e.g., barbiturates, aminopyrine, antipyrine, chlorobutanol) and carcinogens (e.g., 3-methylcholanthrene, benzo-α-pyrene). The stimulation of ascorbic acid biosynthesis that occurs owing to exposure to xenobiotic compounds appears to be due to a general induction of the enzymes of the glucuronic acid pathway, which produces glucuronic acid for conjugating foreign compounds as a means of their detoxification (Fig. 9-1).[4]

Enzyme Deficiency Causes Dietary Need

In the course of evolution, some animal groups appear to have lost the capacity for ascorbic acid biosynthesis.[5] This involves the lost expression of the last enzyme in the biosynthetic pathway, **L-gulonolactone oxidase,**[6,7] the microsomal flavoenzyme that catalyzes the oxidation of L-gulonolactone to L-2-ketogulonolactone, which yields L-ascorbic acid by spontaneous isomerization. Although all species studied appear to have the gene, in some it is so highly mutated[8] that it yields no gene product. The loss of this single enzyme renders ascorbic acid, an otherwise normal

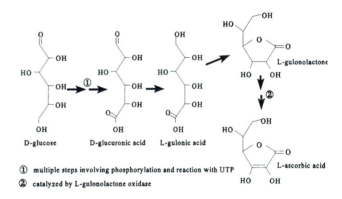

① multiple steps involving phosphorylation and reaction with UTP
② catalyzed by L-gulonolactone oxidase

Fig. 9-1. Biosynthesis of ascorbic acid.

---

[4] Because ascorbic acid synthesis and excretion are increased by exposure to xenobiotic inducers of hepatic, cytochrome P-450-dependent, mixed-function oxidases (MFOs), it has been suggested that the urinary ascorbic acid concentration may be useful as a noninvasive screening parameter of MFO status.

[5] That insects and other invertebrates are incapable of synthesizing L-gulono-1,4-lactone suggests that they do not synthesize ascorbic acid.

[6] This has been established for primates, guinea pigs, and fruit bats; whether the loss of this enzyme activity is the basis of the inabilities of other species to synthesize ascorbic acid is still speculative.

[7] The vitamin C deficiency results from the loss of this enzyme as indicated by the fact that enzyme replacement by injection with the substrate, L-gulonolactone, prevents scurvy in guinea pigs.

[8] This may be due to the presence of retrovirus-like sequences, which have been identified in the human gene, that may have caused the activation of the gene. It has been suggested that mutations in this gene may have been driven by disadvantageous effects of H_2O_2 generated during the oxidation of gulono-1,4-lactone.

metabolite, a vitamin. This occurs in invertebrates, most fishes,[9] and a few species of birds (e.g., **red-vented bulbul**[10]) and mammals (humans, other primates, **guinea pigs, Indian fruit bat**). A mutant strain (ODS-*od/od*) of rat[11] that does not synthesize ascorbic acid has been identified, and it has been said that individual humans and guinea pigs can perform this synthesis. **Scurvy** in humans can correctly be considered a congenital metabolic disease, **hypoascorbemia**. It is apparent that even the species capable of producing this key enzyme may not express it early in development. For example, the fetal rat has been found incapable of ascorbic acid biosynthesis until day 16 of gestation. This developmental lag may account for the perinatal declines in tissue ascorbic acid concentrations that have been observed in the species experimentally.

III. Absorption of Vitamin C

Species without Dietary Needs: Passive Uptake

Species that can synthesize ascorbic acid do not active transport mechanisms. They absorb ascorbic acid strictly by passive diffusion.

Species with Dietary Needs: Active Uptake

Species that do not synthesize ascorbic acid (e.g., humans, guinea pigs) absorb the vitamin by passive diffusion important at high doses, as well as by saturable, carrier-mediated, active transport mechanisms important at low doses. Thus, the efficiency of absorption of physiological doses (e.g., ≤ 180 mg/day for a human adult) of vitamin C is high, 80–90%, and declines markedly at vitamin C doses greater than about 1 g.[12] The reduced and oxidized forms of the vitamin are absorbed by different mechanisms of active transport that occur throughout the small intestine:

- *Ascorbic acid uptake by the sodium-dependent vitamin C transporter (SVCT)*[13]   This carrier moves L-ascorbic acid by an electrogenic, Na+ dependent process with a stoichiometric ratio of two Na^+ ions per ascorbic acid molecule that is inhibited by aspirin.[14] Two isoforms have been identified, SVCT1 and SVCT2, each of which has multiple potential N-glycosylation and protein kinase C (PKC) phosphorylation sites, suggesting regulation via glycosylation and/or PKC pathways. In the absence of ascorbic acid, the SVCTs can facilitate the unitransport of Na^+, allowing that ion to leak from cells. The SVCTs are noncompetitively inhibited by flavonoids. There is evidence that the expression of SVCT1 may be reduced by exposure to high levels of ascorbic acid, at least *in vitro*.[15]
- *Dehydroascorbic acid uptake by glucose transporters*   The uptake of dehydroascorbic acid is 10- to 20-fold faster than that of ascorbic acid[16] and involves isoforms of the glucose transporter, GLUT1,[17] GLUT3, and perhaps GLUT4 as well. Upon entry into the cell, dehydroascorbic acid is quickly reduced to ascorbic acid, probably by glutaredoxine reductase and/or reduced glutathione (GSH).

---

[9] Although some fish appear to be able to synthesize ascorbic acid, only the carp and Australian lungfish appear to be able to do so at rates sufficient to meet their physiologic needs.

[10] The bulbuls (Pycnonotidae) comprise 13 genera and 109 species distributed in Africa, Madagascar, and southern Asia. While the red-vented bulbul is often cited as being unable to biosynthesize ascorbic acid, it is not known how widely distributed the dietary need for vitamin C is in this family as well as in the class Aves.

[11] Derived from the Wistar strain.

[12] The efficiency of vitamin C absorption declines from about 75% of a 1-g dose, to about 40% of a 3-g dose and about 24% of a 5-g dose; net absorption plateaus at 1–1.2 g at doses of at least 3 g.

[13] These are members of the SLC23 human gene family.

[14] For example, in humans a 900-mg dose of aspirin blocks the expected rises in plasma, leukocyte, and urinary levels of ascorbic acid owing to a simultaneous dose of 500 mg of vitamin C.

[15] MacDonald, L. (2002). *Br. J. Nutr.* **87**, 97–100.

[16] Studies with cultured cells have shown that D-isoascorbic acid has only 20–30% of the activity of L-ascorbic acid in stimulating collagen production. The basis of this difference involves the much slower cellular uptake of the D-form, as, once inside the cell, both vitamers behaved almost identically.

[17] Congenital deficiency of GLUT1, a rare condition, is manifest in infancy as seizures and delayed development, presumably due to insufficient supply of glucose to the brain.

Transport of Ascorbic to the Plasma

It is not known how ascorbic acid is transported out of epithelial cells and into the plasma, although it has been suggested that it diffuses through volume-sensitive anion channels in the basolateral membrane.

IV. Transport of Vitamin C

Transport Predominantly in Reduced Form

Vitamin C is transported in the plasma predominantly (80–90%) in the reduced form, ascorbic acid. Also present are small amounts of dehydroascorbic acid, which are thought to be formed by oxidation of ascorbic acid by diffusible oxidants of cellular origin (Fig. 9-2). Plasma ascorbic acid shows a sigmoid relationship with the level of vitamin C intake, saturation in humans being achieved at daily doses of 1000 mg or more.[18] Plasma ascorbic acid levels in healthy humans are typically 30–70 µmol/L and appear to be affected by body fat distribution[19] by mechanisms that may relate to its being a marker for the intake of vitamin C-rich fruits and vegetables.

Cellular Uptake by the Same Mechanisms

Simple diffusion of ascorbic acid and dehydroascorbic acid into cells is negligible owing to the charge of ascorbic acid, which is ionized under physiological conditions, and the oil:water partitioning characteristics of dehydroascorbic acid, which excludes it from lipid bilayers. Nevertheless, cells accumulate in ascorbic acid to levels 5- to 100-fold those of plasma. Human cells become saturated at intakes of about 100 mg/day. The mechanisms of cellular uptake of vitamin C are the same as those responsible for its enteric absorption (Fig. 9-2):

- *Ascorbic acid uptake by sodium-dependent vitamin C transporters (SVCT1 and SVCT2)*   SVCT1 is expressed in epithelial tissues including the intestine,

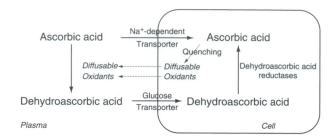

Fig. 9-2.   Redox cycling of ascorbic acid.

liver, and kidney; SVCT2 is expressed in brain, lung, heart, eye, and placenta, in neuroendocrine and exocrine tissues, and in endothelial tissues.
- *Dehydroascorbic acid transport by glucose transporters (GLUT1, GLUT3, GLUT4)*   By interacting at the level of these transporters, **insulin** can promote the cellular uptake of dehydroascorbic acid. By competing for uptake by the transporter, physiological levels of glucose can inhibit dehydroascorbic acid uptake by several cell types (adipocytes, erythrocytes, granulose cells, neutrophils, osteoblasts, and smooth muscle cells). Thus, diabetic patients can have abnormally high plasma levels of dehydroascorbic acid.[20]

Tissue Distribution

Nearly all tissues accumulate vitamin C, including some that lack ascorbic acid-dependent enzymes (Table 9-5). Certain cell types (e.g., peripheral mononuclear leukocytes) can accumulate concentrations as great as several millimolar. Tissue levels are decreased by virtually all forms of stress, which also stimulates the biosynthesis of the vitamin in those animals able to do so.[21] The concentration of ascorbic acid in the adrenals is very high (72–168 mg/100 g in the cow); approximately one-third of the vitamin is concentrated in the reduced form at the site of catecholamine formation in those glands, from which it is released with newly synthesized corticosteroids in response to stress.[22] The ascorbic

---

[18] Levine, M., et al. (1996). *Proc. Natl. Acad. Sci. U.S.A.*, **93**, 14344–14348, found that 200 mg/day doses produced only 80% saturation and that RDA-level doses supported plasma ascorbic acid concentrations on the lower third of the response curve.

[19] Plasma ascorbic acid levels were inversely related to waist-to-hip ratio and to waist and hip circumferences but not to body mass index in a large European cohort (Canoy, D., et al. [2005]. *Am. J. Clin. Nutr.* **82**, 1203–1209).

[20] In fact, it is thought that the impaired cellular uptake of vitamin C, owing to competition with glucose, may be one of the causes of pathology in diabetes.

[21] The ascorbic acid content of brown adipose tissue of rats has been found to increase by about 60% during periods of cold stress.

[22] That is, in response to the release of adrenocorticotropic hormone (ACTH).

Table 9-5. Ascorbic acid concentrations of human tissues

Tissue	Ascorbic acid (mg/100 g)
Adrenals	30–40
Pituitary	40–50
Liver	10–16
Thymus	10–15
Lungs	7
Kidneys	5–15
Heart	5–15
Muscle	3–4
Brain	3–15
Pancreas	10–15
Lens	25–31
Plasma	0.4–1

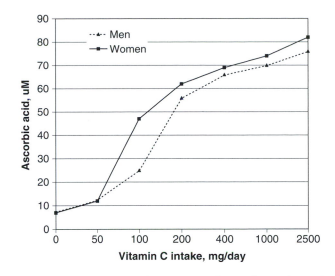

Fig. 9-3. Relationship of plasma ascorbic acid (steady-state) level and vitamin C intake. (*From* Levine, M., et al. [2001]. *Proc. Nat. Acad. Sci. USA* **98**, 9842–9846.)

acid concentration of brain tissue also tends to be high (5–28 mg/100 g); the greatest concentrations are found in regions that are also rich in catecholamines. Brain ascorbic acid levels are among the last to be affected by dietary deprivation of vitamin C in those animals unable to synthesize the vitamin. A relatively large amount of ascorbic acid is also found in the eye, where it is thought to protect critical sulfhydryl groups of proteins from oxidation.[23] The levels of ascorbic acid in plasma reach plateaus at vitamin C doses greater than 2 g/day (Fig. 9-3). White blood cells show similar thresholds, with lymphocytes, platelets, monocytes, and neutrophils showing decreasing plateau levels in that order.[24] Blood cells contain a substantial fraction of the ascorbic acid in the blood; of these, leukocytes have particular diagnostic value, as their ascorbic acid concentrations are regarded as indicative of tissue levels of the vitamin.[25] There is no stable reserve of vitamin C; excesses are quickly excreted. At saturation, the total body pool of the human has been estimated to be 1.5–5 g,[26] the major fractions being found in the liver and muscles by virtue of their relatively large masses.

V. Metabolism of Vitamin C

Oxidation

Ascorbic acid is oxidized *in vivo* by two successive losses of single electrons (Fig. 9-4). The first monovalent oxidation results in the formation of the **ascorbyl free radical**;[27] the ascorbyl radical forms a reversible electrochemical couple with ascorbic acid but can be further oxidized irreversibly to dehydro-L-ascorbic acid.

Subsequent irreversible hydrolysis of dehydroascorbic acid yields 2,3-diketo-L-gulonic acid, which undergoes either decarboxylation to CO_2 and five-carbon fragments (xylose, xylonic acid, lyxonic acid), or oxidation to **oxalic acid** and 4-C fragments

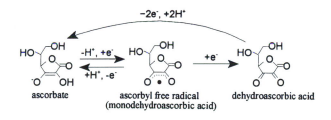

Fig. 9-4. Oxidation-reduction reactions of vitamin C.

---

[23] Lenses of cataract patients have lower lens ascorbic acid concentrations (e.g., 0–5.5 mg/100 g) than those of healthy patients (e.g., 30 mg/100 g).

[24] Levine, M., et al. (2001). *Proc. Nat. Acad. Sci. USA* **98**, 9842–9846.

[25] Leukocyte ascorbic acid concentrations are usually greater in women than in men and normally decrease with age and in some diseases.

[26] The first signs of scurvy are not seen until this reserve is depleted to 300–400 mg.

[27] The ascorbyl radical is also called monodehydroascorbic acid; it is relatively stable, with a rate constant for its decay of about $10^5\ M^{-1}\ sec^{-1}$.

(e.g., threonic acid). In addition, the formation of **L-ascorbic acid 2-sulfate** from ascorbic acid occurs in humans, fishes, and perhaps rats, and the oxidation of the 6-position carbon (C-6) of ascorbic acid to form **L-saccharoascorbic acid** has been demonstrated in monkeys.

Ascorbic acid may also undergo oxidation by reaction with tocopheroxyl or urate radicals (Fig. 9-5). The former interaction, which is discussed in detail in Chapter 7, remains poorly supported by *in vivo* evidence.

Ascorbic Acid Regeneration

Ascorbic acid can also be regenerated in three ways:

- *By recycling of the ascorbic acid-dehydroascorbic acid redox couple*   Because dehydroascorbic acid can be reduced only by intracellular dehydroascorbic acid reductases, the presence of an uptake system specific for the oxidized form effectively establishes a redox cycle whereby plasma intracellular levels of the reduced vitamin are maintained for such functional purposes as the quenching of oxidants (Fig. 9-2). This system may be important in the ascorbate-stimulation of osteoid-forming activity of osteoblasts through the generation by osteoclasts of reactive oxygen species that oxidize ascorbic acid extracellularly. The existence of multiple **dehydroascorbic acid reductase** activities would appear to promote a favorable ascorbate redox potential, indirectly preserving other antioxidants (e.g., tocopherol). That the NADPH-dependent enzyme is found in the intestinal mucosa suggests that this function

may be important in protecting against the many radical species generated there. Although dehydroascorbate appears to have no metabolic function per se, its regeneration to ascorbic renders it biologically active. Impairments in this recycling can occur in uncontrolled diabetes due to excessive plasma glucose, which competes with dehydroascorbic acid for cellular uptake by **glucose transporters**. Reduced cellular uptake of dehydroascorbic acid can lead to diminished intracellular ascorbic acid levels, weakening antioxidant defenses in diabetes.

- *By GSH or dihydrolipoic acid reduction of dehydroascorbic acid*   Dehydroascorbate can react directly with the reduced forms of glutathione (GSH) or lipoic acid (dihydrolipoic acid).

- *By enzymatic reduction of ascorbyl radical*   This is catalyzed by the widely distributed enzyme, semidehydroascorbyl reductase, which uses NADPH as a source of reducing equivalents.

Excretion

Ascorbate is thought to pass unchanged through the glomeruli and to be actively reabsorbed in the tubules by a saturable, carrier-mediated process. Little, if any, ascorbic acid is excreted in the urine of humans consuming less than 100 mg/day and only one-fourth of the dose is excreted at twice that intake. At doses greater than about 500 mg/day (i.e., when blood ascorbic acid concentrations exceed 1.2–1.8 mg/dl), virtually all ascorbic acid above that level is excreted unchanged in the urine, thus producing no further increases in body ascorbate stores. The fractional excretion of a parenteral dose of ascorbic acid approaches 100% at doses greater than 2 g.

The epithelial cells of the renal tubules reabsorb dehydroascorbic acid after it has been filtered from the plasma. Animal species vary in their routes of disposition of dehydroascorbic acid. Guinea pigs and rats degrade it almost quantitatively to CO_2,[28] which is lost across the lungs. Humans, however, normally degrade only a very small amount via that route,[29] excreting the vitamin primarily as various urinary metabolites (mostly ascorbic acid, dehydroascorbic acid, and diketogulonic acid, with small amounts of oxalate and ascorbate 2-sulfate).

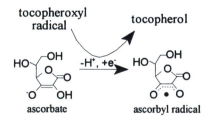

Fig. 9-5. Coupling of ascorbate oxidation to reduction of tocopheroxyl radical.

---

[28] The C-1 carbon of ascorbic acid is the main source of CO_2 derived from the vitamin, whereas C-1 and C-2 are the precursors of oxalic acid.

[29] Degradation by this path is increased greatly in some diseases and can then account for nearly half of ascorbic acid loss.

Humans convert only 1.5% of ingested ascorbic acid to oxalic acid within 24 hours. Nevertheless, the excretion of oxalate is relevant to risk of renal stone formation. It is estimated that, of the oxalate excreted daily (e.g., 30 to 40 mg) by humans consuming physiological amounts of vitamin C, 35 to 50% comes from ascorbic acid degradation (the balance coming from glycine and glyoxylate). Not all humans show increased urinary oxalate excretion in response to ascorbic acid supplementation; about 40% of adults consuming very high doses (1000 mg/day) of vitamin C increased their urinary oxalate levels by more than 16% (Table 9-6). However, as oxalate excretion is not a useful indicator of risk of renal calculi (e.g., a comparison of 75 patients with renal calculi and 50 healthy controls showed the same average oxalate excretion of about 28 mg/day), and as the contributions of high doses of vitamin C to oxalate formation are rather small, the physiological implications of these effects are unclear.

Ascorbic acid is also excreted in the gastric juice, which typically has levels three times that of plasma. Notable exceptions are in patients with atrophic gastritis or *Helicobacter pylori* infection, which shows low gastric juice ascorbic acid.[30]

VI. Metabolic Functions of Vitamin C

Varied Roles

In its various known metabolic functions, vitamin C as ascorbic acid serves as a classic enzyme cofactor (e.g., at the active site of hydroxylating enzymes), as a protective agent (e.g., of hydroxylases in collagen biosynthesis), and as ascorbyl radical in reactions with transition metal ions. Each of these functions of the vitamin appears to involve its redox properties.

Electron Transport

Ascorbic acid loses electrons easily, and, because of its reversible monovalent oxidation to the ascorbyl radical, it can serve as a biochemical redox system.[31] As such, it is involved in many electron transport reactions; these include reactions involved in the synthesis of collagen, the degradation of **4-hydroxyphenylpyruvate**,[32] the synthesis of norepinephrine,[33] and the desaturation of fatty acids. In many of these functions ascorbate is not required per se; that is, it can be replaced by other reductants.[34] However, ascorbate is the most effective *in vitro*. In each, ascorbic acid is regenerated, as the electron acceptor ascorbyl radical is reduced by either of two microsomal enzymes — monodehydroascorbate reductase or ascorbate–cytochrome-b_5 reductase — the latter being part of the fatty acid desaturation system.

Antioxidant Functions

Ascorbic acid can act as an **antioxidant** owing to its ability to react with free radicals, undergoing a single-electron oxidation to yield a relatively poor reactive intermediate, the ascorbyl radical, which disproportionates to ascorbate and dehydroascorbate. Thus, ascorbic acid can reduce toxic, reactive oxygen species

Table 9-6.   Effect of high-level ascorbic acid supplementation on urinary oxalate excretion

Subject group(n)	Treatment[a]	Oxalate, μmoles
Responders (19)	Control	513 ± 97
	Ascorbic acid, 1000 mg/d	707 ± 165[b]
Nonresponders (29)	Control	560 ± 110
	Ascorbic acid, 1000 mg/d	551 ± 129[c]

[a]Each subject experienced alternating 6-day control and ascorbic acid treatments.
[b]Significantly different ($p < 0.05$) from control treatment within responder group.
[c]Significantly different ($p < 0.05$) from other responder group on same treatment.
Source: Massey, L. K., et al. (2005). *J. Nutr.* 135, 1673–1677.

[30] Sobala, G. M., et al. (1993). *Gut* **34,** 1038–1041.

[31] The redox potential of the dehydroascorbic acid–ascorbic acid couple is in the range of 0.06–0.1 V. But that of the ascorbyl radical–ascorbic acid couple is –0.17 V. These redox potentials result in the reduction of many oxidizing compounds.

[32] The first product of tyrosine metabolism.

[33] Noradrenaline.

[34] For example, reduced glutathione, cysteine, tetrahydrofolate, dithiothreitol, and 2-mercaptoethanol.

superoxide anion ($O_2^{\bullet-}$) and hydroxyl radical ($OH^\bullet$), as well as organic ($RO_2^\bullet$) and nitrogen ($NO_2^\bullet$) oxy radicals. Those reactions are likely to be of fundamental importance in all aerobic cells, which must defend against the toxicity of the very element depended on as the terminal electron acceptor for energy production via the respiratory chain enzymes. This type of reaction appears to be the basis of most, if not all, of the essential biological functions of ascorbic acid. One of these functions is important in extending the antioxidant protection to the hydrophobic regions of cells: ascorbic acid appears to be able to reduce the semistable chromanoxyl radical, thus regenerating the metabolically active form of the lipid antioxidant vitamin E.[35] Such quenching of oxidants protects glutathione in its reduced form (Fig. 9-6).

The antioxidant efficiency of ascorbic acid is significant at physiological concentrations of the vitamin (20 to 90 μM). Under those conditions, the predominant reaction is a radical chain-terminating one of ascorbate (AH^-) with a peroxyl radical to yield a hydroperoxide and the ascorbyl radical ($A^{\bullet-}$), which proceeds to reduce a second peroxyl radical and yield the vitamin in its oxidized form, dehydroascorbic acid (A). At low concentrations of the vitamin, 2 mol of peroxyl radical is reduced for every mole of ascorbate consumed:

$$AH^- + RO^\bullet \rightarrow A^{\bullet-} + ROO^\bullet\,(+H^+ \rightarrow ROOH)$$

$$A^{\bullet-} + R'OO^\bullet \rightarrow A + R'OO^-\,(+H^+ \rightarrow R'OOH)$$

In this way, exposure to free radicals can lead to the consumption of vitamin C. *In vitro* studies have confirmed that ascorbic acid is oxidized by free radicals in cigarette smoke.[36] This type of direct effect appears to be moderated by the presence of other antioxidants (e.g., reduced glutathione) but is exacerbated by inflammatory oxidants such as $O_2^\bullet$, H_2O_2, and hypochlorous acid (HOCl) produced by phagocytes recruited and activated in the lungs by cigarette smoke. Accordingly, by exposing themselves to a variety of highly reactive free radicals in tobacco smoke[37,38] (Figs. 9-7 and 9-8), smokers have been found to show a 40% greater turnover of ascorbic acid and higher plasma levels of lipid peroxidation products than do nonsmokers with similar vitamin C intakes.[39] Even nonsmokers exposed passively to tobacco smoke have been found to have lower circulating ascorbic acid levels than nonexposed persons.

At relatively high vitamin C concentrations, a slower radical chain-propagating reaction of ascorbyl radical and molecular oxygen appears to become significant. It yields dehydroascorbic acid and superoxide

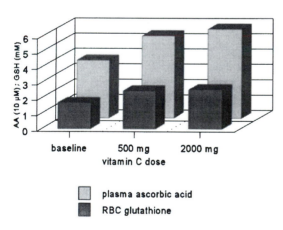

Fig. 9-6. Enhancement of reduced glutathione (GSH) by vitamin C in men. (*From* Johnston, S. C., et al. [1993]. *Am. J. Clin. Nutr.* **58**, 103–105.)

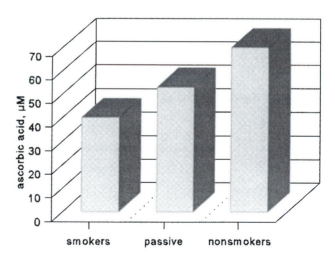
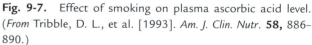

Fig. 9-7. Effect of smoking on plasma ascorbic acid level. (*From* Tribble, D. L., et al. [1993]. *Am. J. Clin. Nutr.* **58**, 886–890.)

[35] Evidence for such an effect comes from demonstrations *in vitro* of the reduction by ascorbic acid of the tocopheroxyl radical to tocopherol, as well as from findings in animals that supplemental vitamin C can increase tissue tocopherol concentrations and spare dietary vitamin E.

[36] See Eiserich, J. P. et al. (1997). In *Vitamin C in Health and Disease* (L. Packer and J. Fuchs, eds.), pp. 399–412. Marcel Dekker, New York.

[37] For example, nitric oxide ($NO^\bullet$); nitrogen dioxide ($^\bullet NO_2$); and alkyl, alkoxyl, and peroxyl radicals.

[38] Free-radical-mediated processes are thought to be involved in the pathobiology of chronic and degenerative diseases associated with cigarette smoking, for example, chronic bronchitis, emphysema, cancer, and cardiovascular disease.

[39] Smith, J. L. et al. (1987). *Ann. N.Y. Acad. Sci.* **498**, 144–151.

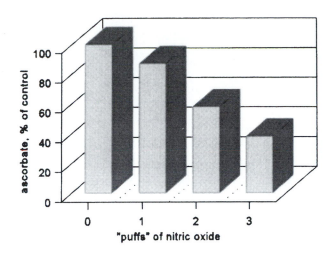

Fig. 9-8. Oxidation of ascorbic acid by nitric oxide. (*From Eiserich, J. P., et al. [1997], in Vitamin C in Health and Disease [Packer, L., and Fuchs, J., eds.], Marcel Dekker, New York, pp. 399–412.*)

radical, which in turn can oxidize ascorbate to return ascorbyl radical:

$$A^{\bullet-} + O_2 \rightarrow A + O_2^{\bullet-}$$

$$O_2^{\bullet-} + AH^- \rightarrow HOO^- + A^{\bullet-}$$

It is thought that, at high vitamin C concentrations, this two-reaction sequence can develop into a radical chain autoxidation process that consumes ascorbate, thus wasting the vitamin. Hence, in aerobic systems, the efficiency of radical quenching of ascorbate is inversely related to the concentration of the vitamin. At physiological concentrations, ascorbic acid thus serves as one of the strongest reductants and radical scavengers; it reduces oxy, nitro, and thyl radicals.

Prooxidant Potential

In the presence of oxidized metal ions (e.g., Fe^{3+}, Cu^{2+}), high concentrations of ascorbic acid can have **prooxidant** functions at least *in vitro*. It does so by donating a single electron to reduce such ions to forms

that, in turn, can react with O_2 to form oxygen radicals (the metal ions being reoxidized in the process):

$$AH^- + Fe^{3+} \rightarrow A^{\bullet-} + Fe^{2+}$$

$$Fe^{2+} + H_2O_2 \rightarrow Fe^{3+} + OH^\bullet + OH^-$$

Thus, ascorbate can react with copper or iron salts *in vitro* and lead to the formation of H_2O_2, $O_2^{\bullet-}$, and $OH^\bullet$, which can damage nucleic acids, proteins, and polyunsaturated fatty acids. Accordingly, iron–ascorbate mixtures are often used to stimulate lipid peroxidation *in vitro*, and such prooxidative reactions with transition metals are likely to be the basis of the cytotoxic and mutagenic effects of ascorbic acid observed in isolated cells *in vitro*. It has been suggested that high serum ascorbic acid may reduce Fe^{3+} in ferritin[40] to the catalytically active form Fe^{2+}.

The physiological relevance of these prooxidative reactions is unclear. Under physiological conditions, tissue concentrations of ascorbic acid greatly exceed those of dehydroascorbic acid, which greatly exceed those of ascorbyl radical. Thus, the redox potentials of the ascorbyl radical/ascorbic acid and dehydroascorbic acid/ascorbyl radical couples are sufficient for the reduction of most oxidizing compounds.

Enzyme Co-Substrate Functions

Ascorbate functions as a co-substrate for at least eight enzymes[41] that are either monooxygenases, which incorporate a single atom of oxygen into a substrate, or dioxygenases, which incorporate both atoms of molecular oxygen, each in a different way (Table 9-7).

Collagen synthesis

The best characterized metabolic role of ascorbic acid is in the synthesis of collagen proteins,[42] in which it is involved in the hydroxylation of specific prolyl and lysyl residues of the unfolded (nonhelical) procollagen chain. These reactions are catalyzed by the enzymes prolyl 4-hydroxylase, prolyl 3-hydroxylase,

---

[40] This would require that ascorbate enter the pores of the ferritin protein shell to react with **iron** on the inner surface.

[41] Three additional ascorbic acid-dependent enzymes have been identified in fungi.

[42] **Collagens,** secreted by fibroblasts and chondrocytes, are the major components of skin, tendons, ligaments, cartilage, the organic substances of bones and teeth, the cornea, and the ground substance between cells. Some 19 types of collagen have been characterized; collectively, they comprise the most abundant type of animal protein, accounting for 25 to 30% of total body protein.

Table 9-7. Enzymes that require ascorbic acid as a cosubstrate

Metabolic role	Enzyme
Collagen synthesis	Prolyl 4-hydroxylase
	Prolyl 3-hydroxylase
	Lysine hydroxylase
Carnitine synthesis	γ-Butyrobetaine 2-oxoglutarate 4-dioxygenase
	Trimethyllysine 2-oxoglutarate dioxygenase
Catecholamine synthesis	Dopamine β-monooxygenase
Peptide hormone synthesis	Peptidylglycine α-amidating monooxygenase
Tyrosine metabolism	4-Hydroxyphenylpyruvate dioxygenase

and **lysyl hydroxylase**. Each is a dioxygenase[43] that requires O_2, Fe^{2+}, and ascorbate, and each is stoichiometrically linked to the oxidative decarboxylation of α-ketoglutarate. It is thought that the role of ascorbate in each reaction is to maintain iron in the reduced state (Fe^{2+}), which dissociates from a critical region (an SH group) of the active site to reactivate the enzyme after catalysis. The post-translational hydroxylation of these procollagen amino acid residues is necessary for folding into the triple helical structure that can be secreted by fibroblasts. Hydroxyproline residues contribute to the stiffness of the collagen triple helix, and hydroxylysine residues bind (via their hydroxyl groups) carbohydrates and form intramolecular cross-links that give structural integrity to the collagen mass. The underhydroxylation of procollagen, which then accumulates[44] and is degraded, appears to be the basis of the pathophysiology of scurvy, and vitamin C-deficient subjects usually show reduced urinary excretion of hydroxyproline.

Studies have indicated some modest effects of vitamin C deficiency on the hydroxylation of proline in the conversion of the soluble **tropoelastin** to the soluble **elastin**.[45] A component of complement, C1q, resembles collagen in containing **hydroxyproline** and **hydroxylysine**. Curiously, vitamin C deprivation reduces overall complement activity but does not affect the synthesis of C1q. A role has been suggested for ascorbate in the synthesis of proteoglycans.

Catecholamine biosynthesis

Ascorbic acid has important roles in several hydroxylases involved in the metabolism of neurotransmitters, steroids, drugs, and lipids. It serves as an electron donor for **dopamine β-monooxygenase**,[46] a copper enzyme located in the chromaffin vesicles[47] of the adrenal medulla and in adrenergic synapses, that hydroxylates dopamine to form the neurotransmitter norepinephrine. In this reaction, ascorbate is oxidized to ascorbyl radical (**monodehydroascorbate**), which is returned to the reduced state by **monodehydroascorbate reductase** (Fig. 9-9).

Peptide hormone biosynthesis

A copper-dependent enzyme, **peptidylglycine α-amidating monooxygenase**, has been identified in the hypopheses of rats and cattle. It catalyzes the α-amidation of peptides and requires ascorbate and O_2. It is thought to be involved in the amidation of the C terminals of physiologically active peptides.[48] That catalase inhibits its activity *in vitro* suggests that H_2O_2 is an intermediate in the reaction.

---

[43] One-half of the O_2 molecule is incorporated into the peptidylprolyl (or peptidyllysyl) residue, and the other half is incorporated into succinate.

[44] Accumulated procollagen also inhibits its own synthesis and mRNA translation.

[45] About 1% of the prolyl residues in elastin are hydroxylated. This amount can apparently be increased by vitamin C, suggesting that normal elastin may by underhydroxylated.

[46] The specific activity of this enzyme has been found to be abnormally low in schizophrenics with anatomical changes in the brain, suggesting impaired norepinephrine and dopamine neurotransmission in those patients.

[47] These vesicles accumulate and store catecholamines in the adrenal medulla; they also contain very high concentrations of ascorbic acid (e.g., 20 mM).

[48] For example, bombesin (human gastrin-releasing peptide), calcitonin, cholecystokinin, corticotropin-releasing factor, gastrin, growth hormone-releasing factor, melanotropins, metorphamide, neuropeptide Y, oxytocin, vasoactive intestinal peptide, vasopressin.

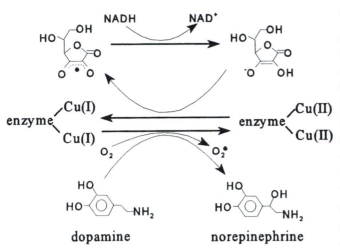

dopamine   norepinephrine

Fig. 9-9. Role of vitamin C in the conversion of dopamine to norepinephrine by dopamine-ß-monooxygenase.

Vitamin C-deficient guinea pigs showed significant increases in the half-lives of phenobarbital, acetanilid, aniline, and antipyrine. Studies in animal models have clearly demonstrated positive correlations between ascorbic acid status, hepatic activity of cytochrome *P*-450, and drug metabolism (hydroxylations, demethylations). The activities of mitochondrial and microsomal steroid hydroxylases of the adrenal have been found to be impaired in scorbutic animals, in which they respond to vitamin C therapy. In these cases, ascorbic acid appears to function as a protective antioxidant. It is thought that reduced synthesis of corticosteroids accounts for the diminished plasma glucocorticoid responses to stress of vitamin C-deficient animals.

Carnitine synthesis

Ascorbic acid is a cofactor of two Fe^{2+}-containing hydroxylases[49] involved in the synthesis of **carnitine**, which is required for the transport of fatty acids into mitochondria for oxidation to provide energy for the cell. Scorbutic guinea pigs show abnormally low carnitine levels in muscle and heart, and it is thought that the fatigue, lassitude, and hypertriglyceridemia observed in scurvy may be due to impaired formation of carnitine.

Drug and steroid metabolism

Ascorbic acid is thought to be involved in microsomal hydroxylation reactions of drug and steroid metabolism—those coupled to the microsomal electron transport chain. For example, the activity of **cholesterol 7α-hydroxylase**, the hepatic microsomal enzyme involved in the biosynthesis of bile acids, is diminished in the chronically vitamin C-deficient guinea pig and is stimulated by feeding that animal high levels of vitamin C.[50] Epidemiologic studies have detected significant positive correlations of ascorbic acid and HDL–cholesterol in the plasma/serum of free-living humans.[51]

The metabolism of drugs and other xenobiotic compounds is similarly affected by ascorbic acid.

Tyrosine metabolism

Vitamin C is involved in the oxidative degradation (which normally proceeds completely to CO_2 and water) of **tyrosine** via two mixed-function oxidases that are dependent on the presence of ascorbic acid. The first is 4-hydroxyphenylpyruvate dioxygenase, which catalyzes the oxidation and decarboxylation of the intermediate of tyrosine degradation, 4-hydroxylphenylpyruvic acid, to homogentisic acid. The second ascorbate-requiring enzyme catalyzes the next step in tyrosine degradation, **homogentisate 1,2-dioxygenase**. By impairing both reactions, vitamin C deficiency can result in tyrosinemia[52] and the excretion of tyrosine metabolites in the urine; both conditions respond to vitamin C supplements.

Nonenzymatic Functions

Ascorbic acid also serves many important physiological functions as chemical antioxidant.

Cellular antioxidation

As the most effective aqueous antioxidant in plasma, interstitial fluids, and soluble phases of cells, ascorbic

---

[49] ε-*N*-trimethyllysine hydroxylase and γ-butyrobetaine hydroxylase.

[50] Guinea pigs fed a diet of 500 mg of ascorbic acid per kilogram show substantial reductions in plasma (about 40%) and liver (about 15%) cholesterol concentrations. Human studies have been inconsistent in showing similar effects.

[51] A study of a healthy, elderly Japanese population found serum ascorbic acid to account for about 5 and 11% of the variation in serum HDL–cholesterol concentrations in men and women, respectively.

[52] Temporary tyrosinemia (serum levels > 4 mg/dl) occurs frequently in premature infants and involves reduced 4-hydroxyphenylpyruvate dioxygenase activity. Low doses of ascorbic acid usually normalize the condition.

acid appears to be the first line of defense against reactive oxygen species arising in those compartments. Those species include superoxide and hydrogen peroxide arising from activated polymorphonuclear leukocytes or other cells, and from gas-phase cigarette smoke,[53] which can promote the oxidation of critical cellular components of proteins and of DNA:

- *Prevention of lipid peroxidation* The LDL-protective action of vitamin E (see Chapter 7) appears to be dependent on the presence of ascorbic acid, which reduces the tocopheroxyl radical, thus preventing the latter from acting prooxidatively by abstracting hydrogen from a cholesteryl-polyunsaturated fatty ester to yield a peroxyl radical.
- *Prevention of protein oxidation* It is clear that, at least *in vitro*, reactive oxygen species can oxidize proteins to produce carbonyl derivatives and other oxidative changes associated with loss of function. Whether ascorbic acid provides such protection *in vivo* is, however, not clear, although this has been suggested as the basis of effects reported for vitamin C in reducing risks to cataracts and other illnesses.
- *Prevention of DNA oxidation* As a physiological antioxidant, ascorbic acid plays a role in the prevention of oxidative damage to DNA, which is elevated in cells at sites of chronic inflammation and in many pre-neoplastic lesions. In fact, the continuing attack of DNA by unquenched reactive oxygen species is believed to contribute to cancer. While most DNA damage is repaired metabolically, the frequency of elevated steady-state levels of oxidized DNA bases is estimated to be sufficient to cause mutational events.[54] The levels of one base damage product, 8-hydroxy-2′-deoxyguanosine, have been found to be elevated in individuals with severe vitamin C deficiency[55] and to be reduced by supplementation with vitamins C and E.[56]

- *Prevention of NO oxidation* Ascorbic acid protects nitric oxide (NO) from oxidation, supporting the favorable effects of nitric acid on vascular epithelial function. This appears to be the basis for the effects of high-level vitamin C intake in lowering blood pressure.

Metal ion metabolism

Ascorbic acid affects the nutritional utilization of iron and other transition elements:

- *Promotion of nonheme iron bioavailability* Ascorbic acid increases the bioavailability of iron in foods. This effect is associated with increased enteric absorption[57] (which is normally low) of the mineral; it affects both nonheme and heme iron. The effect on nonheme iron involves reduction of the ferric form of the element (Fe^{3+}), predominant in the acidic environment of the stomach, to the ferrous form (Fe^{2+}) and then forming a soluble stable chelate that stays in solution in the alkaline environment of the small intestine and is thus rather well absorbed. Studies with iron-deficient rats, which have upregulated enteric iron absorption, have shown ascorbic acid to affect the mucosal uptake of iron but not its mucosal transfer. This effect depends on the presence of both ascorbic acid and iron in the gut at the same time (e.g., the consumption of a vitamin C-containing food with the meal). Thus, the low bioavailability of nonheme iron and the iron-antagonistic effects of polyphenol- or phytate-containing foods, or of calcium phosphate, can be overcome by the simultaneous consumption of ascorbic acid.[58] Similarly, ascorbic acid administered parenterally has been found useful as an adjuvant therapy to erythropoietin in hemodialysis patients.

---

[53] Indeed, genetically scorbutic rats have been found to have elevated levels of LDL lipid peroxidation products (i.e., thiobarbituric-reactive substances, TBARS), which respond to vitamin C supplementation.

[54] About 1 per 10^5 bases (Halliwell, B. [2000]. *Am. J. Clin. Nutr.* **72**, 1082–1087).

[55] Rehman, A., et al. (1998). *Biochim. Biophys. Res. Commun.* **246**, 293–298.

[56] Moller, P., et al. (2004). *Eur. J. Nutr.* **43**, 267–274.

[57] This effect can be 200 to 600%.

[58] Anemia, much of it due to iron deficiency, is an enormous global problem, affecting more than 40% of all women. Yet, iron is the fourth most abundant element in the earth's crust, and few diets do not contain the element at least in nonheme form. The problem of iron-deficiency anemia can be viewed as one of inadequate iron bioavailability; with that in mind, it has been suggested that the problem may be better thought of as one of vitamin C inadequacy.

- *Promotion of heme-iron bioavailability*   Ascorbic acid also promotes the utilization of heme iron, which appears to involve enhanced incorporation of iron into its intracellular storage form, ferritin.[59] This effect involves facilitation of ferritin synthesis: ascorbate enhances the iron-stimulated translation of ferritin mRNA by maintaining the iron-responsive element-binding protein[60] in its enzymatically active form. Studies with cultured cells have shown that ascorbic acid also enhances the stability of ferritin by blocking its degradation through reduced lysosomal autophagy of the protein. Thus, the decline in ferritin and accumulation of *hemosiderin*[61] in scorbutic animals is reversed by ascorbic acid treatment.[62]
- *Interactions with other mineral elements*   Ascorbic acid can also interact with several other metallic elements of nutritional significance. Owing to its activity as a reductant, ascorbic acid reduces the toxicities of elements whose reduced forms are poorly absorbed or more rapidly excreted (e.g., selenium, nickel, lead, vanadium, and cadmium). High dietary levels of the vitamin have been shown to increase tissue levels of manganese but to reduce the efficiency of enteric absorption of copper.[63] The latter effect has been shown to stimulate mechanisms to preserve tissue copper stores, which are required for several enzymes, including two that require ascorbic acid as a co-substrate (dopamine β-monooxygenase, peptidylglycine α-amidating monooxygenase). Ascorbic acid can enhance the utilization of physiologic doses of selenium, increasing the apparent biologic availability of a variety of inorganic and organic forms of that essential nutrient.[64]

Health Effects

Antihistamine reactions

Ascorbic acid is involved in **histamine** metabolism, acting with Cu^{2+} to inhibit its release and enhance its degradation. It does so by undergoing oxidation to dehydroascorbic acid with the concomitant rupture of the histamine imidazole ring. In tissue culture systems, this effect results in reductions of endogenous histamine levels as well as histidine decarboxylase activities, a measure of histamine synthetic capacity. It is also thought that ascorbic acid may enhance the synthesis of the prostaglandin E series (over the F series), members of which mediate histamine sensitivity. Circulating histamine concentration is known to be reduced by high doses of vitamin C, a fact that has been the basis of the therapeutic use of the vitamin to protect against histamine-induced anaphylactic shock. Furthermore, blood histamine concentrations are elevated in several complications of pregnancy that are associated with marginal ascorbic acid status: preeclampsia,[65] abruption,[66] and prematurity. Because blood histamine and ascorbic acid concentrations were negatively correlated in women in preterm labor, it has been suggested that the combined effects of marginal vitamin C status and reduced plasma histaminase may result in the marked elevations of blood histamine levels seen in those conditions.

Immune function

Ascorbic acid has been found to affect immune function in several different ways. It can stimulate the production of interferons, the proteins that protect cells against viral attack. It can stimulate the positive

---

[59] A soluble, iron–protein complex found mainly in the liver, spleen, bone marrow, and reticuloendothelial cells. Containing 23% iron, it is the main storage form of iron in the body. When its storage capacity is exceeded, iron accumulates as the insoluble hemosiderin.

[60] This is a dual-function protein that also has aconitase activity.

[61] A dark yellow, insoluble, granular, iron-storage complex found mainly in the liver, spleen, and bone marrow.

[62] The reverse relationship is apparently not significant; that is, iron loading has been found to have no effect on ascorbic acid catabolism in guinea pigs.

[63] This effect does not appear to be significant at moderate intakes of the vitamin. A study with healthy young men found that intakes up to 605 mg/person/day for 3 weeks had no effects on copper absorption or retention, or on serum copper or ceruloplasmin concentrations (although the oxidase activity of the protein was decreased by 23% in that treatment).

[64] This effect was a surprising finding, as it is known that ascorbic acid can reduce copper compounds to insoluble forms of little or no biological value. The biochemical mechanism of the stimulation of copper bioavailability by ascorbic acid appears to involve enhanced postabsorptive utilization of copper for the synthesis of selenoproteins, perhaps by creating a redox balance of glutathione in favor of its reduced form (GSH).

[65] The nonconvulsive stage of an acute hypertensive disease of pregnant and puerperal (after childbirth) women.

[66] Premature detachment of the placenta.

chemotactic and proliferative responses of neutrophils. It can protect against free-radical-mediated protein inactivation associated with the oxidative burst[67] of neutrophils. It can stimulate the synthesis of humoral thymus factor and antibodies of the IgG and IgM classes. Some studies have found massive oral doses of the vitamin (10 g/day) to enhance delayed-type hypersensitivity responses in humans, although somewhat lower doses (2 g/day) have shown no such effects.

Phagocytic cells of the immune system produce oxidants during infections that may play some role in the appearance of signs and symptoms. Therefore, it can be expected that ascorbic acid, which is present in high concentrations in phagocytes and lymphocytes, will provide some antioxidant protection. Indeed, studies have found that vitamin C increases the proliferative responses of lymphocytes, is associated with enhanced natural killer cell activity, increases the production of interferon, and decreases viral replication in cell culture systems.

Studies have shown protective effects of vitamin C on several infectious diseases:

- *Common cold* A recent meta-analysis[68] of 29 randomized, controlled trials noted a consistent benefit of vitamin C supplementation (=200 mg/ day) in reductions of cold duration by 8% in adults and 13.5% in children (see the section Megadoses of Vitamin C below).
- *Helicobacter pylori* Randomized trials have shown that vitamin C supplementation can reduce seropositivity for *H. pylori*[69] and protect against the progression of gastric atrophy in seropositive patients.[70] This appears to be related to reduced gastric cancer risk for which *H. pylori* is a risk factor.
- *Herpes* Topical application of ascorbic acid reduced the duration of lesions as well as viral shedding in patients with *Herpes simplex* virus infections.[71]

Nevertheless, the results of studies on vitamin C and infections have been inconsistent. Some studies with scorbutic guinea pigs, fishes, and rhesus monkeys have shown vitamin C deficiency to decrease resistance to infections,[72] but several studies have yielded negative results. Studies of ascorbic acid supplementation of species that do not require the vitamin (rodents, birds) have generally shown improved resistance to infection as indicated by increased survival of infected animals, depressed parasitemia, enhanced bacterial clearance, and reduced duration of infection.

Inflammation

A large, cross-sectional study indicated that plasma ascorbic acid was negatively associated with biomarkers of inflammation (C-reactive protein) and endothelial dysfunction (tissue plasminogen activator) (Table 9-8), suggesting that the vitamin has anti-inflammatory effects associated with reduced levels of endothelial dysfunction. Nevertheless, four of five studies of vitamin C in patients reported no anti-inflammatory effects. Therefore, this putative effect of the vitamin remains the subject of investigation.

Cardiovascular disease

The antioxidant characteristics of ascorbic acid allow it to have an anti-atherogenic function in reducing the oxidation of low-density lipoproteins (LDLs), a key early event leading to atherosclerosis.[73] Being rich in both cholesterol and polyunsaturated fatty acids (PUFAs), LDLs are susceptible to lipid peroxidation by the oxidative attack of reactive oxygen species. Research has shown that oxidized LDLs stimulate the recruitment, in the subendothelial space of the vessel wall, of monocyte-macrophages that can take up the oxidized particles via scavenger

---

[67] Neutrophils, when stimulated, take up molecular oxygen (O_2) and generate reactive free radicals and singlet oxygen, which, along with other reactive molecules, can kill bacterial pathogens. This process, called the *oxidative burst* because it can be observed *in vitro* as a rapid consumption of O_2, also involves the enzymatic generation of bactericidal halogenated molecules via *myeloperoxidase*. These killing processes are usually localized in intracellular vacuoles containing the phagocytized bacteria.

[68] Douglas, R. M., et al. (2004). *Cochrane Database Syst. Rev.* **18**(4), CD000980.

[69] Simon, J. A., et al. (2003). *J. Am. Coll. Nutr.* **22**, 283–289.

[70] Sasazuki, S., et al. (2003). *Cancer Sci.* **94**, 378–382.

[71] Hamuy, R., and Berman, B. (1998). *Eur. J. Dermatol.* **8**, 310–319.

[72] For example, *Mycobacterium tuberculosis*, *Rickettsiae* spp., *Endamoeba histolytica*, and other bacteria, as well as *Candida albicans*.

[73] *Atherosclerosis* is the focal accumulation of acellular, lipid-containing material as plaques in the intima of the arteries. The subsequent infiltration of the intima by fatty substances (*arteriosclerosis*) and calcific plaques, and the consequent reduction in the vessel's lumenal cross-sectional area, result in a reduction in blood flow to the organs served by the affected vessel, causing such symptoms as *angina*, *cerebrovascular insufficiency*, and *intermittent claudication*.

Table 9-8. Relationship of vitamin C status and biomarkers of inflammation and endothelial dysfunction

| Biomarker | Quartile[a] of plasma ascorbic acid, µM | | | | |
	<14.44	14.44– < 27.11	27.11– < 40.25	= 40.25	p value
CRP,[b] mg/L	1.88 (1.73–2.03)[c]	1.73 (1.60–1.80)	1.52 (1.40–1.63)	1.34 (1.23–1.44)	<0.001
Fibrinogen, g/L	3.30 (3.26–3.36)	3.29 (3.24–3.34)	3.18 (3.13–3.23)	3.12 (3.07–3.17)	<0.001
t-PA,[d] ng/mL	10.92 (10.63–11.21)	10.66 (10.38–10.93)	10.70 (10.42–10.99)	10.31 (10.03–10.60)	0.01
Blood viscosity, mPa	3.41 (3.39–3.44)	3.41 (3.39–3.43)	3.40 (3.38–3.43)	3.35 (3.33–3.37)	<0.001

[a]3019 subjects.
[b]C-reactive protein.
[c]Mean (95% confidence interval).
[d]Tissue plasminogen activator.
Source: Wannamethee, S. G., et al. (2006). *Am. J. Clin. Nutr.* **83**, 567–574.

receptors[74] to form the lipid-containing foam cells found in the early stages of atherogenesis.

According to this view, atherogenesis can be reduced by protecting LDLs from free-radical attack. The full protection of LDLs appears to involve both ascorbic acid and vitamin E, the latter being important in quenching radicals produced within the hydrophobic interior environment of the LDL particle. That vitamin C deficiency promotes the formation of atherosclerotic lesions in guinea pigs would support the hypothesis that vitamin C can reduce atherogenic risk; however, evidence of such an effect in humans is weak at present. Subjects in the first National Health and Nutrition Examination Survey (NHANES I) with the highest vitamin C intakes showed less cardiovascular death (standardized mortality ratio, 0.66; 95% confidence limits, 0.53–0.83) than subjects with lower estimated vitamin C intakes.[75] Plasma ascorbic acid concentration was found to be highly negatively correlated with both the plasma malonyldialdehyde concentration and the values of several cardiovascular risk factors including blood pressure, total serum cholesterol, and LDL–cholesterol.[76] Similar results have been reported; however, several other large observational studies[77] have not found such relationships.

Resting blood pressure in humans has been found to be inversely related to vitamin C intake or plasma ascorbic acid concentration (Fig. 9-10), and an intervention trial found vitamin C supplementation to

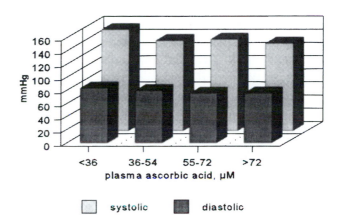

Fig. 9-10. Relationship between blood pressure and plasma ascorbic acid. (*From* Choi, E. S. K., et al. [1991]. *Nutr. Res.* **11**, 1377–1382.)

reduce blood pressure and improve arterial stiffness in patients with non–insulin-dependent diabetes. Although the metabolic basis of this relationship is still unclear, it has been suggested that ascorbic acid may serve to protect cell membrane pumps from oxidative damage in such ways as to promote ion flux and enhance the vasoactive characteristics of blood vessels. The importance of hypertension as a risk factor for cerebrovascular and coronary heart diseases makes the prospective blood pressure-lowering effects of vitamin C supplementation of considerable interest.

---

[74] Monocyte-macrophages have very few LDL receptors, and the few they have are downregulated. Therefore, when incubated with nonoxidized LDLs, they do not form foam cells as the accumulation of cholesterol further reduces LDL receptor activity. On the other hand, these cells have specific receptors for modified LDLs; these are called *scavenger receptors*. It is thought that LDL lipid peroxidation products may react with amino acid side chains of apo B to form epitopes that have affinities for the scavenger receptor.

[75] Enstrom, J. E., et al. (1992). *Epidemiol.* **5,** 255–263.

[76] Toohey, L., et al. (1996). *J. Nutr.* **126,** 121–128.

[77] For example, the National Heart Study (121,700 subjects), the Health Professionals Follow-Up Study (51,529 subjects), a prospective cohort study of 1299 subjects, and the Iowa Women's Health Study (34,486 subjects).

Cohort studies have found high vitamin C intake to be associated with reduced risk to nonfatal ischemic heart disease, and clinical trials have found vitamin C supplementation to enhance the protective effect of aspirin in reducing risk of ischemic stroke and to retard atherosclerotic progression in hypercholesterolemic patients. A recent analysis of nine prospective trials concluded that high-level vitamin C supplements reduced the incidence of major coronary heart disease.[78]

Exercise tolerance

Vigorous physical activity increases ventilation rates and produces oxidative stress, thought to be responsible for perturbations in endothelial function. Studies have shown that antioxidant supplementation can alleviate muscle damage and protein oxidation induced by exercise. That vitamin C may be especially important in such protection is indicated by the finding that vitamin C prevented acute endothelial dysfunction induced by exercise in patients with intermittent claudication[79] (calf pain during walking). This effect is likely due to the protection of nitric oxide (NO), which mediates endothelium-dependent vasodilation.

Diabetes

Diabetic patients typically show lower serum concentrations of ascorbic acid than nondiabetic, healthy controls. Accordingly, reduced serum antioxidant activity has been implicated in the pathogenesis of the disease. That vitamin C supplementation has been found to reduce the glycosylation of plasma proteins (Fig. 9-11) suggests that it may have a role in preventing diabetic complications. Controlled intervention trials have shown that vitamin C supplementation can be effective in reducing erythrocyte sorbitol accumulation[80] (Fig. 9-12) and urinary albumin excretion[81] in non–insulin-dependent diabetics, although one found no effect on microvascular reactivity.[82] Treatment with vitamin C has also been shown to prevent arterial hemodynamic changes induced by hyperglycemia.

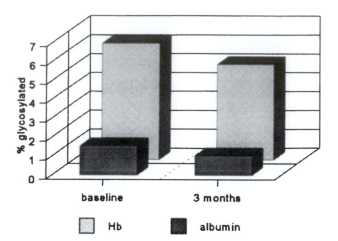

Fig. 9-11. Protein glycosylation reduced by vitamin C (1 g/day). (*From* Davie, S. J., et al. [1992]. *Diabetes* **41**, 167–173.)

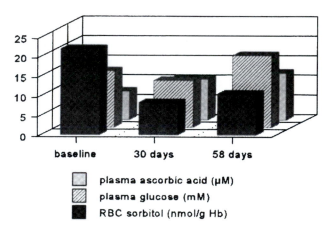

Fig. 9-12. Effects of supplemental vitamin C on patients with diabetes. (*From* Cunningham, J. J., et al. [1994]. *J. Am. Coll. Nutr.* **13**, 344–350.)

Neurologic function

The brain and spinal cord are among the richest tissues in ascorbic acid contents, with concentrations of 100–500 μM. It is estimated that 2% of the ascorbic acid in the brain turns over each hour. Plasma ascorbic acid concentrations have been shown to be positively associated with memory performance in patients that have dementia and with cognitive performance in older subjects. These relationships may

---

[78] Knekt, P., et al. (2004). *Am. J. Clin. Nutr.* **80,** 1508–1520.

[79] Silvetro, A., et al. (2002). *Atherosclerosis* **165,** 277–283.

[80] Because the sorbitol or its metabolites are thought to underlie the pathologic complications of diabetes, reduction of tissue sorbitol accumulation is a strategy for managing diabetes.

[81] Gaede, P., et al. (2001). *Diabetic Med.* **18,** 756–760.

[82] Lu, Q., et al. (2005). *Clin. Sci.* **108,** 507–513.

involve protection from inflammation, as such inflammatory mediators as cytokines and free radicals are important in the pathogenesis of neurodegenerative disease. Controlled intervention trials have not been conducted to evaluate the effects of vitamin C on cognitive function, but oral vitamin C was found to improve psychiatric rating in schizophrenics.

Pregnancy outcomes

Low vitamin C status has been shown to be associated with increased risks of gestational diabetes and premature delivery due to premature rupture of chorioamniotic membranes. The latter responded to vitamin C supplementation.[83]

Skin health

Ascorbic acid is critical for the health of the epidermis, by virtue of its essential role in collagen synthesis. It is well documented that vitamin C-deficient animals show prolonged wound-healing times. This is thought to involve their diminished rates of collagen synthesis as well as their increased susceptibility to infections. Rapid utilization of the vitamin occurs where relatively high levels of ascorbic acid accumulate at wound sites.[84] Greater concentrations of ascorbic acid appear to be required for the maintenance of wound integrity than for collagen development. Topical application of ascorbic acid has been found useful in treating photodamaged skin, as well as inflammatory conditions of the skin such as acne and eczema. That wound repair typically decreases with aging has been suggested as indicative of increasing needs for vitamin C by older individuals.

Dental health

Limited studies have found low vitamin C intake to be associated with slightly increased periodontal disease risk and amount of visible dental plaque.

Cataracts

Cataracts, involving opacification of the ocular lens, is thought to result from the cumulative photo-oxidative effects of ultraviolet light from which the lens is protected by three antioxidants: ascorbic acid, tocopherol, and reduced glutathione. The lens typically contains relatively high concentrations of ascorbic acid (e.g., as much as 30-fold those of plasma), which are lower in aged and cataractous lens.[85] Epidemiological studies have shown inverse associations of ascorbic acid status and cataract incidence (Table 9-9). Scorbutic guinea pigs have been found to develop early cataracts, and ascorbate has been shown to protect against ultraviolet light-induced oxidation of lens proteins.

Pulmonary function

Its redox properties give ascorbic acid an important role in the antioxidant protection of the lung.[86] That role is important to the functional health of that organ, which is exposed consistently to high concentrations of oxygen and inhaled toxic gases,[87] and generates reactive oxygen species via such processes as cytochrome *P*-450-dependent mixed-function oxidase

Table 9-9. Relationship of dietary vitamin C intake and risk to cataracts in humans

Quintile of vitamin C intake (mg/d)	Cataracts risk, odds ratio[a,b]
=102	1
>102–135	0.88
>135–164	0.66
>164–212	0.60
>212	0.70

[a]Ratio of cataracts incidence in each quintile group to that of the lowest (reference) quintile group.
[b]*p* value for trend, 0.04.
Source: Valero, M. P., et al. (2002). *J. Nutr.* **132**, 1299–1306.

[83] Cassaneuva, E., et al. (2005). *Am. J. Clin. Nutr.* **81,** 859–863; Borna, S., et al. (2005). *Internat. J. Gynecol. Obstet.* **90,** 16–20.

[84] Studies with apparently vitamin C-adequate burn patients have shown their plasma ascorbic acid levels to drop to nearly zero after the trauma; this is presumed to reflect the movement of the vitamin to the sites of wound repair.

[85] The ascorbic acid content of the oldest portion of the lens (the nucleus), where most senile cataracts originate, is typically only one-quarter the concentration in the lens cortex.

[86] See review by Brown, L. A. S., and Jones, D. P. (1997). In *Vitamin C in Health and Disease* (L. Packer and J. Fuchs, eds.), pp. 265–278. Marcel Dekker, New York.

[87] For example, ozone, nitric oxide, nitrogen dioxide, and cigarette smoke.

metabolism and exposure to environmental oxidants. Free radicals are also generated in the lung as a result of inflammatory cell invasion in such conditions as asthma or acute respiratory distress syndrome; affected individuals typically show lower than normal concentrations of ascorbic acid in both plasma and leukocytes.

In addition, the function of ascorbic acid in collagen synthesis makes the vitamin important in the synthesis of surfactant apoproteins, which have collagen-like domains that require ascorbic acid-dependent hydroxylation for proper folding and stability. Whether supplemental vitamin C can benefit pulmonary function is not clear. Half of the dozen clinical intervention trials of vitamin C to date have found improvements in parameters of respiratory function of asthma patients; but these studies have been very small (fewer than 160 patients in total). A meta-analysis[88] of randomized, controlled trials revealed no evidence to recommend a role of vitamin C in the management of asthma.

Cancer

Ascorbic acid has been observed to reduce the binding of polycyclic aromatic carcinogens to DNA[89] and to reduce/delay tumor formation in several animal models. This effect is thought to involve quenching of radical intermediates of carcinogen metabolism. Ascorbic acid is also a potent inhibitor of nitrosamine-induced carcinogenesis, functioning as a nitrite scavenger. This action results from the reduction by ascorbate of nitrate (the actual nitrosylating agent of free amines) to NO, thus blocking the formation of nitrosamines.[90] There is evidence that ascorbic acid, normally secreted in relatively high concentrations in gastric juice,[91] is a limiting factor in nitrosation reactions in people. This appears to be particularly true for individuals with gastric

pathologies that affect secretion. Epidemiological studies of human cancer incidence provide evidence of protective roles of vitamin C against cancers of the esophagus, larynx, oral cavity, pancreas, stomach, colon–rectum, and breast.[92] It is possible that ascorbic acid may account for at least a portion of the cancer-protective effects associated with increased intakes of fruits and vegetables.

Other studies have shown ascorbic acid treatment to increase the growth of chemically induced tumors; it has been speculated that such tumor promotion effects may involve the prooxidative characteristics of the vitamin in the presence of oxidizable iron.

Environmental stress

Vitamin C deficiency can have benefits under conditions of environmental stress in which the metabolic demands for ascorbic acid may exceed the rate of its endogenous biosynthesis. This is the case in commercial poultry production. Although the chicken does not require the vitamin in the classic sense, under practical conditions of poultry management, the species frequently benefits from ascorbic acid supplements[93] under stressful environmental conditions (e.g., extreme temperature, prevalent disease, crowding, inadequate ventilation) that stimulate depletion of ascorbic acid from adrenal glands (Table 9-10). Controlled experiments with laying hens have shown that supplemental ascorbic acid can improve egg production and eggshell characteristics in laying hens subjected to heat stress.

VII. Vitamin C Deficiency

Factors Contributing to Vitamin C Deficiency

Vitamin C deficiency can be caused by low dietary intakes, as well as by conditions in which the metabolic

---

[88] Ram, F. S., et al. (2004). *Cochrane Database Syst. Rev.* **3,** CD00993.

[89] Reactions of this type are believed to compose the molecular basis of carcinogenesis. This vitamin C effect probably involves its function as a free-radical scavenger.

[90] Vitamin E also has this effect.

[91] The concentration of ascorbic acid in gastric juice has often been found to exceed those in the plasma.

[92] Statistically significant protective effects of dietary vitamin C have been detected in two-thirds of the epidemiologic studies in which a dietary vitamin C index was calculated. In several cases, high vitamin C intake was associated with half the cancer risk associated with low intake. Protective effects have also been detected in a similarly high proportion of studies in which the intake of fruit, but not vitamin C, was assessed.

[93] For example, inclusion of 150 mg/kg in the diet.

Table 9-10. Adrenal depletion of ascorbic acid in laying hens under simulated adrenal stress

Treatment	Renal ascorbate (μg/g)	Adrenal ascorbate (μg/g)	Adrenal cholesterol (mg/g)	Adrenal corticosterone (μg/g)	Serum corticosterone (μg/liter)
Control	1.41 ± 0.10	1.02 ± 0.05	6.93 ± 0.25	18 ± 2	4.8 ± 0.4
ACTH[a]	1.14 ± 0.14[b]	0.77 ± 0.04[b]	2.57 ± 0.36[b]	32 ± 3[b]	4.4 ± 0.4
Dex[c]	1.30 ± 0.06[b]	0.82 ± 0.08[b]	8.02 ± 0.83[b]	17 ± 2	2.4 ± 0.9[b]

[a]ACTH, Adrenocorticotropic hormone, 2.5 IU/day.
[b]Significantly different ($p < 0.05$) from control value.
[c]Dex, Dexamethasone (a suppressor of adrenal corticosterone production), 50 μg/day.
Source: Rumsey, G. L. (1969). Studies of the Effects of Simulated Stress and Ascorbic Acid upon Avian Adrenocortical Function and Egg Shell Metabolism. Ph.D. Thesis. Cornell University, Ithaca, NY.

demands for ascorbic acid may exceed the rate of its endogenous biosynthesis, thus increasing the turnover of the vitamin in the body. Such conditions include smoking,[94] environmental/physical stress, chronic disease, and diabetes. Indeed, children exposed to environmental tobacco smoke show reduced plasma ascorbic acid concentrations (Table 9-11).

General Signs of Deficiency

In individuals unable to synthesize the vitamin, acute dietary C deficiency is manifest as a variety of signs in the syndrome called scurvy (Table 9-12).

Table 9-11. Effect of environmental tobacco smoke exposure on vitamin C status of children

Age (yrs)	Plasma ascorbic acid, μM[a] Unexposed	Exposed[b]
2–4	53.0 (50.2–55.8)	47.9 (44.4–51.5)
5–8	53.6 (51.4–55.8)	51.0 (48.5–53.5)
9–12	49.7 (47.4–52.0)	47.7 (45.5–49.9)

[a]Mean (95% confidence interval).
[b]A multifactorial ANOVA, with plasma ascorbic acid level adjusted for dietary vitamin C intake, showed the effect of environmental tobacco smoke exposure to be significant across all age groups, $p = 0.002$.
Source: Preston, A.M., et al. (2003). *Am. J. Clin. Nutr.* **77**, 167–172.

Table 9-12. General signs of vitamin C deficiency

Organ system	Signs
General	
Appetite	Decrease
Growth	Decrease
Immunity	Decrease
Heat resistance	Decrease
Muscular	Skeletal muscle atrophy
Vascular	
Vessels	Increased capillary fragility, hemorrhage
Nervous	Tenderness

Deficiency Signs in Humans

Classic scurvy is manifest in human adults after 45–80 days of stopping vitamin C consumption.[95] Signs of the disease occur primarily in mesenchymal tissues. Defects in collagen formation are manifested as impaired wound healing; edema; hemorrhage (due to deficient formation of intercellular substance) in the skin, mucous membranes, internal organs, and muscles; and weakening of collagenous structures in bone, cartilage, teeth, and connective tissues. Scorbutic adults may present with swollen, bleeding gums with tooth loss; but that condition may signify accompanying

[94] The ascorbic acid concentrations of serum and urine of smokers tend to be about 0.2 mg/dl less than those of nonsmokers; these effects have been observed even after correcting for vitamin C intake, which was found to be about 53 mg/day less in smokers. Furthermore, smokers have been found to have lower rates of vitamin C turnover (about 100 mg/day) than nonsmokers (about 60 mg/day). It has been estimated that smokers require 52 to 68 mg of vitamin C per day more than nonsmokers to attain comparable plasma ascorbic acid levels.

[95] Clinical signs/symptoms of scurvy in humans become manifest when the total body pool of vitamin C is reduced to less than about 300 mg, from its normal level of about 1500 mg. At that low level, patients show plasma vitamin C levels of 0.13–0.25 mg/dl (normal levels are 0.8–1.4 mg/dl).

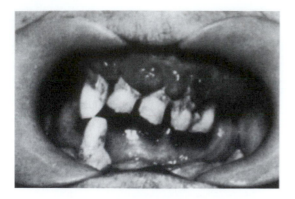

Fig. 9-13. Scurvy in a middle-aged man. Note the swollen, bleeding gums and tooth loss. (*From* J. Marks, Cambridge University.)

periodontal disease (Fig. 9-13). They also show lethargy, fatigue, rheumatic pains in the legs, muscular atrophy, skin lesions, massive sheet hematomas in the thighs, and *ecchymoses*[96] and hemorrhages in many organs, including the intestines, subperiosteal tissues, and eyes. These features are frequently accompanied by psychological changes: hysteria, hypochondria, and depression.

In children, the syndrome is called **Moeller–Barlow disease**; it is seen in non-breastfed infants usually at about 6 months of age (when maternally derived stores of vitamin C have been exhausted)[97] and is characterized by widening of bone–cartilage boundaries, particularly of the rib cage, by stressed epiphyseal cartilage of the extremities, by severe joint pain, and, frequently, by anemia and fever. Scorbutic children may present with a limp or an inability to walk, tenderness of the lower limbs, bleeding of the gums, and petechial hemorrhages. Response to vitamin C is dramatic; clinical improvements are seen within a week of vitamin C therapy.

Deficiency Signs in Animals

In guinea pigs, ascorbic acid deficiency is characterized by intermittent reductions in growth, hematomas (especially of the hind limbs), extremely brittle bones, and abnormalities of epiphyseal bone growth with calcification of bone–cartilage boundaries. Guinea pigs that are deprived of vitamin C also show reduced feed intake and growth, anemia, hemorrhages, altered dentin, and gingivitis. Continued deficiency results in disrupted protein folding and apoptosis in the liver. If not corrected, death usually occurs within 25 to 30 days. Ascorbic acid deficiency in at least some species of fishes (salmonids and carp) results in spinal curvature (scoliosis[98] and lordosis[99] [Fig. 9-14]), reduced survival, reduced growth rate, anemia, and hemorrhaging, especially in the fins, tail, muscles, and eyes. Similar signs have been reported in vitamin C-deficient shrimp and eels.

Subclinical Deficiency

Marginal vitamin status is characterized by oxidative effects in certain tissues, for example, loss of reduced glutathione in lymphocytes, and loss of α-tocopherol with accumulation of lipid peroxidation products in retinal tissues. In addition, elderly people typically show total body vitamin C pools of reduced size, perhaps owing to reduced enteric absorption and

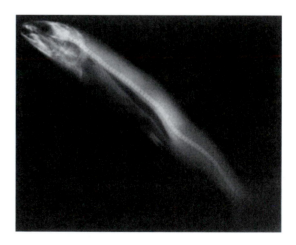

Fig. 9-14. Radiograph of a vitamin C-deficient trout showing lordosis. (*From* G. L. Rumsey, Tunnison Laboratory of Fish Nutrition, USDI.)

---

[96] Bluish patches caused by extravasation of blood into the skin (a "black-and-blue" spot); similar to petechiae except for their larger size.

[97] A retrospective study of the 28 cases diagnosed in at the Queen Sirikit National Institute of Child Health from 1995 to 2002, 93% were 1–4 years of age (Ratanachu-Ek, S., et al. [2003]. *J. Med. Assoc. Thai.* **86,** S734–S740).

[98] Lateral curvature of the spine.

[99] Anteroposterior curvature of the spine.

increased turnover. In humans, marginal vitamin C status characterized by plasma vitamin C level < 0.75 mg/dl and a total body vitamin C pool < 600 mg, results in several nonspecific, pre-scorbutic signs and symptoms: lassitude, fatigue, anorexia, muscular weakness, and increased susceptibility to infection. In the guinea pig, such conditions also result in hypertriglyceridemia, hypercholesterolemia, and decreased vitamin E concentrations in liver and lungs. Epidemiologic data indicate significant associations of low plasma ascorbic acid concentration with increased risk of ischemic heart disease or hypertension in humans.[100]

VIII. Pharmacologic Uses of Vitamin C

Despite the fact that tissue saturation of vitamin C occurs in humans at intakes of about 100 mg/day, higher intakes can result in elevated concentrations of the vitamin in extracellular fluids (plasma, connective tissue fluid, humors of the eye) where pharmacologic action of this antioxidant vitamin may be possible. Accordingly, vitamin C intakes greater than those required to prevent scurvy have been found to promote the bioavailability of dietary iron and, particularly, to counteract the negative effects of dietary fiber on the utilization of that essential mineral. Thus, gram-size doses of vitamin C have been advocated for the prophylaxis/treatment of several conditions including the common cold, *Herpes simplex*, general immune support, cardiovascular diseases, hypercholesterolemia, hypertension, hypertriglyceridemia, diabetes,[101] and some types of cancer.[102]

Most of the clinical studies in which supranutritional doses of vitamin C have been found to be of some benefit have compared treated subjects with controls who did not have tissue saturation with respect to the vitamin. Such studies, therefore, cannot indicate whether the effects of the vitamin C treatments were due simply to achieving tissue saturation or to pharmacologic actions of the vitamin in extracellular fluids. Thus, while there appear to be benefits associated with increasing vitamin C intakes to levels that effect tissue saturation, the evidence in support of benefits of vitamin C doses above that level is not clear.

"Megadose" Vitamin C for Fighting Infections

There are many uncontrolled reports of the beneficial effects of vitamin C supplementation against infections:

- *Common cold* The most widely publicized use of so-called megadoses of vitamin C are in prophylaxis and treatment of the common cold. Large doses (≥ 1 g) of vitamin C have been advocated for prophylaxis and treatment of the common cold, a use that was first proposed some 25 years ago by Dr. Irwin Stone and the Nobel laureate[103] Dr. Linus Pauling. Since that time, many controlled clinical studies have been conducted to test that hypothesis (Table 9-13). Whereas many of these have yielded positive results, until recently few have been appropriately designed with respect to blinding, controls, treatment randomization, and statistical power, to make such conclusions unequivocal. In general, most results have indicated only small positive effects in reducing the incidence, shortening the duration, and ameliorating the symptoms of the common cold.[104] A meta-analysis[105] of six large clinical trials (including more than 5000 episodes) showed no detectable effects of gram doses of vitamin C on cold incidence, but some evidence of small, protective effects in some subgroups of subjects. A more recent meta-analysis[106] of 29 randomized, controlled trials noted a consistent

---

[100] Both effects may indicate relationships of antioxidant status to these diseases, as each is also associated with relatively low status with respect to vitamin E and/or copper. In the case of hypertension, a placebo-controlled, double-blind study showed that vitamin C supplements (1 g/day for 3 months) significantly reduced systolic and diastolic pressures in borderline hypertensive subjects with normal serum ascorbic acid levels.

[101] It is thought that long-term high-plasma ascorbate concentrations may be able to overcome to some degree the competitive inhibition of transport of ascorbic acid into insulin-sensitive tissues by high blood glucose levels, and possibly to allow a reduction of insulin dosage by potentiating the action of the hormone.

[102] Dietary vitamin C appears to be able to inhibit, at least partially, gastric nitrosation of proline (and, presumably, other amines), thus reducing nitrosamine formation and the gastric cancer that it can produce.

[103] Dr. Pauling received the Nobel Prize in Chemistry in 1954 and the Nobel Peace Prize in 1962.

[104] Chalmers, T. C. (1975). *Am. J. Med.* **58**, 532–536.

[105] Hemilä, H. (1997). *Br. J. Nutr.* **77**, 59–72.

[106] Douglas, R. M., et al. (2004). *Cochrane Database Syst. Rev.* **4**, CD000980.

Table 9-13.   Large-scale, placebo-controlled clinical trials do not show vitamin C protection from colds

Study	Vitamin C (g/day)	Duration (months)	Vitamin C group		Placebo group		RR (95% CI)
			n	Colds/person/year	n	Colds/person/year	
1	1	3	407	5.5	411	5.9	0.93 (0.83–1.04)
2	1	3	339	6.7	349	7.2	0.93 (0.84–1.04)
3	3	9	101	1.7	89	1.8	0.93 (0.73–1.20)
4	2	2	331	11.8	343	11.8	1.00 (0.90–1.12)
5	1	3–6	265	1.2	263	1.2	1.03 (0.80–1.32)
6	1	3	304	8.6	311	8.0	1.08 (0.97–1.21)

Source: Hemilä, H. (1997). *Br. J. Nutr.* **77**, 59–72.

benefit of vitamin C supplementation (=200 mg/day) in reductions of cold duration by 8% in adults and 13.5% in children.

- *Other infections*   Ten of 14 randomized, controlled trials found apparent reductions in incidence,[107] and 8 of 10 have found apparent reductions in severity[108] of infections other than colds (Table 9-14).

IX. Vitamin C Toxicity

Recent reviews have identified no significant adverse effects of ascorbic acid and its various salts and esters.[109] Nevertheless, the reported benefits of gram doses of vitamin C have sustained questions concerning the safety of the vitamin. Specifically, it has been

Table 9-14.   Results of placebo-controlled, double-blinded studies of vitamin C and noncold infections

Study	Infection	Vitamin C (g/day)	Cases/total subjects		OR (95% CI)
			Vitamin C	Placebo	
		Studies of infection incidence			
1[a]	Hepatitis	3.2	6/90	8/85	0.69 (0.26–1.80)
2[b]	Pneumonia	2	1/331	7/343	0.15 (0.01–0.74)
3[c]	Bronchitis	1	8/139	13/140	0.60 (0.27–1.30)
4[c]	Pharyngitis, laryngitis, tonsillitis	1	7/139	14/140	0.48 (0.21–1.10)

Study	Infection	Vitamin C (g/day)	Studies of infection severity	Outcome value (n)	
			Outcome	Vitamin C	Placebo
5[d]	Herpes labialis	0.6	Days healing	4.21 ± 7[e] (19)	9.72 ± 8 (10)
		1.0	Days healing	4.4 ± 3.9 (19)	9.72 ± 8 (10)
6[f]	Bronchitis	0.2	Decreased score	3.4 ± 1.8 (28)	2.3 ± 2.5 (29)
7[a]	Hepatitis	3.2	SGOT units	474 ± 386 (6)	759 ± 907 (8)

Abbreviations: SGOT, Serum glutamic-oxaloacetic transaminase; now referred to as aspartate aminotransferase (ALT); an elevated value indicates the possibility of a variety of (nonhepatic) disorders. OR, Odds ratio; CI, confidence interval.
[a]Knodell, R. G., Tate, M. A., Akl, B. F., and Wilson, J. W. (1981). *Am. J. Clin. Nutr.* **34**, 20–23.
[b]Pitt, H. A., and Costrini, A. M. (1996). *J. Am. Med. Assoc.* **241**, 908–911.
[c]Ritzel, G. (1961). *Helv. Med. Acta* **28**, 63–68.
[d]Terzhalmy, T., Chakravorty, M. K., Annan, G., Habibzadeh, N., and Schorah, C. J. (1978). *Oral Surg.* **45**, 56–62.
[e]Significantly different (*p* < 0.05) from control value.
[f]Hunt, C. (1994). *Int. J. Vitam. Nutr. Res.* **64**, 212–219.

---

[107] These involved posttransfusion hepatitis, pneumonia, tuberculosis, pharyngitis, laryngitis, tonsillitis, secondary bacterial infections after a common cold episode, and rheumatic fever.

[108] These involved herpes labialis, bronchitis, tonsillitis, rubella, and tuberculosis.

[109] Hathcock, J. N., et al. (2005). *Am. J. Clin. Nutr.* **81**, 736–745; Elmore, A. R. (2005). *Int. J. Toxicol.* **24**, 51–111.

proposed that megadoses of vitamin C may increase oxalate production and thus increase the formation of renal stones, competitively inhibit the renal reabsorption of uric acid, enhance the destruction of vitamin B_{12} in the gut, enhance the enteric absorption of non-heme iron (thus leading to iron overload), produce mutagenic effects, and increase ascorbate catabolism that would persist after returning to lower intakes of the vitamin. Present knowledge indicates that most, if not all, of these concerns are not warranted.

Perhaps the greatest concern associated with high intakes of vitamin C has to do with increased oxalate production. In humans, unlike other animals, oxalate is a major metabolite of ascorbic acid, which accounts for 35–50% of the 35–40 mg of oxalate excreted in the urine each day.[110] The health concern, therefore, is that increases in vitamin C intake may lead to increased oxalate production and thus to increased risk of formation of urinary calculi. Although metabolic studies indicate that the turnover of ascorbic acid is limited and that high intakes of vitamin C, therefore, should not greatly affect oxalate production, clinical studies have revealed slight oxaluria in patients given daily multiple-gram doses of vitamin C. Whether this effect actually constitutes an increased risk of formation of renal calculi is not clear, however, as its magnitude is low and within normal variation.[111] Nevertheless, prudence dictates the avoidance of doses greater than 1000 mg of vitamin C for individuals with a history of forming renal stones.

Concerns that uricosuria might be induced by megadoses of vitamin C are based on speculation that, because both ascorbic acid and uric acid are reabsorbed by the renal tubules by saturable processes, a common transport system may be involved and thus high levels of ascorbic acid may competitively inhibit uric acid reabsorption. Experimental data, however, do not provide a basis for this concern. A recent, randomized, controlled trial with healthy subjects showed that vitamin C (500 mg/day) significantly reduced serum uric acid concentrations and increased the glomerular filtration rate.[112]

In the 1970s, it was claimed that high levels of ascorbic acid added to test meals that were held warm for 30 min resulted in the destruction (presumed to occur by chemical reduction) of food vitamin B_{12}, thus raising the concern that megadoses of vitamin C may antagonize the utilization of that important vitamin. More recent studies have not supported that claim. In fact, the only form of vitamin B_{12} that is sensitive to reduction and subsequent destruction by ascorbic acid is aquocobalamin, which is not a major form of the vitamin in foods. Furthermore, the results of another study indicate that high doses of vitamin C can, in fact, partially protect rats from vitamin B_{12} deficiency.[113] The results of several clinical investigations have shown clearly that high doses of vitamin C do not affect vitamin B_{12} status.

That ascorbic acid can enhance the enteric absorption of dietary iron has led some to express concern that megadoses of vitamin C may lead to progressive iron accumulation in iron-replete individuals (iron storage disease). Such an effect is not to be expected, however, as optimal iron absorption is effected with rather low doses of vitamin (25 to 50 mg of ascorbic acid per meal). Studies in mice have found that ascorbic acid does not enhance the prooxidative effect induced by dietary iron; nor did high parenteral doses[114] of ascorbic acid increase prooxidative biomarkers in human subjects. Nevertheless, patients with hemochromatosis or other forms of excess iron accumulation should avoid taking vitamin C supplements with their meals.

Persistent, enhanced ascorbic acid catabolism after prolonged intake of large amounts of vitamin C (so-called **systemic conditioning**) has been proposed, on the basis of uncontrolled observations of a few individuals and what is now widely regarded as erroneous interpretations of experimental results.[115] Controlled

---

[110] The balance of urinary oxalate comes mainly from the degradation of glycine (about 40% of the total), but some also can come from the diet (5–10%).

[111] Forty percent of subjects given 2 g of ascorbic acid daily showed increases in urinary oxalate excretion by more than 10% (Chai, W., et al. [2004]. *Am. J. Kidney Dis.* **44**, 1060–1069).

[112] Huang, H. Y., et al. (2005). *Arthritis Rheumatism* **52**, 1843–1847. This finding suggests that vitamin C may be beneficial in the management of gout.

[113] Rats given ascorbic acid (6 g/liter in the drinking water) showed greater hepatic vitamin B_{12} levels and lower urinary methylmalonic acid excretion, both indicators of enhanced vitamin B_{12} status, than controls.

[114] Up to 7500 mg (Mühlhöfer, A., et al. [2004]. *Eur. J. Clin. Nutr.* **58**, 1151–1158).

[115] For example, enhanced $^{14}CO_2$ excretion from guinea pigs with larger body pools of ascorbic acid was taken as evidence of greater catabolism.

studies have not consistently demonstrated such effects. Kinetic studies in humans indicate that high doses of ascorbic acid are mostly degraded to CO_2 by microbes, with major portions also excreted intact in the urine. Although such results would appear to refute the prospect of induced catabolism, a well-controlled study with guinea pigs found plasma ascorbic acid levels to drop transiently in some animals removed from high-level vitamin C treatments; the authors attributed that finding to systemic conditioning.

The suggestion that ascorbic acid might be mutagenic comes from studies with cultured cells that show a dependence on Cu^{2+} for such effects (the vitamin is not intrinsically mutagenic), which apparently involve the production of reactive oxygen radicals. No evidence of mutagenic effects *in vivo* has been produced; doses as great as 5000 mg did not induce mutagenic lesions in mice.[116]

The only consistent deleterious effects of vitamin C megadoses in humans are gastrointestinal disturbances and diarrhea. Little information is available on vitamin C toxicity in animals, although acute LD_{50} (50% lethal dose) values for most species and routes of administration appear to be at least several grams per kilogram of body weight. A single study showed mink to be very sensitive to hypervitaminosis C; with daily intakes of 100 to 200 mg of ascorbic acid, pregnant females developed anemia and had reduced litter sizes.

X. Case Studies

Instructions

Review each of the following case reports, paying special attention to the diagnostic indicators on which the treatments were based. Then answer the questions that follow.

Case 1

A 26-year-old man volunteered for a 258-day experiment of ascorbic acid metabolism. He was 184 cm tall and weighed 84.1 kg. His medical history, physical examination, vital signs, and past diet history revealed a healthy individual with no irregularities. During the experiment, his temperature, pulse, and respiration rates were recorded four times daily, and his blood pressure was measured twice daily. He was examined by an internist daily; periodically, he was examined by an ophthalmologist, and had chest radiograms and electrocardiograms made. Twenty-four-hour collections of urine and feces were made daily in order to determine urinary and fecal nitrogen, and for the radioactive assay of ascorbic acid. Samples of expired air were collected for the measurement of radioactivity.

The subject was fed a control diet consisting of soy-based products. The diet provided 2.5 mg of ascorbic acid per day, which was supplemented by a daily capsule containing an additional 75 mg of ascorbic acid. The subject's body vitamin C pool was labeled with L-[1-^{14}C]ascorbate one week before initiating vitamin C depletion; it was calculated to be 1500 mg. Beginning on day 14, the diet was changed to a liquid formula containing no vitamin C, as ascertained by actual analysis. This diet, based on vitamin-free casein, provided 3300 kcal and supplied protein, fat, and carbohydrate as 15, 40, and 45% of total calories, respectively. It was fed from day 14 to day 104, during which time the subject developed signs of scurvy. Ascorbic acid was not detectable in his urine after 30 days of depletion. He showed **petechiae** on day 45, when his vitamin C pool was 150 mg and his plasma level was 0.19 mg/dl. Spontaneous ecchymoses occurred over days 36–103; these were followed by coiled hairs, gum changes, *hyperkeratosis*,[117] congested follicles and the Sjögren sicca syndrome,[118] dry mouth, and enlarged parotid salivary glands. The subject developed joint pains on day 68 and joint effusions[119] shortly thereafter, when his vitamin C pool was 100 mg and his plasma ascorbic acid level was less than 0.16 mg/dl. He also had the unusual complication of a bilateral femoral neuropathy, which began on day 71, when his vitamin C pool was 80 mg and his plasma ascorbic acid level was 0.15 mg/dl. This, accompanied by the joint effusions, was attributed to hemorrhage into the sheaths of both femoral nerves. On day 80, he experienced a rapid increase in weight, from 81 to 84 kg, in combination with dyspnea[120] on exertion and swelling

---

[116] Vojdani, A., et al. (2000). *Cancer Detect. Prev.* **24,** 508–523.

[117] A mouth disease with clinical characteristics usually of variously sized and shaped, grayish white, flat, adherent patches; having diffuse borders, and a smooth surface with no papillary projections, fissures, erosions, or ulcerations.

[118] Dry eyes due to reduction in tears (i.e., keratoconjunctivitis).

[119] The escape of fluid from the blood vessels or lymphatics into the joint capsule.

[120] Subjective difficulty or distress in breathing, frequently rapid breathing.

of the legs. At this time, his vitamin C pool was 40 mg and his plasma level was 0.15 mg/dl.

Beginning on day 105, the subject was put on a vitamin C-repletion regimen involving daily doses of 4 mg of ascorbic acid. Immediately following this treatment, the edema worsened, urinary output dropped to 340 ml/day, and weight increased to 86.6 kg on day 109. There was no evidence of pulmonary congestion or cardiac failure. The ascorbic acid-repletion dose was increased to 6.5 mg/day on day 111. His edema persisted for 4 days, at which time he had a profound diuresis with complete disappearance of the edema by day 133 at which time his weight was 77.2 kg (he lost 9.4 kg of extracellular fluid). From days 101 to 133, his body ascorbic acid pool increased from 33 to 128 mg. The subject was given 6.5 mg of ascorbic acid per day from day 133 to day 227. During this time, all his scorbutic manifestations disappeared, and his plasma ascorbic acid fluctuated between 0.10 and 0.25 mg/dl. His body pool was restored slowly to an excess of 300 mg. Beginning on day 228, he received 600 mg of ascorbic acid per day, which rapidly repleted his body pool. At the end of the study, his weight was 81 kg, and he was discharged from the metabolic ward in excellent health.

Case 2

A 72-year-old man was admitted to the hospital with symptoms of increasing anorexia, epigastric discomfort unrelated to meals, and nonradiating *precordial*[121] pain. During the year before admission, he had become increasingly weak and easily fatigued, and had lost nearly 13 kg in weight. Six weeks before admission, he began to have sudden attacks of severe substernal pain followed by cough and dyspnea, and 1 month before admission he had a small *hematemesis*[122] and had noted bright red blood in his stools. He had been living alone, and his diet during the past year had consisted chiefly of bread and milk with various soups. For a considerable period, he had noted easy bruising of his skin. His past health had been good except for occasional seizures; these began 2 years before admission and involved loss of consciousness, spasmodic twitching of the limbs, and incontinence preceded by abdominal discomfort.

Physical examination on admission revealed a thin, depressed, lethargic man with a rather gray complexion and numerous petechiae over the arms, legs, and trunk. His blood pressure was 140/80, his pulse 68, his respiration 19, and his temperature 98.8°F. Examination of his head and neck showed an *edentulous*[123] mouth, foul breath, ulcerated palate, and retracted gums without hemorrhage. He had a large ecchymosis (15 cm in diameter) on his right thigh. Neurological examination was negative.

Laboratory findings

Parameter	Patient	Normal range
Hb	13.2 g/dl	15–18 g/dl
WBC	8,000/µl	5,000–9,000/µl
Platelets	140,000/µl	150,000–300,000/µl
Clotting time	5.75 min	5–15 min
Blood urea	48 mg/dl	10–20 mg/dl
Serum protein	7 g/dl	6–8 g/dl
Serum albumin	3.9 g/dl	3.5–5.5 g/dl
Serum ascorbic acid	<0.1 mg/dl	0.4–1.0 mg/dl

His heart was not enlarged and there were no heart murmurs; however, his electrocardiogram showed changes typical of an old myocardial infarction.[124] His chest radiograms showed emphysematous[125] and atheromatous[126] changes. His urine contained occasional pus cells with moderate growth of *Escherichia coli*; no abnormal bacilli were seen in the sputum. Sigmoidoscopy revealed no lesions in the distal 25 cm of the bowel. Because of his anorexia, epigastric discomfort, weight loss, and hematemesis, further investigation of the gastrointestinal tract was made using

---

[121] Relating to the diaphragm and anterior surface of the lower part of the thorax.

[122] Vomiting of blood.

[123] Toothless.

[124] Necrotic changes resulting from obstruction of an end artery.

[125] Emphysema involves dilation of the pulmonary air vesicles, usually due to atrophy of the septa between the alveoli.

[126] *Atheroma* refers to the focal deposit or degenerative accumulation of soft, pasty, acellular, lipid-containing material frequently found in intimal and subintimal plaques in arteriosclerosis (also called *atherosclerosis*).

a barium bolus; this revealed a mass and ulcer crater in the prepyloric area of the stomach, suggesting a gastric neoplasm. A laparotomy[127] was planned. The tentative diagnoses were anterior myocardial infarction, suspected cancer of the stomach, epilepsy, and hemorrhagic diathesis[128] (probably scurvy). Accordingly, the patient was given a high-protein diet and ascorbic acid (1 g/day for 2 weeks, then 150 mg/day for a month).

The patient showed marked improvement following ascorbic acid treatment. He no longer showed an air of lassitude; he gained weight and began to relish his meals. His skin hemorrhages rapidly decreased and no new ones appeared. Three weeks after admission, blood disappeared from his feces. At that time, his epilepsy was satisfactorily controlled using phenobarbital, and his liver function tests and blood chemistry were normal.

Laboratory findings after vitamin C treatment

Parameter	Patient	Normal range
Blood urea	28 mg/dl	10–20 mg/dl
Serum protein	6.3 g/dl	6–8 g/dl
Serum albumin	3.9 g/dl	3.5–5.5 g/dl
Serum ascorbic acid	1.0 mg/dl	0.4–1.0 mg/dl

A second radiological examination, conducted 1 month after ascorbic acid treatment, indicated a normal pylorus; this was confirmed by gastroscopy. A biopsy of the previously involved area showed only a natural glandular pattern, with hemorrhage of the superficial layer of the gastric mucosa. The patient was discharged after 8 weeks of hospitalization and was well when seen later in the outpatient clinic. The gastric lesion did not recur. It was concluded that what had appeared to be a prepyloric tumor and ulcer had actually been a bleeding site with a hematoma.[129]

Case Study Questions

1. What thresholds are suggested by the results of the first case study for total body ascorbic acid pool size and plasma ascorbic acid concentration associated with freedom from signs of scurvy?

2. Compute the rate of reduction in ascorbic acid body pool size from the observations on the subject of the first case. Was it linear throughout the study?

3. What signs/symptoms did the patient in the second case show that indicated a problem related to vitamin C status?

Study Questions and Exercises

1. Construct a concept map illustrating the relationship of the chemical properties and physiological functions of vitamin C.

2. Construct a decision tree for the diagnosis of vitamin C deficiency in humans.

3. What health complications might you expect to be shown by scorbutic individuals?

---

[127] A surgical procedure involving incision through the abdominal wall.

[128] Any of several syndromes showing a tendency to spontaneous hemorrhage, resulting from weakness of the blood vessels and/or a clotting defect.

[129] A localized mass of extravasated blood, usually clotted.

Recommended Reading

Cooke, M. S., Evans, M. D., Mistry, N., and Lunec, J. (2002). Role of dietary antioxidants in the prevention of *in vivo* oxidative DNA damage. *Nutr. Res. Rev.* **15,** 19–41.

Douglas, R., Hemila, H., D'Souza, R., Chalker, E., and Treacy, B. (2004). Vitamin C for preventing and treating the common cold. *Cochrane Database Syst. Rev.* **18,** CD000980.

Duarte, T. L., and Lunee, J. (2005). Review: When is an antioxidant not an antioxidant? A review of novel actions of vitamin C. *Free Radical Res.* **39,** 671–686.

Halliwell, B. (2001). Vitamin C and genomic stability. *Mutation Res.* **475,** 29–35.

Hathcock, J. N., Azzi, A., Blumberg, J., Bray, T., Dickinson, A., Frei, B., Jialal, I., Johnston, C. S., Kelly, F. J., Kraemer, K., Packer, L., Parthasarathy, S., Sies, H., and Traber, M. G. (2005). Vitamins E and C are safe across a broad range of intakes. *Am. J. Clin. Nutr.* **81,** 736–745.

Hemilä, H. (1997). Vitamin C intake and susceptibility to the common cold. *Br. J. Nutr.* **77,** 59–72.

Johnston, C. S., Steinberg, F. M., and Rucker, R. B. (2001). Ascorbic Acid, Chapter 15 in *Handbook of Vitamins*, 3rd ed. (R. B. Rucker, J. W. Suttie, D. B. McCormick, and L. J. Machlin, eds.), pp. 529–568. Marcel Dekker, New York.

Kneckt, P., Ritz, J., Pereira, M. A., O'Reilly, E. J., Augustsson, K., Fraser, G. E., Goldbourt, U., Heitmann, B. L., Hallmans, G., Liu, S., Pietinen, P., Spiegelman, D., Stevens, J., Virtamo, J., Willett, W. C., Rimm, E. B., and Ascherio, A. (2004). Antioxidant vitamins and coronary heart disease risk: A pooled analysis of 9 cohorts. *Am. J. Clin. Nutr.* **80,** 1508–1520.

Lee, K. W., Lee, H. J., Surh, Y. J., and Lee, C. Y. (2003). Vitamin C and cancer chemoprevention: Reappraisal. *Am. J. Clin. Nutr.* **78,** 1074–1078.

Levine, M., Katz, A., and Pakayatty, S. J. (2006). Vitamin C, Chapter 31 in *Modern Nutrition in Health and Disease*, 10th ed. (M. E. Shils, M. Shike, A. C. Ross, B. Caballero, and R. J. Cousins, eds.), pp. 507–524. Lippincott, New York.

May, J. M. (2000). How does ascorbic acid prevent endothelial dysfunction? *Free Radical Biol. Med.* **28,** 1421–1429.

Packer, L., and Fuchs, J. (eds.). (1997). *Vitamin C in Health and Disease*. Marcel Dekker, New York.

Padayatty, S. J., Katz, A., Wang, Y., Eck, P., Kwon, O., Lee, J. H., Chen, S., Corpe, C., Dutta, S. K., and Levine, M. (2003). Vitamin C as an antioxidant: Evaluation of its role in disease prevention. *J. Am. Coll. Nutr.* **22,** 18–35.

Pauling, L. (1970). *Vitamin C and the Common Cold*. W. H. Freeman and Company, San Francisco.

Rice, M. E. (2000). Ascorbate regulation and its neuroprotective role in the brain. *Trends Neurosci.* **23,** 209–216.

Sauberlich, H. E. (1994). Pharmacology of vitamin C. *Ann. Rev. Nutr.* **14,** 371–391.

Smirnoff, N. (2001). L-Ascorbic acid biosynthesis. *Vitamins Hormones* **61,** 241–266.

Wilson, J. X. (2002). The physiological role of dehydroascorbic acid. *FEBS Letts.* **527,** 5–9.

Wilson, J. X. (2005). Regulation of vitamin C transport. *Ann. Rev. Nutr.* **25,** 105–125.

Thiamin

10

There is present in rice polishing a substance different from protein and salts, which is indispensable to health and the lack of which causes nutritional polyneuritis.

—C. Eijkman and C. Grijns

I.	The Significance of Thiamin	266
II.	Sources of Thiamin	266
III.	Absorption of Thiamin	268
IV.	Transport of Thiamin	269
V.	Metabolism of Thiamin	269
VI.	Metabolic Functions of Thiamin	270
VII.	Thiamin Deficiency	274
VIII.	Thiamin Toxicity	278
IX.	Case Studies	278
	Study Questions and Exercises	280
	Recommended Reading	280

Anchoring Concepts

1. Thiamin is the trivial designation of a specific compound, 3-(4-amino-2-methylpyrimidin-5-ylmethyl)-5-(2-hydroxyethyl)-4-methylthiazolium, which is sometimes also called **vitamin B$_1$**.
2. Thiamin is hydrophilic, and its protonated form has a quaternary nitrogen center in the thiazole ring.
3. Deficiencies of thiamin are manifest chiefly as neuromuscular disorders.

Learning Objectives

1. To understand the chief natural sources of thiamin.
2. To understand the means of absorption and transport of thiamin.
3. To understand the biochemical function of thiamin as a coenzyme and the relationship of that function to the physiological activities of the vitamin.
4. To understand the physiologic implications of low thiamin status.

Vocabulary

Acute pernicious beriberi
Alcohol
γ-Aminobutyric acid (GABA)
Anorexia
Ataxia
ATPase
Beriberi
Bradycardia
Branched chain α-keto acid dehydrogenase
Cardiac beriberi
Cardiac hypertrophy
Chastek paralysis
Cocarboxylase
Confabulation
Dry (neuritic) beriberi
Dyspnea
Encephalopathy
Fescue toxicity
Hexose monophosphate shunt
Infantile (acute) beriberi
α-Ketoglutarate dehydrogenase
Maple syrup urine disease
Neuropathy
Nystagmus
Ophthalmoplegia
Opisthotonos
Pantothenic acid
Pentose phosphate pathway
Perseveration
Phosphorylase
Polioencephalomalacia
Polyneuritis
Pyrimidine ring
Pyrithiamin
Pyruvate dehydrogenase
Shoshin beriberi
Star-gazing
Sulfate

Sulfite
Tachycardia
Thiaminases
Thiamin-binding protein (TBP)
Thiamin disulfide
Thiamin monophosphate (TMP)
Thiamin monophosphatase
Thiamin pyrophosphatase
Thiamin pyrophosphate (TPP)
Thiamin pyrophosphokinase
Thiamin-responsive megaloblastic anemia (TRMA)
Thiamin triphosphate (TTP)
Thiazole ring
Thiochrome
Transketolase
TTP-ATP phosphoryltransferase
Vitamin B$_1$
Wernicke–Korsakoff syndrome
Wernicke's encephalopathy
Wet (edematous) beriberi

I. The Significance of Thiamin

Thiamin is essential in carbohydrate metabolism and neural function. Severe thiamin deficiency results in the nerve and heart disease *beriberi*; less severe deficiency results in nonspecific signs: malaise, loss of weight, irritability, and confusion. Thiamin-deficient animals show inanition and poor general performance and, in severe cases, *polyneuritis*, making thiamin status economically important in livestock production.

Historically, thiamin deficiency has been prevalent among peoples dependent on polished rice as the predominant, if not sole, source of food. Demographic trends indicate that for many people dependence on rice is likely to increase in the future. Rice and rice/wheat crop rotations are now the basis of the food systems currently supporting a fifth of the world's people—those in East, South, and Southeast Asia where human numbers are expected to more than double within the next four decades. The irony is that whole-grain rice and other cereals are not particularly deficient in thiamin. However, the removal of their thiamin-containing aleurone cells renders the polished grains, which consist of little more than the carbohydrate-rich endosperm, nearly devoid of thiamin as well as other vitamins and essential inorganic elements. In fact, thiamin-containing rice polishings

are often used to fuel the parboiling of the thiamin-deficient grain. Thus, efforts are needed to reduce the need to polish rice[1] such that increased reliance on the new, high-yielding cultivars of rice will not lead to expansions of thiamin deficiency among the poor of southern Asia.

II. Sources of Thiamin

Distribution in Foods

Thiamin is widely distributed in foods, but most contain only low concentrations of the vitamin. The richest sources are yeasts (e.g., dried brewer's and baker's yeasts) and liver (especially pork liver); however, cereal grains comprise the most important dietary sources of the vitamin in most human diets. Food sources of thiamin are considered to be readily available to healthy subjects except in cases of exposure to certain antagonists (see Thiamin antagonists below).

Whole grains are typically rich in thiamin; however, the vitamin is distributed unevenly in grain tissues. The greatest concentrations of thiamin in grains are typically found in the scutellum (the thin layer between the germ and the endosperm) and the germ. The endosperm (the starchy interior) is quite low in the vitamin. Therefore, milling to degerminate grain, which, because it removes the highly unsaturated oils associated with the germ, yields a product that will not rancidify and, thus, has a longer storage life, also results in very low thiamin content. It is estimated that more than a third of thiamin in the U.S. food supply is provided by grains and grain products, with meats providing about a quarter.

In foods derived from plants, thiamin occurs predominantly as free thiamin (Table 10-1). In contrast, thiamin occurs in animal tissues almost entirely (95–98%) in phosphorylated forms (*thiamin mono-, di-,* and *triphosphates*), the predominant form (80–85%) being the coenzyme thiamin diphosphate also called **thiamin pyrophosphate (TPP)**.

Stability in Foods

Thiamin is susceptible to destruction by several factors including neutral and alkaline conditions, heat, oxidation, and ionizing radiation (Table 10-2). It is stable at low pH (pH < 7), but decomposes when

---

[1] Rice aleurone cells are rich in a highly polyunsaturated oil, which is prone to oxidative rancidity.

Table 10-1.   Thiamin contents of foods

Food	Thiamin (mg/100 g)	Food	Thiamin, (mg/100 g)
Grains		Fruits	
Cornmeal	0.20	Apples	0.04
Oatmeal	0.55	Apricots	0.03
Rice		Bananas	0.05
Brown	0.29	Grapes	0.05
White	0.07	Oranges	0.10
White, cooked	0.02	Pears	0.02
Rye		Pineapples	0.08
Whole-grain	0.30	Meats	
Degerminated	0.19	Beef	0.08
Wheat		Duck	0.10
Whole-grain	0.55	Pork	1.10
White	0.06	Cured ham	0.74
Vegetables		Veal	0.18
Asparagus	0.18	Trout	0.09
Beans, green	0.07	Salmon	0.17
Broccoli	0.10	Heart, veal	0.60
Cabbage	0.05	Liver	
Carrots	0.06	Beef	0.30
Cauliflower	0.11	Pork	0.43
Kale	0.16	Dairy products and eggs	
Peas, green	0.32	Cheese	0.02–0.06
Potatoes	0.11	Milk	0.04
Tomatoes	0.06	Eggs	0.12
Other			
Brewer's yeast	15.6		
Human milk	0.01		

Table 10-2.   Thiamin losses in food processing

Procedure	Food	Loss (%)
Convection cooking	Meats	25–85
Baking	Bread	5–35
Heating with water	Vegetables	0–60
Pasteurization	Milk	9–20
Spray drying	Milk	~10
Canning	Milk	~40
Room temperature storage	Fruits, vegetables	0–20

heated, particularly under nonacidic conditions.[2] Protein-bound thiamin, found in animal tissues, is more stable to such losses. Thiamin is stable during frozen storage; substantial losses occur during thawing, however, owing mainly to removal via drip fluid.

Thiamin Antagonists

Thiamin in foods can be destroyed by *sulfites* added in processing and by *thiamin-degrading enzymes* (**thiaminases**) and other antithiamin compounds that may occur naturally (Table 10-3). Many cases of

---

[2] Therefore, the practice of adding sodium bicarbonate to peas or beans for retention of their color in cooking or canning results in large losses of thiamin.

Table 10-3. Types of thiaminases

Type	Present in:	Mechanism
I	Fresh fish, shellfish, ferns, some bacteria	Displaces pyrimidine methylene group with a nitrogenous base or SH compound, to eliminate the thiazole ring
II	Certain bacteria	Hydrolytic cleavage of methylene–thiazole–nitrogen bond to yield the pyrimidine and thiazole moieties

thiamin deficiency have been found to be related to the ingestion of food containing such thiamin antagonists (Table 10-4).[3] Sulfites react with thiamin to cleave its methylene bridge between the **pyrimidine ring** and **thiazole ring**; the reaction is slow at high pH, but is rapid in neutral and acidic conditions. Because rumen microbes can reduce sulfate to sulfite, high dietary levels of sulfate can have thiamin-antagonistic activities for ruminants. Thiamin-destroying enzymes occur in a variety of natural products. Bacterial thiaminases are *exoenzymes*; that is, they are bound to the cell surface; their activities depend on their release from the cell surface. This can occur under acidotic conditions in ruminants. The thiaminases are heat labile but can be effective antagonists of the vitamin when consumed without heat treatment. Heat-stable thiamin antagonists occur in several plants (e.g., ferns, tea, betel nut). These include *o- and p-hydroxypolyphenols* (e.g., caffeic acid, chlorogenic

acid, tannic acid),[4] which react with thiamin to oxidize the thiazole ring, yielding the nonabsorbable form **thiamin disulfide**. In addition, some *flavonoids* (quercetin, rutin) have been reported to antagonize thiamin, and *hemin*[5] in animal tissues is thought to bind the vitamin.

III. Absorption of Thiamin

Two Means of Uptake

Thiamin released by the action of phosphatase and pyrophosphatase in the upper small intestine is absorbed in two ways. At low luminal concentrations ($<2\,\mu M$) the process is carrier-mediated; at higher concentrations (e.g., a 2.5-mg dose for a human) passive diffusion also occurs. The active transport mechanism is greatest in the proximal regions of the small intestine (jejunum and ileum); therefore, thiamin produced by the lower gut microflora is not utilized by noncoprophagous animals. The cells of the intestinal mucosa have a **thiamin pyrophosphokinase** activity, with a K_m about the same as that of the carrier-mediated absorption process. However, it is not clear whether that enzyme is linked to the active absorption of the vitamin.[6] Although most of the thiamin present in the intestinal mucosa is in phosphorylated form, thiamin arriving on the serosal side of the intestine is largely in the free (nonphosphorylated) form. Therefore, the uptake of thiamin by the mucosal cell may be coupled in some way to its phosphorylation/dephosphorylation. Evidence indicates that the serosal discharge of thiamin by those cells is dependent on an Na⁺-dependent **ATPase** on that

Table 10-4. Thiaminase activities in seafoods

Seafood	Thiamin destroyed (mg/100 g/hr)
Marlin	0
Yellowfin tuna	265
Red snapper	265
Skipjack tuna	1000
Mahi mahi	120
Ladyfish	35
Clam	2640

Source: Hilker, D. M., and Peter, G. F. (1966). *J. Nutr.* **89**, 419–421.

---

[3] Perhaps the best known of these is the condition referred to as **Chastek paralysis**, which is a neurological disorder in commercially raised foxes fed a diet containing raw carp. The syndrome, named for the fox producer, was found to be a manifestation of thiamin deficiency brought on by a thiaminase present in fish gut tissue. Cooking the fish before feeding them to Mr. Chastak's foxes did not produce the syndrome, apparently because heat denatured the intestinal thiaminase.

[4] These and related compounds are found in blueberries, red currents, red beets, Brussels sprouts, red cabbage, betel nuts, coffee, and tea.

[5] Ferriprotoporphyrin, the nonprotein, Fe^{3+}-containing portion of hemoglobin.

[6] Both processes follow Michaelis–Menton kinetics, with half-maximal rates at 0.1–$0.4\,\mu M$ concentrations of thiamin. This finding led to the assumption that the two processes may be closely associated.

side of the cell.[7] Because adrenalectomized rats have been found to absorb thiamin poorly, it is thought that enteric absorption of the vitamin may also be subject to control by corticosteroid hormones.

IV. Transport of Thiamin

Thiamin Bound to Serum Proteins

Most of the thiamin in serum is bound to protein, chiefly albumin. About 90% of the total thiamin in blood (typically, 5–12 μg/dl) is in erythrocytes.[8] A specific binding protein, **thiamin-binding protein (TBP)**,[9] has been identified in rat serum.[10] It is believed that TBP is a specific, hormonally regulated carrier protein that is essential for the distribution of thiamin to critical tissues.

Cellular Uptake

Thiamin is taken up by cells of the blood and other tissues by active transport. Intracellular thiamin occurs predominantly (80%) in phosphorylated form, most of which is bound to proteins. Thiamin uptake and secretion, at least in some tissues, appears to be mediated by a soluble thiamin transporter that is dependent on Na$^+$ and a transcellular proton gradient. The transporter has been cloned[11] and mapped to the human chromosome 1q24. This 497-amino acid protein has a high sequence homology with the reduced folate transporter, for which reason it is considered a member of that transporter family.[12] The greatest amounts of the transporter have been found in skeletal muscle, heart, and placenta, with low or nondetectable amounts in liver, kidney, brain, and intestine. Mutations in the transporter are associated with the condition of **thiamin-responsive megaloblastic anemia (TRMA, see)**.[13]

Tissue Distribution

The adult human stores only 25 to 30 mg thiamin, most of which is in skeletal muscle, heart, brain, liver, and kidneys. Plasma, milk, and cerebrospinal fluid, and probably all extracellular fluids, contain free (unesterified) thiamin and **thiamin monophosphate (TMP)**, which, unlike the more highly phosphorylated forms (**thiamin diphosphate [TPP], thiamin triphosphate [TTP]**), appear capable of crossing cell membranes. Tissue levels of thiamin vary within and between species, with no appreciable storage in any tissue.[14] In infants, blood thiamin levels decline after birth, owing initially to a decrease in free thiamin, followed by a decrease in phosphorylated forms. In thiamin-deficient chickens fed the vitamin, heart tissues take up thiamin at much greater rates than liver or brain. In general, the thiamin contents of human tissue tend to be less than those of analogous tissues in other species, particularly the pig, which has relatively high tissue thiamin stores.

V. Metabolism of Thiamin

Role of Phosphorylation

Thiamin is phosphorylated in the tissues by two enzymes (Fig. 10-1):

- **Thiamin pyrophosphokinase** catalyzes the formation of TPP using ATP.
- **TTP-ATP phosphoryltransferase** catalyzes the formation of TTP from TPP and ATP.

---

[7] The ingestion of alcohol can inhibit the enteric absorption of thiamin. That parenterally administered alcohol can also inhibit thiamin utilization suggests that the basis of the antagonism may be in the absorption process itself, probably at the level of the Na$^+$-dependent ATPase, which is known to be inhibited by alcohol.

[8] Several children who died of SIDS (sudden infant death syndrome) have been found to have had extraordinarily high plasma thiamin concentrations (e.g., fivefold those of infants who died of other diseases). The physiological basis of this effect is unknown, although thiamin deficiency is not thought to be a cause of death in SIDS.

[9] TBP has a molecular mass of about 38kDa. It binds 1 mol of free thiamin per mole and forms a 1:1 complex with the riboflavin-binding protein. Like the latter, TBP appears to be regulated by estrogens (i.e., it is inducible in male or ovariectomized rats by parenterally administered estrogen).

[10] TBP has also been identified in rat liver and hens' eggs (in both the yolk and albumen).

[11] Ganapathy, V., et al. (2004). *Pflugers Arch.* **447**, 641–646.

[12] The SLC19 family of transporters includes the folate transporter (SLC19A1), the thiamin transporter (SLC19A2), and at least one other protein capable of binding thiamin (SLC19A3).

[13] Lagarde, W. H. et al. (2004). *Am. J. Med. Genet. A* **266**, 299–309.

[14] Thiamin concentrations are generally greatest in the heart (0.28–0.79mg/100g), kidneys (0.24–0.58mg/100g), liver (0.20–0.76mg/100g), and brain (0.14–0.44mg/100g), and are retained longest in the brain.

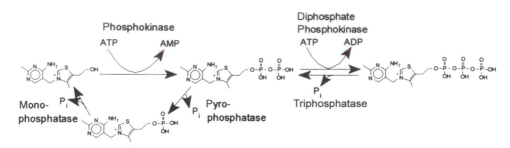

Fig. 10-1. Metabolic activation of thiamin.

Each of these esters is catabolized by **thiamin pyrophosphatase** which yields the monophosphorylated product thiamin monophosphate (TMP).

Catabolism

The turnover of thiamin varies between tissues, but it is generally high.[15] Thiamin in excess of that which binds in tissues is rapidly excreted. With an estimated half-life of 10 to 20 days in humans, thiamin deficiency states can deplete tissue stores within a couple of weeks. Studies with fasting and undernourished soldiers have shown that food restriction increases the rate of thiamin excretion.[16] Declines in tissue thiamin levels are thought to involve enhanced degradation of TPP-dependent enzymes in the absence of the vitamin. Numerous metabolites of thiamin have been identified (see the following subsection).

Urinary Excretion

Thiamin is excreted in the urine, chiefly as free thiamin and thiamin monophosphate, but also in small amounts as the diphosphate ester and other metabolites (e.g., **thiochrome**, thiamin disulfide, and some two dozen other metabolites, a few of which are of quantitative importance: thiamin acetic acid, 2-methyl-4-amino-5-pyrimidine carboxylic acid, 4-methylthiazole-5-acetic acid, 2-methyl-4-aminopyrimidine-5-carboxylic acid, 2-methyl-4-amino-5-hydroxymethylpyrimidine, 5-(2-hydroxyethyl)-4-methylthiazole, 3-(2′-methyl-4-amino-5′-pyrimidinylmethyl)-4-methylthiazole-5-acetic acid and 2-methyl-4-amino-5-formylaminomethylpyrimidine). Thiamin metabolites retaining the pyrimidine–thiazole ring linkage account for increasing proportions of total thiamin excretion as thiamin status declines.

VI. Metabolic Functions of Thiamin

Cocarboxylase

The metabolically functional form of thiamin is its diphosphate ester, **thiamin pyrophosphate (TPP)**, also called **cocarboxylase**. Several enzymes use TPP as an essential cofactor for the cleavage of the C–C bond of α-keto acids (e.g., pyruvate) to yield products subsequently transferred to an acceptor. In each case, TPP serves as a classic coenzyme, binding covalently to the holoenzyme by apoenzymic recognition of both the substituted pyrimidyl and thiazole moieties. Each TPP-dependent enzyme also requires Mg^{2+} or some other divalent cation for activity.

The general mechanism of the coenzyme action of TPP involves its deprotonation to form a carbanion at C-2 of the thiazole ring, which reacts with the polarized 2-carbonyl group of the substrate (an α-keto acid or α-keto sugar) to form a covalent bond. This bond formation results in the labilization of certain C–C bonds to release CO_2, with the remaining adduct reacting by

- Protonation to give an active aldehyde addition product (e.g., decarboxylases)
- Direct oxidation with suitable electron acceptors to yield a high-energy, 2-acyl product
- Reaction with oxidized lipoic acid to yield an acyldihydrolipoate product (e.g., oxidases or dehydrogenases)
- Addition to an aldehyde carbonyl to yield a new ketol (e.g., *transketolase*)

In higher animals, the decarboxylation is oxidative (producing a carboxylic acid). These involve the transfer of the aldehyde from TPP to lipoic acid

---

[15] Thiamin turnover in rat brain was 0.16–.055 μg/g/hr, depending on the region (Rindi, G., et al. [1980]. *Brain Res.* **181**, 369–380.

[16] Consolazio, C. F., et al. (1971). *Am. J. Clin. Nutr.* **24**, 1060–1067.

(forming a 6-*S*-acylated dihydrolipoic acid and free TPP) from which it is transferred to coenzyme A.[17]

Several effective thiamin antagonists are analogs of the vitamin, differing from it with respect to the chemical structure of the thiazole ring. Some involve substitutions on either the pyrimidine or thiazole ring;[18] loss of catalytic activity occurs with any change that disturbs the peculiar environment of the thiazole ring system, which is required to make the C-2 atom reactive. Most have hydroxyethyl groupings, which allow them to compete with the vitamin for phosphorylation (via thiamin **pyrophosphorylase**). In addition, members of a large group of synthetic thiamin antagonists with anticoccidial activity have a thiamin-like pyrimidine ring combined through a methylene bridge to a quaternary nitrogen of a pyridine ring.[19] These, not having a hydroxyethyl group, cannot be phosphorylated. They inhibit the carrier-mediated cellular uptake of thiamin.

α-Keto Acid Dehydrogenases

In animals, TPP functions in the oxidative decarboxylation of α-keto acids by serving as an essential cofactor in multienzyme α-keto acid dehydrogenase complexes. There are three classes of this type of TPP-dependent enzyme:

- **Pyruvate dehydrogenase**, converting pyruvate to acetyl-CoA
- **α-Ketoglutaric dehydrogenase** converting α-ketoglutarate to succinyl-CoA
- **Branched-chain α-keto acid dehydrogenase**, converting branched-chain α-keto acids to the corresponding acyl-CoAs

Each of these complexes is composed of a decarboxylase (which binds TPP), a core enzyme (which binds lipoic acid), and a flavoprotein dihydrolipoamide dehydrogenase (which regenerates lipoamide). Each also contains one or more regulatory components. Those of pyruvate dehydrogenase include a kinase and a phosphatase that regulate the activity of the enzyme complex by interconversion between active nonphosphorylated and inactive phosphorylated forms.

A rare (1 per 100,000 births) genetic defect in the TPP enzyme branched-chain keto acid dehydrogenase results in the condition called **maple syrup urine disease**. The disorder is manifested in infancy as lethargy, seizures, and, ultimately, mental retardation. It can be detected by the maple syrup odor of the urine, resulting from the presence of the keto acid leucine. Some cases respond to high doses (10–200 mg/day) of thiamin.

Transketolase

Thiamin functions in the form of TPP as an essential cofactor for **transketolase**, which catalyzes the cleavage of a C–C bond in α-keto sugars (xylulose 5-phosphate, sedoheptulose 7-phosphate, fructose 6-phosphate, D-xylulose, D-fructose), transferring the resulting 2-C fragment (the so-called active glycoaldehyde) to an aldolase[20] acceptor (Fig. 10-2). Transketolase functions at two steps in the **hexose monophosphate shunt** for the oxidation of glucose.[21]

Transketolase is found in the cytosol of many tissues, particularly liver blood cells that rely on carbohydrate metabolism. Although the synthesis

---

[17] Coenzyme A is the metabolically active form of the vitamin **pantothenic acid**.

[18] Another group of derivatives includes the amprolium-type thiamin antagonists, which resemble pyrithiamin but have no hydroxyethyl group and, therefore, are not substrates for thiamin pyrophosphokinase.

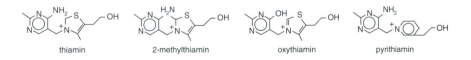

thiamin   2-methylthiamin   oxythiamin   pyrithiamin

These compounds are valuable in the protection of young poultry from coccidial infections by inhibiting the cellular uptake of thiamin by enteric coccidia. At low doses, this inhibition affects chiefly thiamin transport, but at higher doses it can affect the enteric absorption of the vitamin, producing clinical thiamin deficiency.

[19] An example is the following:

amprolium

[20] A sugar aldehyde.

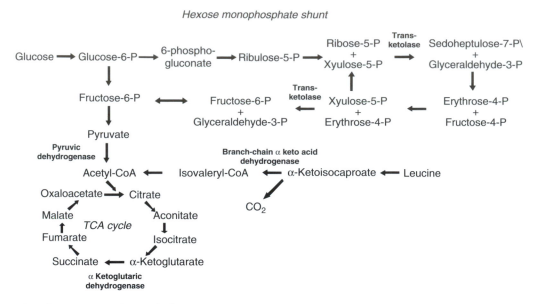

Fig. 10-2. Roles of TPP-enzymes in metabolism.

of the enzyme is not affected by thiamin status, its catalytic activity depends on its binding TPP. Transketolase responses to thiamin do not necessarily involve an immediate activation of an *apoenzyme*, suggesting that thiamin may have a direct effect on the genetic expression of the enzyme.

In subjects adequately nourished with respect to thiamin, TPP-binding is at least 85% of saturation, whereas in thiamin deficiency the percentage of transketolase bound to TPP is much less. This phenomenon is exploited in the clinical assessment of thiamin status; the increase, on addition of exogenous TPP, in the activity of erythrocyte transketolase *in vitro* can be used to determine the percentage TPP saturation of the enzyme and, hence, thiamin status. The percentage stimulation in erythrocyte transketolase activity by the addition of TPP is called the *transketolase activity coefficient*. Subjects with activity coefficients < 1.15 are considered to be at low risk of thiamin deficiency, whereas those with activity coefficients of 1.15–1.25 or >1.25 are considered to be at moderate and high risk, respectively.

Transketolase isolated from fibroblasts of patients with *Wernicke–Korsakoff syndrome* was found to have an abnormally low binding affinity for TPP (K_m = 195 μM versus K_m = 16 μM for control subjects). That this difference persisted after many passages in tissue culture indicates a hereditary defect in this enzyme in these patients.

Role of Thiamin in Nervous Function

It is clear that thiamin has a vital role in nerve function, although the biochemical nature of that role is still unclear. That thiamin is required by nervous tissue is evidenced by the localization of signs of thiamin deprivation, which are mainly neurologic. Furthermore, thiamin has been identified in mammalian brain, in synaptosomal membranes, and in cholinergic nerves. Studies have shown that brain thiamin concentrations tend to be resistant to change by dietary thiamin deprivation or parenteral thiamin administration, a finding suggesting homeostasis of the vitamin in that organ. Nervous stimulation by either electrical or chemical means has been found to result in the release of thiamin (as free thiamin and the monophosphate ester) that is associated with the dephosphorylation of its higher phosphate esters (thiamin di- and triphosphates). The antagonist **pyrithiamin**[22] can displace thiamin from nervous tissue and change the electrical activity of the tissue. Irradiation with ultraviolet (UV) light at wavelengths absorbed by thiamin destroys the electrical potential of nerve fibers in a manner corrected by thiamin treatment, suggesting a direct function

---

[21] This pathway, also called the *pentose pathway*, is an important alternate to the glycolysis–Krebs cycle pathway, especially for the production of pentoses for RNA and DNA synthesis and NADPH for the biosynthesis of fatty acids, and so on.

of thiamin in nervous tissue. TTP also stimulates chloride transport, perhaps by phosphorylating an ion channel.[23]

Because the oxidative decarboxylation of pyruvate and α-ketoglutarate represents essential steps in energy production via the Krebs cycle (also called the tricarboxylic acid [TCA] cycle), which plays an important role in the energy metabolism of the brain, it has been suggested that the neurological signs of thiamin deficiency may be due to failure of this system by the absence of sufficient amounts of its essential cofactor, TPP. However, several experiments have indicated that the depressions of pyruvate and α-ketoglutarate dehydrogenase activities that occur in thiamin-deficient animals (Table 10-5)

are not of sufficient magnitude to produce the neurological dysfunction associated with the deficiency. Nevertheless, it has also been found that brain ATP levels are unaffected by thiamin deprivation, suggesting that the metabolic flux though the alternative pathway, the so-called **γ-aminobutyric acid (GABA)** shunt,[24] is considerably increased in the brains of thiamin-deficient individuals, suggesting that, in addition to its role in the synthesis of that neurotransmitter (GABA), it may also serve to yield energy under conditions of thiamin deprivation (Fig. 10-3). This phenomenon may explain the anorexia that is characteristic of thiamin deficiency, as increased GABA flux through the hypothalamus has been shown to inhibit feeding in animals.

Table 10-5. Effects of thiamin deficiency on brain metabolism of 3-week-old rats

Parameter	Thiamin fed	Thiamin deficient
Body weight (g)	135 ± 4	96 ± 5
Erythrocyte transketolase (nmol hexose/min/mg)		
Basal activity	6.4 ± 0.6	2.9 ± 0.4[a]
+ TPP	6.9 ± 1.4	4.7 ± 0.8
Activation coefficient	1.08 ± 0.08	1.63 ± 0.12[a]
Liver thiamin (nmol/g)	132.0 ± 8.2	6.0 ± 0.7[a]
Brain analytes		
Thiamin (nmol/g)	12.6 ± 0.6	6.2 ± 0.3[a]
ATP (μmol/g)	2.8 ± 0.1	2.9 ± 0.1
Glutamate (μmol/g)	13.8 ± 0.3	11.3 ± 0.2[a]
α-Ketoglutarate (μmol/g)	0.14 ± 0.01	0.09 ± 0.0[a]
GABA (μmol/g)	1.67 ± 0.05	1.58 ± 0.03[a]

[a] $p < 0.05$.

Source: Page, M. G., Ankoma-Sey, V., Coulson, W. F., and Bender, D. A. (1989). *Br. J. Nutr.* **62**, 245–253.

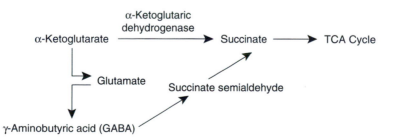

Fig. 10-3. Flux through GABA shunt is increased to maintain ATP levels in thiamin deficiency.

---

[22] Pyrithiamin (see footnote 19) is an analog of thiamin in which a pyridine moiety replaces the thiazole ring.

[23] Bettendorf, L., et al. (1993). *J. Membr. Biol.* **136**, 281–288.

Transketolase has also been found to be highly responsive to thiamin deprivation; however, it is not clear whether the **pentose phosphate pathway** is important in brain metabolism. It has also been suggested that thiamin may be involved in the synthesis of myelin, but the fact that the turnover of myelin is much slower (its half-time is 4 to 5 days) than the response of thiamin therapy (full recovery within 24 hours) does not appear to support that possibility.

Therefore, it has been proposed that thiamin has another function, that is, a nonmetabolic role related to nerve transmission. Currently, two hypotheses for such a role have been presented: that thiamin has a catalytic activity in the mechanism of Na^+ permeability; and that thiamin, probably as TPP, is involved in maintaining the fixed negative charge on the inner surface of the membrane.

Other Signs

Thiamin deficiency has been implicated in cases of sleep apnea as well as in sudden infant death syndrome (SIDS). Although this relationship is not elucidated, it would appear reasonable to expect thiamin to have a role in maintaining the brainstem function that governs automatic respiration.

VII. Thiamin Deficiency

General Signs

Thiamin deficiency in humans and animals is characterized by a predictable range of signs/symptoms (see Table 10-6), including loss of appetite (**anorexia**) and cardiac and neurologic signs. Underlying these are a number of metabolic effects including increased plasma concentrations of pyruvate, lactate, and, to a lesser extent, α-ketoglutarate (especially after a glucose meal), as well as decreased activities of erythrocyte transketolase. These effects result from diminished activities of TPP-dependent enzymes.

Increased production of reactive species of oxygen and nitrogen has been reported in the brains of thiamin-deficient animals. This, and the finding that antioxidants can attenuate the neurologic effects of thiamin

Table 10-6. General signs of thiamin deficiency

Organ system	Signs
General	
Appetite	Severe decrease
Growth	Decrease
Dermatologic	Edema
Muscular	Cardiomyopathy, bradycardia, heart failure, weakness
Gastrointestinal	Inflammation, ulcer
Vital organs	Hepatic steatosis
Nervous	Peripheral neuropathy
	Opisthotonos

deficiency,[25] suggests that oxidative stress plays a role in the clinical manifestation of the nutritional deficiency.

The presentation of thiamin deficiency is variable, apparently affected by such factors as the subject age, caloric (especially carbohydrate) intake, and presence/absence of other micronutrient deficiencies.[26]

Animals: Polyneuritis

The most remarkable sign of thiamin deficiency in most species is anorexia, which is so severe and more specific than any associated with other nutrient deficiencies (apart from that of sodium) that it is a useful diagnostic indicator for thiamin deficiency. Other signs include the secondary effects of reduced total feed intake: weight loss, impaired efficiency of feed utilization, weakness, and hypothermia. The appearance of anorexia correlates with the loss of transketolase activity and precedes changes in pyruvate or α-ketoglutarate dehydrogenase activities.

Animals axlso show neurologic dysfunction due to thiamin deficiency; birds, in particular, show a tetanic retraction of the head called **opisthotonos**, also **stargazing** (Fig. 10-4).[27] Other species generally show **ataxia** and incoordination, which progresses to convulsions and death. These conditions are generally referred to as **polyneuritis**.

---

[24] *GABA* is synthesized by the decarboxylation of glutamate, which is produced by transamination of α-ketoglutarate. GABA, in turn, can be transaminated to form succinic semialdehyde, which is oxidized to succinate before entering the TCA cycle.

[25] Pannunzio, P., et al. (2000). *J. Neurosci. Res.* **62**, 286–292.

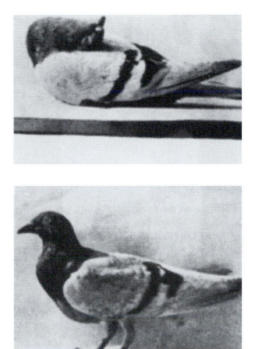

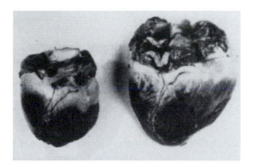

Fig. 10-5. Hearts from normal (*left*) and thiamin-deficient (*right*) pigs. (Courtesy of T. Cunha, University of Florida.)

Fig. 10-4. Opisthotonus in a thiamin-deficient pigeon before (*top*) and after (*bottom*) thiamin treatment. (Courtesy of Cambridge University Press.)

Most species, but especially dogs and pigs, show **cardiac hypertrophy**[28] in thiamin deficiency (Fig. 10-5) with slowing of the heart rate (**bradycardia**) and signs of congestive heart failure, including labored breathing and edema. Some species also show diarrhea and achlorhydria (rodents), gastrointestinal hemorrhage (pigs), infertility (chickens[29]), high neonatal mortality (pigs), and impaired learning (cats).

The rumen microflora are important sources of thiamin for ruminant species. Nevertheless, thiamin deficiency can occur in ruminants if their microbial yield of the vitamin is impaired. Such cases have occurred owing either to depressed thiamin synthesis due to a change in diet that disturbs rumen fermentation, or to enhanced thiamin degradation due to an alteration in the microbial population that increases total thiaminase activity. Increased ruminal degradation of thiamin is usually associated with the presence of certain microbial species, including *Bacteroides thiaminolyticus, Clostridium sporogenes, Megasphaera elsdenii*, and *Streptococcus bovis*.[30] These species and other *Clostridium* spp., *Bacillus* spp., and gram-negative cocci have thiaminases bound to their cell surfaces as exoenzymes. These can become significant sources of thiamin destruction when they are released into the rumen fluid, which can happen under conditions of sharply declining rumen pH. Therefore, signs of thiamin deficiency have been observed in animals fed high-concentrate diets. Ruminants can also experience thiamin deficiency by consuming thiamin antagonists such as excess **sulfate** (which rumen microbes reduce to **sulfite**), excess amprolium, or factors contained in bracken fern or endophyte-infected fescue. Thiamin treatment has been found to reduce the signs of summer **fescue toxicity** (reduced performance, elevated body temperature, rough hair coat) in grazing beef cattle.

The clinical manifestation of thiamin deficiency in young ruminants is the neurologic syndrome called **polioencephalomalacia**,[31] a potentially fatal condition involving inflammation of brain gray matter and presenting as opisthotonos (Figs. 10-5 and 10-6); it readily responds to thiamin treatment.[32]

---

[26] For example, deprivation of magnesium was shown to aggravate the signs of thiamin deficiency in the rat (Dyckner, T., et al. [1985]. *Acta Scand.* **218**, 129–131).

[27] This sign occurs in young mammals, but it is not usual.

[28] Enlargement of the heart.

[29] Thiamin deficiency impairs the fertility of both roosters (via testicular degeneration) and hens (via impaired oviductal atrophy).

[30] Of these, *B. thiaminolyticus* appears to be of greatest pathogenic importance, as it appears to occur routinely in the ruminal contents and feces of all cases of polioencephalomalacia.

[31] Cerebrocortical necrosis.

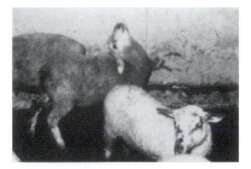

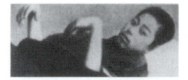

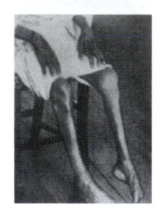

Fig. 10-6. Opisthotonos in a thiamin-deficient sheep. (Courtesy of M. Hidiroglou, Agricultural Canada, Ottawa, Ontario, Canada.)

Humans: Beriberi

The classic syndrome resulting from thiamin deficiency in humans is **beriberi**. This disease is prevalent in Southeast Asia, where polished rice is the dietary staple. It appears to be associated with the consumption of diets high in highly digestible carbohydrates but marginal or low in micronutrients. The general symptoms of beriberi are anorexia, cardiac enlargement, lassitude, muscular weakness (with resulting ataxia), paresthesia,[33] loss of knee and ankle jerk responses (with subsequent foot and wrist droop), and **dyspnea** on exertion (Fig. 10-7). Beriberi occurs in three clinical types:

- **Dry (neuritic) beriberi** occurs primarily in adults; it is characterized by peripheral neuropathy consisting of symmetrical impairment of sensory and motor nerve conduction affecting the distal (more than proximal) parts of the arms and legs. It usually does not have cardiac involvement.
- **Wet (edematous) beriberi** involves as its prominent signs edema, tachycardia,[34] cardiomegaly, and congestive heart failure; in severe cases, heart failure is the outcome.[35] The onset of this form of beriberi can vary from chronic to acute, in which case it is called **shoshin beriberi**[36] and is characterized by greatly elevated lactic acid concentrations in the blood.

Fig. 10-7. Neurologic signs of beriberi. (Courtesy of Cambridge University Press.)

- **Infantile (or acute) beriberi** occurs in breastfed infants of thiamin-deficient mothers, most frequently at 2–6 months of age. It has a rapid onset and may have both neurologic and cardiac signs, with death due to heart failure, usually within a few hours. Affected infants are anorectic and milk is regurgitated; they may experience vomiting, diarrhea, cyanosis, tachycardia, and convulsions. Their mothers may show no signs of thiamin deficiency.

Wernicke–Korsakoff Syndrome

Owing to the fortification of rice and wheat with thiamin, frank thiamin deficiency is rare in industrialized countries but continues to be prevalent in countries without such fortification programs. Nevertheless, subclinical thiamin insufficiency appears to occur in industrialized countries. When such conditions are associated with excessive **alcohol** consumption,[37] they produce an **encephalopathy**

---

[32] Polioencephalomalacia is thought to be a disease of thiamin deficiency that is induced by thiaminases such as those synthesized by rumen bacteria or present in certain plants. Affected animals are listless and have uncoordinated movements; they develop progressive blindness and convulsions. The disease is ultimately fatal but responds dramatically to thiamin.

[33] An abnormal spontaneous sensation, such as burning, pricking, or numbness.

[34] In contrast to thiamin-deficient animals, which show *bradycardia* (slow heart beat), beriberi patients show *tachycardia* (rapid heart rate, >100 beats/min).

[35] Wet beriberi is also called **cardiac beriberi**.

[36] Shoshin beriberi is also called **acute pernicious beriberi**.

called the **Wernicke–Korsakoff syndrome**.[38] The signs of this syndrome range from mild confusion to coma; they include **ophthalmoplegia**[39] with lateral or vertical **nystagmus**,[40] cerebellar ataxia, psychosis, **confabulation**,[41] and severely impaired retentive memory and cognitive function. The pathology is limited to the central nervous system.

Chronic alcohol consumption can lead to thiamin deficiency in several ways:

- Reduced thiamin intake due to the displacement of foods rich in thiamin (and other nutrients) by alcohol
- Impaired absorption of thiamin from the small intestine
- Impaired cellular uptake and utilization of thiamin

The risk of Wenicke's–Korsakoff syndrome is not limited to heavy alcohol users. The thiamin-responsive syndrome has been diagnosed in nonalcoholic patients with hyperemesis gravidarum[42] or undergoing dialysis.

Patients with Wernicke–Korsakoff syndrome frequently have a transketolase that has an abnormally low binding affinity for TPP. In most cases, it appears that this low affinity can be overcome by using high intramuscular doses of thiamin, to which most affected patients respond. While a quarter of Wernicke–Korsakoff syndrome patients are cured by thiamin treatment, it has been suggested that those who fail to respond may have yet another aberrant transketolase (or other TPP-dependent enzyme) incapable of binding TPP.

Epidemic Neuropathy

Widespread thiamin depletion in Cuba in 1992–1993 was reported during an epidemic of optic and peripheral **neuropathy** that affected some 50,000 people in a population of some 11 million.[43] Large percentages (30–70% by various parameters) of the affected population showed signs of low thiamin status. However, the incidences of low thiamin indicators were comparable in affected and nonaffected groups, and other risk factors were present. The incidence of new cases subsided with the institution of multivitamin supplementation in 1993. Still, it is not clear that thiamin deficiency, while widespread in that population, was the cause of the epidemic neuropathy.

Other Neurodegenerative Diseases

Alzheimer's disease

Comparisons of Alzheimer's disease patients and healthy controls have revealed modest (20%) reductions in the TPP contents of patients' brains, but dramatic differences in the brain activities of TPP-dependent enzymes: 55% less α-ketoglutaric dehydrogenase,[44] 70% less pyruvic dehydrogenase,[45] markedly reduced transketolase.[46] It has been suggested that these associations reflect genetic variations in genes encoding portions of one or more of these enzymes. A very limited number of small trials have been conducted to test the therapeutic value of thiamin for Alzheimer's disease; results have been inconclusive.

Parkinson's disease

Limited studies have suggested that patients with Parkinson's disease may have lower cerebrospinal fluid levels of free thiamin (but not TPP or TMP) and reduced activities of less α-ketoglutaric dehydrogenase.[47] In addition, α-ketoglutaric dehydrogenase was found to be inhibited by dopamine oxidation products,[48] which are known to be elevated in Parkinson's disease. A polymorphism in the E2K

---

[37] Excessive alcohol intake appears to be antagonistic to adequate thiamin status in two ways. First, the diets of alcoholics are frequently low in thiamin, a large percentage of the daily energy intake being displaced by nutrient-deficient alcoholic beverages. Second, alcohol can inhibit the intestinal ATPase involved in the enteric absorption (and, probably, the cellular uptake) of thiamin.

[38] This is also called **Wernicke's encephalopathy**. It has been seriously underdiagnosed, missing as much as 80% of cases (Harper, C. G., [1979]. *J. Neurol. Neurosurg. Psychiatry* **46,** 593–598).

[39] Paralysis of one or more of the motor nerves of the eye.

[40] Rhythmical oscillation of the eyeballs, either horizontally, rotary, or vertically.

[41] Readiness to answer any question fluently with no regard whatever to facts.

[42] Hyperemesis gravidarum is a severe and intractable form of nausea and vomiting in pregnancy.

[43] Macias-Matos, C., et al. (1996). *Am. J. Clin. Nutr.* **64,** 347–353.

[44] Gibson, G. E. (1998). *Ann. Neurol.* **44,** 676–681.

[45] Gibson, G. E. (1981). *Am. J. Med.* **70,** 1247–1254.

gene of α-ketoglutaric dehydrogenase has been suggested as the basis of this association.

Thiamin-Responsive Megaloblastic Anemia

Thiamin-responsive megaloblastic anemia (TRMA) with diabetes and deafness is a rare, autosomal recessive disorder reported in fewer than three dozen families. The disorder presents early in childhood with any of the above signs, plus optic atrophy, cardiomyopathy, and stroke-like episodes. The anemia responds to high doses of thiamin.[49] Defects in thiamin transport were reported in TRMA patients.[50] These have been found to be due to mutations of the SLC19A2 gene encoding the high-affinity thiamin transporter.

Thiamin Dependency

A few cases of apparent thiamin dependency have been reported. These have involved cases of intermittent episodes of cerebral ataxia, pyruvate dehydrogenase deficiency, branched chain keto-aciduria, and abnormal transketolase, all of which responded to very high doses of thiamin.[51]

Other Disorders

Thiamin deficiency has been reported in more than a fifth of nonalcoholic HIV-positive or AIDS patients.[52] Pregnant women with hyperemesis gravidarum are known to be at risk of developing low thiamin status. In women with gestational diabetes, maternal thiamin deficiency correlates with macrosomia (abnormally high infant body weight).[53]

VIII. Thiamin Toxicity

Little information is available concerning the toxic potential of thiamin for livestock or humans. Most of the published information pertains to the toxicity of the vitamin administered in the form of thiamin hydrochloride. From those studies it is clear that at least that form can be fatal, apparently by suppressing the respiratory center, at levels approximately 1000-fold those required to prevent signs of thiamin deficiency. Such doses of the vitamin to animals produce curare[54]-like signs, suggestive of blocked nerve transmission: restlessness, epileptiform convulsions, cyanosis, and dyspnea. In humans, parenteral doses of thiamin at 100-fold the recommended intake have been found to produce headache, convulsions, weakness, paralysis, cardiac arrhythmia, and allergic reactions.

IX. Case Studies

Instructions

Review each of the following case reports, paying special attention to the diagnostic indicators on which the treatments were based. Then answer the questions that follow.

Case 1

A 35-year-old man with a history of high alcohol intake for 18 years was admitted to the hospital complaining of massive swelling and shortness of breath on exertion. For several months, he had subsisted almost entirely on beer and whiskey, taking no solid food. He was grossly edematous, slightly jaundiced, and showed transient *cyanosis*[55] of the lips and nail beds. His heart showed *gallop rhythm*.[56] His left pleural cavity contained fluid. His liver was enlarged with notable *ascites*.[57] He had a coarse tremor of the hands and reduced tendon reflexes. His electrocardiogram showed sinus **tachycardia**.[58] His radiogram showed pulmonary edema and cardiac enlargement. He was evaluated by cardiac catheterization.

---

[46] Butterworth, R. F., and Besnard, A. M. (1990). *Metab. Brain Dis.* **5,** 179–184.

[47] Mizuno, Y. (1995). *Biochim. Biophys. Acta* **1271,** 265–274.

[48] Cohen, G., et al. (1997). *Proc. Nat. Acad. Sci.* **94,** 4890–4894.

[49] 20–60 times higher than RDA levels.

[50] Poggi, V., et al. (1984). *J. Inherit. Metab. Dis.* **7,** 153–154.

[51] Lonsdale, D. (2006). e*CAM* **3,** 49–59.

[52] Butterworth, R. F., et al. (1991). *Metab. Brain Dis.* **6,** 207–212.

[53] Baker, H. (2000). *Int. J. Vit. Nutr. Res.* **70,** 317–320.

[54] Curare is an extract of various plants (e.g., *Strychnos toxifera, S. castelraei, S. crevauxii, Chondodendron tomentosum*). Practically inert when administered orally, it is a powerful muscle relaxant when administered intravenously or intramuscularly, exerting its effect by blocking nerve impulses at the myoneural junction. Curare is used experimentally and clinically to produce muscular relaxation during surgery. It was originally used as an arrow poison by indigenous hunters of South America to kill prey by inducing paralysis of the respiratory muscles.

[55] Dark bluish discoloration of the skin resulting from deficient oxygenation of the blood in the lungs or abnormally reduced flow of blood through the capillaries.

The patient was given thiamin intravenously (10 mg every 6 hr) for several days. Improvement was evident by 48 hr and continued for 2 weeks. Thirty days later, he was free of edema, dyspnea, and cardiomegaly. Cardiac catheterization at that time showed that his blood, systemic venous, and all intracardiac pressures, as well as cardiac output, had all returned to normal.

Case 2

Fibroblasts were cultured from skin biopsies from four patients with Wernicke–Korsakoff syndrome and from four healthy control subjects. The properties of transketolase were studied (Table 10-7). The first patient was a 50-year-old woman with a history of chronic alcoholism. She had been admitted to the hospital with disorientation, nystagmus, sixth-nerve weakness,[59] ataxia, and malnutrition. Treatment with intravenous thiamin and large oral doses of multivitamins had improved her neurologic signs over a few months, but her mental state had deteriorated. She was readmitted with disorientation in both place and time, impaired short-term memory, nystagmus, ataxia, and signs of peripheral neuropathy. She was treated with parenteral thiamin and enteral B vitamins with thiamin; this had improved her general health but had not affected her mental status. The second patient, a 48-year-old man with a 20-year history of chronic alcoholism, was admitted in a severe confusional state. He was disoriented, had severe impairment of recent memory, confabulation, **perseveration**,[60] delusions, nystagmus, and ataxia. Treatment with thiamin and B vitamins had improved his behavior, without

Table 10-7. Characteristics of transketolase from Wernicke–Korsakoff patients

Parameter	Patients	Controls
V_{max} (nmol/min/mg protein)	27 ± 3	17 ± 1
K_m (μM) TPP	195 ± 31	16 ± 2

Laboratory results

Parameter	Patient	Normal value/range
Systemic arterial pressure (mmHg)	100/55	120/80
Systemic venous pressure (cmH$_2$O)	300	<140
Pulmonary artery pressure (mmHg)	64/36	<30/<13
Right ventricular pressure (mmHg)	65/17	<30/<5
O$_2$ consumption (ml/min)	259	200–250
Peripheral blood O$_2$ (ml/liter)	148	170–210
Pulmonary arterial blood O$_2$ (ml/liter)	126	100–160
Cardiac output (liters/min)	11.8	5–7
Blood hemoglobin (g/dl)	11.0	14–19
Cyanide circulation time (sec)	12	20
Femoral arterial pyruvate (mg/dl)	1.5	0.8
Femoral arterial lactate (mg/dl)	14.1	4.7
Femoral arterial glucose (mg/dl)	86	74

affecting his memory. These results show that the affinity of transketolase for its coenzyme (TPP) in Wernicke–Korsakoff patients was less, by an order of magnitude, than that of controls. Furthermore, this biochemical abnormality persisted in fibroblasts cultured for >20 generations in medium containing excess thiamin and no ethanol. The characteristics of pyruvate and α-ketoglutarate dehydrogenases were similar in fibroblasts from patients and controls.

Case Questions

1. What factors would appear to have contributed to the thiamin deficiencies of these patients?
2. What defect in cardiac energy metabolism would appear to be the basis of the high-output cardiac failure observed in the first case?
3. What evidence suggests that the transketolase abnormality of these patients was hereditary? Would you expect such patients to be more or less susceptible to thiamin deprivation? Explain.

---

[56] Triple cadence to the heart sounds at rates of ≥100 beats/min, indicative of serious myocardial disease.
[57] Accumulation of serous fluid.
[58] Rapid beating of the heart (≥100 beats/min), originating in the sinus node.
[59] The sixth cranial nerve is the nervus abducens, the small motor nerve to the lateral rectus muscle of the eye.
[60] The constant repetition of a meaningless word or phrase.

Study Questions and Exercises

1. Construct a schematic map of intermediary metabolism showing the enzymatic steps in which TPP is known to function as a coenzyme.
2. Construct a decision tree for the diagnosis of thiamin deficiency in humans or animals.
3. How does the chemical structure of thiamin relate to its biochemical function?
4. What parameters might you measure to assess the thiamin status of a human or an animal?
5. Construct a concept map illustrating the possible interrelationships of excessive alcohol intake and thiamin status.

Recommended Reading

Bates, C. J. (2001). Thiamin. Chapter 17 in *Present Knowledge in Nutrition*, 8th ed. (B. A. Bowman, and R. M. Russell, eds.), pp. 184–190. ILSI Press, Washington, DC.

Butterworth, R. F. (2003). Thiamin deficiency and brain disorders. *Nutr. Res. Rev.* **16**, 277–283.

Butterworth, R. F. (2006). Thiamin. Chapter 23 in *Modern Nutrition in Health and Disease* (M. E. Shils, M. Shike, A. C. Ross, B. Caballero, and R. Cousins, eds.), 10th ed., pp. 426–433.

Flodin, N. W. (1988). *Pharmacology of Micronutrients*, pp. 103–116. Alan R. Liss, New York.

Friedrich, W. (1988). *Vitamins*, pp. 339–401. Walter de Gruyter, New York.

Gibson, G. E., and Zhang, H. (2002). Interactions of oxidative stress with thiamine homeostasis promote neurodegeneration. *Neurochem. Internat.* **40**, 493–504.

Gregory, J. F., III. (1997). Bioavailability of thiamin. *Eur. J. Clin. Nutr.* **51**, S34–S37.

Harmeyer, J., and Kollenkirchen, U. (1989). Thiamin and niacin in ruminant nutrition. *Nutr. Res. Rev.* **2**, 201–225.

Lonsdale, D. (2006). A review of the biochemistry, metabolism and clinical benefits of thiamin(e) and its derivatives. *eCAM* **3**, 49–59.

Martin, P. R., Singleton, C. K., and Hiller-Sturmhöfel, S. (2003). The role of thiamine deficiency in alcoholic brain disease. *Alcohol Res. Health* **27**, 134–142.

Pohl, M., Sprenger, G. A., and Müller, M. (2004). *Curr. Opin. Biotechnol.* **15**, 335–342.

Rindi, G., and Laforenza, U. (2000). Thiamine intestinal transport and related issues: Recent aspects. *Proc. Soc. Exp. Biol. Med.* **224**, 246–255.

Schenk, G., Duggleby, R. G., and Nixon, P. F. (1998). Properties and functions of thiamin diphosphate dependent enzyme transketolase. *Internat. J. Biochem. Cell Biol.* **30**, 1297–1318.

Tanphaichitr, V. (2001). Thiamine, Chapter 8 in *Handbook of Vitamins*, 3rd ed. (R. B. Rucker, J. W. Suttie, D. B. McCormick, and L. J. Machlin, eds.), pp. 275–316. Marcel Dekker, New York.

Riboflavin

11

In retrospect—the discovery of riboflavin may be considered a scientific windfall. It opened the way to the unraveling of the truly complex vitamin B_2 complex. Perhaps even more significantly, it bridged the gap between an essential constituent and cell enzymes and cellular metabolism. Today, with the general acceptance of this idea, it is not considered surprising that water-soluble vitamins represent essential parts of enzyme systems.

— P. György

I.	The Significance of Riboflavin	282
II.	Sources of Riboflavin	282
III.	Absorption of Riboflavin	283
IV.	Transport of Riboflavin	284
V.	Metabolism of Riboflavin	285
VI.	Metabolic Functions of Riboflavin	287
VII.	Riboflavin Deficiency	288
VIII.	Riboflavin Toxicity	293
IX.	Case Study	293
	Study Questions and Exercises	294
	Recommended Reading	294

Anchoring Concepts

1. Riboflavin is the trivial designation of a specific compound, 7,8-dimethyl-10-(1′-D-ribityl)-isoalloxazine, sometimes also called **vitamin B_2.**
2. Riboflavin is a yellow, hydrophilic, tricyclic molecule that is usually phosphorylated (to FMN and FAD) in biological systems.
3. Deficiencies of riboflavin are manifested chiefly as dermal and neural disorders.

Learning Objectives

1. To understand the chief natural sources of riboflavin.
2. To understand the means of enteric absorption and transport of riboflavin.
3. To understand the biochemical function of riboflavin as a component of key redox coenzymes, and the relationship of that function to the physiological activities of the vitamin.
4. To understand the physiologic implications of low riboflavin status.

Vocabulary

Acyl-CoA dehydrogenase
Adrenodoxin reductase
Alkaline phosphatase
Cheilosis
Curled-toe paralysis
Dehydrogenase
Electron transfer flavoprotein (ETF)
Erythrocyte glutathione reductase
FAD-pyrophosphatase
FAD-synthase
Flavin adenine dinucleotide (FAD)
Flavin mononucleotide (FMN)
Flavokinase
Flavoprotein
FMN-phosphatase
Geographical tongue
Glossitis
L-Gulonolactone oxidase
Hypoplastic anemia
Leukopenia
Lumichrome
Monoamine oxidase
NADH-cytochrome *P*-450 reductase
NADH dehydrogenase
Normocytic hypochromic anemia
Ovoflavin
Oxidase
Reticulocytopenia
Riboflavin-binding proteins (RfBPs)
Riboflavin-5′-phosphate
Riboflavinuria
Stomatitis
Subclinical riboflavin deficiency
Succinate dehydrogenase
Thrombocytopenia

Thyroxine
Ubiquinone reductase

I. The Significance of Riboflavin

Riboflavin is essential for the intermediary metabolism of carbohydrates, amino acids, and lipids, and it also supports cellular antioxidant protection. The vitamin discharges these functions as coenzymes that undergo reduction through two sequential single-electron transfer steps. This allows the reactions catalyzed by **flavoproteins** (i.e., *flavoenzymes*) to involve single- as well as dual-electron transfers. This versatility means that flavoproteins serve as switching sites between obligate two-electron donors such as the pyridine nucleotides and various obligate one-electron acceptors. Because of these fundamental roles of riboflavin in metabolism, a deficiency of the vitamin first manifests itself in tissues with rapid cellular turnover, such as skin and epithelium.

II. Sources of Riboflavin

Distribution in Foods

Riboflavin is widely distributed in foods (Table 11-1), where it is present almost exclusively bound to proteins, mainly in the form of **flavin mononucleotide (FMN)** and **flavin adenine dinucleotide (FAD)**.[1,2] Rapidly growing, green, leafy vegetables are rich in the vitamin; however, meats and dairy products are the most important contributors of riboflavin to American diets, with milk products providing about one-half of the total intake of the vitamin.[3] Animal tissues have been found to contain small amounts of riboflavin-5′α-D-glucoside, which appears to be as well utilized as free riboflavin.

Stability

Riboflavin is stable to heat; therefore, most means of heat sterilization, canning, and cooking do not affect the riboflavin contents of foods. Exposure to light (e.g., sun drying, sunlight exposure of milk in glass bottles, cooking in an open pot) can result in substantial losses, for the vitamin is very sensitive to destruction by light.[4] Riboflavin photodegradation can be exacerbated by sodium bicarbonate, which is used to preserve vegetable colors. Also, because riboflavin is water soluble, it leaches into water used in cooking and into the drippings of meats. As riboflavin in cereal grains is located primarily in the germ and bran, the milling of such materials,[5] which removes those tissues, results in considerable losses in their contents of the vitamin. For example, about half of the riboflavin in whole-grain rice, and more than a third of riboflavin in whole wheat, are lost when these grains are milled. Parboiled ("converted") rice contains most of the riboflavin of the parent grain, as the steam processing of whole brown rice before milling this product drives vitamins originally present in the germ and aleurone layers into the endosperm, where they are retained.

Bioavailability

The noncovalently bound forms of riboflavin in foods, FMN, FAD, and free riboflavin appear to be well absorbed, where as covalently bound flavin complexes, such as are found in plant tissues, are stable to digestion and thus unavailable. In general, riboflavin in animal products tends to have a greater bioavailability than that in plant products.

Role of Hindgut Microflora

Riboflavin is synthesized by the bacteria populating the hindgut. It has been suggested that microfloral

---

[1] Notable exceptions are milk and eggs, which contain appreciable amounts of free riboflavin.

[2] Strictly speaking, FMN is not a nucleotide, nor is FAD a dinucleotide, because each is a D-ribityl derivative; nevertheless, these names have been accepted.

[3] It is estimated that milk and milk products contribute about 50% of the riboflavin in the American diet, with meats, eggs, and legumes contributing a total of about 25%, and fruits and vegetables each contributing about 10%.

[4] Irradiation of food results in the production of reactive free-radical species of oxygen (e.g., superoxide radical anion, hydroxyl radical) that react with riboflavin to destroy it. Thus, exposure of milk in glass bottles to sunlight can result in the destruction of more than one-half of its riboflavin within a day. The short exposure of meat to sterilizing quantities of γ radiation destroys 10–15% of its riboflavin content.

[5] It is the practice in many countries to enrich refined wheat products with several vitamins, including riboflavin, which results in their actually containing *more* riboflavin than the parent grains (e.g., 0.20 mg/100 g versus 0.11 mg/100 g). However, rice is usually *not* enriched with riboflavin to avoid coloring the product yellow by this intensely colored vitamin.

Table 11-1.   Riboflavin contents of foods

Food	Riboflavin (mg/100 g)	Food	Riboflavin (mg/100 g)
Dairy products		Vegetables	
Milk	0.17	Asparagus	0.18
Yogurt	0.16	Broccoli	0.20
Cheese		Cabbage	0.06
American	0.43	Carrots	0.06
Cheddar	0.46	Cauliflower	0.08
Cottage	0.28	Corn	0.06
Ice cream	0.21	Lima beans	0.10
Meats		Potatoes	0.04
Liver, beef	3.50	Spinach	0.14
Beef	0.24	Tomatoes	0.04
Chicken	0.19	Fruits	
Lamb	0.22	Apples	0.01
Pork	0.27	Bananas	0.04
Ham, cured	0.19	Oranges	0.03
Cereals		Peaches	0.04
Wheat, whole	0.11	Strawberries	0.07
Rye	0.08	Other	
Oat meal	0.02	Eggs	0.30
Rice	0.01		

riboflavin can be absorbed across the colon to contribute to nutritional riboflavin status of the host.

III. Absorption of Riboflavin

Hydrolysis of Coenzyme Forms

Because riboflavin occurs in most foods as protein complexes of the coenzyme forms FMN and FAD, the utilization of the vitamin in foods depends on their hydrolytic conversion to free riboflavin. This occurs by the proteolytic activity of the intestinal lumen, which releases the riboflavin coenzymes from their protein complexes, and the subsequent hydrolytic activities of several brush border phosphatases that liberate riboflavin in free form. These include the relatively nonspecific alkaline phosphatase,[6] as well as FAD-pyrophosphatase (which converts FAD to FMN) and FMN-phosphatase (which converts FMN to free riboflavin).

Active Transport of Free Riboflavin

Riboflavin is absorbed in the free form by means of carrier-mediated processes in the proximal small intestine and colon. This process has been found to be at least partially dependent on Na^+ and may also involve the Ca^{+2}/calmodulin-, protein kinase A and G pathways.[7] The upper limit of intestinal absorption has been estimated to be about 25 mg—an order of magnitude greater than the requirement. Riboflavin absorption is enhanced riboflavin deficiency, bile salts,[8] and psyllium gum, and downregulated by high doses of the vitamin. The last-named effect appears to involve decreased activity of the riboflavin carrier induced by increased intracellular concentrations of cyclic AMP.

---

[6] Alkaline phosphatase appears to have the greatest hydrolytic capacity of the brush border phosphatases.

[7] Huang, S. N., and Swaan, P. (2001). *J. Pharmacol. Exp. Ther.* **298,** 264–271.

[8] Children with *biliary atresia* (a congenital condition involving the absence or pathological closure of the bile duct) show reduced riboflavin absorption.

Absorption Linked to Phosphorylation

The free form of riboflavin is transported into the intestinal mucosal cell; however, much of that form is quickly trapped within the enterocyte by phosphorylation to FMN. This is accomplished by an ATP-dependent **flavokinase**. Thus, riboflavin enters the portal circulation as both the free vitamin and FMN.

IV. Transport of Riboflavin

Protein Binding

Riboflavin is transported in the plasma as both free riboflavin and FMN, both of which are bound in appreciable amounts (e.g., about half of the free riboflavin and 80% of FMN) to plasma proteins. This includes tight binding to globulins[9] and fibrinogen, and weak binding to albumin. These proteins bind riboflavin and FMN by hydrogen bonding; the vitamin can be displaced readily by boric acid[10] or several drugs,[11] which thus inhibit its transport peripheral tissues.

Pregnancy-Specific Binding Proteins

Riboflavin-binding proteins (RfBPs) have been identified in the plasma of the laying hen and pregnant cows, mice, rats, monkeys, and humans. The plasma RfBP of the hen has been well characterized; it is not found in the immature female, but is synthesized in the liver under the stimulus of estrogen with the onset of sexual maturity or with induction by estrogen treatment. The avian plasma RfBP is a 32-kDa phosphoglycoprotein with a single binding site for riboflavin. It appears to be one of three products of a single gene, which are variously modified post-translationally to yield the RfBPs in egg white and yolk. The hen plasma RfBP is antigenically similar to the RfBPs of pregnant mice and rats. In both species

RfBP has vital functions in the transplacental/transovarian movement of riboflavin[12] and in the uptake of riboflavin by spermatozoa, as immunoneutralization of the protein terminates pregnancy in females and reduced sperm fertility in males.[13]

Cellular Uptake

Riboflavin uptake appears to occur by a manner similar to its enteric absorption, by a Na^+-dependent, carrier-mediated process probably also involving the Ca^{+2}/calmodulin-, protein kinase A and G pathways. Receptor-mediated endocytosis has also been implicated, particularly in the transport of riboflavin across the placental barrier.[14]

Tissue Distribution

Riboflavin is transported into cells in its free form. However, in the tissues, riboflavin is converted to the coenzyme form, predominantly as FMN (60–95% of total flavins) but also as FAD (5–22% of total flavins in most tissues but about 37% in kidney), both of which are found almost exclusively bound to specific flavoproteins. The greatest concentrations of the vitamin are found in the liver, kidney, and heart. In most tissues, free riboflavin comprises <2% of the total flavins. Significant amounts of free riboflavin are found only in retina, urine, and cow's milk,[15] where it is loosely bound to casein. Although the riboflavin content of the brain is not great, the turnover of the vitamin in that tissue is high and the concentration of the vitamin is relatively resistant to gross changes in riboflavin nutriture. These findings suggest a homeostatic mechanism for regulating the riboflavin content of the brain; such a mechanism has been proposed for the chorioid plexus,[16] in which riboflavin transport has been found to be inhibited by several of its catabolic products and analogs. It has been estimated that the

---

[9] Notably, the immunoglobulins IgA, IgG, and IgM.

[10] The feeding of boric acid to humans and rats has been shown to produce riboflavinuria and to precipitate riboflavin deficiency. In addition, some effects of boric acid toxicity can be overcome by feeding riboflavin.

[11] For example, ouabain, theophylline, and penicillin.

[12] Hens that do not express RfBP produce eggs that lack the normal faint yellow tinge of their otherwise clear albumen. This observation led to the discovery of RfBP as being essential to transferring riboflavin to the egg (Winter, W. P., et al. [1967]. *Comp. Biochem. Physiol.* **22,** 889–896).

[13] Plasma RfBP or fragments have been suggested as having potential utility as a vaccine to regulate fertility in both sexes (Adiga, P. R. [1997]. *Human Reprod. Update* **3,** 325–334).

[14] Foraker, A. M., et al. (2002). *Adv. Drug Deliv. Rev.* **55,** 1467–1483.

[15] Cow's milk differs from human milk in both the amount and form of riboflavin. Cow's milk typically contains 1160–2020 µg of riboflavin per liter, which (like the milk of most other mammals studied) is present mostly as the free vitamin. In contrast, human milk typically contains 120–485 µg of riboflavin per liter (depending on the riboflavin intakes of the mother), which is present mainly as FAD and FMN.

[16] The anatomical site of the blood–cerebrospinal fluid barrier.

total body reserve of riboflavin in the adult human is equivalent to the metabolic demands for 2 to 6 weeks. Riboflavin is found in much lower concentrations in maternal plasma than in cord plasma (in humans, this ratio has been found to be 1:4.7), suggesting the presence of a transplacental transport mechanism.

Tissue RfBPs have been identified in the liver, egg albumen,[17] and egg yolk of the laying hen. Each is similar to the plasma RfBP[18] in that species, differing only in the nature of their carbohydrate[19] contents.[20] A hereditary abnormality in the chicken results in the production of defective RfBPs (in plasma as well as liver and egg). Affected hens show **riboflavinuria** and produce eggs with about half the normal amount of riboflavin and embryos that fail to develop.[21]

V. Metabolism of Riboflavin

Conversion to Coenzyme Forms

After it is taken up by the cell, free riboflavin is converted to its coenzyme forms (Fig. 11-1) in two steps, both of which appear to be regulated by thyroid hormones:

1. *Conversion to FMN*   The ATP-dependent phosphorylation yields **riboflavin-5′-phosphate** (flavin mononucleotide, FMN). This occurs in the cytoplasm of most cells and is catalyzed by the enzyme *flavokinase*.[22] FMN so produced can be complexed with specific apoproteins to form several functional flavoproteins.

2. *Conversion to FAD*   Most FMN is converted to the other coenzyme form, **flavin adenine dinucleotide (FAD),** by a second ATP-dependent enzyme, **FAD-synthase**.[23] This step appears to be feedback-inhibited by FAD, which is complexed in tissues with a variety of dehydrogenases and oxidases mostly by noncovalent associations in discrete dinucleotide-binding domains apparently facilitated by a protein factor. This includes associations via hydrogen bonding with purines,[24] phenols, and indoles (e.g., to

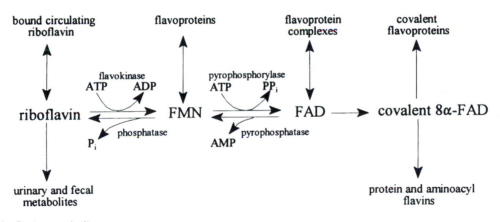

Fig. 11-1.   Riboflavin metabolism.

---

[17] This is the flavoprotein formerly called **ovoflavin**. Comprising nearly 1% of the total protein in egg white, it is the most abundant of any vitamin-binding protein. Unlike the plasma RfBP, which is normally saturated with its ligand, the egg white RfBP is normally less than half-saturated with riboflavin, even when hens are fed diets high in the vitamin. Still, its bound riboflavin is responsible for the faint yellow tinge of egg albumen.

[18] It appears that the plasma RfBP, produced and secreted by the liver in response to estrogens, is the precursor to these other binding proteins found in tissues.

[19] Primarily in their contents of sialic acid, which occurs in many polysaccharides.

[20] It is interesting to note that egg white RfBP forms a 1:1 complex with the thiamin-binding protein (TBP) from the same source.

[21] Embryos from hens that are homozygous recessive for the mutant *rd* allele die of riboflavin deficiency on days 13–14 of incubation. They can be rescued by injecting riboflavin or FMN into the eggs.

[22] Also called riboflavin kinase, the activity of this enzyme is regulated by **thyroxine**, which stimulates its synthesis. Therefore, hypothyroidism is associated with reduced flavokinase activity and, accordingly, reduced tissue levels of FMN and FAD. Hyperthyroidism, in contrast, results in increased flavokinase activity, although tissue levels of FMN and FAD, which appear to be regulated via degradation, do not rise.

[23] The activity is also increased by thyroxine.

[24] In FAD, the riboflavin and adenine moieties are predominantly (85%) hydrogen bonded in an intramolecular complex.

peptidyltryptophan in RfBPs). Less than 10% of FAD is covalently attached to certain apoenzymes (Table 11-2). Linkages of this type involve the riboflavin 8-methyl group, which can form a methylene bridge to the peptide histidyl imidazole function (e.g., in succinic dehydrogenase and sarcosine oxidase), or to the thioether function of a former cysteinyl residue (e.g., in **monoamine oxidase**).[25]

Glycosylation

The capacity to glycosylate riboflavin to yield riboflavin 5'-α-D-glucoside has been demonstrated in rat liver. This metabolite has been shown to be comparable to riboflavin as a cellular source of the vitamin; it has also been identified in the urine of riboflavin-fed rats. These findings suggest that riboflavin 5'-α-D-glucoside is a metabolically significant metabolite.

Catabolism of FAD and FMN

Flavins that are bound to proteins are resistant to degradation; however, when those proteins are saturated with flavins, the unbound forms are subject to catabolism. Both FAD and FMN are catabolized by intracellular enzymes in ways directly analogous to the breakdown of these forms in foods during their absorption across the intestinal mucosal cell. Thus, FAD is converted to FMN by **FAD-pyrophosphatase** (releasing AMP), and FMN is degraded to free riboflavin by **FMN-phosphatases**. Both FAD and FMN are split to yield free riboflavin by **alkaline phosphatase**.

Table 11-2. Covalent flavoproteins in animals

Linkage	Enzyme
Histidinyl(N^3)-8α-FAD	Succinate dehydrogenase
	Dimethylglycine dehydrogenase
	Sarcosine dehydrogenase
Histidinyl (N^1)-8α-FAD	**L-Gulonolactone oxidase**
Cysteinyl(s)-8α-FAD	Monoamine oxidase

Catabolism of Riboflavin

The degradation of riboflavin per se initially involves its hydroxylation at the 7α- and 8α-positions of the isoalloxazine ring by hepatic microsomal cytochrome *P*-450-dependent processes. It is thought that catabolism proceeds by the oxidation and then removal of the methyl groups. The liver, in at least some species, has the ability to form riboflavin α-glycosides. As a result of this metabolism, human blood plasma contains FAD and FMN as the major riboflavin metabolites, as well as small amounts of 7α-hydroxyriboflavin.[26] Side-chain oxidation has been observed in bacterial systems, but not in higher animals.

Excretion

Riboflavin is rapidly excreted; therefore, dietary needs for the vitamin are determined by its rate of excretion, not metabolism. Riboflavin is excreted primarily in the urine. In a riboflavin-adequate human adult, nearly all of a large oral dose of the vitamin will be excreted, with peak concentrations showing in the urine within about 2 hr. Studies in the rat show riboflavin to be turned over with a half-life of about 16 days in adequately nourished animals and much longer in riboflavin-deficient animals. In normal human adults, the urinary excretion of riboflavin is about 200 μg/24 hr, whereas riboflavin-deficient individuals may excrete only 40–70 μg/24 hr. Studies with a diabetic rat model[27] have shown riboflavin excretion to be significantly greater in diabetic individuals than in controls. Riboflavin excretion at <27 μg/mg creatinine is generally considered to indicate riboflavin deficiency in adults; however, this parameter tends to reflect current intake of the vitamin rather than total flavin stores.

The vitamin is excreted mainly (60–70%) as the free riboflavin, with smaller amounts of 7α-[21] and 8α-hydroxyriboflavin,[28] 8α-sulfonylriboflavin, 5'-riboflavinylpeptide, 10-hydroxyethylflavin, riboflavin 5'-α-D-glucoside, **lumichrome**,[29] and 10-formylmethylflavin. Small amounts of riboflavin degradation products are found in the feces (<5% of an oral dose). As only about 1% of an oral dose of the vitamin is excreted

---

[25] Another type of linkage involving the 8-methyl group (i.e., a thiohemiacetal linkage) is found in a microbial FAD-containing cytochrome.

[26] This compound is also called *7-hydroxymethylriboflavin*.

[27] Streptozocin-induced diabetes.

[28] This compound is also called *8-hydroxymethylriboflavin*.

[29] 7,8-Dimethylalloxazine, an irradiation product of riboflavin believed also to be produced by intestinal microbes.

in the bile by humans, most fecal metabolites are thought to be predominantly of gut microbial origin. Little, if any, riboflavin is oxidized to CO_2.[30] Ingestion of boric acid, which binds to the riboflavin sidechain, increases the urinary excretion of the vitamin.

Riboflavin is secreted into mammalian milk mostly as free riboflavin and FAD, and the antagonistic metabolite 10-(2′-hydroxyethyl)flavin, the amounts of which depend on the riboflavin intake of the mother. Milk also contains small amounts of other metabolites including 7- and 8-hydroxymethylriboflavins, 10-formylmethylflavin, and lumichrome.

VI. Metabolic Functions of Riboflavin

Coenzyme Functions

Riboflavin functions metabolically as the essential component of the coenzymes FMN and FAD, which act as intermediaries in transfers of electrons in biological oxidation–reduction reactions. More than 100 enzymes are known to bind FAD or FMN in animal and microbial systems. Most of these enzymes bind the flavinyl cofactors tightly but noncovalently; however, some[31] bind FAD covalently via histidinyl or cysteinyl linkages to the 8α-position of the isoalloxazine ring. These enzymes, called flavoproteins or flavoenzymes, include **oxidases**, which function aerobically, and **dehydrogenases**, which function anaerobically. Some involve one-electron transfers, whereas others involve two-electron transfers. This versatility allows

flavoproteins to serve as switching sites between obligate two-electron donors (e.g., NADH, succinate) and obligate one-electron acceptors (e.g., iron–sulfur proteins, heme proteins). Flavoproteins serve this function by undergoing reduction through two single-electron transfer steps (Fig. 11-2) involving a riboflavinyl radical or semiquinone intermediate (with the unpaired electron localized at N-5). Because the radical intermediate can react with molecular oxygen, flavoproteins can also serve as cofactors in the two-electron reduction of O_2 to H_2O, and in the four-electron activation and cleavage of O_2 in monooxygenase reactions.

Collectively, the flavoproteins show great versatility in accepting and transferring one or two electrons with a range of potentials. This feature can be attributed to the variation in the angle between the two planes of the isoalloxazine ring system (intersecting at N-5 and N-10), which is modified by specific protein binding. The flavin-containing dehydrogenases or reductases (their reduced forms) react slowly with molecular oxygen, in contrast to the fast reactions of the flavin-containing oxidases and monooxygenases. In the former reactions, hydroperoxide derivatives of the flavoprotein are cleaved to yield superoxide anion ($O_2\bullet^-$), but in the latter a heterolytic cleavage of the hydroperoxide group occurs to yield the peroxide ion (OOH^-). Many flavoproteins contain a metal (e.g., iron, molybdenum, zinc), and the combination of flavin and metal ion is often involved in the adjustments of these enzymes in transfers between single- and double-electron donors. In some flavoproteins, the means for multiple-electron transfers is provided by the presence of multiple flavins as well as metals.

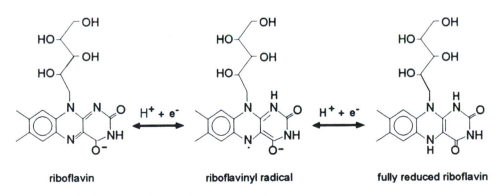

Fig. 11-2. Two-step, single-electron, redox reactions of riboflavin.

---

[30] Rats have been found to oxidize less than 1% of an oral dose of the vitamin.
[31] For example, succinate dehydrogenase, monoamine oxidase, and monomethylglycine dehydrogenase.

Metabolic Roles

The flavoproteins, which are a large group of enzymes involved in biological oxidations and reductions, are essential for the metabolism of carbohydrates, amino acids, and lipids (Table 11-3). Some are also essential for the activation of the vitamins pyridoxine and folate to their respective coenzyme forms.[32]

Health Effects

Oxidative stress

Flavoenzymes participate in protection of erythrocytes and other cells against oxidative stress. This includes the support of intracellular levels of reduced glutathione via glutathione reductase and the direct reduction of oxidized forms of hemoproteins by methemoglobin reductases.

Vascular disease

Riboflavin is essential in the metabolism of homocysteine, as FAD is a required coenzyme of methyltetrahydrofolate reductase, the enzyme responsible for converting N-5,10-methylenetetrahydrofolate to N-5-methyltetrahydrofolate (see Chapter 16, Folic Acid). Impairments in that conversion are manifest as homocysteinemia, which has been associated with increased risks to occlusive vascular disease, total and cardiovascular disease-related mortality, stroke, dimentia, Alzheimer's disease, fracture, and chronic heart failure.[33] The Framingham Offspring study found elevated plasma homocysteine levels in subjects with relatively low plasma riboflavin levels (Table 11-4).

Congenital defects in fat metabolism

As essential coenzymes for **acyl-CoA dehydrogenase** and **NADH dehydrogenase**, riboflavin plays essential roles in lipid metabolism. Accordingly, riboflavin therapy has been found useful in treating cases of deficient expression of these enzymes that otherwise involve recurrent hypoglycemia and lipid storage myopathy. FAD-dependent pathways are involved in the oxidative folding, due to the formation of disulfide bonds, of secretory proteins in the endoplasmic reticulum such as apolipoprotein B-100, the *in vitro* secretion of which has been shown to be impaired by riboflavin deprivation.

Mineral utilization

Riboflavin has the capacity to form complexes with divalent cations such as iron (Fe^{+2}) and zinc (Zn^{+2}). That correction of riboflavin deficiency has been shown to improve significantly the enteric absorption of iron and zinc in the mouse model[34] suggests that riboflavin can be a determinant of the bioavailability of such minerals.

VII. Riboflavin Deficiency

Many tissues are affected by riboflavin deficiency (Table 11-5). Therefore, deprivation of the vitamin causes in animals such general signs as loss of appetite, impaired growth, and reduced efficiency of feed utilization, all of which constitute significant costs in animal agriculture. In addition, both animals and humans experiencing riboflavin deficiency show specific epithelial lesions and nervous disorders. These manifestations are accompanied by abnormally low activities of a variety of flavoenzymes. The most rapid and dramatic loss of activity involves **erythrocyte glutathione reductase**, making this enzyme a useful marker of riboflavin status.[35] Substantial losses also occur in the activities of flavokinase and FAD-synthetase; thus, the biosynthesis of flavoproteins is lost under conditions of riboflavin deprivation. In summary, then, riboflavin deficiency results in impairments in the metabolism of energy, amino acids, and lipids. These metabolic impairments are manifested morphologically as arrays of both general and specific signs/symptoms.

---

[32] Riboflavin has been found to play a role in the regulation of gene expression in bacteria by forming mRNA structures called "riboswitches" that repress conformation to cause premature termination of transcription or inhibit the initiation of translation. Analogous function in higher animals has not been reported.

[33] Selhub, J. (2006). *J. Nutr.* **136,** 1726S–1730S.

[34] Agte, V. V., et al. (1998). *Biol Trace Elem. Res.* **65,** 109–115.

[35] Estimation of the degree of saturation of erythrocyte glutathione reductase (*EGR*) by FAD has proven extremely useful in assessing riboflavin status, in a manner analogous to the use of erythrocyte transketolase saturation by thiamin pyrophosphate (TPP) to assess thiamin status.. Studies have shown that *in vitro* EGR activities of normal, riboflavin-adequate individuals is stimulated ≤20% by the addition of exogenous FAD. Individuals showing activity coefficients (native EGR activity/EGR activity with added FAD) of 20–30% and >30% are considered to be at moderate and high risk, respectively, of riboflavin deficiency.

Table 11-3.   Important flavoproteins of animals[a]

Flavoprotein	Flavin	Metabolic function
One-electron transfers		
Mitochondrial **electron transfer flavoprotein (ETF)**	FAD	e^- acceptor for acyl-CoA, branched-chain acyl-CoA, glutaryl-CoA, and sarcosine and dimethylyglycine dehydrogenases; links primary flavoprotein dehydrogenases with respiratory chain via ETF-ubiquinone reductase
Ubiquinone reductase	FAD	1-e^- transfer from ETF and coenzyme Q of respiratory chain
NADH-cytochrome *P*-450 reductase[b]	FMN	1-e^- transfer from FMN to cytochrome *P*-450 (monooxygenase)
Pyridine-linked dehydrogenases		
NADP-cytochrome *P*-450 reductase[b]	FAD	2-e^- transfer from NADP to FAD
Adrenodoxin reductase	FAD	2-e^- transfer from NADP to adrenodoxin[c] in steroid hydroxylation by adrenal cortex
NADP dehydrogenase	FMN	2-e^- transfer from NADP to FMN, then to ubiquinone[d]
NADP-dependent methemoglobin reductase	FAD	2-e^- transfer from NADP to FAD, then to methemoglobin
Nonpyridine nucleotide-dependent dehydrogenases		
Succinate dehydrogenase	FAD	Transfer reducing equivalents from succinate to ubiquinone yielding fumarate
Acyl-CoA dehydrogenases	FAD	2-e^- transfer from substrate to flavin, in oxidation of the *N*-methyl groups of choline and sarcosine
Pyridine nucleotide oxidoreductases		
Glutathione reductase	FAD	Reduction of GSSG to GSH using NADPH
Lipoamide dehydrogenase[e]	FAD	Oxidation of dihydrolipoamide to lipoamide using NAD⁺
Reactions of reduced flavoproteins with oxygen		
D-Amino acid oxidase	FAD	Dehydrogenation of D-amino acid substrates to imino acids, which are hydrolyzed to α-keto acids
L-Amino acid oxidase	FMN	Dehydrogenation of L-amino acid substrates to imino acids, which are hydrolyzed to α-keto acids
Monoamine oxidase	FAD	Dehydration of biogenic amines[f] to their corresponding imines with hydrogen transfer to O_2, forming H_2O_2
Xanthine oxidase	FAD	Oxidation of hypoxanthine and xanthine to uric acid with formation of H_2O_2
L-Gulonolactone oxidase	FAD	Oxidation of L-gulonolactone to ascorbic acid
Flavoprotein monooxygenase		
Microsomal flavoprotein monooxygenase	FAD	Oxidation of N, S, Se, and I centers of various substrates in drug metabolism

[a]Key enzymes are indicated in boldface.
[b]A component of microsomal cytochrome *P*-450, it contains one molecule each of FAD and FMN.
[c]An iron-sulfur protein.
[d]Also has NADH-ubiquinone reductase activity, reductively releasing iron from ferritin.
[e]A component of the pyruvate dehydrogenase and α-ketoglutarate dehydrogenase complexes.
[f]For example, serotonin, noradrenaline, benzylamine.

Table 11-4. Relationship of plasma riboflavin and homocysteine levels among subjects in the Framingham offspring cohort study

	Plasma riboflavin tertile, nmol/L		
	< 6.89	6.89–10.99	=11.0
Subjects	147	151	152
Plasma			
homocysteine			
Mean	10.3	9.5	9.5
95% C.I.	9.8–10.8	9.1–10.0	9.1–10.0
P-value	—	0.02	0.03

Source: Jacques, P. F., et al. (2002). *J. Nutr.* **132**, 283–288.

Table 11-5. Signs of riboflavin deficiency

Organ system	Sign(s)
General	
Appetite	Decrease
Growth	Decrease
Dermatologic	Cheilosis, stomatitis
Muscular	Weakness
Gastrointestinal	Inflammation, ulcer
Skeletal	Deformities
Vital organs	Hepatic steatosis
Vascular	
Erythrocytes	Anemia
Nervous	Ataxia, paralysis
Reproductive	
Male	Sterility
Female	Decreased egg production
Fetal	Malformations, death
Ocular	
Retinal	Photophobia
Corneal	Decreased vascularization

Riboflavin deficiency produces in the small intestine a hyperproliferative response of the mucosa, characterized by reductions in number of villi, increases in villus length, and increases in the transit rates of enterocytes along the villi. These morphological effects are associated with reduced enteric absorption of dietary iron, resulting in secondary impairments in nutritional iron status in riboflavin-deprived individuals.

Factors Contributing to Riboflavin Deficiency

Several factors can contribute to riboflavin deficiency:

- *Inadequate diet* Inadequate diet is the most important cause of riboflavin deficiency. Frequently, this involves the low consumption of milk,[36] which is the most important source of the vitamin available in most diets. In industrialized countries, riboflavin deficiency occurs most frequently among alcoholics, whose dietary practices are often faulty, leading to this and other deficiencies.
- *Enhanced catabolism* Catabolic conditions associated with illness or vigorous physical exercise and involving nitrogen loss increase riboflavin losses.
- *Alcohol* High intakes of alcohol appear to antagonize the utilization of FAD from foods.
- *Phototherapy* Phototherapy of infants with hyperbilirubinemia often leads to riboflavin deficiency (by photodestruction of the vitamin)[37] if such therapy does not also include the administration of riboflavin.[38]
- *Exercise* Physical exercise can produce abnormalities in a variety of biochemical markers of riboflavin status such as increased erythrocyte glutathione reductase activity coefficient and reduced urinary riboflavin. Nevertheless, there is no evidence that such abnormalities lead to impairments in physiological performance.
- *Other factors* Although earlier studies purported to show reduced riboflavin status among some women using oral contraceptive agents, more recent critical studies have failed to detect any such interaction. Patients receiving diuretics or undergoing hemodialysis experience enhanced loss of riboflavin (as well as other water-soluble vitamins).

---

[36] Children consuming less than a cup of milk per week are likely to be deficient in riboflavin.

[37] Phototherapy can be an effective treatment for infants with mild hyperbilirubinemia; however, the mechanism by which it leads to the degradation of bilirubin (to soluble substances that can be excreted) necessarily leads also to the destruction of riboflavin. It is the photoactivation of riboflavin in the patient's plasma that generates singlet oxygen, which reacts with bilirubin. Thus, plasma riboflavin levels of such patients have been found to drop as the result of phototherapy. Riboflavin supplementation prevents such a drop and has been shown to enhance bilirubin destruction.

[38] For example, 0.5 mg of riboflavin sodium phosphate per kilogram body weight per day.

Deficiency Disorders in Animals

Riboflavin deficiency in animals is potentially fatal. In addition to the general signs already mentioned, animals show other signs that vary with the species. Riboflavin-deficient rodents show dermatologic signs (alopecia, seborrheic inflammation,[39] moderate epidermal hyperkeratosis[40] with atrophy of sebaceous glands) and a generally ragged appearance. Red, swollen lips and abnormal papillae of the tongue are seen. Ocular signs may also be seen (blepharitis,[41] conjunctivitis,[42] and corneal opacity). Feeding a high-fat diet can increase the severity of deficiency signs; high-fat-fed rats showed anestrus, multiple fetal skeletal abnormalities (shortening of the mandible, fusion of ribs, cleft palate, deformed digits and limbs), paralysis of the hind limbs (degeneration of the myelin sheaths of the sciatic nerves[43]), hydrocephalus,[44] ocular lesions, cardiac malformations, and hydronephrosis.[45]

The riboflavin-deficient chick also experiences myelin degeneration of nerves, affecting the sciatic nerve in particular. This results in an inability to extend the digits, a syndrome called **curled-toe paralysis** (see Fig. 11-3). In hens, the deficiency involves reductions in both egg production and embryonic survival (decreased hatchability of fertile eggs). Riboflavin-deficient turkeys show severe dermatitis. The deficiency is rapidly fatal in ducks.

Riboflavin-deficient dogs are weak and ataxic. They show dermatitis (chest, abdomen, inner thighs, axillae, and scrotum) and **hypoplastic anemia**,[46] with fatty infiltration of the bone marrow. They can have bradycardia and sinus arrhythmia[47] with respiratory failure. Corneal opacity has been reported. The deficiency can be fatal, with collapse and coma. Swine fed a riboflavin-deficient diet grow slowly and develop a scaly dermatitis with

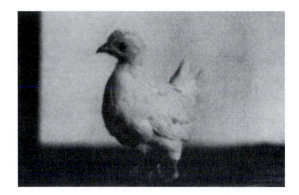

Fig. 11-3. Curled-toe paralysis in a riboflavin-deficient chick.

alopecia. They can show corneal opacity, cataracts, adrenal hemorrhages, fatty degeneration of the kidney, inflammation of the mucous membranes of the gastrointestinal tract, and nerve degeneration. In severe cases, deficient individuals can collapse and die.

Riboflavin deficiency in the newborn calf[48] is manifested as redness of the buccal mucosa,[49] angular **stomatitis**,[50] alopecia, diarrhea, excessive tearing and salivation, and inanition. Signs of riboflavin deficiency appear to develop rather slowly in rhesus monkeys. The first signs seen are weight loss (6–8 weeks), followed by dermatologic changes in the mouth, face, legs, and hands and a **normocytic hypochromic anemia**[51] (2–6 months) and, ultimately, collapse and death with fatty degeneration of the liver. Similar signs have been produced in baboons made riboflavin-deficient for experimental purposes.

Deficiency Signs in Humans

Uncomplicated riboflavin deficiency becomes manifest in humans only after 3 to 4 months of deprivation

---

[39] Involving excess oiliness due to excess activity of the sebaceous glands.

[40] Hypertrophy of the horny layer of the epidermis.

[41] Inflammation of the eyelids.

[42] Inflammation of the mucous membrane covering the anterior surface of the eyeball.

[43] The nerve situated in the thigh.

[44] A condition involving the excessive accumulation of fluid in the cerebral ventricles, dilating these cavities, and, in severe cases, thinning the brain and causing a separation of the cranial bones.

[45] Dilation of one or both kidneys owing to obstructed urine flow.

[46] Progressive nonregenerative anemia resulting from depressed, inadequate functioning of the bone marrow.

[47] Irregular heart beat, with the heart under control of its normal pacemaker, the sino-atrial (S-A) node.

[48] Ruminants do not normally require a dietary source of riboflavin, as the bacteria in their rumens synthesize the vitamin in adequate amounts. However, newborn calves and lambs, whose rumen microflora is not yet established, require riboflavin in their diets. This is normally supplied by their mothers' milk or by supplements in their milk-replacer formula diets.

[49] The mucosa of the cheek.

[50] Lesions in the corners of the mouth.

[51] Anemia involving erythrocytes of normal size but low hemoglobin content.

of the vitamin. Signs include **cheilosis**,[52] angular stomatitis, **glossitis** (see Fig. 11-4),[53] hyperemia,[54] and edema[55] of the oral mucosa, seborrheic dermatitis around the nose and mouth and scrotum/vulva, and a normocytic, normochromic anemia with **reticulocytopenia**,[56] **leukopenia**,[57] and **thrombocytopenia**.[58] Riboflavin-deficient humans also experience neurological dysfunction involving peripheral neuropathy of the extremities characterized by hyperesthesia,[59] coldness and pain, as well as decreased sensitivity to touch, temperature, vibration, and position.

Subclinical Deficiency

Although clinical signs of riboflavin deficiency are rarely seen in the industrialized world, **subclinical riboflavin deficiency**—that is, conditions wherein a subject's intake of the vitamin may be sufficient to prevent clinical signs but not to keep the flavoproteins saturated for optimal metabolism—is not uncommon. It has been estimated that as much as 27% of urban American teenagers of low socioeconomic status have subclinical riboflavin deficiency.

Riboflavin deficiency has been reported to enhance carcinogenesis.[60] This effect is thought to be due to diminished antioxidant protection, increasing the activation of carcinogens and oxidative damage to DNA, and/or diminished folate metabolism, reducing DNA synthesis, repair, and methylation.

Subclinical riboflavin deficiency may actually be beneficial under certain conditions:

- *Protection against malaria* Because growth of the malarial parasite (*Plasmodium* sp.) in the erythrocytes of infected hosts causes oxidative stress in those cells, riboflavin deficiency is protective against propagation of the infection. This has been demonstrated in both humans and animal models. Similarly, flavin analog[61] that antagonize riboflavin and inhibit glutathione reductase have been shown to have antimalarial activities. The metabolic basis of this protection is thought to involve erythrocytes of riboflavin-deficient individuals being vulnerable to destructive lipid peroxidation due to their lost antioxidant protection. Hence, they tend to autolyze before the plasmodia they contain can mature, reducing the parasitemia and decreasing the symptoms of infection. In addition, malarial parasites have been shown to be even more susceptible than erythrocytes to reactive oxygen species. The infected erythrocyte has been found to have an increased need for riboflavin,[62] suggesting that marginal riboflavin status may be selectively debilitating to the infected cell.
- *Protection against tryptophan deficiency-induced cataract* Riboflavin deficiency has been shown to protect the rat from the cataractogenic effect of a low-tryptophan diet. The metabolic basis of this effect may involve the lack of formation of a riboflavinyl tryptophan adduct that accelerates the photo-oxidation of the amino acid to a prooxidative form.

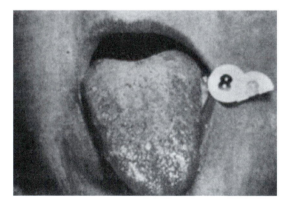

Fig. 11-4. Geographical tongue in riboflavin deficiency. (Courtesy of Cambridge University Press.)

---

[52] Lesions of the lips.

[53] Inflammation of the tongue. This can involve disappearance of filiform papillae and enlargement of fungiform papillae, with the tongue color changing to a deep red. Subjects with this condition, called **geographical tongue**, have soreness of the tongue and loss of taste sensation.

[54] Increased amount of blood present.

[55] Accumulation of excessive fluid in the tissue.

[56] Abnormally low number of immature red blood cells in the circulating blood.

[57] Abnormally low number of white blood cells in the circulating blood (<5000/ml).

[58] Abnormally low number of platelets in the circulating blood.

[59] Excessive sensibility to touch, pain, etc.

[60] Webster, R. P., et al. (1973). *Cancer Res.* 33, 1997.

[61] Galactoflavin, 10-(4′-chlorophenyl)-3-methylflavin and some isoalloxazine derivatives.

[62] Dutta, P. (1991). *J. Protozool.* **38,** 479–483.

VIII. Riboflavin Toxicity

The toxicity of riboflavin is *very low*, and thus problems of hypervitaminosis are not expected. Probably because it is not well absorbed, high oral doses of riboflavin are essentially nontoxic. Oral riboflavin doses as great as 2–10 g/kg body weight produce no adverse effects in dogs and rats. The vitamin is somewhat more toxic when administered parenterally. The LD_{50} (50% lethal dose) values for the rat given riboflavin by the intraperitoneal, subcutaneous, and oral routes have been estimated to be 0.6, 5, and >10 g/kg, respectively.

IX. Case Study

Instructions

Review the following summary of a research report, paying special attention to the diagnostic indicators on which the treatments were based. Then answer the questions that follow.

Case

An experiment was conducted to determine the basis of protection by riboflavin deficiency against malarial infection. An animal model, which previously showed such protection against *Plasmodium berghei*, was used. It involved depleting 3-week-old male rats of riboflavin by feeding them a sucrose-based purified diet containing <1 mg of riboflavin per kilogram. A control group was pair-fed[63] the same basal diet supplemented with 8.5 mg of riboflavin per kilogram.[64] At 6 weeks of age, several biochemical characteristics of erythrocytes (RBCs) were measured: reduced glutathione levels, activities of antioxidant enzymes, stabilities of erythrocytes to hemolysis (measured by incubating 0.5% suspensions of RBCs with prooxidants [500 μM

H_2O_2 or 2.5 μM ferriprotoporphyrin IX] or in a hypotonic medium [151 mOsm] for 1 hr at 37°C). Oxidative damage was assessed by measuring H_2O_2-induced production of malonyldialdehyde (MDA). Other studies with this and similar animal models have shown that the riboflavin-deficient group, when infected with the parasite, *grows better* and shows *reduced parasitemia* than pair-fed controls.

Results of biochemical studies of erythrocytes

Parameter	Riboflavin deficient	Control	p Value
Reticulocytes (% total RBCs)	1.50 ± 0.29	1.26 ± 0.37	NS[a]
Hemoglobin (g/dl blood)	14.7 ± 0.6	14.9 ± 0.3	NS
GSH (mmol/g Hb)	7.97 ± 2.89	6.19 ± 2.52	<0.001
Glutathione reductase (mU[b]/mg protein)	42 ± 6	124 ± 16	<0.001
Glutathione reductase activity coefficient	2.37 ± 0.19	1.20 ± 0.08	<0.01
Glutathione peroxidase (mU[b]/g Hb)	918 ± 70	944 ± 62	NS
In vitro hemolysis (%)			
H_2O_2-induced	32 ± 9	55 ± 9	<0.05
Hypotonicity	69 ± 4	53 ± 7	<0.01
Ferriprotoporphyrin IX	42 ± 3	29 ± 4	<0.001
MDA (nmol/g Hb)			
Before incubation	25.5 ± 3.8	25.9 ± 3.4	NS
Incubated with H_2O_2	34.8 ± 1.2	42.7 ± 1.8	<0.01

[a]NS = Not significant.
[b]1 mU = 1 nmol of NADPH oxidized per minute.

---

[63] *Pair-feeding* is a method of controlling for the effects of reduced food intake that may be secondary to the independent experimental variable (e.g., a nutrient deficiency). It involves the matching of one animal from the experimental treatment group with one of similar body weight from the control group, and the feeding of the latter individual a measured amount of feed equivalent to the amount of feed consumed by the former individual on the previous day. In experiments of more than a few days' duration, this approach normalizes the feed intake of both the experimental and control groups.

[64] This level is about three times the amount normally required by the rat.

Case Questions

1. What dependent variables did the investigators measure to confirm that riboflavin deficiency had been produced in their experimental animals?
2. Propose a hypothesis to explain the apparently discrepant results regarding the effects of riboflavin deficiency on erythrocyte stability.
3. Propose a hypothesis for the protective effect of riboflavin deficiency against malarial infection. What other nutrients might you expect to influence susceptibility to this erythrocyte-attacking parasite?

Study Questions and Exercises

1. Diagram the general roles of FAD- and FMN-dependent enzymes in various area of metabolism.
2. Construct a decision tree for the diagnosis of riboflavin deficiency in humans or in animal species.
3. What key feature of the chemistry of riboflavin relates to its biochemical functions in flavoproteins?
4. What diet and lifestyle factors would you expect to affect dietary riboflavin needs? Justify your answer.
5. What parameters might you measure to assess the riboflavin status of a human or animal?

Recommended Reading

Bates, C. J. (1997). Bioavailability of riboflavin. *Eur. J. Clin. Nutr.* **51,** S38–S42.

Decker, K. F. (1993). Biosynthesis and function of enzymes with covalently bound flavin. *Annu. Rev. Nutr.* **13,** 17–41.

Foraker, A. B., Khantwal, C. M., and Swaan, P. W. (2003). Current perspectives on the cellular uptake and trafficking of riboflavin. *Adv. Drug Deliv. Rev.* **55,** 1467–1483.

Hefti, M. H., Vervoot, J., and van Berkel, W. J. H. (2003). Deflavination and reconstitution of flavoproteins. Tackling fold and function. *Eur. J. Biochim.* **270,** 4227–4242.

McCormick, D. B. (2002). Micronutrient cofactor research with extensions to applications. *Nutr. Res. Rev.* **15,** 245–262.

McCormick, D. B. (2006). Riboflavin, Chapter 24 in *Modern Nutrition in Health and Disease,* 10th ed. (M. E. Shils, M. Shike, A. C. Ross, B. Caballero, and R. J. Cousins, eds.), pp. 434–441. Lippincott, New York.

Mewies, M., McIntire, W. S., and Scrutton, N. S. (1998). Covalent attachment of flavin adenine dinucleotide (FAD) and flavin mononucleotide (FMN) to enzymes: The current state of affairs. *Protein Sci.* **7,** 7–20.

Powers, H. J. (2003). Riboflavin (vitamin B-2) and health. *Am. J. Clin. Nutr.* **77,** 1352–1360.

Rivlin, R. S. (2001). Riboflavin. Chapter 18 in *Present Knowledge in Nutrition,* 8th ed. (B. A. Bowman and R. M. Russell, eds.), pp. 191–198. ILSI Press, Washington, DC.

Rivlin, R. S., and Pinto, J. T. (2001). Riboflavin, Chapter 7 in *Handbook of Vitamins* 3rd ed. (R. B. Rucker, J. W. Suttie, D. B. McCormick, and L. J. Machlin, eds.), pp. 255–274. Marcel Dekker, New York.

Vitreschak, A. G., Rodionov, D. A., Mironov, A. A., and Gelfand, M. S. (2004). Riboswitches: The oldest mechanism for the regulation of gene expression? *Trends Genet.* **20,** 44–50.

White, H. B., and Merrill, A. J., Jr. (1988). Riboflavin-binding proteins. *Annu. Rev. Nutr.* **8,** 279–299.

Winkler, W. C., and Breaker, R. R. (2003). Genetic control by metabolite-binding riboswitches. *Chem. Bio. Chem.* **4,** 1024–1032.

Niacin

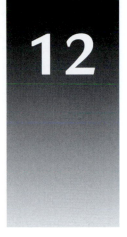

12

So far as they have been studied, the foodstuffs that appear to be good sources of the black tongue preventive also appear to be good sources of the pellagra preventive.... Considering the available evidence as a whole, it would seem highly probable, if not certain, that experimental black tongue and pellagra are essentially identical conditions and, thus, that the preventive of black tongue is identical with the pellagra preventive, or factor P-P. On the basis of the indications afforded by the test in the dog, liver, salmon and egg yolk are recommended for use in the treatment and prevention of pellagra in humans.

—J. Goldberger

I.	The Significance of Niacin	296
II.	Sources of Niacin	296
III.	Absorption of Niacin	298
IV.	Transport of Niacin	298
V.	Metabolism of Niacin	299
VI.	Metabolic Functions of Niacin	303
VII.	Niacin Deficiency	304
VIII.	Pharmacologic Uses of Niacin	307
IX.	Niacin Toxicity	309
X.	Case Study	309
	Study Questions and Exercises	310
	Recommended Reading	311

Anchoring Concepts

1. Niacin is the generic descriptor for pyridine 3-carboxylic acid and derivatives exhibiting qualitatively the biological activity of nicotinamide.
2. The two major forms of niacin, nicotinic acid and nicotinamide, are active metabolically as the pyridine nucleotide coenzymes NAD(H) and NADP(H).
3. Deficiencies of niacin are manifest as dermatologic, gastrointestinal, and neurologic changes and can be fatal.

Learning Objectives

1. To understand the chief natural sources of niacin.
2. To understand the means of enteric absorption and transport of niacin.
3. To understand the biochemical function of niacin as a component of coenzymes of a variety of metabolically important redox reactions, and the relationship of that function to the physiological activities of the vitamin.

4. To understand the factors that can affect low niacin status, and the physiological implications of that condition.

Vocabulary

Acetyl-CA
α-Amino-β-carboxymuconic-ϵ-semialdehyde (ACS)
α-Aminomuconic-ϵ-semialdehyde
Anthranilic acid
Black tongue disease
Casal's collar
Flushing
Formylase
N-Formylkynurenine
Glucose tolerance factor
Hartnup disease
3-Hydroxyanthranilic acid (3-OH-AA)
3-Hydroxyanthranilic acid oxygenase (3-HAAO)
3-Hydroxykynurenine (3-OH-Ky)
Kynurenic acid
Kynurenine
Kynurenine 3-hydroxylase
Leucine
1-Methylnicotinamide
1-Methylnicotinic acid
1-Methyl-6-pyridone 3-carboxamide
NAD⁺ kinase
NAD⁺ synthetase
NAD(P)⁺ glycohydrolase
Niacytin
Nicotinate phosphoribosyltransferase
Nicotinamide (NAm)
Nicotinamide-adenine dinucleotide (NAD(H))
Nicotinamide-adenine dinucleotide phosphate (NADP(H))
Nicotinamide methylase

Nicotinamide *N*-methyltransferase
Nicotinamide riboside (NR)
Nicotinic acid (NA)
Pellagra
Perosis
Phosphodiesterase
Picolinic acid
Picolinic acid carboxylase (PAC)
Poly(ADP-ribose) polymerase
Pyridine nucleotide
Pyridoxal phosphate
Quinolinate phosphoribosyltransferase
Quinolinic acid (QA)
Schizophrenia
Transaminase
Transhydrogenase
Trigonelline
Tryptophan
Tryptophan pyrrolase
Xanthurenic acid

I. The Significance of Niacin

Niacin is required for the biosynthesis of the **pyridine nucleotides NAD(H)** and **NADP(H)**, through which the vitamin has key roles in virtually all aspects of metabolism. Historically, niacin deficiency was prevalent among people who relied on maize (corn) as their major food staple; before the availability of inexpensive supplements, the deficiency was also a frequent problem of livestock fed maize-based diets.

Great irony characterizes niacin deficiency. Unlike thiamin deficiency (which also involves a cereal-based diet), niacin deficiency more frequently results from poor bioavailability rather than scarcity per se. Hence, paradoxical questions have been asked:

- Why does niacin deficiency occur among individuals who can biosynthesize the vitamin?
- Why did pellagra occur among people eating corn, whereas in the Americas, where maize was a historically important part of the diet, the disease was unknown?

- Why do corn-based diets produce pellagra, although corn contains an appreciable amount of niacin?
- Why does milk, which contains little niacin, prevent pellagra?
- Why does rice, which contains less niacin than corn, not produce pellagra?

More recently, interest in niacin has moved to its apparent value as a pharmacologic agent at multigram-dose levels. Understanding the bases of the physiologic and pharmacologic activities of niacin calls for an appreciation of its complexities, which are manifested differently in various species.

II. Sources of Niacin

Distribution in Foods

Niacin occurs in greatest quantities in brewers' yeasts and meats, but significant amounts are also found in many other foods (Table 12-1). The vitamin is distributed unevenly in grains, being present mostly in the bran fractions. Niacin occurs predominantly in bound forms, for example, in plants mostly as protein-bound **nicotinic acid (NA)** and in animal tissues mostly as **nicotinamide (NAm)** in **nicotinamide-adenine dinucleotide (NAD(H))** and **nicotinamide-adenine dinucleotide phosphate (NADP(H))**. Niacin is added by law to wheat flour and other grain products in the United States.[1]

Stability

Niacin in foods is very stable to storage and to normal means of food preparation and cooking (e.g., moist heat).

Bioavailability

Niacin is found in many types of foods in forms from which it is not released on digestion, thereby rendering it unavailable to the eater. In grains, niacin is present in covalently bound complexes with small peptides and carbohydrates, collectively referred to as **niacytin**.[2] The esterified niacin in these complexes is not normally available; however, its bioavailability

---

[1] Fortification is mandated for niacin, thiamin, riboflavin, folate, and iron.

[2] A polysaccharide extracted from wheat bran has been found to contain more than 1% nicotinic acid bound via an ester linkage to glucose in a complex also containing arabinose, galactose, and xylose. Although NAD^+ and $NADP^+$, both of which are biologically available to humans and animals, are present in early-stage corn, those levels decline as the grain matures and are replaced by nicotinamide and nicotinic acid as well as forms of very low bioavailability such as bound niacin and trigonelline.

Table 12-1.   Niacin contents of foods

Food	Niacin (mg/100 g)	Food	Niacin (mg/100 g)
Dairy products		Vegetables	
Milk	0.2	Asparagus	1.5
Yogurt	0.1	Beans	0.5–2.4
Cheeses	1.2	Broccoli	0.9
Meats		Brussels sprouts	0.9
Beef	4.6	Cabbage	0.3
Chicken	4.7–14.7	Carrots	0.6
Lamb	4.5	Cauliflowr	0.7
Pork	0.8–5.6	Celery	0.3
Turkey	8.0	Corn	1.7
Calf heart	7.5	Kale	2.1
Calf kidney	6.4	Lentils	2.0
Herring	3.6	Onions	0.2
Cod	2.2	Peas	0.9–25.0
Flounder	2.5	Peppers	1.7–4.4
Haddock	3.0	Potatoes	1.5
Tuna	13.3	Soy beans	1.4
Cereals		Spinach	0.6
Barley	3.1	Tomatoes	0.7
Buckwheat	4.4	Fruits	
Cornmeal	1.4–2.9	Apples	0.6
Rice		Bananas	0.7
Polished	1.6	Grapefruit	0.2
Unpolished	4.7	Oranges	0.4
Rye	0.9–1.6	Peaches	1.0
Wheat		Strawberries	0.6
Whole grain	3.4–6.5	Nuts	
Wheat bran	8.6–33.4	Most nuts	0.6–1.8
Other		Peanuts	17.2
Eggs	0.1		
Mushrooms	4.2		
Yeast	50.1		

can be improved substantially by treatment with base to effect the alkaline hydrolysis of those esters. The tradition in Central American cuisine of soaking corn in lime[3]-water before the preparation of tortillas effectively renders available the niacin in that grain. This practice appears to be responsible for effective protection against pellagra in that part of the world. In other foods, niacin is present as a methylated derivative (**1-methylnicotinic acid**, also called **trigonelline**) that functions as a plant hormone but is also not biologically available to animals. This form, however, is heat labile and can be converted to NA by heating.[4]

---

[3] Calcium oxide.

[4] Thus, the roasting of coffee beans effectively removes the methyl group from trigonelline, increasing the nicotinic acid content of that food from 20 to 500 mg/kg. This practice, too, appears to have contributed to the rarity of pellagra in the maize-eating cultures of South and Central America.

Importance of Dietary Tryptophan

A substantial amount of niacin can be synthesized from the indispensable amino acid **tryptophan.** Therefore, the niacin adequacy of diets involves not only the level of the preformed vitamin, but also that of its potential precursor (Table 12-2).

III. Absorption of Niacin

Digestion of NAD/NADP

The predominant forms of niacin in most animal-derived foods, NAD(H) and NADP(H), appear to be digested to release NAm, in which form the vitamin is absorbed (Fig. 12-1). Both coenzyme forms can be degraded by the intestinal mucosal enzyme **NAD(P)⁺ glycohydrolase**, which cleaves the pyridine nucleotides into NAm and ADP-ribose. Nicotinamide can also be cleaved at the pyrophosphate bond to yield **nicotinamide mononucleotide (NMN)** and 5'-AMP, or by a **phosphodiesterase** to yield **nicotinamide riboside (NR)** and ADP. The dephosphorylation of NMN also yields NR, which can be converted to NAm either by hydrolysis (yielding ribose) or phosphorylation (yielding ribose 1-phosphate). The cleavage of NAm to free NA appears to be accomplished by intestinal microorganisms and is believed to be of quantitative importance in niacin absorption.

Table 12-2. Niacin-equivalent contents of several foods

Food	Preformed niacin (mg/ 1000 kcal)	Tryptophan (mg/ 1000 kcal)	Niacin equivalents[a] (mg/ 1000 kcal)
Cow's milk	1.21	673	12.4
Human milk	2.46	443	9.84
Beef	2.47	1280	23.80
Eggs (whole)	0.60	1150	19.80
Pork	1.15	61	2.17
Wheat flour	2.48	297	7.43
Corn meal	4.97	106	6.74
Corn grits	1.83	70	3.00
Rice	4.52	290	9.35

[a]Based on a conversion efficiency of 60:1 for humans.

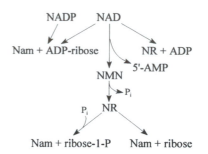

Fig. 12-1. Metabolic disposition of absorbed niacin.

Facilitated Diffusion

Niacin is absorbed in the stomach and small intestine. Studies using everted intestinal sacs prepared from rats have demonstrated that both NA and NAm are absorbed at low concentrations via Na⁺-dependent, carrier-mediated facilitated diffusion. Both forms of the vitamin are absorbed across the human buccal mucosa by the same mechanism. The rate of diffusion of NA is about half that of NAm. At high concentrations, however, each is absorbed via passive diffusion. Therefore, at pharmacologic concentrations the vitamin is absorbed nearly completely.[5] The presence or absence of food in the gut appears to have no effect on niacin absorption. Because NR is not found in plasma, it appears not to be absorbed per se, but is first converted to NAm.

IV. Transport of Niacin

Free in Plasma

Niacin is transported in the plasma as both NA and NAm in unbound forms. Because the NA is converted to NAD(H) and subsequently to Nam, in the intestine and liver, circulating levels of NAm tend to exceed those of NA.

Cellular Uptake

Both NA and NAm are taken up by most peripheral tissues through passive diffusion; however, some tissues have transport systems that facilitate niacin uptake. Erythrocytes take up NA by the anion transport system. Renal tubules do so by an Na⁺-dependent, saturable transport system. The brain takes up the vitamin by energy-dependent transport systems; the site of the blood–cerebrospinal fluid barrier, the choroid plexus,

---

[5] In humans at steady state, consuming 3 g of nicotinic acid per day, 85% of the vitamin is excreted in the urine.

appears to have separate systems for the accumulation/release of NA and NAm. In addition, brain cells also have a high-affinity transport system for NAm. These two levels of control effect the homeostasis of niacin in the brain, with NAm but not NA entering readily. A high-affinity, G protein-coupled receptor for NA has been identified in adipose tissue.[6]

Tissue Storage

Niacin is retained in tissues that take it up as NA and/or NAm by being trapped by conversion to the pyridine nucleotides NAD(H) and NADP(H) (see Table 12-3). By far the greater amount is found as NAD(H), most of which, in contrast to NADP(H), is found in the oxidized form (NAD⁺).

V. Metabolism of Niacin

Niacin Biosynthesis

Tryptophan-niacin conversion

All animal species (including humans) appear to be capable, to varying degrees, of the *de novo* synthesis of the metabolically active forms of niacin, NAD(H) and NADP(H), from quinolinic acid, a metabolite of the indispensable amino acid tryptophan (Fig. 12-2). This conversion involves several steps:

Table 12-3. Pyridine nucleotide contents of various organs of rats

Organ	NAD⁺ (mg/kg)	NAD(H) (mg/kg)	NADP⁺ (mg/kg)	NADP(H) (mg/kg)
Liver	370	204	6	205
Heart	299	184	4	33
Kidney	223	212	3	54
Brain	133	88	<2	8
Thymus	116	35	<2	12
Lung	108	52	9	18
Pancreas	80	78	<2	12
Testes	80	71	<2	6
Blood	55	36	5	3

Source: Offermanns, H. E., Kleemann, A., Tanner, H., Beschke, H., and Friedrich, H. (1984). *Kirk-Othmer Encycl. Chem. Technol.* **24,** 59.

1. Oxidative cleavage of the tryptophan pyrrole ring by **tryptophan pyrrolase**, which yields *N*-**formylkynurenine**
2. The removal of the formyl group by **formylase** to form **kynurenine**
3. Ring-hydroxylation of kynurenine by the FAD-dependent **kynurenine 3-hydroxylase** to yield **3-hydroxykynurenine (3-OH-Ky)**
4. Deamination of 3-OH-Ky by a zinc-activated enzyme, pyridoxal phosphate-dependent **transaminase**, to yield **xanthurenic acid** which can be excreted in the urine or further metabolized
5. The xanthurenic acid side chain's cleaving of the amino acid alanine by the pyridoxal phosphate-dependent enzyme **kynureninase**, to yield **3-hydroxyanthranilic acid (3-OH-AA)**.[7]
6. Oxidative ring-opening of 3-OH-AA by an Fe²⁺-dependent dioxygenase, **3-hydroxyanthranilic acid oxygenase (3-HAAO),** to yield the semistable α-**amino-β-**

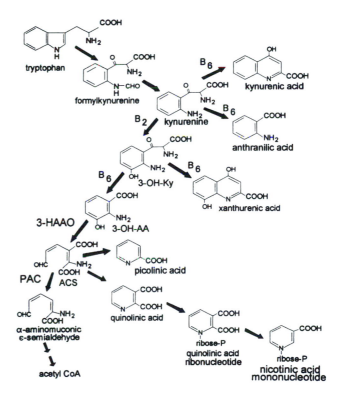

Fig. 12-2. Metabolic interconversion of tryptophan to niacin.

---

[6] Lorensen, A., et al. (2001). *Mol. Pharmacol.* **59,** 349–357.

[7] Kynureninase can also convert kynurenine to another urinary metabolite **anthranilic acid.**

carboxymuconic-ε-semi-aldehyde (ACS). ACS is a branch-point intermediate in the pathway:

a. *Catabolism to inactive metabolites* ACS can spontaneously cyclize and undergo decarboxylation to yield **picolinic acid**, or it can be converted by **picolinic acid carboxylase (PAC)** to α-aminomuconic-ε-semialdehyde, which is reduced and further decarboxylated to yield **acetyl-CoA**.

b. *Conversion to* **NAD⁺** ACS can spontaneously cyclize to form **quinolinic acid (QA)** (with dehydration but not decarboxylation), which can be decarboxylated and phosphoribosylated to yield NMN by **quinolinate phosphoribosyltransferase**. NMN is phosphoadenylated by the ATP-dependent **NAD⁺ synthetase** to yield NAD⁺.

Three sources of NAD(H) and NADP(H)

The metabolically active forms of niacin, the pyridine nucleotides NAD(H) and NADP(H), are synthesized from three precursors: NA, NAm, and tryptophan (see Fig. 12-3). Whereas NA and NAm are formal intermediates in the biosynthesis of NAD⁺ from tryptophan, that step (quinolinate phosphoribosyltransferase) actually leads directly to NAD⁺ via NMN. Both NA and NAm are converted to NAD⁺ by the same pathway after the latter is deamidated to yield NA. As the nicotinamide deamidase activities of animal tissues are low, this step is thought to be carried out by the intestinal microflora. The resulting NA is then phosphoribosylated (by **nicotinate phosphoribosyltransferase**), adenylated (by deamido-NAD⁺ pyrophosphorylase), and amidated (by NAD synthetase) ultimately to yield NAD⁺, which can be phosphorylated by an ATP-dependent **NAD⁺ kinase** to yield NADP⁺.

Although the various tissues of the body are each apparently capable of synthesizing their own pyridine nucleotides, there is clearly an exchange between the tissues that occurs primarily at the level of NAm, which is rapidly transported between tissues. In the rat, NA appears to be the most important precursor of these coenzymes in the liver, kidneys, brain, and erythrocytes; but in the testes and ovaries NAm appears to be a better precursor. Studies with chickens have shown that NAm can be a better dietary source of niacin than NA.[8]

Determinants of tryptophan-niacin conversion efficiency

The conversion of tryptophan to NAD is a generally inefficient process. Humans appear normally to convert 60 mg of tryptophan to 1 mg of niacin;[9] this ratio is also wide for the chick (45:1) and the rat (50:1) and extremely wide for the duck (175:1). This conversion efficiency has been found in chicks to be depressed under conditions of iron deficiency and in several species to be improved under conditions of niacin deficiency. For example, niacin-deficient humans are estimated to use nearly 3% of dietary tryptophan for niacin biosynthesis, and thus are able to satisfy two-thirds of their requirement for the vitamin from the metabolism of this amino acid.

Higher niacin-biosynthetic efficiencies (i.e., low tryptophan:niacin ratios) are associated with *high* activities of 3-HAAO (enhancing production of ACS, the branch-point intermediate in the pathway), and *low* activities of PAC (removing that intermediate). Thus, the ratio of the hepatic activity of 3-HAAO to that of PAC and, in particular, the hepatic activity of PAC vary greatly between animal species and are inversely correlated with their dietary requirements for preformed niacin (see Tables 12-4 and 12-5).

Role of protein turnover

It would appear that protein turnover may preempt niacin synthesis under conditions of limiting tryptophan. In such circumstances the amount of tryptophan available for niacin synthesis would be expected to be low, rendering the calculation of niacin equivalents inaccurate.

Role of vitamin B₆

Pyridoxal phosphate-dependent enzymes are involved at four points in the tryptophan–niacin pathway: two transaminases (which catalyze the conversions of kynurenine to **kynurenic acid** and of

---

[8] Ohuho, M., and Baker, D. (1993). *J. Nutr.* **123**, 2201–2206, showed NAm to be utilized some 24% better than NA by broiler chickens.

[9] Hence, food niacin value is defined in terms of niacin equivalents, one unit of which is defined as 1 mg niacin + 1/60 mg tryptophan.

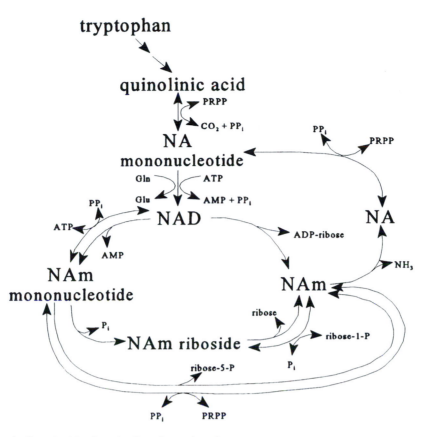

Fig. 12-3. Niacin metabolism. PRPP, phosphoribosylpyrophosphate.

Table 12-4. Relationship between the 3-HAAO:PAC ratio and dietary niacin requirement

Animal	3-HAAO:PAC ratio	Niacin requirement[a] (mg/kg diet)
Rat	273	0
Chick		
Low-niacin requirement strain	48	5
High-niacin requirement strain	27	15
Duck	5.3	40
Cat	5	45
Brook trout, lake trout	2.5	88
Turkey	1.6	70
Rainbow trout, Atlantic salmon	1.3	88
Coho salmon	3.4	175

[a]Animals fed tryptophan.

Source: Poston, H. A., and Combs, G. F., Jr. (1980). *Proc. Soc. Exp. Biol. Med.* **163,** 452.

Table 12-5. Variation in hepatic picolinic acid carboxylase in animals

Animal	PAC activity (IU/g)
Cat	50,000
Lizard	29,640
Duck	17,330
Frog	13,730
Turkey	9,230
Cow	8,300
Pig	7,120
Pigeon	6,950
Chicken	
High-niacin requirement strain	5,380
Low-niacin requirement strain	3,200
Rabbit	4,270
Mouse	4,200
Guinea pig	3,940
Human	3,180
Hamster	3,140
Rat	1,570

Source: DiLorenzo, R. N. (1972). Studies of the Genetic Variation in Tryptophan–Nicotinic Acid Conversion in Chicks. Ph.D. thesis. Cornell University, Ithaca, NY.

3-hydroxykynurenine to xanthurenic acid) and *kynureninase* (which catalyzes the conversion of kynurenine to anthranilic acid as well as that of 3-hydroxykynurenine to 3-hydroxyanthranilic acid). Thus, the conversion efficiency of tryptophan to niacin is reduced under conditions of pyridoxine deficiency. Despite the dependence of each on the active form of pyridoxine (**pyridoxal phosphate**), only the latter is affected by deficiency of that vitamin. The affinity of kynureninase for pyridoxal phosphate, as measured by its K_m,[10] is about 10^{-3} M, whereas that for transaminases is typically on the order of 10^{-8} M. Accordingly, the deprivation of pyridoxal phosphate that occurs in pyridoxine deficiency reduces kynureninase activity in most cases without affecting the activities of the transaminases, which themselves require only 10^{-5} as much of the cofactor. Thus, pyridoxine deficiency impairs the overall conversion of tryptophan to niacin by blocking the production of 3-hydroxyanthranilic acid.[11] It does not, however, block the excretion of the urinary metabolites kynurenic acid and xanthurenic acid. This phenomenon has been exploited for the assessment of pyridoxine status by monitoring the urinary excretion of xanthurenic acid after a tryptophan load.

Catabolism

The pyridine nucleotides are catabolized by hydrolytic cleavage of their two β-glycosidic bonds, primarily the one at the nicotinamide moiety, by $NAD(P)^+$ glycohydrolase. Nicotinamide so released can be deamidated to form NA, in which form it can be reconverted to NAD^+. Alternatively, it can be methylated (mainly in the liver) by **nicotinamide *N*-methyltransferase** to yield **1-methylnicotinamide**,[12,13] which can be oxidized to a variety of products that are excreted in the urine.

Excretion

Niacin is excreted in appreciable amounts under conditions of supranutritional intake, as both vitamers are actively reabsorbed by the renal glomerulus. Excretion involves a variety of water-soluble metabolites in the urine. At typical levels of intake of the vitamin, the major urinary metabolites are **1-methylnicotinamide**[14] and its oxidation product **1-methyl-6-pyridone-3-carboxamide**. Under such conditions, intact NA and NAm, as well as other oxidation products, are also excreted, but in much smaller amounts. Most mammals excrete several metabolites: nicotinamide 1-oxide, 1-methyl-4-pyridone-3-carboxamide, 1-methyl-6-pyridone-3-carboxamide, 6-hydroxynicotinamide, and 6-hydroxynicotinic acid; some species also excrete nicotinic acid/nicotinamide conjugates of ornithine (2,5-dinicotinyl ornithine by birds only) or glycine (nicotinuric acid by rabbits, guinea pigs, sheep, goats, and calves).

The major urinary metabolite in the rat is 1-methyl-4-pyridone-3-carboxamide. This metabolite is also found in human urine, but at levels substantially less than 1-methylnicotinamide and 1-methyl-2-pyridone-5-carboxamide. The urinary metabolite profile can be changed by dietary deprivation of protein and/or amino acids, and it has been suggested that the ratio of the pyridone metabolites to 1-methylnicotinamide may have utility as a biomarker for adequate amino acid intake.

At high rates of niacin intake, the vitamin is excreted predominantly (65–85% of total) in unchanged form. At all rates of intake, however, NAm tends to be excreted as its metabolites more extensively than is NA. Furthermore, the biological turnover of each vitamer is determined primarily by its rate of excretion; thus, at high intakes, the half-life of NAm is shorter than that of NA.

---

[10] Michaelis constant; in this case, the concentration of pyridoxal phosphate necessary to support half-maximal enzyme activity.

[11] It has also been suggested that the deficiency of zinc, an essential cofactor of pyridoxal kinase (see Chapter 13), may also impair tryptophan–niacin conversion by reducing the production of pyridoxal phosphate.

[12] **Nicotinamide methylase** activity is very low in fetal rat liver, increasing only in mature animals or in animals in which hepatocyte proliferation has been stimulated (e.g., after partial hepatectomy or treatment with thioacetamide). Such increases in enzyme activity are accompanied by drops in tissue NAD^+ concentrations, as 1-methylnicotinamide reduces NAD^+ synthesis either by inhibiting NAD^+ synthetase and/or stimulating $NAD(P)^+$ glycohydrolase. Thus, it is thought that nicotinamide methylase and its product may be involved in the control of hepatocyte proliferation.

[13] Nicotinic acid does not appear to be methylated by animals. Trigonelline (1-methylnicotinic acid) does appear, however, in the urine of coffee drinkers, owing to its presence in that food.

[14] Humans normally excrete daily up to 30 mg of total niacin metabolites, of which 7–10 mg is 1-methylnicotinamide.

VI. Metabolic Functions of Niacin

Coenzyme Functions

Niacin functions metabolically as the essential component of the enzyme co-substrates NAD(H)[15] and NADP(H).[16] The most central electron transport carriers of cells, each acts as an intermediate in most of the hydrogen transfers in metabolism, including more than 200 reactions in the metabolism of carbohydrates, fatty acids, and amino acids according to the general reaction:

$$\text{substrate} + \text{NAD(P)}^+ \rightarrow \text{product} + \text{NAD(P)H} + \text{H}^+$$

The hydrogen transport by the pyridine nucleotides is accomplished by two-electron transfers in which the hydride ion (H^-) serves as a carrier for both electrons. The transfer is stereospecific, involving C-4 of the pyridine ring. The two hydrogen atoms at C-4 of NAD(H) and NADP(H) are not equivalent; each is stereospecifically transferred by the enzymes to the corresponding substrates.[17] In general, stereospecificity is independent of the nature of the substrate and the source of the enzyme, and few regularities are apparent except that dehydrogenases with phosphorylated and non-phosphorylated substrates tend to show opposite stereospecificities.[18]

The reactions catalyzed by the pyridine nucleotide-dependent dehydrogenases occur by the abstraction of the proton from the alcoholic hydroxyl group of the donor substrate, and the transfer of hydride ion from the same carbon atom to the C-4 of NAm. In many cases, this reaction is coupled to a further reaction, such as phosphorylation or decarboxylation.

Metabolic Roles

Despite their similarities of mechanism and structure,[19] NAD(H) and NADP(H) have quite different metabolic roles and most dehydrogenases have specificity for one or the other.[20]

NAD in numerous redox reactions

The oxidized form NAD^+ serves as a hydrogen acceptor at the C-4 position of the pyridine ring, forming NAD(H) which, in turn, functions as a hydrogen donor to the mitochondrial respiratory chain (TCA cycle) for ATP production (Table 12-6). These reactions include

- Glycolytic reactions
- Oxidative decarboxylations of pyruvate
- Oxidation of acetate in the TCA cycle
- Oxidation of ethanol
- ß-oxidation of fatty acids
- Other cellular oxidations

NADP(H) in reduction reactions

The phosphorylation of NAD^+ facilitates the separation of oxidation and reduction pathways of niacin cofactors by allowing NADP(H) to serve as a codehydrogenase in the oxidation of physiological fuels.[21] Thus, NADP(H) is maintained in the reduced state, NADPH[22] by the pentose phosphate pathway such that reduction reactions are favored. Many of these also involve flavoproteins.[23] These reactions involve reductive biosyntheses, such as those of fatty acids and steroids (Table 12-6). In addition, NADPH also serves as a co-dehydrogenase for the oxidation of glucose 6-phosphate in the pentose phosphate pathway.

---

[15] Historically known as coenzyme I, or diphosphopyridine nucleotide (DPN).

[16] Historically known as coenzyme II, or triphosphopyridine nucleotide (TPN).

[17] Because of this phenomenon, the pyridine nucleotide-dependent enzymes are classified according to the side of the dihydropyridine ring to which each transfers hydrogen (i.e., class A and class B).

[18] Dehydrogenases with phosphorylated substrates tend to be B-stereospecific (see footnote 15), whereas those with small (i.e., no more than three carbon atoms), nonphosphorylated substrates tend to be A-stereospecific.

[19] For example, each contains adenosine, which appears to serve as a hydrophobic *anchor*.

[20] A small number of dehydrogenases can use either NAD(H) or NADP(H).

[21] For example, glyceraldehyde-3-phosphate, lactate, alcohol, 3-hydroxybutyrate, pyruvate, and α-ketoglutarate dehydrogenases.

[22] The NADP+/NADPH couple is largely reduced in animal cells, owing to the **transhydrogenase** activity that catalyzes the energy-dependent exchange of hydride between the pyridine nucleotides coupled to proton transport across the mitochondrial membrane in which it resides (the so-called *redox-driven proton pump*).

[23] The first step in most biological redox reactions is the reduction of a flavoprotein by NADPH.

Table 12-6. Some important pyridine nucleotide-dependent enzymes of animals

	Enzyme	
Role	NAD(H) dependent	NADP(H) dependent
Carbohydrate metabolism	3-Phosphoglyceraldehyde dehydrogenase	Glucose-6-phosphate dehydrogenase
	Lactate dehydrogenase	6-Phosphogluconate dehydrogenase
	Alcohol dehydrogenase	
Lipid metabolism	α-Glycerophosphate dehydrogenase	3-Ketoacyl ACP reductase
	β-Hydroxyacyl-CoA dehydrogenase	Enoyl-ACP reductase
		3-Hydroxy-3-methylglutaryl-CoA reductase
Amino acid metabolism	Glutamate dehydrogenase	Glutamate dehydrogenase
Other	NADH dehydrogenase/NADH-ubiquinone reductase complex	Glutathione reductase
		Dihydrofolate reductase
	Poly(ADP-ribose) polymerase	Thioredoxin-NADP reductase
		4-Hydroxybenzoate hydroxylase
		NADPH-cytochrome *P*-450 reductase

Abbreviation: ACP, Acyl carrier protein.

Genomic Stability

The niacin metabolite NAD(H) functions in the post-translational modification of nuclear proteins by **poly(ADP-ribose) polymerase** (Table 12-6). Unlike the other coenzyme functions of the vitamin, wherein its active forms serve as reductants/oxidants, this enzyme uses NAD$^+$ as a direct substrate to provide the ribosyl moiety that is added to the receptor protein. Poly-ADP-ribosylated proteins function in signal transduction by modulating the activities of G protein and p53, thus playing a role in DNA repair and replication, and in cell differentiation and apoptosis. This activity has been found in the rat to be very sensitive to niacin deprivation. It increases during growth and cell differentiation. This effect is thought to underlie the increase in spontaneous mutation rate that is seen in niacin deficiency. Poly(ADP-ribosylaton) causes extensive turnover of NAD$^+$ with concomitant production of NAm.

Glucose Tolerance Factor

Niacin has been identified as part of the chromium-containing **glucose tolerance factor** of yeast, which enhances the response to insulin. Its role, if any, in that factor is not clear, as free niacin is without effect. It is possible that this activity involves a metal-chelating capacity of NA such as has been reported for zinc and iron.[24]

VII. Niacin Deficiency

General Signs

Niacin deficiency in animals is characterized by a variety of species-specific signs that are usually accompanied by loss of appetite and poor growth (Table 12-7). The general progression of signs is captured as the four Ds of niacin deficiency:

- Dermatitis
- Diarrhea
- Delirium
- Death

Deficiency Disorders in Animals

Most niacin-deficient animals show poor growth and reduced efficiency of feed utilization. Pigs and ducks are particularly sensitive to niacin deficiency. Pigs show diarrhea, anemia, and degenerative

---

[24] Agte, W., et al. (1997). *Biometals* **10**, 271–276.

Table 12-7. Signs of niacin deficiency

Organ system	Signs
General	
Appetite	Decrease
Growth	Decrease
Dermatologic	Dermatitis, photosensitization
Gastrointestinal	Inflammation, diarrhea, glossitis
Skeletal	Perosis
Vascular	
Erythrocytes	Anemia
Nervous	Ataxia, dementia

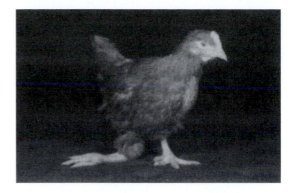

Fig. 12-4. Perosis (left leg) in niacin-deficient chick.

changes in the intestinal mucosa and nervous tissue;[25] ducks show severely bowed and weakened legs and diarrhea. Niacin-deficient dogs show necrotic degeneration of the tongue with changes of the buccal mucosa and severe diarrhea.[26] Rodents show alopecia and nerve cell histopathology. Chickens show inflammation of the upper gastrointestinal tract, dermatitis of the legs, reduced feather growth, and **perosis** (Fig. 12-4).[27]

It has been thought that ruminants are not susceptible to niacin deficiency, owing to the synthesis of the vitamin by their rumen microflora. Although that appears to be true for most ruminant species, evidence indicates that fattening beef cattle and some high-producing dairy cows can benefit from niacin supplements under some circumstances. Studies have shown niacin treatment of lactating cows to depress circulating levels of ketones, apparently by reducing lipolysis in adipocytes by a process involving increased cyclic 3',5'-adenosine monophosphate (cAMP) and, consequently, the concentrations of nonesterified fatty acids in the plasma. That ruminal synthesis of the vitamin may not meet the nutritional needs of the host would appear most likely in circumstances wherein rumen fermentation

is altered to enhance energy utilization, with associated reductions in rumen microbial growth.

Deficiency Signs in Humans

Niacin deficiency in humans results in changes in the skin, gastrointestinal tract, and nervous system. The dermatologic changes, which are usually most prominent (being called **pellagra**), are most pronounced in the parts of the skin that are exposed to sunlight (face, neck,[28] backs of the hands and forearms) (Figs. 12-5 and 12-6). In some patients, lesions resemble early sunburn; in chronic cases the symmetric lesions feature cracking, desquamation,[29] hyperkeratosis, and hyperpigmentation. Lesions of the gastrointestinal tract include angular stomatitis, cheilosis, and glossitis as well as alterations of the buccal mucosa, tongue, esophagus, stomach (resulting in achlorhydria[30]), and intestine (resulting in diarrhea).[31] Pellagra almost always involves anemia.[32] Early neurological symptoms associated with pellagra include anxiety, depression, and fatigue;[33] later symptoms include depression, apathy, headache, dizziness, irritability, and tremors.

---

[25] The syndrome is called *pig pellagra*.

[26] **Black tongue disease**.

[27] Inflammation and misalignment of the tibiotarsal joint (*hock*), in severe cases involving slippage of the Achilles tendon from its condyles, which causes crippling due to an inability to extend the lower leg.

[28] This is referred to as **Casal's collar**.

[29] The shedding of the epidermis in scales.

[30] The absence of hydrochloric acid from the gastric juice, usually due to gastric parietal cell dysfunction.

[31] Many of these gastrointestinal changes also occur in schizophrenia.

[32] The anemia associated with pellagra is of the macro- or normocytic, hypochromic types.

[33] Many of these symptoms also occur in schizophrenia.

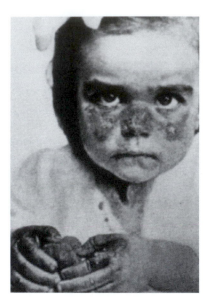

Fig. 12-5. Pellagra: Affected child with facial *butterfly wing.* (Courtesy of Cambridge University Press.)

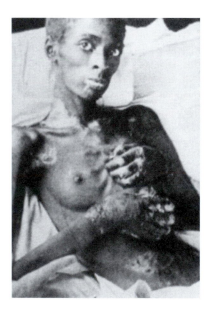

Fig. 12-6. Pellagra: Affected woman with *pellagra glove.* (Courtesy of Cambridge University Press.)

Determinants of Niacin Status

Because a substantial amount of niacin can be synthesized from tryptophan, nutritional status with respect to niacin involves not only the level of intake of the preformed vitamin, but also that of its potential amino acid precursor. Accordingly, the clinical manifestation of niacin deficiency includes evidence of an unbalanced diet with respect to both of these essential nutrients and, frequently, pyridoxine. Thus, the occurrence of pellagra, as well as niacin-deficiency diseases in animals, is properly viewed as the result of a multifactorial dietary deficiency rather than of insufficient intake of niacin per se.

In addition to tryptophan and pyridoxine[34] supplies being important determinants of niacin status, it has been suggested that excess intake of the branched-chain amino acid **leucine** may antagonize niacin synthesis and/or utilization and thus may also be a precipitating factor in the etiology of pellagra. Excess leucine has been shown to inhibit the production of quinolinic acid from tryptophan by isolated rat hepatocytes. However, the magnitude of this effect is small in comparison with the K_m of quinolinate phosphoribosyltransferase for quinolinate, indicating that excess leucine (and/or its metabolites) is unlikely to affect the rate of NAD^+ biosynthesis by the liver. Some studies with intact animals (rats) have produced results supporting the view that excess leucine can impair the synthesis of NAD^+ from tryptophan (either by inhibiting the enzymatic conversion itself, or the cellular uptake of the amino acid). Other studies, however, have yielded negative results in this regard. Therefore, the role that high leucine intakes may have in the etiology of pellagra is not clear at present.

It has been suggested that zinc plays some role in the pyridoxine-dependent metabolic interconversion of tryptophan to niacin. Pellagra patients have been found to have low-plasma zinc levels, and zinc supplementation increases their urinary excretion of 1-methylnicotinamide and 1-methyl-2-pyridone-5-carboxamide. Studies with rats have shown that treatment of niacin-deficient animals with the metabolic intermediate picolinic acid increases circulating zinc levels.

---

[34] Zinc, which is required by the enzyme *pyridoxal phosphokinase*, is also related to the function of pyridoxine in this system. Alcoholics, who typically have low zinc status, have been shown to excrete high levels of the niacin metabolites 1-methyl-6-pyridone-3-carboxamide and 1-methylnicotinamide. The excretion of these metabolites was increased by zinc supplementation, presumably owing to increased pyridoxal phosphokinase activities and the consequent activation of pyridoxine to the form (pyridoxal phosphate) that facilitates tryptophan–niacin conversion. It has also been suggested that zinc deficiency may reduce the availability of tryptophan for niacin biosynthesis by enhancing its oxidation, as has been shown for several other amino acids.

Hereditary Disorders of Niacin Metabolism

Two hereditary disorders of humans involve impaired niacin function and are successfully treated with high doses of niacin: **schizophrenia** and **Hartnup disease**. Schizophrenia appears to be an NAD-deficiency disease involving a failure to provide sufficient amounts of that pyridine nucleotide to critical areas of the brain. Affected individuals apparently oxidize NAm more readily than do healthy people, as they excrete greater amounts of *1-methyl-6-pyridone-3-carboxamide* than do healthy controls. Because the excretion of this methylated product is increased by treatment with methylated hallucinogens (e.g., methylated indoles) and is decreased by treatment with tranquilizers, it has been suggested that the high endogenous production of methylated hallucinogenic substances[35] in schizophrenics results in a depletion of NAm (via its methylation and excretion), resulting in a substrate limitation of NAD^+ synthesis. Indeed, schizophrenics respond to high oral doses (e.g., 1 g day) of NA.[36] Patients with a rare familial disorder, **Hartnup disease**,[37] which involves malabsorption of tryptophan (and other amino acids), also respond to treatment with NA. That hereditary disease is characterized by hyperaminoaciduria,[38] a pellagra-like skin rash (precipitated by psychological stress, sunlight, or fever), and neurological changes including attacks of ataxia and psychiatric disorders ranging from emotional instability to delirium. Patients appear to have abnormally low capacities to convert tryptophan to niacin, which appears to result from reduced enteric absorption and renal reabsorption of monoamino monocarboxylic acids (including tryptophan). In these patients, nonreabsorbed tryptophan appears to be degraded by microbial tryptophanase to pyruvate and indole, the latter of which is reabsorbed from the intestine and is neurotoxic.

Health Benefits of Niacin

Niacin has been associated with a number of health effects unrelated to the signs of frank niacin deficiency. These include:

- *Skin injury* Niacin deficiency produces photosensitivity of the skin, a sign common in pellagra. This may relate to the function of niacin as a vasodilator in the skin. Niacin supplementation has been shown to protect skin from DNA damaging agents in animal models.
- *Oxidant lung injury* Hyperoxia has been shown to induce poly(ADP-ribose) synthesis in the lung. While this synthesis is limited by dietary deprivation of niacin, it is not stimulated by niacin supplementation of nondeficient subjects.
- *Cancer risk* Epidemiological studies have associated marginal niacin intake with increase risk of esophageal cancer,[39] although no associations of cancer risk and niacin status have been reported.

VIII. Pharmacologic Uses of Niacin

Nicotinic Acid

High doses of NA can cause several effects:

- *Vasodilation* NA has been used as an agent to stimulate tooth eruption, to increase gastric juice flow, and to increase intestinal motility.
- *Skin flushing* High doses of NA can cause skin **flushing** due to the release of prostaglandin D2 in the skin followed by the release of its metabolites.
- *Antihyperlipidemic effects* High doses of NA have been used in treating humans for their antihyperlipidemic effects. Results show reductions in all major lipids and lipoproteins, with increases in HDL-cholesterol (Table 12-8). These effects appear to be better in response to extended release forms of NA. These effects appear to be unrelated to the pyridine nucleotides and are thought to involve direct binding of NA to a putative G-protein receptor[40] and perhaps adenylate cyclase, exerting several actions:
  - *Inhibition of lipolysis in adipose tissue* Inhibition of adenylate cyclase leads to increased

---

[35] For example, methylated derivatives of norepinephrine, dopamine, and epinephrine such as the so-called *pink factor* (3,4-dimethoxyphenylethylamine).

[36] It is also likely that, at such high doses of nicotinic acid, the enhanced metabolic production of nicotinamide will further increase NAD(H) levels (by retarding its turnover), as the latter vitamer can inhibit NADase, whose activity is high in brain.

[37] The disease was named for the first case, described in 1951, involving a boy thought to have pellagra. Since that time, some 50 proved cases involving 28 families have been described.

[38] The presence of abnormally high concentrations of amino acids in the urine.

[39] Franceschi, S., et al. (1990). *J. Nat. Cancer Inst.* **82**, 1407–1411.

[40] Karpe, F., and Frayn, J. N. (2004). *Lancet* 363, 1892–1894.

Table 12-8. Serum lipid responses to niacin

Parameter	Trials	Effect of niacin treatment[a]
Triglycerides	27	20
Total cholesterol	27	10
LDL cholesterol	27	21
HDL cholesterol	27	16

[a]% less than control.
Source: Birjmohum, R. S., et al. (2005). *J. Am. Coll. Cardiol.* **45,** 185–190.

levels of cAMP, which activates a protein kinase that phosphorylates a hormone-sensitive lipase that mobilizes fatty acids from triglycerides.

○ *Reduced synthesis of very low-density lipoproteins (VLDLs)* The reduced release of fatty acids from adipose tissue is responsible for at least part of the reduction of hepatic synthesis and secretion of VLDLs.

○ *Reduced plasma cholesterol levels* Decreased amounts of VLDLs in the plasma are associated with decreased plasma concentrations of triglycerides and cholesterol. Also contributing to reduced cholesterol levels is a decrease in cholesterol biosynthesis by NA-inhibition of 3-hydroxy-3-methylglutaryl CoA reductase.[41]

○ *Lowering the plasma concentrations of low-density lipoproteins (LDLs) and VLDLs* Decreased synthesis of VLDLs, from which LDLs are derived, lead to reduced plasma levels of the latter.

○ *Increasing plasma high-density lipoproteins (HDLs)* These effects involve increases in HDL–cholesterol and as much as a threefold increase in the ratio of $HDL_2:HDL_3$.[42]

These effects, in aggregate, are associated with reduced risk of atherosclerosis and provide the basis of current interest in nicotinic acid in the prophylaxis of coronary artery disease. Reviews of the clinical use of high doses of nicotinic acid show it to be among the most useful drugs for the treatment of hypercholesterolemia and for the prevention of coronary disease.[43]

Nicotinamide

Nicotinamide does *not* show the antihyperlipidemic effects of NA. Although the results of clinical trials have been generally inconsistent, NAm has been used successfully for the treatment of several conditions:

- *Clinical depression* NAm enhances the effect of tryptophan in supporting brain serotonin levels. NAm, which reduces the urinary excretion of tryptophan metabolites in patients treated with the amino acid, appears to block the tryptophan–niacin pathway and thus increase the availability of tryptophan for the synthesis of serotonin, the effect of which is antidepressive.

- *Diabetes* When used prophylactically in animal models, NAm has been found to delay or prevent the development of diabetic signs in the non-obese diabetic mouse model,[44] to decrease the severity of diabetic signs associated with β–cell proliferation induced by partial pancreatectomy,[45] and to protect against diabetes induced by agents[46] that cause DNA strand breakage in β–cells. In clinical trials, NAm has been found to protect high-risk children from developing clinically apparent insulin-dependent diabetes.[47] These actions of NAm are thought to involve support of pancreatic β–cell function through the maintenance of both NAD^+ and DNA-protective enzyme poly(ADP-ribose) polymerase activity. The question has been raised whether these effects might also enhance cancer risks by virtue of increased β–cell survival under conditions of autoimmune attack. This hypothesis has not been tested.

---

[41] DiPalma, J. R., and Thayer, W. S. (2001). *Ann. Rev. Nutr.* **11,** 169–187.

[42] Alderman, J. D., et al. (1989). *Am. J. Cardiol.* **64,** 725–729.

[43] A retrospective evaluation of results from the U.S. Coronary Drug Project showed nicotinic acid treatment to have reduced lethal coronary events, resulting in highly significant reduction of mortality from all causes by 11% (versus a placebo).

[44] Reddy, S., et al. (1990). *Diabetes Res.* **15,** 95–102.

[45] Yonemura, Y., et al. (1984). *Diabetes* **33,** 401–404.

[46] Alloxan, streptozotocin.

[47] Elliott, R.B., et al. (1991). *Diabetologia* **34,** 362–365; Manna, R., et al. (1992). *Br. J. Clin. Pract.* **46,** 177–179.

- *Anxiety*   A high dose (1 g/day) of NAm has been reported to reduce anxiety in at least one case. Whether this effect may be due to the modulation of neurotransmitters is not clear.

IX. Niacin Toxicity

Low Toxicity

In general, the toxicity of niacin is low. Nonruminant animals can tolerate oral exposures of at least 10- to 20-fold their normal requirements for the vitamin. The toxic potential of NAm appears to be greater than that of NA, probably by a factor of four. Side effects appear to result from metabolic disturbances due to the depletion of methyl groups as the result of the metabolism of the vitamin in high doses. These include:

Nicotinic Acid

Short-term effects   High doses of NA have been reported to cause **skin flushing,**[48] itching urticaria (hives), and gastrointestinal discomfort (heartburn, nausea, vomiting, rarely diarrhea) in humans. Animal studies have shown that high levels of NAm can raise circulating homocysteine levels, particularly on a high-methionine diet.

Chronic effects   The longer term effects of high NA doses include cases of altered glucose tolerance and hyperuricemia.[49] A few cases of transient elevations in the plasma activities of liver enzymes without associated hepatic dysfunction have been reported, and chronic doses of NA have been reported to cause hepatic damage.[50]

Nicotinamide

Short-term effects   While acute adverse effects of NAm have not been reported for doses used to treat insulin-dependent diabetes (ca. 3 g/day), larger doses (10 g/day) have been found to cause hepatic damage.

Chronic effects   It is possible that chronic, high intakes of NAm may deplete methyl groups due to the increased demand for methylation to excrete the vitamin. Such effects would be exacerbated by low intakes of methyl donors, methionine, and choline. In principle, this could increase the risk of carcinogenesis.

X. Case Study

Instructions

Review the following report, paying special attention to the responses to the experimental treatments. Then answer the questions that follow.

Case

Fourteen patients with alcoholic pellagra and 7 healthy controls, all ranging in age from 21 to 45 years, were studied in the metabolic unit of a hospital. None had severe hepatic dysfunction on the basis of medical history, clinical examination, and routine laboratory tests. The nutritional status of each subject was evaluated at the beginning of the study by clinical examination, anthropometric measurements [body mass index (BMI; weight divided by the square of the height), triceps skinfold thickness, arm and muscle circumference], biochemical tests [24-hr urinary creatinine, serum albumin, total iron-binding capacity (TIBC)], and 24-hr recalls of food consumption. Results indicated that, before admission, the patients with alcoholic pellagra consumed a daily average of 270 g of ethanol. Each showed signs of protein-calorie malnutrition (reduced BMI, skinfold thickness, arm and muscle circumference, serum albumin, and TIBC). In addition, their plasma zinc concentrations were significantly lower than those of controls, although their urinary zinc concentrations were not different from those of the control group.

The pellagra patients were assigned to one of two experimental treatment groups and the healthy controls to another (three treatments, each with $n = 7$). During the 7-day study, each group received enteral diets prepared from 10% crystalline amino acids (adequate amounts of each, except for tryptophan) and 85% sucrose, which supplied daily amounts of 0.8 g of protein per kilogram of body weight and 200 kcal/gN. In addition, each patient was given weekly by vein 500 ml of an essential fatty acid emulsion as well as a vitamin–mineral supplement. The diets were administered

---

[48] Skin flushing in response to niacin is attenuated in many individuals with schizophrenia, suggesting that such patients may have abnormal prostaglandin signaling.

[49] NAm can inhibit uricase, thereby depressing intestinal microbial uricolysis.

[50] Rader, J. I., et al. (1992). *Am. J. Med.* **92,** 77–81.

by intubation directly to the midportion of the duodenum. The control diet was supplemented with tryptophan, and the vitamin–mineral supplement contained both niacin and zinc. The diets provided to each group of pellagra patients contained no tryptophan; neither did their vitamin supplement contain niacin. One group of pellagra patients received supplemental zinc (220 mg of $ZnSO_4$) whereas the other did not. Several biochemical measurements were made at the beginning of the experiment and, again, after 4 days. Each of the biochemical measurements was repeated after 7 days of treatment. In most cases, the results showed the same effects but of greater magnitudes.

Case Questions

1. What signs support the diagnosis of protein-calorie malnutrition in these alcoholic patients with pellagra?
2. Propose an hypothesis for the mechanism of action of zinc in producing the responses that were observed in these patients with alcoholic pellagra. Outline an experiment (using either pellagra patients or a suitable animal model) to test that hypothesis.
3. List the probable contributing factors to the pellagra observed in these patients.

Results

Subject group	Parameter	Initial value	Day 4 value
Healthy controls	Plasma zinc (mmol/liter)	14.2 ± 1.5	16.0 ± 2.2
	Plasma tryptophan (mmol/liter)	50.8 ± 12.5	74.3 ± 18.5
	Urine zinc (mmol/day)	7.34 ± 1.38	9.18 ± 2.91
	Urine 6-pyridone[a] (mmol/day)	70 ± 22	640 ± 235
	Urine CH_3-NAm[b] (mmol/day)	78 ± 32	143 ± 48
Pellagra patients	Plasma zinc (mmol/liter)	9.9 ± 1.1	9.6 ± 2.0
	Plasma tryptophan (mmol/liter)	33.3 ± 15.3	29.5 ± 6.1
	Urine zinc (mmol/day)	9.79 ± 3.06	11.93 ± 10.55
	Urine 6-pyridone[a] (mmol/day)	16 ± 10	19 ± 12
	Urine CH_3-NAm[b] (mmol/day)	6 ± 3	9 ± 6
Pellagra patients fed zinc	Plasma zinc (mmol/liter)	9.8 ± 1.0	15.8 ± 3.2
	Plasma tryptophan (mmol/liter)	37.3 ± 17.8	23.7 ± 7.6
	Urine zinc (mmol/day)	9.80 ± 3.10	24.02 ± 8.11
	Urine 6-pyridone[a] (mmol/day)	16 ± 11	55 ± 18
	Urine CH_3-NAm[b] (mmol/day)	6 ± 3	33 ± 20

[a]1-Methyl-6-pyridone-3-carboxamide.
[b]1-Methylnicotinamide.

Study Questions and Exercises

1. Diagram the several general areas of metabolism in which NAD(H)- and NADP(H)-dependent enzymes are involved.
2. In general, how do the pyridine nucleotides interact with the flavoproteins in metabolism? What is the fundamental metabolic significance of this interrelationship?
3. Construct a decision tree for the diagnosis of niacin deficiency in humans or an animal species.
4. What key feature of the chemistry of nicotinamide relates to its biochemical functions as an enzyme cosubstrate?
5. What parameters might you use to assess niacin status of a human or animal?

Recommended Reading

Bourgeois, C., Cervantes-Laurean, D., and Moss, J. (2006). Niacin, Chapter 25 in *Present Knowledge in Nutrition*, 10th ed. (M. E. Shils, M. Shike, A. C. Ross, B. Caballero, and R. J. Cousins, eds.), pp. 442–451. Lippincott, New York.

Capuzzi, D. M., Morgan, J. M, Brusco, O. A., Jr., and Intenzo, C. M. (2000). Niacin dosing: Relationship to benefits and adverse effects. *Cutt. Atheroscler. Rep.* **2,** 64–71.

DiPalma, J. R., and Thayer, W. S. (1991). Use of niacin as a drug. *Annu. Rev. Nutr.* **11,** 169–187.

Harmeyer, J., and Kollenkirchen, U. (1989). Thiamin and niacin in ruminant nutrition. *Nutr. Res. Rev.* **2,** 201–225.

Hegyi, J., Schwarts, R. A., and Hegyi, V. (2004). Pellagra: Dermatitis, dementia and diarrhea. *Internat. J. Dermatol.* **43,** 1–5.

Jacob, R. A. (2001). Niacin, Chapter 19, in *Present Knowledge in Nutrition,* 8th ed. (B. A. Bowman and B. M. Russell, eds.), pp. 199–206. ILSI Press, Washington, D.C.

Kirkland, J. B., and Rawling, J. M. (2001). Niacin, Chapter 6, in *Handbook of Vitamins*, 3rd ed. (R. B. Rucker, J. W. Suttie, D. B. McCormick, and L. J. Machlin, eds.), pp. 213–254. Marcel Dekker, New York.

Vitamin B$_6$

13

Had we been able to afford Monel metal or stainless steel cages, we would have missed xanthurenic acid.

— S. Lepkovsky

I.	The Significance of Vitamin B$_6$	314
II.	Sources of Vitamin B$_6$	314
III.	Absorption of Vitamin B$_6$	316
IV.	Transport of Vitamin B$_6$	316
V.	Metabolism of Vitamin B$_6$	317
VI.	Metabolic Functions of Vitamin B$_6$	318
VII.	Vitamin B$_6$ Deficiency	323
VIII.	Pharmacologic Uses of Vitamin B$_6$	326
IX.	Vitamin B$_6$ Toxicity	327
X.	Case Studies	327
	Study Questions and Exercises	329
	Recommended Reading	329

Anchoring Concepts

1. Vitamin B$_6$ is the generic descriptor for all 3-hydroxy-2-methylpyridine derivatives exhibiting qualitatively the biological activity of pyridoxine [3-hydroxy-4,5-*bis*(hydroxymethyl)-2-methylpyridine].
2. The metabolically active form of vitamin B$_6$ is pyridoxal phosphate, which functions as a coenzyme for reactions involving amino acids.
3. Deficiencies of vitamin B$_6$ are manifested as dermatologic, circulatory, and neurologic changes.

Learning Objectives

1. To understand the chief natural sources of vitamin B$_6$.
2. To understand the means of absorption and transport of vitamin B$_6$.
3. To understand the biochemical function of vitamin B$_6$ as a coenzyme of a variety of reactions in the metabolism of amino acids, and the relationship of that function to the physiological activities of the vitamin.
4. To understand the physiological implications of low vitamin B$_6$ status

Vocabulary

Acrodynia
Aldehyde dehydrogenase (NAD$^+$)
Aldehyde (pyridoxal) oxidase
Alkaline phosphatase
γ-Aminobutyric acid (GABA)
Cheilosis
Cystathionuria
Epinephrine
Glossitis
Glycogen phosphorylase
Hemoglobin
Histamine
Homocysteinuria
Isonicotinic acid hydrazide (INH)
Kynureninase
Methionine load
Norepinephrine
Premenstrual syndrome
Pyridoxal
Pyridoxal dehydrogenase
Pyridoxal kinase
Pyridoxal oxidase
Pyridoxal phosphate
Pyridoxamine
Pyridoxamine phosphate
Pyridoxamine phosphate oxidase
4-Pyridoxic acid
Pyridoxine
Pyridoxine hydrochloride
Pyridoxol
Schiff base
Schizophrenia

Selenocysteine ß-lyase
Selenocysteine γ-lyase
Serotonin
Sideroblastic anemia
Stomatitis
Transaminases
Tryptophan load
Xanthurenic acid

I. The Significance of Vitamin B$_6$

The biological functions of the three naturally occurring forms of vitamin B$_6$, **pyridoxal, pyridoxine**, and **pyridoxamine**, depend on the metabolism of each to a common coenzyme form, **pyridoxal phosphate**. That coenzyme plays critical roles in several aspects of metabolism, giving the vitamin importance in such diverse areas as growth, cognitive development, depression, immune function, fatigue, and steroid hormone activity. Vitamin B$_6$ is fairly widespread in foods of both plant and animal origin; therefore, problems of primary deficiency are not prevalent. Still, vitamin B$_6$ status can be antagonized by alcohol and other factors that displace the coenzyme from its various enzymes to increase the rate of its metabolic degradation.

II. Sources of Vitamin B$_6$

Distribution in Foods

Vitamin B$_6$ is widely distributed in foods, occurring in greatest concentrations in meats, whole-grain products (especially wheat), vegetables, and nuts (Table 13-1). In the cereal grains, vitamin B$_6$ is concentrated primarily in the germ and aleuronic layer. Thus, the refining of grains in the production of flours, which removes much of these fractions, results in substantial reductions in vitamin B$_6$ content. White bread, therefore, is a poor source of vitamin B$_6$ unless it is fortified.

The chemical forms of vitamin B$_6$ tend to vary among foods of plant and animal origin; plant tissues contain mostly pyridoxine (the free alcohol form, **pyridoxol**), whereas animal tissues contain mostly pyridoxal and pyridoxamine. A large portion of the vitamin B$_6$ in many foods is phosphorylated or bound to proteins via the ε-amino groups of lysyl residues or the sulfhydryl groups of cysteinyl residues. The vitamin is also found in glycosylated forms such as 5'-O-(β-D-glucopyranosyl) pyridoxine. Vitamin B$_6$ glycosides are found in varying amounts in different foods but little, if at all, in animal products.

Stability

Vitamin B$_6$ in foods is stable under acidic conditions, but unstable under neutral and alkaline conditions, particularly when exposed to heat or light. Of the several vitamers, pyridoxine is far more stable than either pyridoxal or pyridoxamine. Therefore, the cooking and thermal processing losses of vitamin B$_6$ tend to be highly variable (0–70%), with plant-derived foods (which contain mostly pyridoxine) losing little, if any, of the vitamin and with animal products (which contain mostly pyridoxal and pyridoxamine) losing substantial amounts. Milk, for example, can lose 30–70% of its inherent vitamin B$_6$ on drying. The storage losses of naturally occurring vitamin B$_6$ from many foods and feedstuffs, although they occur at slower rates, can also be substantial (25–50% within a year). Because it is particularly stable, **pyridoxine hydrochloride** is used for food fortification and in multivitamin supplements.

Bioavailability

The bioavailability of vitamin B$_6$ in most commonly consumed foods appears to be in the range of 70–80%. However, appreciable amounts of the vitamin in some foods is not biologically available. The determinants of the bioavailability of vitamin B$_6$ in a food include:

- *Pyridoxine glycoside content* The pyridoxal-5-β-D-glycosides are poorly digested. Compared to free pyridoxine, the bioavailability of the glycoside has been estimated to be 20–30% in the rat and about 60% in humans. In addition, the presence of pyridoxine glycosides has been found to reduce the utilization of co-ingested free pyridoxine.
- *Peptide adducts* Vitamin B$_6$ can condense with peptide lysyl and/or cysteinyl residues during food processing, cooking, or digestion; such products are less well utilized than the free vitamin. The reductive binding of

Table 13-1.   Vitamin B$_6$ contents of foods

Food	Vitamin B$_6$ (mg/100 g)	Glycosylated (%)	Food	Vitamin B$_6$ (mg/100 g)	Glycosylated (%)
Dairy products			Vegetables		
Milk	0.04	—	Asparagus	0.15	—
Yogurt	0.05	—	Beans	0.08–0.18	15–57
Cheeses	0.04–0.08	—	Broccoli	0.17	66
Meats			Brussels sprouts	0.18	—
Beef	0.33	—	Cabbage	0.16	46
Chicken	0.33–0.68	—	Carrots	0.15	51–86
Lamb	0.28	—	Cauliflower	0.21	66
Pork	0.35	—	Celery	0.06	—
Ham	0.32	—	Corn	0.20	—
Calf liver	0.84	—	Onions	0.13	—
Herring	0.37	—	Peas	0.16	15
Haddock	0.18	—	Potatoes	0.25	32
Tuna	0.43	—	Spinach	0.28	50
Oysters	0.05	—	Fruits		
Shrimp	0.10		Apples	0.03	—
Cereals			Grapefruit	0.03	—
Corn meal	0.20	—	Oranges	0.06	47
Rice			Peaches	0.02	22
Polished	0.17	20	Strawberries	0.06	—
Unpolished	0.55	23	Tomatoes	0.10	46
Wheat, whole	0.29	28	Nuts		
Other			Peanuts	0.40	—
Eggs	0.19	—	Pecans	0.18	—
Human colostrum	0.001–0.002	—	Walnuts	0.73	7
Human milk	0.010–0.025	—			

Source: USDA data; Leklem, J. E. (1996). In: *Present Understanding in Nutrition* (E. E. Ziegler and L. J. Filer, Jr., eds.), 7th ed., p. 175. ILSI Press, Washington, DC.

pyridoxal and pyridoxal 5′-phosphate to ε-amino groups of lysyl residues in proteins or peptides produces adducts that not only are biologically unavailable but that also have vitamin B$_6$-antagonist activity.[1] For example, wheat bran contains vitamin B$_6$ in largely unavailable form(s), the presence of which reduces the bioavailability of the vitamin from other foods consumed at the same time.[2] Because plants generally contain complexed forms of pyridoxine, bioavailability of the vitamin of plant foods tends to be greater than that of foods derived from animals.

Hindgut Microbial Synthesis

Although the microflora of the colon synthesize vitamin B$_6$, it is not absorbed there, and noncoprophagous animals derive no benefit from this microbial source of the vitamin. In contrast, ruminants benefit

---

[1] Gregory, J. F. (1980). *J. Nutr.* **110**, 995–1005.

[2] Owing to the poor availability of vitamin B$_6$ from the bran fraction of the grain, the bioavailability of the vitamin from whole-wheat bread is less than that of pyridoxine-fortified white bread.

from their rumen microflora, which produce vitamin B$_6$ in adequate amounts to meet their needs, proximal to where it is absorbed.

III. Absorption of Vitamin B$_6$

Diffusion Linked to Phosphorylation

The various forms of vitamin B$_6$ are absorbed via passive diffusion primarily in the jejunum and ileum. The capacity for absorption is therefore very large; animals have been found to be able to absorb quantities of the vitamin two to three orders of magnitude greater than their physiological needs demand. The enteric absorption of pyridoxal phosphate and pyridoxamine phosphate involves their obligate dephosphorylation catalyzed by a membrane-bound **alkaline phosphatase**. Those products and the non-phosphorylated vitamers in the digesta are absorbed by diffusion driven by trapping of the vitamin as 5′-phosphates through the action of phosphorylation by a **pyridoxal kinase** in the jejunal mucosa. Pyridoxine and pyridoxamine that have been thus trapped are then oxidized to **pyridoxal phosphate** in that tissue.

IV. Transport of Vitamin B$_6$

Plasma Vitamin B$_6$

Only a small portion (<0.1%) of total body vitamin B$_6$ is present in blood plasma. Pyridoxal phosphate comprises more than 90% of the vitamin in plasma bound to albumin, which protects it from hydrolysis. Most of the vitamer in plasma is derived from the liver after metabolism by hepatic flavoenzymes. The plama pyridoxal phosphate concentration typically is less than 1 mmol. Smaller amounts of other vitamers are also found. The circulating vitamin is tightly bound to proteins (primarily albumin in the plasma and **hemoglobin** in erythrocytes[3]) via **Schiff base** linkages.[4]

In humans and other animals, plasma pyridoxal phosphate concentrations decline during pregnancy; this appears to result from a shift in the distribution of the vitamer in the blood to favor erythrocytes over the plasma, as neither the enteric absorption, excretion, or hepatic uptake of the vitamin is affected. Renal failure has been found to reduce the plasma pyridoxal phosphate level,[5] whereas submaximal exercise has been shown to increase it.

Role of Phosphorylation in Tissue Uptake

Pyridoxal crosses cell membranes more readily than pyridoxal phosphate; thus, it appears to be the form taken up by the tissues, suggesting the roles of phosphatases in the cellular retention and, perhaps, also the uptake of the vitamin. After being taken into the cell, the vitamin is again phosphorylated by pyridoxal kinase to yield the predominant tissue form, pyridoxal phosphate. Small quantities of vitamin B$_6$ are stored in the body, mainly as pyridoxal phosphate but also as **pyridoxamine phosphate.** The greatest levels are found in the liver, brain, kidney, spleen, and muscle, where the vitamin is bound to various proteins (Table 13-2). In muscle, pyridoxal phosphate is bound mostly to **glycogen phosphorylase**; in other tissues it is bound to various enzymes with which it has coenzyme functions. Protein-binding of pyridoxal phosphate in the tissues is thought to protect the vitamin from hydrolysis as well as to provide storage of the vitamin.

The total body pools of vitamin B$_6$ in the human adult is estimated to be 40–150 mg, constituting a supply sufficient to satisfy the body's needs for 20–75 days. This amount appears to be composed of two pools: one with a rapid (0.5 day) turnover and a second with a longer (25–33 days) turnover.[6] Muscle contains most (70–80%) of the body's vitamin B$_6$, in the form of pyridoxal 5′-phosphate bound to glycogen phosphorylase.[7]

---

[3] Vitamin B$_6$ binds via the amino group of the N-terminal valine residue of the hemoglobin α chain. This binding, like that of pyridoxine and pyridoxamine, is twice as strong as that of albumin, appearing to drive uptake by erythrocytes, which normally contain more than six times more vitamin than the plasma. These levels are relatively high in infants, but decline to adult levels by about 5 years of age. The pyridoxal phosphate content of erythrocytes is often used as a parameter of vitamin B$_6$ status.

[4] Schiff bases are condensation products of aldehydes and ketones with primary amines; they are stable if there is at least one aryl group on either the nitrogen or the carbon that is linked. Vitamin B$_6$ forms Schiff base linkages with proteins by the bonding of the keto-carbon of pyridoxal phosphate to a peptidyl amino group. The vitamin also forms a Schiff base with the amino acid substrates of the enzymes for which it functions as a coenzyme; this occurs by the bonding of the amino nitrogen of pyridoxal phosphate and the α-carbon of the substrate.

[5] One study showed this depression to be greater than 40% in rats.

[6] Shane, B. (1978). *Human Vitamin B$_6$ Requirements*, pp. 111–128. *Nat. Acad*. Press, Washington, DC.

[7] Glycogen phosphorylase-binding accounts for only 10% of the vitamin B$_6$ in the liver.

Table 13-2. Concentrations (nM) of vitamers B$_6$ in the plasma of several species

Species	PalP	Pal	Pol	Pam	PamP	Pac
Pig	29	139	167	—	—	139
Human	62	13	33	6	<3	40
Calf	308	96	50	—	9	91
Sheep	626	57	43	—	466	318
Dog	417	268	66	—	65	109
Cat	2443	139	93	44	271	17

Abbreviations: PalP, Pyridoxal phosphate; Pal, pyridoxal; Pol, pyridoxol; Pam, pyridoxamine; PamP, pyrodoxamine phosphate; Pac, pyridoxic acid.

Moderate exercise in humans has been found to increase plasma pyridoxal phosphate concentrations by 23% within 20 min. This appears to be related to the increased need for gluconeogenesis, which results in the release of pyridoxal phosphate from glycogen phosphorylase. That plasma pyridoxal phosphate levels increase so quickly under such conditions indicates either that the vitamer rapidly undergoes hydrolysis, discharge from the muscle, and then rephosphorylation in the liver, or that it is released intact through interstial fluid.[8]

V. Metabolism of Vitamin B$_6$

Interconversion of Vitamers

The vitamers B$_6$ are readily interconverted metabolically by reactions involving phosphorylation/dephosphorylation, oxidation/reduction, and amination/deamination (Fig. 13-1). Because the nonphosphorylated vitamers cross membranes more readily than their phosphorylated analogs, phosphorylation appears to be an important means of retaining the vitamin intracellularly. Three enzymes are involved in this metabolism:

- **Pyridoxal kinase**[9] This hepatic enzyme catalyzes the phosphorylation of pyridoxine, pyridoxal, and pyridoxamine, yielding the corresponding phosphates. It requires a zinc–ATP complex, the formation of which is facilitated by zinc-metallothioneine (MT), and is stimulated by potassium ion (K$^+$). The role of MT in pyridoxal kinase activity suggests that zinc status may be important in the regulation of vitamin B$_6$ metabolism.
- **Alkaline phosphatases** Phosphorylated forms of the vitamin can be dephosphorylated by

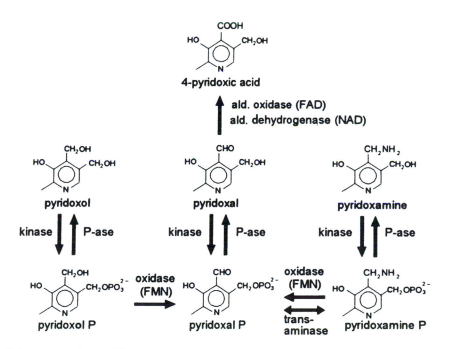

Fig. 13-1. Metabolic interconversions of vitamin B$_6$.

---

[8] Crozier, P., et al. (1994). *Am. J. Clin. Nutr.* **40**, 552–558.

[9] Erythrocyte pyridoxal kinase activity in black Americans has been reported to be about half that of white Americans, although lymphocytes, granulocytes, and fibroblasts show no such differences. This difference suggests that the retention of vitamin B$_6$ by erythrocytes, which appears to depend on the phosphorylation, may be lower in blacks.

membrane-bound alkaline phosphatases in many tissues (e.g., liver, brain, and intestine).

- **Pyridoxamine phosphate oxidase** This enzyme catalyzes the limiting step in vitamin B$_6$ metabolism. It requires flavin mononucleotide (FMN); therefore, deprivation of riboflavin may reduce the conversion of pyridoxine and pyridoxamine to the active coenzyme pyridoxal phosphate.
- **Pyridoxal dehydrogenase** The reduced forms (pyridoxine or pyridoxol phosphate) can be oxidized by pyridoxal dehydrogenase to yield pyridoxal or pyridoxal phosphate, either of which can be aminated by transaminases.

The liver is the central organ for vitamin B$_6$ metabolism, containing all of the enzymes involved in its interconversions. The major forms of the vitamin in that organ are pyridoxal phosphate and pyridoxamine phosphate, which are maintained at fairly constant intracellular concentrations in endogenous pools that are not readily accessible to newly formed molecules of those species. Instead, the latter, comprise a second pool that is readily mobilized for metabolic conversion (mostly to pyridoxal phosphate, pyridoxal, and pyridoxic acid) and release to the blood.

Catabolism

Pyridoxal phosphate is dephosphorylated and oxidized primarily in the liver, probably by the FAD-dependent **aldehyde (pyridoxal) oxidase** as well as the NAD-dependent **aldehyde dehydrogenase** to yield **4-pyridoxic acid**. Pyridoxic acid is excreted in the urine, accounting for half of the daily consumption of the vitamin.

Effects of Alcohol and Other Drugs

Several drugs can antagonize vitamin B$_6$. Among these is alcohol; its degradation product, acetaldehyde, displaces pyridoxal phosphate from proteins, resulting in enhanced catabolism of the coenzyme. Acetaldehyde also stimulates the activity of alkaline phosphatase, enhancing the dephosphorylation of **pyridoxal phosphate**. The antituberculosis drug **isonicotinic acid hydrazide (INH)** also antagonizes vitamin B$_6$; it does so by binding the vitamin directly. For this reason, vitamin B$_6$ must be given to patients treated with INH. Pyridoxal kinase binds the antianxiety drug benzodiazepine and can be inhibited by the antiasthmatic drug theophylline. Short-term theophylline therapy induces biochemical signs of vitamin B$_6$ deficiency due to this effect.

Excretion

The products of vitamin B$_6$ metabolism are excreted in the urine, the major one being 4-pyridoxic acid. It has been estimated that humans oxidize 40–60% of ingested vitamin B$_6$ to 4-pyridoxic acid. In the rat, the urinary excretion of 4-pyridoxic acid increases with age in parallel with increases in the hepatic activities of pyridoxal oxidase and pyridoxal dehydrogenase. Small amounts of pyridoxal, pyridoxamine, and pyridoxine and their phosphates, as well as the lactone of pyridoxic acid and a ureido–pyridoxyl complex,[10] are also excreted when high doses of the vitamin have been given.[11]

Urinary levels of 4-pyridoxic acid are inversely related to protein intake (Table 13-3); this effect appears to be greater for women than for men. However, 4-pyridoxic acid is not detectable in the urine of vitamin B$_6$-deficient subjects, making it useful in the clinical assessment of vitamin B$_6$ status.[12,13]

VI. Metabolic Functions of Vitamin B$_6$

Mechanisms of Action

The metabolically active form of vitamin B$_6$ is pyridoxal phosphate, which serves as a coenzyme

---

[10] This is formed by the reaction of an amino group of urea with a hydroxyl group of the hemiacetal form of the aldehyde at position 4 of pyridoxal.

[11] For example, humans given 100 mg of pyridoxal excrete about 60 mg of 4-pyridoxic acid and about 2 mg of pyridoxal over the next 24 hr.

[12] In humans, excretion of less than 0.5 mg/day (men) or 0.4 mg/day (women) is considered indicative of inadequate intake of the vitamin. Typical excretion of total vitamin B$_6$ by adequately nourished humans is 1.2–2.4 mg/day. Of that amount, 0.5–1.2 mg (men) or 0.4–1.1 mg (women) is in the form of 4-pyridoxic acid.

[13] Although no explanation has been offered for the correlation, it is of interest that excretion of relatively low amounts (< 0.81 mg/24 hr) of 4-pyridoxic acid is associated with increased risk of relapse after mastectomy.

Table 13-3.   Effect of protein intake on vitamin B_6 status

Treatment			
Protein intake (g/kg/day)	0.5	1.0	2.0
Vitamin B_6 intake (mg/g protein)	0.04	0.02	0.01

Parameter (adequate value)	Percentage of subjects with low values		
Urinary 4-pyridoxic acid (>3 mmol/day)	11	22	78
Urinary total vitamin B_6 (>0.5 mmol/day)	56	56	67
Plasma pyridoxal phosphate (>30 nmol/liter)	33	67	78
Urinary xanthurenic acid (<65 mmol/day)	11	11	44

Source: Hansen, C. M., Leklem, J. E., and Miller, L. T. (1996). *J. Nutr.* **126,** 1891–1901.

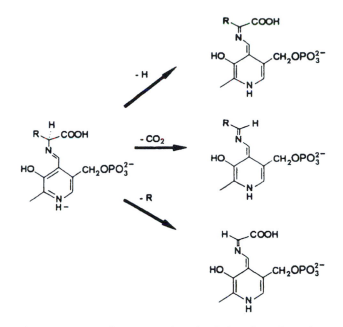

Fig. 13-2.   General reactions of pyridoxal phosphate-dependent enzymes in amino acid metabolism.

of numerous enzymes, most of which are involved in the metabolism of amino acids (Fig. 13-2). That vitamer functions through the following general mechanisms:

- Decarboxylations
- Transamination, racemization, elimination, and replacement reactions
- β-group interconversions

In each of these reactions the cofactor remains tightly bound to the enzyme, pyridoxal phosphate more so than pyridoxamine phosphate. Binding occurs by the formation of a Schiff base between the keto-carbon of the coenzyme and the ε-amino group of a specific lysyl residue of the apoenzyme. Thus, vitamin B_6-dependent enzymes tend to have structural similarities in the coenzyme-binding region. The mechanisms of the reactions catalyzed by the vitamin B_6-dependent enzymes also tend to be similar. Each involves the binding of an α-carbon of an α-amino acid substrate to the pyridine nitrogen of pyridoxal phosphate. The delocalization of the electrons from the α-carbon by the action of the protonated pyridine nitrogen as an *electron sink*

results in the conversion of the α-carbon to a carbanion at the α-carbon and the labilization of its bonds. This results in the heterolytic cleavage of one of the three bonds to the α-carbon (Table 13-4 and Fig. 13-2). The particular bond to be cleaved is determined by the particular pyridoxal phosphate-dependent enzyme; each involves the loss of the cationic ligand of an amino acid.

Metabolic Roles

Vitamin B_6 is widely involved in metabolism (Table 13-4).

Amino acid metabolism

Pyridoxal phosphate is involved in practically all amino acid metabolism reactions, in both their biosynthesis and their catabolism.

- *Transaminations*   Pyridoxal phosphate-dependent **transaminases** catabolize most amino acids.[14] The response of erythrocyte aspartate aminotransferase (EAAT) to *in vitro* additions of pyridoxal phosphate has been used as a biochemical maker of vitamin B_6 status.[15]

---

[14] The only amino acids that are *not* substrates for pyridoxal phosphate-dependent transaminases are threonine, lysine, proline, and hydroxyproline.

[15] However, EAAT activity coefficients can be affected by factors unrelated to vitamin B_6 status (e.g., intake of protein and alcohol, differences in body protein turnover, certain drugs, and genetic polymorphism of the enzyme), which can compromise its use without careful controls.

Table 13-4. Important pyridoxal phosphate-dependent enzymes of animals

Type of reaction	Enzyme
Decarboxylations	Aspartate 1-decarboxylase
	Glutamate decarboxylase
	Ornithine decarboxylase
	Aromatic amino acid decarboxylase
	Histidine decarboxylase
R-group interconversions	Serine hydroxymethyltransferase
	δ-Aminolevulinic acid synthase
Transaminations	Aspartate aminotransferase
	Alanine aminotransferase
	γ-Aminobutyrate aminotransferase
	Cysteine aminotransferase
	Tyrosine aminotransferase
	Leucine aminotransferase
	Ornithine aminotransferase
	Glutamine aminotransferase
	Branched-chain amino acid aminotransferase
	Serine-pyruvate aminotransferase
	Aromatic amino acid transferase
	Histidine aminotransferase
Racemization	Cystathionine β-synthase
α, β-Elimination	Serine dehydratase
γ-Elimination	Cystathionine γ-lyase
	Kynureninase

- *Transsulfuration* Pyridoxal phosphate-dependent enzymes cystathionine synthase and cystathionase catalyze the transsulfuration of methionine to cysteine. Vitamin B$_6$ deprivation, therefore, reduces the activities of these enzymes. Affected individuals show **homocysteinuria** (due to the impaired conversion to cystathionine) and **cystathionuria** (due to the impaired cleavage of cystathionine to cysteine and α-ketobutyrate). These conditions can be exacerbated for diagnostic purposes by the use of an oral methionine load. Plasma homocysteine concentrations, however, usually do not change in vitamin B$_6$ deficiency and are therefore not suitable for assessment of vitamin B$_6$ status.

- *Selenoamino acid metabolism* Vitamin B$_6$ is essential for the utilization of selenium from the major dietary form, selenomethionine; after that selenium is transferred to selenohomocysteine. Pyridoxal phosphate is a cofactor for two enzymes, **selenocysteine β-lyase** and **selenocysteine γ-lyase**, which catalyze the elimination of the selenium atom from selenohomocysteine to yield hydrogen selenide. Selenide is the obligate precursor for the incorporation of selenium into selenoproteins in the form of selenocysteinyl residues produced during translation.[16]

Tryptophan–niacin conversion

Vitamin B$_6$ is required, as a cofactor for **kynureninase**, for the removal of an alanyl residue from 3-hydroxykynurenine in the metabolism of tryptophan to the branch-point intermediate α-amino-β-carboxymuconic-ε-semialdehyde in the tryptophan–niacin conversion pathway. In addition, kynureninase catalyzes the analogous reaction (removal of alanine) using nonhydroxylated kynurenine as substrate and yielding the nonhydroxylated analog of 3-hydroxykynurenine, anthranilic acid. Vitamin B$_6$-dependent transaminases are also able to metabolize kynurenine and 3-hydroxykynurenine, yielding kynurenic and **xanthurenic acids**, respectively. However, because the transaminases have much greater binding affinities for pyridoxal phosphate than does kynureninase,[17] vitamin B$_6$ deprivation usually reduces the latter activity preferentially to the former ones. The result is a blockage in the tryptophan–niacin pathway, with an accumulation of 3-hydroxykynurenine that continues to be transaminated, resulting in increased production of xanthurenic acid. Vitamin B$_6$ deficiency, therefore, impairs the metabolic conversion of tryptophan to niacin, diverting it instead to xanthurenic

---

[16] These include the selenium-dependent glutathione peroxidases and thioredoxin reductases, which have antioxidant functions; the iodothyronine 5′-deiodinases, which are involved in thyroid hormone metabolism; selenophosphate synthase, which is involved in selenoprotein synthesis; selenoproteins P and W, which are major selenium-containing proteins in plasma and muscle, respectively; and at least a dozen other proteins, with unclear functions.

[17] The Michaelis constants (K_m) for the transaminases are on the order of $10^{-8} M$, whereas that for kynureninase is on the order of $10^{-3} M$.

acid, which appears in the urine.[18] This phenomenon is exploited in the assessment of vitamin B_6 status: deficiency is indicated by urinary excretion of xanthurenic acid after a tryptophan load.

Gluconeogenesis

Vitamin B_6 has two roles in gluconeogenesis:

- *Transaminations* Amino acid catabolism depends on pyridoxal phosphate and is a cofactor for transaminases (see Amino Acid Metabolism above).
- *Gycogen utilization* Vitamin B_6 is required for the utilization of glycogen to release glucose by serving as a coenzyme of glycogen phosphorylase, to which it is bound (as pyridoxal phosphate) via a Schiff base linkage to a peptidyllysine residue. Unlike the other pyridoxal phosphate enzymes, it is the coenzyme's phosphate group that is catalytically important, participating in the transfer of inorganic phosphate to the glucose units of glycogen to produce glucose-1-phosphate, which is released. That it is essential for enzymatic activity is clear; the shift of the enzyme from its inactive form to its active form involves an increase in the binding (2–4 mol per mole of enzyme) of the coenzyme. This role accounts for more than half of the vitamin B_6 in the body, owing to the abundance of both muscle and glycogen phosphorylase (5% of soluble muscle protein).

Neurotransmitter synthesis

Pyridoxal phosphate-dependent enzymes function in the biosynthesis of the neurotransmitters **serotonin** as a cofactor for tryptophan decarboxylase, of **epinephrine** and **norepinephrine** as a cofactor for tyrosine carboxylase, as a source of energy for the brain, **γ-aminobutyric acid (GABA)**, and as a cofactor for glutamate decarboxylase.[19]

Histamine synthesis

Pyridoxal phosphate functions in the metabolism of the vasodilator and gastric secretagogue **histamine** as a cofactor for histidine decarboxylase.

Hemoglobin synthesis and function

Pyridoxal phosphate functions in the synthesis of heme from porphyrin precursors as a cofactor for δ-aminolevulinic acid synthase. The vitamin also binds to hemoglobin at two sites on the β chains: the N-terminal valine and Lys-82 residues. Pyridoxal also binds at the N-terminal valine residues of the α chains. The binding of pyridoxal and pyridoxal phosphate enhances the O_2-binding capacity of that protein and inhibits sickling in sickle-cell hemoglobin. The catalytic properties of other enzymes are also affected (some stimulated,[20] others inhibited[21]) by interactions with pyridoxal phosphate (usually via valine, histidine, or lysine residues), suggesting that vitamin B_6 status may have effects beyond those involving its classic coenzyme function.

Lipid metabolism

Changes in lipid metabolism have been reported in response to vitamin B_6 deprivation. Vitamin B_6 is required for the biosynthesis of sphingolipids via the pyridoxal phosphate-dependent serine palmitoyltransferase and other enzymes in phospholipid synthesis. Diminution in the activities of these enzymes is thought to account for the changes observed in phospholipid contents of linoleic and arachidonic acids in vitamin B_6-deficient animals. Such effects may be involved in other putative effects of vitamin B_6 in lipid metabolism manifest as decreased

---

[18] Xanthurenic acid was discovered quite unexpectedly by Dr. Sam Lepkovsky (University of California), who during the Great Depression sought to elucidate the nature of rat *adermin*. Lepkovsky wrote of his surprise in finding that the urine voided by his vitamin B_6-deficient rats was green, whereas that of his controls was the normal yellow color. In pursuing this observation, he found that urine from deficient animals was normally colored as it was voided, but that it turned green only on exposure to the rusty dropping pans their limited budget had forced them to use. Thus, he recognized that vitamin B_6-deficient rats excreted an unidentified metabolite that reacted with an iron salt to form a green derivative. This small event, which might have been missed by someone "too busy" to observe the experimental animals, resulted in Lepkovsky's identifying the metabolite as xanthurenic acid and discovering the role of vitamin B_6 in the tryptophan–niacin conversion pathway. His message: "*The investigator has to do more than sit at his desk, outline experiments and examine data.*"

[19] It has been shown *in vitro* that pyridoxal phosphate can inhibit the binding of GABA to brain synaptic membranes.

[20] For example, thymidylate synthase, vitamin K-dependent carboxylase/epoxidase.

[21] For example, glucose-6-phosphate dehydrogenase, glycerol-3-phosphate dehydrogenase, ribulose bisphosphate carboxylase, ribosomal peptidyltransferase.

carcass fat, hepatic steatosis, dermatitis, arteriosclerosis, hypertriglyceridemia, and hypercholesterolemia. The metabolic basis of such effects remains unclear. Best evidence suggests that such effects on fatty acids and phospholipids are secondary to vitamin B$_6$-dependent changes in methionine metabolism and, perhaps, on carnitine biosynthesis.

Gene expression

Pyridoxal phosphate has been shown to modulate gene expression. Instances recognized to date include:

- *Steroid hormone receptor-induced enzymes* Elevated intracellular levels of the vitamin are associated with decreased transcription in responses to glucocorticoid hormones (progesterone, androgens, estrogens). Such diminished responses include hydrocortisone-induction of rat liver cytosolic aspartate aminotransferase. Inhibition is caused by the formation of Schiff base linkages of the vitamin to the DNA-binding site of the receptor–steroid complex. This inhibits the ligand binding to the glucocorticoid-responsive element in the regulatory region of the gene.
- *Serum albumin* Vitamin B$_6$ deficiency increases the expression of albumin mRNA sevenfold. The effect appears due to the action of pyridoxal phosphate inactivating tissue-specific transcription factors by directly interacting with DNA ligand-binding sites.[22]
- *Glycoprotein IIb* Pyridoxal phosphate appears to modulate glycoprotein IIb gene expression by interacting directly with tissue-specific transcription factors.[23] This results in inhibition of platelet aggregation due to impaired binding of fibrinogen or other adhesion proteins to glycoprotein complexes.
- *Other proteins* Pyridoxal phosphate has been shown to suppress mRNA levels for glycogen

phosphorylase, apolipoprotein A-1, phenylalanine hydroxylase, glyceraldehyde-3-phosphate dehydrogenase, and ß-actin, but to decrease mRNA levels for RNA polymerases I and II in the rat model.[24] The effect on glycogen phosphorylase appears to be tissue-specific, as deprivation of the vitamin was found to reduce phosphorylase mRNA levels in muscle but to increase them in liver.[25]

Health Effects

Vascular disease

Low vitamin B$_6$ status results in homocyteinemia as a result of lost capacity to convert that metabolite to cystathionine due to impaired activities of the pyridoxal phosphate-dependent enzyme cystathionine ß-synthase. Homocysteinemia has been associated with increased risks to occlusive vascular disease, total and cardiovascular disease-related mortality, stroke, dimentia, Alzheimer's disease, fracture, and chronic heart failure.[26] Low plasma pyridoxal phosphate levels have been associated with increased risk to vascular disease independent of plasma homocysteine level.[27] A recent study suggested that treatment with high doses of vitamin B$_6$ and folic acid were effective in reducing both plasma homocysteine and the incidence of abnormal exercise electrocardxiography tests, suggesting reductions in risk of atherosclerotic disease.[28] However, a meta-analysis of 12 randomized trials of vitamin (folate, vitamin B$_6$, vitamin B$_{12}$) supplements to lower homocysteine levels in free-living people found no evidence of effectiveness for vitamin B$_6$ supplements.[29]

Neurologic function

Vitamin B$_6$ has been shown to affect the postnatal development of a glutamate receptor in the brain that is thought to have an important role in learning. Animal studies of long-term potentiation, a synaptic model of learning and memory, have revealed that

---

[22] See review: Oka, T. (2001). *Nutr. Res. Rev.* **14,** 257–265.

[23] Chang, S. J., et al. (1999). *J. Nutr. Sci. Vitaminol.* **45,** 471–479.

[24] Oka, T., et al. (1993). *FEBS Letts.* **331,** 162–164.

[25] Oka, T., et al. (1994). *Experientia* **50,** 127–129.

[26] Selhub, J. (2006). *J. Nutr.* **136,** 1726S–1730S.

[27] Robinson, K., et al. (1998). *Circulation* **97,** 437–443.

[28] Vermuelen, E. G. J., et al. (2000). *Lancet* **355,** 517–522.

[29] Folic acid produced an average 25% reduction, and vitamin B$_{12}$ produced an average 7% reduction (Clarke, R., and Armitage, J. [2000]. *Semin. Thromb. Hemost.* **26,** 341–348).

maternal deprivation of the vitamin during gestation and lactation specifically reduces the development of the *N*-methyl-D-aspartate receptor subtype in the young. Although the metabolic basis for this lesion is not understood, it is clear that these effects are related to the loss of dendritic arborization in vitamin B$_6$ deficiency. These lesions are thought to underlie reported effects of impaired learning among the progeny of vitamin B$_6$-deficient animals and humans. There is no evidence for vitamin B$_6$ affecting mood, depression, or cognitive functions.

Immune function

Vitamin B$_6$ has a role in the support of immune competence that has not been elucidated. Animal and human studies have demonstrated effects of vitamin B$_6$ deprivation on both humoral (diminished antibody production) and cell-mediated immune responses (increased lymphocyte proliferation, reduced delayed-type hypersensitivity responses, reduced T cell-mediated cytotoxicity, reduced cytokine production), and suboptimal status of the vitamin has been linked to declining immunologic changes among the elderly (Table 13-5), persons with human immunodeficiency virus (HIV), and patients with uremia or rheumatoid arthritis. These effects may relate to reduced activities of such pyridoxal phosphate enzymes as serine transhydroxymethylase and thymidylate synthase, which would be expected to impair single-carbon metabolism and reduce DNA synthesis. The vitamin has also been shown to bind to a histamine-like T lymphocyte receptor, by which it affects photoimmunosuppression, and to noncompetitively inhibit HIV-1 reverse transcriptase.[30]

Cancer

Epidemiological studies have demonstrated inverse associations of projected vitamin B$_6$ intake and colon cancer risk. Recent studies in animal models have found that supranutritional doses of the vitamin can reduce tumorigenesis through effects on cell proliferation, production of reactive oxygen and nitrogen species, and angiogenesis.[31]

Table 13-5.   Effects of vitamin B$_6$ status on mitogenic responses and interleukin 2 production by peripheral blood mononucleocytes of elderly humans

Parameter	Baseline	B$_6$ deprived	B$_6$ supplemented
Mitogenic response			
Concanavalin A	120	70	190
Phytohemagglutinin	100	70	100
Staphylococcus aureus	115	60	200
IL-2 production (kU/liter)	105	40	145

Source: Meydani, S. N., Ribaya-Meradi, J. D., Russel, R. M., Sahyoung, N., Morrow, F. D., and Gershoff, S. N. (1991). *Am. J. Clin. Nutr.* **53,** 1275–1280.

VII. Vitamin B$_6$ Deficiency

Severe vitamin B$_6$ deficiency results in dermatologic and neurologic changes in most species. Less obvious are the metabolic lesions associated with insufficient activities of the coenzyme pyridoxal phosphate. The most prominent of these lesions is impaired tryptophan–niacin conversion, which can be detected on the basis of urinary excretion of xanthurenic acid after an oral **tryptophan load**. Vitamin B$_6$ deficiency also results in impaired transsulfuration of methionine to cysteine, which can be detected as homocysteinuria and cystathionuria after an oral **methionine load**. The pyridoxal phosphate-dependent transaminases and glycogen phosphorylase give the vitamin a role in gluconeogenesis. Deprivation of vitamin B$_6$, therefore, impairs glucose tolerance, although it may not affect fasting glucose levels.

Deficiency Syndromes in Animals

Vitamin B$_6$ deficiency in animals is generally manifest as symmetrical scaling dermatitis. In rodents, the condition is called **acrodynia** and is characterized by hyperkeratotic[32] and acanthotic[33] lesions on the tail, paws, face, and upper thorax, as well as by muscular weakness, hyperirritability, anemia, hepatic steatosis,[34] increased urinary oxalate excretion, insulin

---

[30] Mitchell, L. L. W., and Cooperman, B. S. (1992). *Biochem.* **31,** 7707–7713.

[31] Komatsu, S., et al. (2003). *Biochem. Biophys. Acta* **1647,** 127–130.

[32] Involving hypertrophy of the horny layer of the epidermis.

[33] Involving an increase in the prickle cell layer of the epidermis.

[34] This can be precipitated by feeding a vitamin B$_6$-deficient diet rich in protein.

insufficiency,[35] hypertension, and poor growth. Neurological signs include convulsive seizures (epileptiform type) that can be fatal.[36] Reproductive disorders include infertility, fetal malformations,[37] and reduced fetal survival. Some reports indicate effects on blood cholesterol levels and immunity. That tissue carnitine levels are depressed in vitamin B$_6$-deficient animals has been cited as evidence of a role of the vitamin in carnitine synthesis.

Similar changes are observed in vitamin B$_6$-deficient individuals of other species. Chickens and turkeys show reduced appetite and poor growth, dermatitis, marked anemia, convulsions, reduced egg production, and low fertility. Pigs show paralysis of the hind limbs, dermatitis, reduced feed intake, and poor growth. Monkeys show an increased incidence of dental caries and altered cholesterol metabolism with arteriosclerotic lesions. Vitamin B$_6$ deficiency has been reported to cause hyperirritability, hyperactivity, abnormal behavior, and performance deficits in several species. These signs accompany an underlying neuropathology that reduces axonal diameter and dendritic arborization and thus impairs nerve conduction velocity.

Ruminants are rarely affected by vitamin B$_6$ deficiency, as their rumen microflora appear to satisfy their needs for the vitamin. Exceptions are lambs and calves, which, before their rumen microfloras are established, are susceptible to dietary deprivation of vitamin B$_6$, showing many dermatologic and neurologic changes observed in nonruminant species.

Deficiency in Humans

Vitamin B$_6$-deficiency occurs in free-living populations. Prevalences in the range of 0.8 to 68% have been reported for signs of vitamin B$_6$ deficiency in developed countries.

Vitamin B$_6$-deficient humans exhibit symptoms that can be quickly corrected by administration of the vitamin: weakness, sleeplessness, nervous disorders (peripheral neuropathies), **cheilosis,**[38] **glossitis,**[39] **stomatitis**, and impaired cell-mediated immunity (Table 13-6). Behavioral differences have been associated with low vitamin B$_6$ status: a study in Egypt found that mothers of marginal (subclinical) vitamin B$_6$ status were less responsive to their infants' vocalizations, showed less effective response to infant distress, and were more likely to use older siblings as caregivers than were mothers of better vitamin B$_6$ status. In addition, studies with volunteers fed a vitamin B$_6$-free diet or a vitamin B$_6$ antagonist[40] have shown elevated urinary xanthurenic acid concentrations[41] and increased susceptibility to infection. Because plasma concentrations of pyridoxal phosphate decrease with age, it is expected that elderly people may be at greater risk of vitamin B$_6$ deficiency than younger people.

Table 13-6. Signs of vitamin B$_6$ deficiency

Organ system	Signs
General	
Appetite	Decrease
Growth	Decrease
Dermatologic	Acrodynia, cheilosis, stomatitis, glossitis
Muscular	Weakness
Skeletal	Dental caries
Vital organs	Hepatic steatosis
Vascular	
Vessels	Arteriosclerosis
Erythrocytes	Anemia
Nervous	Paralysis, convulsions, peripheral neuropathy
Reproductive	
Female	Decreased egg production
Fetal	Malformations, death

---

[35] This is believed to be due to reduced pancreatic synthesis of the hormone.

[36] Nervous dysfunction is believed to be due to nerve tissue deficiencies of γ-aminobutyric acid (GABA) resulting from decreased activities of the pyridoxal phosphate-dependent *glutamate decarboxylase*. The seizures of vitamin B$_6$-deficient animals can be controlled by administering either the vitamin or GABA.

[37] For example, omphalocele (protrusion of the omentum or intestine through the umbilicus), exencephaly (defective skull formation with the brain partially outside of the cranial cavity), cleft palate, micrognathia (impaired growth of the jaw), and splenic hypoplasia.

[38] The lesion is morphologically indistinguishable from that produced by riboflavin deficiency.

[39] The lesion is morphologically indistinguishable from that produced by niacin deficiency.

[40] For example, 4'-deoxypyridoxine.

[41] After tryptophan loading, vitamin B$_6$-deficient subjects also had elevated urinary concentrations of kynurenine, 3-hydroxykynurenine, kynurenic acid, acetylkynurenine, and quinolinic acid.

Infants consuming less than 100 mg of vitamin B$_6$ per day are at risk of developing seizures, which are thought to result from insufficient activities of the pyridoxal phosphate-dependent enzyme glutamate carboxylase required for the synthesis of GABA.

Congenital Disorders

Several rare familial disorders of vitamin B$_6$ metabolism have been identified, each thought to be caused by the expression of deficient amounts or dysfunctional forms of pyridoxal phosphate-dependent enzyme (Table 13-7).

Homocysteinuria

Hereditary deficiency of the cystathionine β-synthase occurs at a rate of 3/1,000,000. The resulting impairment in homocysteine catabolism is manifest as elevations in plasma levels of homocysteine, methionine, and cysteine, with dislocation of the optic lens,[42] osteoporosis and abnormalities of long bone growth, mental retardation, and thromboembolism. The condition is treated with a low-methionine diet. Half of cases respond to high doses (250–500 mg/day) of pyridoxine.[43] Of more than a hundred alleles that have been studied, mutations of the cystathionine β-synthase associated with disease phenotypes have been found in almost a third.[44] Some mutations, including some of the most frequent ones in the human populations studied to date,[45] have been shown to correlate with pyridoxine-responsiveness; these would appear to involve the expression of a mutant enzyme with low affinity for pyridoxal phosphate.

Pyridoxine-responsive seizures

This is a rare,[46] autosomal recessive disorder involving impaired synthesis of the inhibitory neurotransmitter, γ-aminobutyric acid (GABA). The defect was originally thought to involve the inability of an abnormal form of glutamic acid decarboxylase, GAD-65, in the nerve terminal[47] to bind pyridoxal phosphate. Recent studies have shown that the defect instead involves mutations in pyridoxine/pyridoxamine oxidase.[48] The disorder is manifest as intractable seizures appearing within hours after birth. Patients show normal circulating levels of pyridoxal phosphate, but their seizures stop immediately upon administration of high levels (100–500 mg) of pyridoxine intravenously and are controlled using daily oral doses of pyridoxine (0.2–3 mg/kg body weight).[49] If untreated, progressive cerebral atrophy ensues.

Hyperoxaluria

Type 1 primary hyperoxaluria has been found to be due to a mutant hepatic alanine glyoxylate transferase with abnormally low pyridoxal phosphate-binding capacity. In such cases high doses of vitamin B$_6$ (e.g., 400 mg/day) reduce hyperoxaluria and thus the risk of formation of oxalate stones and renal injury.

Table 13-7.   Congenital disorders of vitamin B$_6$-dependent metabolism

Disorder	Enzyme deficiency	Clinical manifestations
Homocysteinuria[a]	Cystathionine β-synthase	Dislocation of lenses, thromboses, malformation of skeletal and connective tissue, mental retardation
Cystathionuria	Cystathionine γ-lyase	Mental retardation
GABA deficiency	Glutamate decarboxylase	Neuropathies
Sideroblastic anemia	δ-Aminolevulinic acid synthase	Anemia, cystathionuria, xanthurenic aciduria

[a]Another form is caused by impaired vitamin B$_{12}$-dependent methionine synthesis.

---

[42] *Ectopia lentis.*

[43] Berber, G., and Spaeth, G. (1969). *J. Pediatr.* **75**, 463–478.

[44] Kraus, J. P., et al. (1999). *Human Mutation* **13**, 362–375.

[45] To date, such studies have been conducted only in some parts of Europe; no information is available for other populations.

[46] By 2001, only a hundred cases had been reported, but the disorder is likely underreported.

[47] Another, nonpyridoxal phosphate-dependent glutamic acid decarboxylase, GAD-67, is present in neuronal soma and dendrites.

[48] Gospe, S. M., Jr. (2006). *Curr. Opin. Neurol.* **19**, 148–153.

[49] Gupta, V., et al. (2001). *J. Pediatr. Child Health* **37**, 592–596; Gospe, S. M., Jr. (2002). *Ped. Neurol.* **26**, 181–185.

VIII. Pharmacologic Uses of Vitamin B$_6$

Vitamin B$_6$ has been used at supranutritional doses for the management of a variety of human disorders:

- *Sideroblastic anemia* Dosages as great as 200 mg/day (usually as pyridoxine HCl) have been found effective in stimulating hematopoiesis (δ-aminolevulinic acid synthase) in sideroblastic anemia patients.
- *Sickle cell anemia* A small study found patients to have lower plasma pyridoxal phosphate levels than controls, which responded to oral supplementation (100 mg/day) of pyridoxine within two months. Both pyridoxine and pyridoxal phosphate have been found to protect sickle cells in vitro,[50] but it is not clear whether supplementation with the vitamin may benefit sickle-cell anemia patients.
- *Iron storage disease* Complexes of pyridoxal, which chelate iron (e.g., the isonicotinyl and benzoyl hydrazones), are effective in stimulating the excretion of that mineral in patients with iron-storage disease.
- *Suppression of lactation* A few studies have reported vitamin B$_6$ as effective in suppressing lactation, probably through the stimulation of dopaminergic activity in the hypothalamus and thus the suppression of prolactin.
- *Adverse drug effects* The vitamin is used (3–5 mg/kg body weight) to counteract adverse effects of several types of drugs:
  - *Hydrazines* The antituberculin drug isonicotinic acid hydrazide (isoniazid) produces a peripheral neuropathy similar to that of vitamin B$_6$ deficiency. It inhibits pyridoxal phosphate-dependent glutamate-decarboxylase and γ-aminobutyrate aminotransferase which produce and degrade GABA, respectively, in nerve tissue.
  - *Antibiotics* Two antibiotics have been found to antagonize vitamin B$_6$ by reacting with pyridoxal phosphate to form inactive products. Cycloserine reacts with the coenzyme to produce an oxime. Penicillamine produces thiazolidine.
  - *L-DOPA* L-3,4-dihydroxyphenylalanine antagonizes vitamin B$_6$ by reacting with pyridoxal phosphate to form tetrahydroquinolines.
  - *Ethanol* Ethanol increases the catabolism of pyridoxal phosphate.
  - *Oral contraceptives* Synthetic estrogens can alter tryptophan–niacin conversion by increasing the synthesis of pyridoxal phosphate-dependent enzymes in that pathway and thus the need for vitamin B$_6$ in some subjects.
- *Schizophrenia* Vitamin B$_6$ is recommended (0.1–1 g/day alone or in combination with tryptophan or magnesium) for the treatment of **schizophrenia,** and to reduce the incidence of seizures in alcoholics.
- *Asthma* Low circulating pyridoxal phosphate levels have been reported in patients with asthma, and one small study found vitamin B$_6$ treatment (100 mg/day) to reduce the severity and frequency of attacks.[51] These effects may be secondary to those of theophylline, which inhibits pyridoxal kinase.
- *Herpes* Pyridoxine has been used to treat *herpes gestationis* at doses of 400–4000 mg/day.
- *Carpal tunnel syndrome* This disorder, involving pain and paresthesia of the hand, is caused by irritation and compression of the medial nerve by the transverse ligaments of the wrist in ways that are exacerbated by redundant motions. The condition has been associated with low circulating levels of pyridoxal phosphate and low erythrocyte glutamic-oxaloacetic transaminase activities. It has been suggested that such deficiencies lead to edematous changes to and proliferation of the synovia, causing compression of the nerve in the carpal tunnel. Some investigators have reported high doses (50–300 mg/day for 12 weeks) of pyridoxine to be effective as treatment;[52] however, there is no evidence from randomized clinical trials supporting such use of the vitamin.

[50] Kark, J. A., et al. (1983). *J. Clin. Invest.* **71,** 1224–1229.

[51] Simon, R. A., and Reynolds, R. D. (1988) in *Clinical and Physiological Applications of Vitamin B$_6$* (J. E. Leklem and R. D. Reynolds, eds.), pp. 307–315. Alan R. Liss, New York.

[52] Aufiero, E., et al. (2004). *Nutr. Rev.* **62,** 96–104; Goodyear-Smith, F., and Arroll, B. (2004). *Ann. Fam. Med.* **2,** 267–273; Ellis, J. M., and Pamplin, J. (1999). *Vitamin B$_6$ Therapy*, pp. 47–56. Avery Publ. Group.

- *Chinese restaurant syndrome* The syndrome, which involves headache, sensation of heat, altered heart beat, nausea, and tightness of the neck induced by oral intake of monosodium glutamate, has been reported to respond to vitamin B_6 (50 mg/day).
- *Premenstrual syndrome* **Premenstrual syndrome** occurs in an estimated 40% of women 2–3 days before their menstrual flow. It involves tension of the breasts, pain in the lumbar region, thirst, headache, nervous irritability, pelvic congestion, peripheral edema, and, usually, nausea and vomiting. Premenstrual syndrome has been reported to respond to vitamin B_6, presumably by affecting levels of the neurotransmitters, serotonin, and γ-aminobutyric acid, which control depression, pain perception, and anxiety. Women experiencing premenstrual symptoms appear to have circulating pyridoxal phosphate levels comparable to those of unaffected women. Nevertheless, high doses of the vitamin have been found to alleviate at least some symptoms in many cases. A review of randomized, clinical trials concluded that pyridoxine doses of up to 100 mg/day are likely to be of benefit in treating these symptoms.[53]
- *Morning sickness* A randomized clinical trial showed that the use of pyridoxine (25 mg every eight hours for three days) significantly reduced vomiting and nausea in pregnant women.[54] However, there is no evidence that women who experience nausea and vomiting in pregnancy are of abnormal vitamin B_6 status.

IX. Vitamin B_6 Toxicity

The toxicity of vitamin B_6 appears to be relatively low, although high doses of the vitamin (several grams per day) have been shown to induce sensory neuronopathy marked by changes in gait and peripheral sensation. Thus, the primary target, appears to be the peripheral nervous system; although massive doses of the vitamin have produced convulsions in

rats, central nervous abnormalities have not been reported frequently in humans. The potential for toxicity resulting from the therapeutic or pharmacologic uses of the vitamin for human disorders (which rarely exceed 50 mg/day) must be considered small. Reports of individuals taking massive doses of the vitamin (>2 g/day) indicate that the earliest detectable signs were ataxia and loss of small motor control. Many of the signs of vitamin B_6 toxicity resemble those of vitamin B_6 deficiency; it has been proposed that the metabolic basis of each condition involves the tissue-level depletion of pyridoxal phosphate. Doses up to 250 mg/day for extended periods of time appear safe.

In doses of 10–25 mg, vitamin B_6 increases the conversion of L-dopa to dopamine,[55] which, unlike its precursor, is unable to cross the blood–brain barrier. The vitamin can therefore interfere with L-dopa in the management of Parkinson's disease; it should not be administered to individuals taking L-dopa without the concomitant administration of a decarboxylase inhibitor.

X. Case Studies

Instructions

Review the following case reports, paying special attention to the diagnostic indicators on which the treatments were based. Then, answer the questions that follow.

Case 1

A 16-year-old boy was admitted with *dislocated lenses* and *mental retardation*. Four years earlier, an ophthalmologist had found dislocation of the lenses. On the present occasion, he was thin and blond-headed, with *ectopia lentis*,[56] an anterior thoracic deformity (*pectus excavatum*[57]), and normal vital signs. His palate was narrow with crowding of his teeth. He had mild scoliosis[58] and genu valgum,[59] which caused him to walk with a toe-in, *Chaplin-like* gait. His neurological examination was within normal limits. On radiography,

[53] Wyatt, K. M., et al. (1999). *Br. Med. J.* **318,** 1375–1381.
[54] Sahakian, V., et al. (1991). *Obstet. Gynecol.* **78,** 33–36.
[55] It has been claimed that, through its effect on dopamine, vitamin B_6 can inhibit the release of prolactin, thus inhibiting lactation in nursing mothers. Although this proposal is still highly disputed, their is no evidence that daily doses of less than about 10 mg of the vitamin (in multivitamin preparations) has any such effect on lactation.
[56] Dislocated lenses.
[57] Funnel chest.
[58] Lateral curvature of the spine.
[59] Knock-knee.

his spine appeared osteoporotic. His performance on the Stanford–Binet Intelligence Scale gave him a development quotient of 60. His hematology, blood glucose, and blood urea nitrogen values were all within normal limits. His plasma *homocystine* level (undetectable in normal patients) was 4.5 mg/dl, and his blood *methionine* level was 10-fold normal; the levels of all other amino acids in his blood were within normal limits. Both homocystine and methionine were increased in his urine, which also contained traces of *S-adenosylhomocystine*.

The patient was given oral *pyridoxine HCl* in an ascending dose regimen. Doses up to 150 mg/day were without effect but, after the dose had been increased to 325 mg/day for 200 days, his plasma and urinary homocystine and methionine levels decreased to normal. These changes were accompanied by a striking change in his hair pigmentation: dark hair grew out from the scalp (the cystine content of the dark hair was nearly double that of the blond hair, 1.5 versus 0.8 mEq/mg). On maintenance doses of pyridoxine, he attained relatively normal function, although the connective tissue changes were irreversible.

Case 2

A 27-year-old woman had experienced increasing difficulty in walking. Some 2 years earlier, she had been told that vitamin B$_6$ prevented premenstrual edema, and she began taking 500 mg/day of *pyridoxine HCl*. After a year, she had increased her intake of the vitamin to 5 g/day. During the period of this increased vitamin B$_6$ intake, she noticed that flexing her neck produced a tingling sensation down her neck and to her legs and soles of her feet.[60] During the 4 months immediately before this examination, she had become progressively unsteady when walking, particularly in the dark. Finally, she had become unable to walk without the assistance of a cane. She had also noticed difficulty in handling small objects, and changes in the feeling of her lips and tongue, although she reported no other positive sensory symptoms and was not aware of any weaknesses. Her

gait was broad-based and stamping, and she was not able to walk at all with her eyes closed. Her muscle strength was normal, but all of her limb reflexes were absent. Her sensations of touch, temperature, pin-prick, vibration, and joint position were severely impaired in both the upper and lower limbs. She showed a mild subjective alteration of touch-pressure and pin-prick sensation over her cheeks and lips, but not over her forehead. Laboratory findings showed the spinal fluid and other clinical tests to be normal. Electrophysiologic studies revealed that no sensory nerve action potentials could be elicited in her arms and legs, but that motor nerve conduction was normal.

The patient was suspected of having vitamin B$_6$ intoxication and was asked to stop taking that vitamin. Two months after withdrawal, she reported some improvement and a gain in sensation. By 7 months, she could walk steadily without a cane and could stand with her eyes closed. Neurologic examination at that time revealed that, although her strength was normal, her tendon reflexes were absent. Her feet still had severe loss of vibration sensation, despite definite improvements in the senses of joint position, touch, temperature, and pin-prick. Electrophysiologic examination revealed that her sensory nerve responses were still absent.

Case Questions

1. Propose a hypothesis consistent with the findings in Case 1 for the congenital metabolic lesion experienced by that patient.
2. Would you expect supplements of methionine and/or cystine to have been effective in treating the patient in Case 1? Defend your answer.
3. If the toxicity of pyridoxine involves its competition, at high levels, with pyridoxal phosphate for enzyme-binding sites, which enzymes would you propose as potentially being affected in the condition described in Case 2? Provide a rationale for each of the candidate enzymes on your list.

---

[60] Lhermitte's sign.

Study Questions and Exercises

1. Diagram schematically the several steps in amino acid metabolism in which pyridoxal phosphate-dependent enzymes are involved.
2. Construct a decision tree for the diagnosis of vitamin B_6 deficiency in humans or an animal species.
3. What key feature of the chemistry of vitamin B_6 relates to its biochemical functions as a coenzyme?
4. What parameters might you measure to assess vitamin B_6 status of a human or animal?
5. What factors might be expected to affect the dietary need for vitamin B_6?

Recommended Reading

Aufiero, E., Stitk, T. P., Foye, P. M., and Chen, B. (2004). Pyridoxine hydrochloride treatment of carpal tunnel syndrome: A review. *Nutr. Rev.* **62,** 96–104.

Baxter, P. (2003). Pyridoxine-dependent seizures: A clinical and biochemical conundrum. *Biochim. Biophys. Acta* **1647,** 36–41.

Bender, D. A. (1999). Non-nutritional uses of vitamin B_6. *Br. J. Nutr.* **81,** 7–20.

Dakshinamurti, K. (ed.). (1990). Vitamin B_6. *Ann. N.Y. Acad. Sci.* **585,** 241–249.

Driskell, J. A. (1994). Vitamin B-6 requirements of humans. *Nutr. Res.* **14,** 293–324.

Gregory, J. F. (1997). Bioavailability of vitamin B-6. *Eur. J. Clin. Nutr.* **51,** S43–S48.

Gregory, J. F. (1998). Nutritional properties and significance of vitamin glycosides. *Ann. Rev. Nutr.* **18,** 277–296.

Guilarte, T. R. (1993). Vitamin B_6 and cognitive development: Recent research findings from human and animal studies. *Nutr. Rev.* **51,** 193–198.

Leklem, J. E. (2001). Vitamin B_6, Chapter 10 in *Handbook of Vitamins*, 3rd ed. (R. B. Rucker, J. W. Suttie, D. B. McCormick, and L. J. Machlin, eds.), pp. 339–396. Marcel Dekker, New York.

Lheureux, R., Penaloza, A., and Gris, M. (2005). Pyridoxine in clinical toxicology: A review. *Eur. J. Emerg. Med.* **12,** 78–85.

Mackey, A. D., Davis, S. R., and Gregory, J. F. (2006). Vitamin B. Chapter 26 in *Modern Nutrition in Health and Disease*, 10th ed. (M. E. Shils, M. Shike, A. C. Ross, B. Caballero, and R. Cousins, eds.), pp. 452–461. Lippincott, New York.

McCormick, D. B. (2001). Vitamin B-6, Chapter 20 in *Present Knowledge in Nutrition*, 8th ed. (B. A. Bowman and R. M. Russell, eds.), pp. 207–213. ILSI, Washington, DC.

McCormick, D. B., and Chen, H. (1999). Update on interconversions of vitamin B-6 with its coenzyme. *J. Nutr.* **129,** 325–327.

Oka, T. (2001). Modulation of gene expression by vitamin B_6. *Nutr. Res. Rev.* **14,** 257–265.

Rall, L. C., and Meydani, S. N. (1993). Vitamin B_6 and immune competence. *Nutr. Rev.* **51,** 217–225.

Schneider, G., Kack, H., and Lindquist, Y. (2000). The manifold of vitamin B6 dependent enzymes. *Structure* **8,** R1–R6.

Biotin

We started with a bushel of corn, and at the end of the purification process, when the solution was evaporated in a small beaker, nothing could be seen, yet this solution of nothing greatly stimulated growth (of propionic acid bacteria). We now know that the factor was biotin, which is one of the most effective of all vitamins.

—H. G. Wood

I.	The Significance of Biotin	331
II.	Sources of Biotin	332
III.	Absorption of Biotin	334
IV.	Transport of Biotin	334
V.	Metabolism of Biotin	335
VI.	Metabolic Functions of Biotin	336
VII.	Biotin Deficiency	338
VIII.	Biotin Toxicity	341
IX.	Case Studies	341
	Study Questions and Exercises	343
	Recommended Reading	344

Anchoring Concepts

1. Biotin is the trivial designation of the compound hexahydro-2-oxo-1*H*-thieno[3,4-*d*]imidazole-4-pentanoic acid.
2. Biotin functions metabolically as a coenzyme for carboxylases, to which it is bound by the carbon at position 2 (C-2) of its thiophene ring via an amide bond to the ε-amino group of a peptidyllysine residue.
3. Deficiencies of biotin are manifested predominantly as dermatologic lesions.

Learning Objectives

1. To understand the chief natural sources of biotin.
2. To understand the means of absorption and transport of biotin.
3. To understand the biochemical function of biotin as a component of coenzymes of metabolically important carboxylation reactions.
4. To understand the metabolic bases of biotin-responsive disorders, including those related to dietary deprivation of the vitamin and those involving inherited metabolic lesions.

Vocabulary

Acetyl-CoA carboxylase
Achromotrichia
Alopecia
Apocarboxylase
Avidin
Biocytin
Biotin-binding proteins
Biotin holoenzyme synthetase
Biotin sulfoxide
Biotinidase
Biotinyl 5'-adenylate
Bisnorbiotin
Egg white injury
Fatty liver and kidney syndrome (FLKS)
Glucokinase
Holocarboxylases
3-Hydroxyisovaleric acid
Kangaroo gait
3-Methylcrotonoyl-CoA carboxylase
Monocarboxylate transporter (MCT1)
Multiple carboxylase deficiencies
Ornithine transcarbamylase
Phospho*enol*pyruvate carboxykinase (PEPCK)
Propionyl-CoA carboxylase
Pyruvate carboxylase
Sodium-dependent vitamin transporter (SMVT)
Spectacle eye
Streptavidin
Sudden infant death syndrome (SIDS)
Transcarboxylase

I. The Significance of Biotin

Biotin was discovered in the search for the nutritional factor that prevents *egg white injury* in experimental animals, and the use of the biotin antagonist in egg white, the biotin-binding protein **avidin**, remains useful in producing biotin deficiency in animal models. Practical cases of biotin deficiency were encountered with the advent of total parenteral nutrition before the vitamin was routinely added to tube-feeding solutions, and biotin-responsive cases of *foot pad dermatitis* remain problems in commercial poultry production. Biotin deficiency manifests itself differently in different species, but most often involves dermatologic lesions to some extent. In addition to primary deficiencies of the vitamin, genetic disorders in biotin metabolism have been identified; some of these respond to large doses of biotin. A key feature of biotin metabolism is that it is recycled by proteolytic cleavage from the four biotinyl carboxylases by the enzyme **biotinidase**. This recycling, and the prevalent hind gut microbial synthesis of the vitamin, allow quantitative dietary requirements for biotin to be relatively small. Nevertheless, inborn errors of metabolism have been identified which are associated with impaired absorption of, and increased need for, the vitamin.

II. Sources of Biotin

Distribution in Foods

Biotin is widely distributed in foods and feedstuffs, but mostly in very low concentrations (Table 14-1). Only a couple of foods (royal jelly[1] and brewers' yeast) contain biotin in large amounts. Milk, liver, egg (egg yolk), and a few vegetables are the most important natural sources of the vitamin in human nutrition; the oilseed meals, alfalfa meal, and dried yeasts are the most important natural sources of the vitamin for the feeding of nonruminant animals. The biotin contents of foods and feedstuffs can be highly variable;[2] for the cereal grains at least, it is influenced by such factors as plant variety, season, and yield (endosperm-to-pericarp ratio). Biotin is found in human milk at concentrations in the range of 30–70 nM; it occurs almost exclusively as free biotin in the skim fraction.[3] Most foods contain the vitamin as free biotin and as **biocytin**, that is, biotin covalently bound to protein lysyl residues.

Stability

Biotin is unstable to oxidizing conditions and, therefore, is destroyed by heat, especially under conditions that support simultaneous lipid peroxidation.[4] Therefore, such processing techniques as the canning of foods and the heat curing and solvent extraction of feedstuffs can result in substantial losses of biotin. These losses can be reduced by the use of an antioxidant (e.g., vitamin C, vitamin E, butylated hydroxytoluene [BHT], butylated hydroxyanisole [BHA]).

Bioavailability

Studies of the bioavailability of food biotin to humans have not been conducted. However, biotin bioavailability has been determined experimentally using two types of bioassay: healing of skin lesions in avidin-fed rats; and support of growth and maintenance of **pyruvate carboxylase** activity in chicks. The results of such assays have shown that the nutritional availability of biotin can be low and highly variable among different foods and feedstuffs (Table 14-2). In general, less than one-half of the biotin present in feedstuffs is biologically available. Although all of the biotin in corn is available, only 20–30% of that in most other grains and none in wheat is available. Biotin in meat products also tends to be very low.

Differences in biotin bioavailability appear to be due to differential susceptibilities to digestion of the various biotin–protein linkages in which the vitamin occurs in foods and feedstuffs. Those linkages involve the formation of covalent bonds between the carboxyl group of the biotin side chain with free amino

---

[1] Royal jelly is a substance produced by the labial glands of worker honeybees and has been found to contain more than 400 μg of biotin per 100 g. Female honeybee larvae that are fed royal jelly develop reproductive ability as *queens*, whereas those fed a mixture of honey and pollen fail to develop reproductive ability and become *workers*. Although the active factor in royal jelly has not been identified, it appears to be associated with the lipid fraction of that material (one known component, 10-hydroxy-Δ^2-decenoic acid, has been suggested). It is interesting to speculate about the apparent survival value to the honeybee colony of biotin as a component of this unique food that is necessary for the sexual development of the female.

[2] In one study, the biotin contents of multiple samples of corn and meat meal were found to be 56–115 μg/kg ($n = 59$) and 17–323 μg/kg ($n = 62$), respectively.

[3] These levels are 20- to 50-fold greater than those found in maternal plasma. Human milk also contains biotinidase, which is presumed to be important in facilitating infant biotin utilization.

[4] About 96% of the pure vitamin added to a feed was destroyed within 24 hr after the addition of partially peroxidized linolenic acid.

Table 14-1. Biotin contents of foods

Food	Biotin (µg/100 g)	Food	Biotin (µg/100 g)
Dairy products		Vegetables (Cont'd)	
Milk	2	Brussels sprouts	0.4
Cheeses	3–5	Cabbage	2
Meats		Carrots	3
Beef	3	Cauliflower	17
Chicken	11	Corn	6
Pork	5	Kale	0.5
Calf kidney	100	Lentils	13
Cereals		Onions	4
Barley	14	Peas	9
Cornmeal	7.9	Potatoes	0.1
Oats	24.6	Soybeans	60
Rye	8.5	Spinach	7
Sorghum	28.8	Tomatoes	4
Wheat	10.1	Fruits	
Wheat bran	36	Apples	1
Oilseed meals		Bananas	4
Rapeseed meal	98.4	Grapefruit	3
Soybean meal	27	Grapes	2
Other		Oranges	1
Eggs	20	Peaches	2
Brewers' yeast	80	Pears	0.1
Alfalfa meal	54	Strawberries	1.1
Molasses	108	Peanuts	34
Vegetables		Walnuts	37
Asparagus	2	Watermelons	4

Source: USDA National Nutrient Database for Standard Reference, Release 18 (http://www.nal.usda.gov/fnic/foodcomp/search/)

groups of proteins. Such amide linkages constitute the means by which biotin binds to the enzymes for which it serves as an essential prosthetic group, in which cases they involve the ε-amino group of a peptidyl lysine residue. That form, biotinyl lysine, is referred to as biocytin. The utilization of biotin bound in such forms thus depends on the hydrolytic digestion of the proteins and/or the hydrolysis of those amide bonds. Biotin from purified preparations, such as are used in dietary supplements, should be well utilized.

Synthesis by Intestinal Microflora

In both rats and humans it has been found that total fecal excretion of biotin exceeds the amount consumed in the diet. This is due to the biosynthesis of significant amounts of biotin by the microflora of the proximal colon. Whether hind gut microbial biotin can be a determinant of the biotin status of the host is not clear. That biotin can be absorbed across the colon is indicated by the demonstration of transport capacity at levels as great as 25% that of the rat jejunum,[5] and

5 Bowman, B. B., and Rosenberg, I. H. (1987). *J. Nutr.* **117,** 2121–2126.

Table 14-2. Biotin availability in several feedstuffs

Feedstuff	Total biotin[a] (µg/100 g)	Available biotin[b] (µg/100 g)	Bioavailability (%)
Barley	10.9	1.2	11
Corn	5.0	6.5	133
Wheat	8.4	0.4	5
Rapeseed meal	93.0	57.4	62
Sunflower seed meal	119.0	41.5	35
Soybean meal	25.8	27.8	108

[a]Determined by microbiological assay.
[b]Determined by chick growth assay.
Source: Whitehead, C. C., Armstrong, J. A., and Waddington, D. (1982). *Br. J. Nutr.* **48,** 81.

the dietary requirement of the rat for biotin has been determined only under gnotobiotic (germ-free) conditions or with avidin feeding. That hindgut sources may not make significant contributions to biotin nutriture is indicated by findings that the intracecal treatment of pigs with antibiotics to inhibit microbial growth or with lactulose to stimulate microbial growth failed to affect plasma biotin.[6]

III. Absorption of Biotin

Liberation from Bound Forms

In the digestion of food proteins, protein-bound biotin is released by the hydrolytic action of the intestinal proteases to yield the ε-N[1]-biotinyllysine adduct, biocytin, from which free biotin is liberated by the action of an intestinal biotin amide aminohydrolase, biotinidase.

Two Types of Transport

Little is known about the mechanism of enteric biotin absorption. Free biotin is absorbed in the proximal small intestine by what appears to be two mechanisms, depending on its lumenal concentration:

- *Facilitated transport* At low concentrations, it is absorbed by a saturable, facilitated mechanism dependent on Na$^+$. This process has been found to be inhibited by certain anticonvulsant drugs[7] and chronic ethanol exposure. The inhibitory effect of ethanol has been demonstrated with solutions

Table 14-3. Inhibition of enteric biotin transport by ethanol

Ethanol (%, v/v)	Biotin transport (pmol/g tissue/15 min)
0	16.89 ± 0.80
0.5	15.16 ± 1.02
1	12.56 ± 1.03[a]
2	11.59 ± 1.16
5	6.61 ± 0.42[a]

[a]$p > 0.05$.
Source: Said, H. M., Sharifian, A., Bagharzadeh, A., and Mock, D. (1990). *Am. J. Clin. Nutr.* **52,** 1083–1086.

as dilute as 1% (v/v); it has also been shown for the major metabolite of ethanol, acetaldehyde, at similar concentrations (Table 14-3). Similar inhibition has been demonstrated for ethanol against biotin transport in human placental basolateral membrane vesicles, which also occurs by an Na$^+$-dependent, carrier-mediated process.

- *Passive diffusion* At high lumenal concentrations, free biotin is also absorbed by nonsaturable, simple diffusion.

IV. Transport of Biotin

Unbound Biotin

Less than half of the total biotin present in plasma appears to be free biotin, the balance being composed of **bisnorbiotin, biotin sulfoxide,** and other biotin metabolites yet to be identified. Most of this

---

[6] Kopinski, J. S., et al. (1989). *Br. J. Nutr.* **62,** 781–789.
[7] Carbamazepine, primidone.

total is not protein bound; only 12% of the total biotin in human plasma is covalently bound.

Protein-Bound Biotin

Some 7% of plasma biotin is reversibly and nonspecifically bound to plasma proteins including α- and ß-globulins. The only biotin-binding protein in human plasma appears to be biotinidase, which has two high-affinity binding sites for the vitamin and thus has been proposed to function in its transport. Biotinidase also occurs in human milk, where it may have important functions in the transport of biotin by the mammary gland and/or its utilization by the infant.

Cellular Uptake

Biotin is taken up by cells via multiple mechanisms

- The **sodium-dependent vitamin transporter (SMVT)**   A Na^+-dependent, carrier-mediated process that is not specific for the vitamin, but that functions in the cellular uptake of biotin, pantothenic acid, and lipoic acid with similar affinities. Biotin uptake by intestinal cells is inhibited by the activation of protein kinase C, apparently through phosphorylation of SMVT.[8]
- A **monocarboxylate transporter (MCT1)**   That this member of the monocarboxylate tansporter family can facilitate the cellular uptake of biotin into peripheral blood mononuclear cells explained the facts that biotin is taken up by those cells by process with a K_m three orders of magnitude less than that for SMVT-mediated transport, and is not competitively inhibited by either pantothenic or lipoic acids. It remains to be seen whether MCT1 is expressed in other tissues and whether other members of this family of transporters may be involved in biotin uptake.

The routing of biotin within cells would appear to be related to the activity of transporters as well as its binding to proteins and its incorporation into biotin-dependent carboxylases. In fact, the intracellular distribution of biotin closely parallels that of its carboxylases: primarily in the cytoplasm (the primary location of acetylCoA carboxylase) and mitochondria (in which MCT1 has been detected). A small amount (<1%) is found in the nucleus;[9] because this fraction has been found to increase (to ca. 1% of total cellular biotin) in response to proliferation, it would appear to be associated with the binding of the vitamin to histones.

Tissue Distribution

Appreciable storage of the vitamin appears to occur in the liver, where concentrations of 800–3000 ng/g have been found in various species.[10] Most of this appears to be in mitochondrial acetyl CoA carboxylase. Hepatic stores, however, appear to be poorly mobilized during biotin deprivation and thus do not show the reductions measurable in plasma under such conditions. **Biotin-binding proteins** have been identified in the egg yolks of many species of birds and in a few species of mammals and reptiles. These are believed to function in the transport of the vitamin into the oocyte, as their binding to it is weak enough to be reversible.[11] The yolk biotin-binding protein also occurs in the plasma of the laying hen.

V. Metabolism of Biotin

Linkage to Apoenzymes

Free biotin is attached to its apoenzymes via the formation of an amide linkage to the ε-amino group of a specific lysine residue. In each of the four biotin-dependent enzymes, this binding occurs in a region containing the same amino acid sequence (-Ala-Met-biotinyl-Lys-Met-. It is catalyzed by **biotin holoenzyme synthetase**.[12]

---

[8] Said, H. M. (1999). *J. Nutr.* **129**, 490S–493S.

[9] Stanley, J. S., et al. (2001). *Eur. J. Biochem.* **268**, 5424–5429.

[10] These levels contrast with those of plasma/serum, which, in humans and rats, are typically about 300 ng/liter.

[11] The yolk biotin-binding protein is a glycoprotein with a molecular mass of 74.3 kDa and a homologous tetrameric structure, each subunit of which binds a biotin molecule. This protein is not to be confused with avidin, the biotin-binding protein of egg white, which irreversibly binds biotin with an affinity three orders of magnitude greater than that of the yolk protein.

[12] Several holoenzyme synthetases have been characterized in microorganisms; but among animals these have been observed only in birds. It is presumed, however, that such an enzyme may also exist in animals (including humans), which, after all, have biotin bound in the same way in their biotin-dependent carboxylases.

Recycling the Vitamin

The normal turnover of the biotin-containing **holocarboxylases** involves their degradation to yield biocytin. The biotinyl lysine bond is not hydrolyzed by cellular proteases; however, it is cleaved by biotinidase to yield free biotin. Biotinidase is the major biotin-binding protein in plasma; it is also present in breast milk, in which its activity is particularly high in colostrum. The proteolytic liberation of biotin from its bound forms is essential for the reutilization of the vitamin, which is accomplished by its reincorporation into another holoenzyme. Congenital deficiencies of biotinidase have been described. These are characterized by deficiencies of the multiple biotin-dependent carboxylases; in some cases, they can be corrected with pharmacologic doses of the vitamin.

A storage system for biotinyl enzymes has been suggested. This would involve the mitochondrial biotinyl acetyl-CoA carboxylase serving as a reservoir to maintain hepatic acetyl-CoA at appropriate levels in the cytosol. This would provide biotin indirectly to support other biotinyl mitochondrial enzymes under low-biotin conditions.

Catabolism

Little catabolism of biotin seems to occur in mammals. A small fraction is oxidized to biotin D- and L-*sulfoxides*, but the ureido ring system is not otherwise degraded. The side chain of a larger portion is metabolized via mitochondrial β-oxidation to yield bisnorbiotin and its degradation products. Biotin catabolism appears to be greater in smokers than in nonsmokers.[13]

Excretion

Biotin is rapidly excreted in the urine (Fig. 14-1). Studies have shown the rat to excrete about 95% of a single oral dose (5 mg/kg) of the vitamin within 24 hr. Half of urinary biotin occurs as free biotin, the balance being composed of bisnorbiotin, bisnorbiotin methyl ketone, biotin sulfone, tetranorbiotin-*L*-sulfoxide, and various side-chain products.[14] Although unabsorbed biotin appears in the feces, much fecal biotin is of gut microbial origin and benefits the host by way of hind gut absorption. Thus, at low dietary levels of the vitamin, urinary excretion of biotin can exceed intake. Only a small amount (<2% of an intravenous dose) of biotin is excreted in the bile.

VI. Metabolic Functions of Biotin

Metabolic Roles

Biotin functions in intermediary metabolism in the transfer of covalently bound, single-carbon units in the most oxidized form, CO_2. This function is implemented by a number of biotin-dependent carboxylases and in a

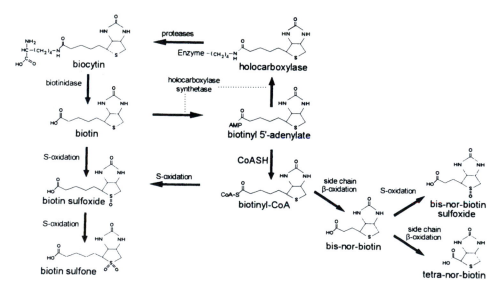

Fig. 14-1. Biotin metabolism and recycling.

---

13 Sealey, W. M., et al. (2004). *Am. J. Clin. Nutr.* **80,** 932–935.

14 The urinary excretion of patients with achlorhydria is very low. It is thought that this reflects impaired release of bound biotin for absorption.

number of other carboxylases, transcarboxylases,[15] and decarboxylases in microorganisms. Biotin also has additional metabolic functions: as a regulator of gene expression, and as a substrate for the modification of proteins by biotinylation, and in the regulation of the cell cycle.

Biotin holoenzyme synthetase

This enzyme catalyzes the formation of the linkage of the biotin prosthetic group to each apoenzyme covalently to the ε-amino group of a lysyl residue (Fig. 14-2) in two steps:

1. Activation of the vitamin as **biotinyl 5′-adenylate**
2. Covalent attachment of the vitamin to the **apocarboxylase** with the release of AMP

Carboxylases

The catalytic action of each of the biotin-dependent carboxylases of animals proceeds by way of a non-classic, two-site, *ping-pong* mechanism, with partial reactions being performed by dissimilar subunits:

1. The first reaction (*biotin carboxylase*) occurs at the carboxylase subsite; it involves the

enzymatic carboxylation of biotin using the bicarbonate/ATP system as the carboxyl donor.
2. The following step (*carboxyl transferase*) occurs at the carboxyl transferase subsite; it involves transfer of the carboxyl group from carboxybiotin to the acceptor substrate.

These two subsites appear to be spatially separated in each enzyme. The physicochemical mechanisms proposed for these reactions entail the transfer of biotinyl CO_2 between subsites via movement of the prosthetic group back and forth by virtue of rotation of at least one of the 10 single bonds (probably C-2–C-6) on the valeryl lysyl side chain.

Biotin-dependent carboxylases

The biotin-containing carboxylases have important functions in the metabolism of lipids, glucose, some amino acids, and energy (Table 14-4).

- **Pyruvate carboxylase** is a key enzyme in gluconeogenesis, along with **phospho*enol*pyruvate carboxykinase (PEPCK)**, to catalyze the formation of phospho*enol*pyruvate from three-carbon precursors. It also served to replenish the mitochondrial supply of oxaloacetate to support the citric acid cycle as well as the formation of citrate for transport to the cytosol for lipogenesis. Thus, biotin deficiency can lead to fasting hypoglyecemia and ketosis.
- **Acetyl-CoA carboxylase** catalyzes the first committed step in the synthesis and elongation of fatty acids. Therefore, biotin deficiency results in

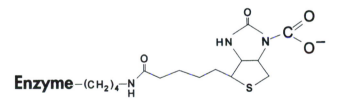

Fig. 14-2. Biotin is bound covalently to its apocarboxylases.

Table 14-4. Biotin-dependent carboxylases of animals

Enzyme	Location	Metabolic function
Pyruvate carboxylase	Mitochondria	Formation of oxaloacetate from pyruvate; requires acetyl-CoA
Acetyl-CoA carboxylase	Cytosol	Formation of malonyl-CoA from acetyl-CoA for carboxylase fatty acid synthesis; requires citrate
Propionyl-CoA carboxylase	Mitochondria	Formation of methylmalonyl-CoA from propionyl-CoA produced by catabolism of some amino acids (e.g., isoleucine) and odd-chain fatty acids
β-Methylcrotonoyl-CoA carboxylase	Mitochondria	Part of the leucine degradation pathway

---

[15] **Transcarboxylase** is called by those working with it the "Mickey Mouse enzyme," as the electron micrograph of the purified bacterial enzyme, with its large single subunit and two smaller subunits flanking to one side, resembles the head of the famous rodent.

impaired lipid metabolism (see Table 14-6 later in this chapter).

- **Propionyl-CoA carboxylase** catalyzes the oxidation of odd-chain fatty acids produced by the degradation of the branched-chain amino acids as well as methionine and threonine, and by the ruminal and/or gastrointestinal microflora. The enzyme produces methylmalonyl-CoA, which is used for energy and glucose production.
- **3-Methylcrotonoyl-CoA carboxylase** degrades the ketogenic amino acid, leucine. Loss of the latter activity results in the shunting of the leucine degradation product 3-methylcrotonyl CoA through an alternate catabolic pathway to **3-hydroxyisovaleric acid**, which is excreted in the urine.[16]

Gene expression

That biotin may have a role in the regulation of gene expression was first suggested by evidence of major reduction (40–45%) in the expression of **ornithine transcarbamylase** and **glucokinase** in the biotin-deficient rat. Subsequent studies have revealed that some 2000 human genes, aligned in clusters, depend on biotin for expression. The expression of these gene clusters appears to involve the following cell signals and transcription factors:

- *Biotinyl AMP and cGMP* It has been suggested that biotinyl AMP activates a soluble guanylate cyclase, which increases the synthesis of cGMP, stimulating protein kinase G and leading to phosphorylation and activation of proteins that increase the transcription of genes encoding biotin holoenzyme synthetase and some carboxylases.
- *Nuclear factor (NF)-κB* Biotin deprivation has been shown to increase the nuclear translocation, binding and transcriptional activity of NF-κB, and increasing the nuclear contents of p50 and p65 and activities of IκBa kinases.
- *Sp1 and Sp3* Biotin appears necessary for the expression of these transcription factors, which are associated with the expression of a cytochrome P450 gene and decreased transcription

of the sarco/endoplasmic reticulum ATPase 3 gene.

- *Receptor tyrosine kinases* Biotin deficiency has been shown to activate the signaling by tyrosine kinases, which may contribute to increasing SMVT-mediated biotin uptake.

Biotinylation of proteins

The addition of biotin to DNA-binding, histone proteins[17] appears to involve a biotin transferase function of biotinidase, which uses biocytin for this purpose.[18] This suggests that biotin may play a role in the packaging, transcription and/or replication of DNA to effect epigenetic regulation of gene function. Among the gene products affected by biotin status are cytokines and their receptors, oncogenes, genes involved in glucose metabolism, and genes that play a role in cellular biotin homeostasis.

Cell cycle

Biotin has been shown to be necessary for the normal progression of cells through the cell cycle, with biotin-deficient cells arresting in the G1 phase. In fact, proliferating lymphocytes increase their activities of ß-methylcrotonyl-CoA carboxylase and propionyl-CoA carboxylase as well as their biotin uptake.

VII. Biotin Deficiency

Because biotin is rather widespread among foods and feedstuffs and is synthesized by the intestinal microflora,[19] simple deficiencies of biotin in animals or humans are rare (Table 14-5). However, biotin deficiency can be induced by certain antagonists.

Egg White Injury

When, in the mid-1930s, it was found that biotin supplements prevented the dermatitis and alopecia produced in experimental animals by feeding uncooked egg white, the damaging factor was isolated and named *avidin*. Avidin is a water-soluble, basic glycoprotein with a molecular mass of 67kDa. It is a homologous

---

[16] Urinary 3-hydroxyisovalerate has, therefore, been proposed as a screening parameter for the detection of biotin deficiency.

[17] Histones regulate the transcription, replication, and repair of DNA.

[18] Hymes, J., et al. (1995). *Biochem. Mol. Med.* **56,** 76–83.

[19] Although it is clear that the gut microflora synthesize biotin, the quantitative importance of this source to the biotin nutrition of humans and other nonruminant species is highly speculative.

Table 14-5. Signs of biotin deficiency

Organ system	Signs
General	
Appetite	Decrease
Growth	Decrease
Dermatologic	Dermatitis, alopecia, achromotrichia
Skeletal	Perosis
Vital organs	Hepatic steatosis, FLKS

Abbreviation: FLKS, fatty liver and kidney syndrome.

tetramer, each 128-amino acid subunit of which binds a molecule of biotin apparently by linking to two to four tryptophan residues and an adjacent lysine in the subunit binding site. The binding of biotin to avidin is the strongest known noncovalent bond in nature.[20] Avidin is secreted by the oviductal cells of birds, reptiles, and amphibians and is thus found in the whites of their eggs, which is thought to function as a natural antibiotic, because it is resistant to a broad range of bacterial proteases. It antagonizes biotin by forming with the vitamin a noncovalent complex[21] that is also resistant to pancreatic proteases, thus preventing the absorption of biotin.[22] The avidin–biotin complex is unstable to heat; heating to at least 100°C denatures the protein and releases biotin available for absorption. Therefore, although raw egg white is antagonistic to the utilization of biotin, the cooked product is without effect. The consumption of raw or undercooked whole eggs is probably of little consequence to biotin nutrition, as the biotin-binding capacity of avidin in the egg white is roughly comparable to the biotin content of the egg yolk. However, as a tool to produce experimental biotin deficiency, avidin in the form of dried egg white has been very useful.[23]

Deficiency Syndromes in Animals

Avidin-induced biotin deficiency causes the syndrome originally referred to as **egg white injury**. The major lesions appear to involve impairments in lipid metabolism and energy production. In rats and mice, this is characterized by seborrheic dermatitis and **alopecia**, a hind-limb paralysis that results in **kangaroo gait**. In mice and hamsters it involves congenital malformations (cleft palate, micrognathia,[24] micromelia[25]). Fur-bearing animals (mink and fox) show general dermatitis with hyperkeratosis, circumocular alopecia (**spectacle eye**), **achromotrichia** of the underfur, and unsteady gait. Pigs and kittens show weight loss, digestive dysfunction, dermatitis, alopecia, and brittle claws. Guinea pigs and rabbits show weight loss, alopecia, and achromotrichia. Monkeys show severe dermatitis of the face, hands, and feet, alopecia, and watery eyes with encrusted lids. The dermatologic lesions of biotin deficiency relate to impairments of lipid metabolism; affected animals show reductions in skin levels of several long-chain fatty acids (16:0—that is, a 16-carbon fatty acid with no double bonds—16:1, 18:0, 18:1, and 18:2) with concomitant increases in certain others (in particular, 24:1 and 26:1). All species show depressed activities of the biotin-dependent carboxylases, which respond rapidly to biotin therapy.

Biotin deficiency can be produced in chicks by dietary deprivation and seems to occur from time to time in practical poultry production, particularly in northern Europe.[26] This results in impaired growth and reduced efficiency of feed utilization, and is characterized by dermatitis (mainly at the corners of the beak). In some instances, death occurs suddenly without gross lesions. This condition usually involves hepatic and renal steatosis with hypoglycemia, lethargy, paralysis, and hepatomegaly, and is thus referred to as **fatty liver and kidney syndrome (FLKS)**. The etiology of FLKS appears to be complex, involving such other factors as choline, but it seems to involve a marginal deficiency of biotin that impairs gluconeogenesis by limiting the activity of pyruvate carboxylase, especially under circumstances of glycogen depletion brought on by stress.

---

[20] $K_a = 10^{15}$ mol/L.

[21] Two very similar biotin-binding proteins have been identified, both of which show considerable sequence homology with avidin at the biotin-binding site. One, from *Streptomyces avidinii*, is called **streptavidin**. The other is an epidermal growth factor homolog found in the purple sea urchin *Strongylocentrotus purpuratus*.

[22] Some cultured mammalian cells (e.g., fibroblasts and HeLa cells) are able to absorb the biotin–avidin complex, using it as a source of the vitamin.

[23] Other structural analogs of biotin are also antagonistic to its function: α-dehydrobiotin, 5-(2-thienyl)valeric acid, acidomycin, α-methylbiotin, and α-methyldethiobiotin, several of which are antibiotics.

[24] Underdevelopment of the jaw (usually the lower jaw).

[25] Undergrowth of the limbs.

[26] In that part of the world, barley and wheat, each of which has little biologically available biotin, are frequently used as major ingredients in poultry diets.

Deficiency Signs in Humans

Clinical deficiency

Few cases of biotin deficiency have been reported in humans, and most of these have involved nursing infants whose mothers' milk contained inadequate supplies of the vitamin,[27] or patients receiving incomplete parenteral nutrition. One case involved a child fed raw eggs for 6 years. The signs and symptoms included dermatitis, glossitis, anorexia, nausea, depression, hepatic steatosis, and hypercholesterolemia. The impairments of lipid metabolism respond to biotin therapy (Table 14-6).

It is thought that marginal biotin status may play a role in the etiology of **sudden infant death syndrome (SIDS)**, which occurs in human infants at 2–4 months of age. In many ways, SIDS resembles FLKS in the chick; marginal biotin status coupled with stress is thought to be an important cause of each disease. Studies have shown that infants who died of SIDS had significantly lower hepatic concentrations of biotin than did infants who died of unrelated causes.[28]

Subclinical deficiency

The frequency of marginal biotin status (deficiency without clinical manifestation) is not known, but the incidence of low circulating biotin levels has been found to be substantially greater among alcoholics than the general population.[29] Relatively low levels of biotin (versus healthy controls) have also been reported in the plasma or urine of patients with partial gastrectomy or other causes of achlorhydria, burn patients, epileptics,[30] elderly individuals, and athletes. Because animal products figure prominently as dietary sources of biotin, it has been suggested that vegetarians may be at risk for deficiency. Studies have failed to support that hypothesis; in fact, both plasma and urinary biotin levels of strict vegetarians (vegans) and lactoovovegetarians[31] have been found to exceed that of persons eating mixed diets, indicating that the biotin status of the former groups was not impaired relative to the latter group.

Studies with validated biomarkers of biotin status indicate that subclinical biotin deficiency may be common in pregnancy—perhaps as frequently as one-third of pregnancies. The increased urinary excretion

Table 14-6. Effect of biotin treatment on abnormalities in serum fatty acid concentrations in a biotin-deficient human

Fatty acid	Normal values	Biotin-deficient patient values	
		Before biotin	After biotin
18:2ω6	21.56 ± 6.65	9.85[a]	5.36[a]
18:3ω6	0.21 ± 0.27	0.45	0.40
20:3ω6	3.67 ± 1.39	8.66[a]	10.62[a]
20:4ω6	12.49 ± 3.79	9.26	11.72
22:4ω6	1.87 ± 1.01	0.52[a]	0.71[a]
20:3ω9	1.30 ± 1.25	1.05	1.67
18:3ω3	0.21 ± 0.19	0.33	0.18
Total ω6 acids	41.08 ± 5.86	29.42[a]	29.61[a]
Total ω3 acids	5.23 ± 2.16	5.24	4.97
Total ω9 acids	13.14 ± 3.98	17.59[a]	16.4

[a]$p > 0.05$.

Source: Mock, D. M., Johnson, S. B., and Holman, R. T. (1988). *J. Nutr.* **118,** 342–348.

---

[27] The biotin content of human milk, particularly early in lactation, is often insufficient to meet the demands of infants. Therefore, it is recommended that nursing mothers take a biotin supplement. When this is done, substantial increases in the biotin concentrations of breast milk are observed (e.g., a 3-mg/day supplement increases milk biotin concentrations from 1.2–1.5 µg/dl to >33 µg/dl).

[28] Johnson, A. R., et al. (1980). *Nature* **285,** 159–160.

[29] About 15% of alcoholics have plasma biotin concentrations less than 140 pmol/liter, whereas only 1% of randomly selected hospital patients have plasma biotin levels that low.

[30] This may be due to anticonvulsant drug therapy, known side effects of which are dermatitis and ataxia. Some anticonvulsants (e.g., carbamazepine and primidone) have been shown to be competitive inhibitors of biotin transport across the intestinal brush border.

[31] Individuals eating plant-based diets that include dairy products and eggs.

of **3-hydroxyisovaleric acid**, which can occur late in pregnancy, has been found to respond to biotin supplementation.[32] This finding, and the detection of increases in the urinary excretion of bisnorbiotin, biotin sulfoxide, and other biotin metabolites, suggests that pregnant women may experience marginal biotin deficiency due to increased catabolism of the vitamin. On the basis of findings in the mouse model (Table 14-7), it has been suggested that subclinical biotin deficiency may be teratogenic.

Congenital Disorders

Genetic defects in all of the known biotin enzymes have been identified in humans (Table 14-8). These are rare, affecting infants and children, and usually have serious consequences. Some, in which the defect involves the absence of a biotin apoenzyme, do not respond to supplements of the vitamin and are treated by limiting the production of metabolites upstream of the metabolic lesion through restriction of dietary protein. Other congenital disorders (the **multiple carboxylase deficiencies**) respond to high doses of biotin.

VIII. Biotin Toxicity

The toxicity of biotin appears to be very low. No cases have been reported of adverse reactions by humans to high levels (doses as high as 200 mg orally or 20 mg intravenously) of the vitamin, as are used in treating seborrheic dermatitis in infants, egg white injury, or inborn errors or metabolism. Animal studies have revealed few, if any, indications of toxicity, and it is probable that animals, including humans, can tolerate the vitamin at doses at least an order of magnitude greater than their respective nutritional requirements. Biotin excess appears to provide effective therapy to reduce the diabetic state, lowering postprandial glucose and improving glucose tolerance.

IX. Case Study

Instructions

Review the following case report, paying special attention to the diagnostic indicators on which the treatments were based. Then, answer the questions that follow.

Case

A 12-month-old girl had experienced malrotation[33] and midgut volvulus,[34] resulting in extensive infarction[35] of the small and large bowel, at 4 months of age. Her bowel was resected, after which her clinical course was complicated by failure of the anastomosis[36] to heal, peritoneal infection, and intestinal obstruction. After several subsequent surgeries, she was left with only 30 cm of jejunum, 0.5 cm of ileum, and approximately 50% of colon. By 5 months of

Table 14-7.   Effect of egg white injury on fetal malformations in pregnant mice

Malformation	Dietary egg white, %						
	0	1	2	3	5	10	25
Cleft palate	0.10 ± 0.13	0.25 ± 0.25	2 ± 2	4 ± 2	10 ± 1	11 ± 1	12 ± 0.4
Micrognathia	0	0	0.2 ± 0.2	3 ± 2	9 ± 1	11 ± 1	12 ± 1
Microglossia	0	0	0	0.5 ± 0.5	2 ± 1	6 ± 2	9 ± 3
Hydrocephaly	0	0	0	0.3 ± 0.2	2 ± 1	3 ± 1	3 ± 2
Open eye	0	0	0	0	0.8 ± 0.5	4 ± 1	5 ± 2
Forelimb hypoplasia	0	0	0	7 ± 2	9 ± 2	11 ± 1	12 ± 0.4
Hindlimb hypoplasia	0	0	0	5 ± 2	9 ± 2	10 ± 0.8	12 ± 0.4
Pelvic girdle hypoplasia	0	0	0	5 ± 2	9 ± 2	10 ± 1	12 ± 0.5

Source: Mock, D. M., et al. (2003). *J. Nutr.* **133,** 2519–2525.

---

[32] Mock, D. M., et al (1997). *J. Nutr.* **127,** 710–716.
[33] Failure of normal rotation of the intestinal tract.
[34] Twisting of the intestine, causing obstruction.
[35] Necrotic changes resulting from obstruction of an end artery.
[36] An operative union of two hollow or tubular structures—in this case the divided ends of the intestine.

Table 14-8. Congenital disorders of biotin enzymes

Defect	Metabolic basis	Physiological effect	Treatment
Propionyl CoA carboxylase deficiency	Autosomal recessive lack of enzyme[a]	Propionate accumulation: acidemia, ketoacidosis, hyperammonemia; high urine citrate, 3-OH-propionate, propionyl glycine *Symptoms*[b]: Vomiting, lethargy, hypotonia, mental retardation, cramps	Restrict protein biotin
Pyruvate carboxylase deficiency	Autosomal recessive lack of enzyme[c]	Changes in energy production, gluconeogenesis, and other pathways *Symptoms*: Metabolic acidosis (lactate), hypotonia, mental retardation	None
3-Methylcrotonyl-CoA carboxylase deficiency	Defective enzyme (basis unknown[d])	High urine 3-CH₃-crotonylglycine and 3-OH-isovaleric acid *Symptoms*: Cramps	Restrict protein
Acetyl-CoA carboxylase deficiency	Lack of enzyme (basis unknown[e])	Aciduria *Symptoms*: Myopathy, neurologic changes	None
Multiple carboxylase deficiency			
Neonatal type	Autosomal recessive lack of holoenzyme synthase[f]	Deficiencies of all biotin-containing holocarboxylases; acidosis and aciduria *Symptoms*: Vomiting, lethargy, hypotonia	None[g]
Juvenile type	Autosomal recessive lack of biotinidase[h]	Deficiencies of all biotin-containing holocarboxylases; acidosis and aciduria *Symptoms*: Skin rash, alopecia, conjunctivitis, ataxia, developmental anomalies, neurological signs	Massive doses of biotin

[a]Incidence: 1 in 350,000.
[b]There is a wide variation in the clinical expression.
[c]Fewer than two dozen patients described.
[d]Three confirmed cases.
[e]One case described.
[f]Involves failure to link biotin to the apocarboxylases to produce active holoenzymes.
[g]Fatal early in life.
[h]Involves failure to release biotin from its bound forms in the holocarboxylases; this reduces use of biotin in foods and blocks endogenous recycling of the vitamin.

age, she had lost 1.5 kg in weight, and total parenteral nutrition[37] (TPN) was initiated (providing 125 kcal/kg/day). By the third month of TPN, she had gained 2.9 kg; thereafter, her energy intake was reduced to 60 kcal/kg/day, which sustained her growth within the normal range. Soybean oil emulsion[38] was administered parenterally at least twice weekly in amounts that provided 3.9% of total calories as linoleic acid. Repeated attempts at feeding her orally failed because of vomiting and rapid intestinal transit;

therefore, her only source of nutrients was TPN. She had repeated episodes of sepsis and wound infection; broad-spectrum antibiotics were administered virtually continuously from 4 to 11 months of age. Multiple enteroenteric and enterocutaneous fistulas[39] were formed; over 8 months, they provided daily fluid losses >500 ml.

During the third month of TPN, an erythematous[40] rash was noted on the patient's lower eyelids adjacent to the outer canthi.[41] Over the next 3 months

---

[37] Feeding via means other than through the alimentary canal, referring particularly to the introduction of nutrients into veins.
[38] For example, Intralipid.
[39] Passages created between one part of the intestine and another (an *enteroenteric* fistula) or between the intestine and the skin of the abdomen (an *enterocutaneous* fistula).
[40] Marked by redness of the skin owing to inflammation.
[41] Corners of the eye.

the rash spread, became more exfoliative, and exuded clear fluid. New lesions appeared in the angles of the mouth, around the nostrils, and in the perineal region.[42] This condition did not respond to topical application of various antibiotics, cortisone, and safflower oil.

During the fifth and sixth months of TPN, the patient lost all body hair, developed a waxy pallor, irritability, lethargy, and mild hypotonia.[43] That she was not deficient in essential fatty acids was indicated by the finding that her plasma fatty acid triene-to-tetraene ratio was normal (0.11). During the period from the third to the sixth month, the patient was given parenteral zinc supplements at 7, 30, and 250 times the normal requirement (0.2 mg/day). Her serum zinc concentration increased from 35 to 150 µg/dl (normal, 50–150 µg/dl) and, finally, to greater than 2000 µg/dl without any beneficial effect. Intravenous zinc supplementation was then reduced to 0.4 mg/day. Biotin was determined by a bioassay using *Ochromonas danica*; urinary organic acids were determined by HPLC[44] and GC/MS[45]:

Treatment with biotin (10 mg/day) was initiated and, after 1 week, the plasma biotin concentration increased to 11,500 pg/ml and organic acid excretion dropped to <0.01 µmol/mg creatinine. After 7 days of biotin supplementation, the rash had improved strikingly, and the irritability had resolved. After 2 weeks of supplementation, new hair growth was noted, the waxy pallor of the skin was less pronounced, and hypotonia improved. During the next 9 months of biotin therapy, no symptoms and signs of deficiency recurred. The patient's rapid transit time and vomiting did not improve.

Case Questions

1. What signs were first to indicate a problem related to biotin utilization by the patient?
2. What is the relevance of aciduria to considerations of biotin status?
3. How were problems involving essential fatty acids and zinc ruled out in the diagnosis of this condition as biotin deficiency?

Laboratory results

Parameter	Patient	Normal range
Plasma biotin	135 pg/ml	215–750 pg/ml
Urinary biotin excretion	<1 µg/24 hr	6–50 µg/24 hr
Urinary organic acid excretion		
Methylcitrate	0.1 µmol/mg creatinine	<0.01 µmol/mg creatinine
3-Methylcrotonylglycine	0.7 µmol/mg creatinine	<0.2 µmol/mg creatinine
3-Hydroxyisovalerate	0.35 µmol/mg creatinine	<0.2 µmol/mg creatinine

Study Questions and Exercises

1. Diagram the areas of metabolism in which biotin-dependent carboxylases are involved.
2. Construct a decision tree for the diagnosis of biotin deficiency in humans or an animal species.
3. What key feature of the chemistry of biotin relates to its biochemical function as a carrier of active CO_2?
4. What parameters might you measure to assess biotin status of a human or animal?

---

[42] The area between the thighs extending from the coccyx to the pubis.

[43] A condition of reduced tension of any muscle, leading to damage by overstretching.

[44] High-performance liquid–liquid partition chromatography.

[45] Gas–liquid partition chromatography with mass spectrometric detection.

Recommended Reading

Brownsey, R. W., Boone, A. W., Elliot, J. E., Kulpa, J. E., and Lee, W. M. (2006). Regulation of acetyl-CoA carboxylase. *Biochem. Soc. Trans.* **34,** 223–227.

Chapman-Smith, A., and Cronan, J. E., Jr. (1999). Molecular biology of biotin attachment to proteins. *J. Nutr.* **129,** 477S–484S.

Cronan, J. E., Jr., and Waldrop, G. L. (2002). Multi-subunit acetyl-CoA carboxylases. *Progr. Lipid Res.* **41,** 407–435.

Dakshinamurti, K. (2005). Biotin—a regulator of gene expression. *J. Nutr. Biochem.* **16,** 419–423.

Fernandez-Mejia, C. (2005). Pharmacological effects of biotin. *J. Nutr. Biochem.* **16,** 424–427.

Jitrapakdee, S., and Wallace, J. S. (1999). Structure, function and regulation of pyruvate carboxylase. *Biochem. J.* **340,** 1–16.

McMahan, R. J. (2002). Biotin in metabolism and molecular biology. *Ann. Rev. Nutr.* **22,** 221–239.

Mock, D. M. (2006). Biotin, Chapter 30 in *Modern Nutrition in Health and Disease*, 10th ed. (M. E. Shils, M. Shike, A. C. Ross, B. Caballero, and R. J., Cousins, eds.), pp. 498–506. Lippincott, New York.

Rodrigues-Melendez, M., and Zemplini, J. (2003). Regulation of gene expression by biotin. *J. Nutr. Biochem.* **14,** 680–690.

van den Berg, H. (1997). Bioavailability of biotin. *Eur. J. Clin. Nutr.* **51,** S60–S61.

Wolf, B. (2005). Biotinidase: Its role in biotinidase deficiency and biotin metabolism. *J. Nutr. Biochem.* **16,** 441–445.

Zemplini, J. (2001). Biotin, Chapter 23 in *Present Knowledge in Nutrition*, 8th ed. (B. A. Bowman and R. M. Russell, eds.), pp. 241–252. ILSI Press, Washington, D.C.

Zemplini, J. (2005). Uptake, localization and noncarboxylase roles of biotin. *Ann. Rev. Nutr.* **25,** 175–196.

Pantothenic Acid

15

A pellagrous-like syndrome in chicks has recently been obtained ... in an experiment which was originally designed to throw added light upon an unusual type of leg problem occurring in chicks fed semi-synthetic rations.... The data obtained in this experiment demonstrate the requirement in another species of the vitamin or vitamins present in auto-claved yeast, occasionally called vitamin B_2, vitamin G or the P-P factor, and indicate that the chick may be a more suitable animal than the white rat for delineating the quantities of this vitamin present in feedstuffs.

—L . C. Norris and A. T. Ringrose

I.	The Significance of Pantothenic Acid	345
II.	Sources of Pantothenic Acid	346
III.	Absorption of Pantothenic Acid	347
IV.	Transport of Pantothenic Acid	347
V.	Metabolism of Pantothenic Acid	348
VI.	Metabolic Functions of Pantothenic Acid	350
VII.	Pantothenic Acid Deficiency	352
VIII.	Pantothenic Acid Toxicity	353
IX.	Case Study	353
	Study Questions and Exercises	354
	Recommended Reading	354

Anchoring Concepts

1. Pantothenic acid is the trivial designation for the compound dihydroxy-β,β-dimethylbutyryl-β-alanine.
2. Pantothenic acid is metabolically active as the prosthetic group of coenzyme A (CoA) and the acyl-carrier protein.
3. Deficiencies of pantothenic acid are manifested as dermal, hepatic, thymic, and neurologic changes.

Learning Objectives

1. To understand the chief natural sources of pantothenic acid.
2. To understand the means of absorption and transport of pantothenic acid.
3. To understand the biochemical functions of pantothenic acid as components of coenzyme A and the acyl-carrier protein.
4. To understand the physiological implications of low pantothenic acid status.

Vocabulary

Acetyl-CoA
Acyl-carrier protein (ACP)
Acyl-CoA synthase
Burning feet syndrome
Coenzyme A (CoA)
Dephospho-CoA kinase
Fatty acid synthase
Malonyl CoA
ω-Methylpantothenic acid
Pantetheine
Pantetheinase
Pantothenate kinase
Pantothenic acid
4'-Phosphopantetheine
4'-Phosphopantothenic acid
Phosphopantetheine adenyltransferase
4'-Phosphopantothenylcysteine
Phosphopantothenylcysteine decarboxylase
Phosphopantothenylcysteine synthase
Propionyl-CoA

I. The Significance of Pantothenic Acid

Pantothenic acid is widely distributed in many foods. Therefore, problems of deficiency of the vitamin are rare. The vitamin has critical roles in metabolism, being an integral part of the acylation factors **coenzyme-A (CoA)** and **acyl-carrier protein (ACP)**. In these forms, pantothenic acid is required for the normal metabolism of fatty acids, amino acids, and carbohydrates, and has important roles in the acylation of proteins. Because pantothenic acid is required for the synthesis of CoA, it has been a surprising observation that the rates of tissue CoA synthesis are not affected by deprivation of the vitamin. From such observations it can be inferred that the vitamin is recycled metabolically; however, the regulation of pantothenic acid remains to be elucidated.

II. Sources of Pantothenic Acid

Distribution in Foods

As its name implies, pantothenic acid is widely distributed in nature (Table 15-1). It occurs mainly in bound forms (CoA, CoA esters, acyl-carrier protein). A glycoside has been identified in tomatoes. Therefore, it must be determined in foods and feedstuffs after enzymatic hydrolysis to liberate the vitamin from CoA. This is done in a two-step procedure using alkaline phosphatase followed by avian hepatic pantotheinase, yielding "total" pantothenic acid.

The most important food sources of pantothenic acid are meats (liver and heart are particularly rich). Mushrooms, avocados, broccoli, and some yeasts are also rich in the vitamin. Whole grains are also good sources; however, the vitamin is localized in the outer layers; thus, it is largely removed by milling. The most important sources of pantothenic acid for animal feeding are rice and wheat brans, alfalfa, peanut meal, molasses, yeasts, and condensed fish solubles. The richest sources of the vitamin in nature are coldwater fish ovaries,[1] which can contain more than 2.3 mg/g, and royal jelly,[2] which can contain more than 0.5 mg/g.

Table 15-1. Pantothenic acid contents of foods

Food	Pantothenic acid (mg/100 g)	Food	Pantothenic acid (mg/100 g)
Dairy products		Vegetables	
Milk	0.2	Avocado	1.1
Cheeses	0.1–0.9	Broccoli	1.2
Meats		Cabbage	0.1–1.4
Beef	0.3–2	Carrots	0.27
Pork	0.4–3.1	Cauliflower	1.0
Calf heart	2.5	Lentils	1.4
Calf kidney	3.9	Potatoes	0.3
Chicken liver	9.7	Soybeans	1.7
Pork liver	7.0	Tomatoes	0.3
Cereals		Fruits	
Cornmeal	0.9	Apples	0.1
Rice, unpolished	1.1	Bananas	0.2
Oatmeal	0.9	Grapefruits	0.3
Wheat	1.0	Oranges	0.2
Wheat bran	2.9	Strawberries	0.3
Barley	1.1	Nuts	
Other		Walnuts	0.7
Eggs	2.9	Cashews	1.3
Mushrooms	2.1	Peanuts	2.8
Bakers' yeast	5.3–11		

---

[1] Tuna, cod.

[2] Royal jelly, the food responsible for the diet-induced reproductive development of the queen honeybee, is also the richest natural source of biotin.

Stability

Pantothenic acid in foods and feedstuffs is fairly stable to ordinary means of cooking and storage. It can, however, be unstable to heat and either alkaline (pH > 7) or acid (pH < 5) conditions.[3] Reports indicate losses of 15 to 50% from cooking meat, and of 37 to 78% from heat-processing vegetables. The alcohol derivative, pantothenol, is more stable; for this reason it is used as a source of the vitamin in multivitamin supplements.

Bioavailability

The biologic availability of pantothenic acid from foods and feedstuffs has not been well investigated. One single study in this area indicated that "average" bioavailability of the vitamin in the American diet in the range of 40–60%;[4] similar results were obtained for maize meals in another study.[5]

III. Absorption of Pantothenic Acid

Hydrolysis of Coenzyme Forms

Because pantothenic acid occurs in most foods and feedstuffs as CoA and the acyl-carrier protein, the utilization of the vitamin in foods depends on the hydrolytic digestion of these protein complexes to release the free vitamin. Both CoA and ACP are degraded in the lumen of the intestine to release the vitamin as **4′-phosphopantetheine** (Fig. 15-1). That form is dephosphorylated to yield **pantetheine**, which is rapidly converted by the intestinal **pantetheinase** to **pantothenic acid**.

Carrier-Mediated Uptake

Pantothenic acid is absorbed by a saturable, Na^+-dependent, energy-requiring process[6] that shows highest rates in the jejunum. At high levels, it is also absorbed by simple diffusion throughout the small intestine.[7] The alcohol form, *panthenol*, which is oxidized to pantothenic acid *in vivo*, appears to be absorbed somewhat faster than the acid form.

IV. Transport of Pantothenic Acid

Free in Plasma; as Coenzyme A in Blood Cells

Pantothenic acid is transported in both the plasma and erythrocytes. Plasma contains the vitamin only in the free acid form, which erythrocytes take up by

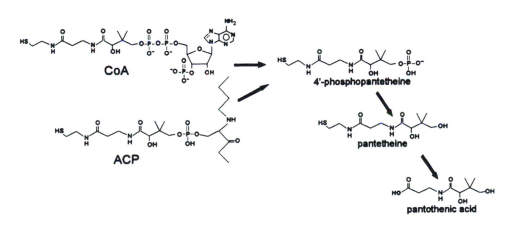

Fig. 15-1.   Liberation of pantothenic acid from coenzyme forms in foods.

[3] Pasteurization of milk, owing to its neutral pH, does not affect its content of pantothenic acid.

[4] Tarr, J. B., et al. (1981). *Am. J. Clin. Nutr.* **34,** 1328–1337.

[5] Yu, B. H., et al. (1993). *Plant Food Hum. Nutr.* **43,** 87–95.

[6] The intestinal pantothenic acid transporter has been demonstrated in the rat, chick, and mouse.

[7] Earlier studies in which unphysiologically high concentrations of the vitamin were employed failed to detect the carrier-mediated mechanism of its enteric absorption. This led to the conclusion that the vitamin is absorbed only by simple diffusion.

passive diffusion. While erythrocytes carry some of the vitamin unchanged, they convert some of the vitamin to 4'-phosphopantothenic acid and pantetheine. Erythrocytes carry most of the vitamin in the blood.[8,9]

Cellular Uptake

Pantothenic acid is transported into other cells in its free acid form by a Na^+ co-transporter,[10] apparently the same mechanism involved in enteric absorption. The pantothenic acid transport also appears to transport biotin and to be influenced by hormonal status, and to be mediated by protein kinase C[11] and calmodulin; however, the mechanisms are not clear. Upon cellular uptake, most of the vitamin is converted to CoA, the predominant tissue form.

Tissue Distribution

The greatest concentrations of CoA are found in the liver,[12] adrenals, kidneys, brain, heart, and testes. Much of this (70% in liver and 95% in heart) is located in the mitochondria. Tissue CoA concentrations are not affected by deprivation of the vitamin. This surprising finding has been interpreted as indicating a mechanism for conserving the vitamin by recycling it from the degradation of pantothenate-containing molecules.

There appear to be two renal mechanisms for regulating the excretion of pantothenic acid: at physiological concentrations of the vitamin in the plasma, pantothenic acid is reabsorbed by active transport; at higher concentrations, tubular secretion of pantothenic acid occurs. Tubular reabsorption appears to be the only mechanism for conserving free pantothenic acid in the plasma. Pantothenic acid is taken up in the choroid plexus by a specific transport process, which, at low concentrations of the vitamin,

involves the partial phosphorylation of the vitamin. The cerebrospinal fluid, because it is constantly renewed in the central nervous system, requires a constant supply of pantothenic acid, which, as CoA, is involved in the synthesis of the neurotransmitter acetylcholine in brain tissue.

V. Metabolism of Pantothenic Acid

Coenzyme A Biosynthesis

All tissues have the ability to synthesize CoA from pantothenic acid of dietary origin. At least in rat liver, all of the enzymes in the CoA biosynthetic pathway are found in the cytosol. Four moles of ATP are required for the biosynthesis of a mole of CoA from a single mole of pantothenic acid. The process (Fig. 15-2) is initiated in the cytosol and is completed in the mitochondria:

In the cytosol:

1. **Pantothenate kinase** catalyzes the ATP-dependent phosphorylation of pantothenic acid to yield **4'-phosphopantothenic acid.** This is the rate-limiting step in CoA synthesis; under normal conditions, it appears to function far below its maximal capacity. It can be induced[13] and appears to be feedback inhibited by 4'-phosphopantothenic acid, CoA esters (**acetyl-CoA, malonyl-CoA** and **propionyl-CoA**) and more weakly by CoA and long-chain acyl-CoAs, all of which appear to act as allosteric effectors of pantothenate kinase. Inhibition by CoA esters appears to be reversed by carnitine. The ethanol metabolite acetaldehyde also inhibits the conversion of pantothenic acid to CoA, although the mechanism of this effect is not clear.[14]

---

[8] For example, in the human adult, whole blood contains 1120–1960 ng of total pantothenic acid per milliliter; of that, the plasma contains 211–1096 ng/ml. The pantothenic acid concentration of liver is about 15 μM; that of heart is about 150 μM.

[9] Blood pantothenic acid levels are generally lower in elderly individuals (e.g., 500–700 ng/ml).

[10] Pantothenic acid transporters have been identified in *Escherichia coli* and *Haemophilus influenzae*; these are members of the SGLT Na^+ cotransporter family.

[11] Treatment of cells with a PKC activator has been shown to inhibit pantothenic acid uptake.

[12] The human liver typically contains about 28 mg of total pantothenic acid.

[13] Pantothenate kinase is induced by the antilipidemic drug clofibrate. Treatment with clofibrate increases hepatic concentrations of CoA, apparently owing to increased synthesis.

[14] Alcoholics have been reported to excrete in their urine large percentages of the pantothenic acid they ingest, a condition corrected on ethanol withdrawal.

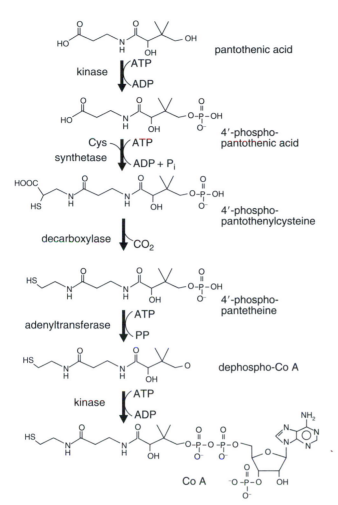

Fig. 15-2.   Biosynthesis of coenzyme A.

2. **Phosphopantothenylcysteine synthase** catalyzes the ATP-dependent condensation of 4'-phosphopantothenic acid with cysteine to yield **4'-phosphopantothenylcysteine.**
3. **Phosphopantothenylcysteine decarboxylase** catalyzes the decarboxylation of 4'-phosphopantothenylcysteine to yield **4'-phosphopantetheine** in the cytosol, whereupon it is transported into the mitochondria.

In the mitochondrial inner membrane:

4. **Phosphopantetheine adenyltransferase** catalyzes the ATP-dependent adenylation of 4'-phosphopantetheine to CoA to yield **dephospho-CoA**. Because this reaction is reversible, at low ATP levels dephospho-CoA can be degraded to yield ATP.
5. **Dephospho-CoA kinase** catalyzes the ATP-dependent phosphorylation of dephospho-CoA to yield CoA.

It was previously thought that CoA cannot cross the inner mitochondrial membrane and that the ability of 4-phosphopantetheine to enter mitochondria constituted the way to move the vitamin from the cytosol for CoA synthesis in the mitochrondia. It appears, however, that CoA can indeed enter the mitochondria. Such movement of radiolabeled CoA has been characterized. It involves both an energy-independent process driven by nonspecific membrane-binding and an energy-dependent process involving a membrane transporter.[15]

Acyl-Carrier Protein Biosynthesis

The acyl-carrier protein (ACP) is synthesized as the apoprotein lacking the prosthetic group. That group, 4'-phosphopantetheine, is transferred to ACP from CoA by the action of 4'-phosphopantetheine-apoACP transferase (Fig. 15-3). The prosthetic group is bound to the apo-ACP via a phosphoester linkage at a serinyl residue.

Catabolism of Coenzyme A and Acyl-Carrier Protein

The pantothenic acid components of both CoA and ACP are released metabolically ultimately in the free acid form of the vitamin. An ACP hydrolase has been identified that releases 4'-phosphopantetheine

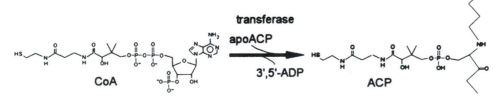

Fig. 15-3.   Coenzyme A provides 4-phosphopantetheine in the biosynthesis of the acyl-carrier protein.

[15] Tahiliani, A. G., and Neely, J. R. (1987). Mitochondrial synthesis of coenzyme A is on the external surface. *J. Mol. Cell Cardiol.* **19,** 1161–1168.

from holo-ACP to yield apo-ACP. The catabolism of CoA appears to be initiated by a nonspecific, phosphate-sensitive, lysosomal phosphatase, which yields dephospho-CoA. That metabolite appears to be degraded by a pyrophosphatase in the plasma membrane. 4'-Phosphopantetheine produced from either source is degraded to 4'-pantothenylcysteine and, finally, to pantothenic acid by microsomal and lysosomal phosphatases.

Excretion

No catabolic products of pantothenic acid are known. The vitamin is excreted mainly in the urine as free pantothenic acid, as well as some 4'-phosphopantethenate. The renal tubular secretion of pantothenic acid, probably by a mechanism common to weak organic acids, results in urinary excretion of the vitamin correlating with dietary intake. An appreciable amount (~15% of daily intake) is oxidized completely and is excreted across the lungs as CO_2. Humans typically excrete in the urine 0.8–8.4 mg of pantothenic acid per day.

VI. Metabolic Functions of Pantothenic Acid

General Functions

Both CoA and ACP/4'-phosphopantetheine function metabolically as carriers of acyl groups and activators of carbonyl groups in a large number of vital metabolic transformations, including the tricarboxylic acid (TCA) cycle[16] and the metabolism of fatty acids. In each case, the linkage with the transported acyl group involves the reactive sulfhydryl of the 4'-phosphopantetheinyl prosthetic group.

Coenzyme A

Coenzyme A serves as an essential cofactor for some 4% of known enzymes, including at least 100 in intermediary metabolism. In these reactions CoA forms high-energy thioester bonds with carboxylic acids, the most important of which is acetic acid, which can come from the metabolism of fatty acids, amino acids, or carbohydrates (Fig. 15-4). Coenzyme A functions widely in metabolism in reactions involving either the carboxyl group (e.g., formation of acetylcholine, acetylated amino sugars, acetylated sulfonamides[17]) or the methyl group (e.g., condensation with oxaloacetate to yield citrate) of an acyl CoA:

- As acetyl CoA, the so-called *active acetate* group can enter the TCA cycle and be used for the synthesis of fatty acids[18] or isopranoid compounds (e.g., cholesterol, steroid hormones).
- Acetyl CoA is used in acetylations of alcohols, amines, and amino acids (e.g., choline, sulfonamides, *p*-aminobenzoate, proteins[19]).
- Acetyl CoA is used in the oxidation of amino acids.
- Acetyl CoA participates in the N-terminal acetylation in more than half of eukaryotic proteins. This includes the processing of certain peptide hormones from their polyprotein precursors, such as the processing of ACTH to α-melanocyte-stimulating hormone and ß-lipotropin to ß-endorphin as well as the subsequent tissue-dependent acetylation of those products.
- Acetyl CoA participates in the internal acetylation of proteins, including histones[20] and α-tubulin[21] internal lysinyl, residues of which are reversibly acetylated.
- Acyl CoAs are used to modify a large number of proteins (GTP-binding proteins, protein kinases, membrane receptors, cytoskeletal proteins, mitochrondial proteins) through the addition of long-chain fatty acids. These reactions most frequently involve palmitic acid,[22] which is added post-translationally in a reversible ester bond, and myristic acid,[23] which is added co-translationally in an irreversible amide linkage.

---

[16] Often called the *citric acid cycle* or the *Krebs cycle*.

[17] Coenzyme A was discovered as an essential factor for the acetylation of sulfonamide by the liver and for the acetylation of choline in the brain; hence, *coenzyme A* stands for *coenzyme for acetylations*.

[18] Studies with liver slices *in vitro* have demonstrated a correlation between hepatic CoA content and lipid biosynthetic capacity, suggesting that CoA may be a limiting factor in lipogenesis.

[19] Many CoA-dependent reactions modify protein structure and function via acetylations at N termini or at internal sites (particularly, at the ε-amino groups of lysyl residues).

[20] Acetylated histones are enriched in genes that are being actively transcribed.

[21] Acetylation occurs in the α-tubulin after it has been incorporated into the microtubule. It can be induced by such agents as taxol. Acetylated microtubules are more stable to depolymerizing agents such as colchicines.

[22] *n*-hexadecanoic acid, C16:0.

[23] *n*-tetradecanoic acid, C14:0.

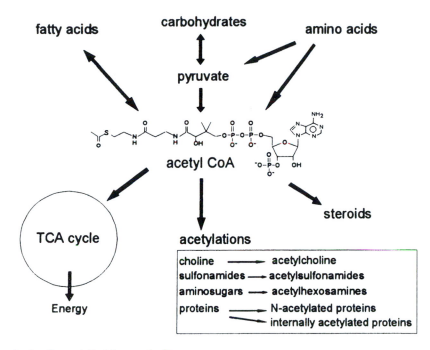

Fig. 15-4. The central role of acetyl-CoA in metabolism.

- Acyl CoAs are used to activate fatty acids for incorporation into triglycerides, membrane phospholipids, and regulatory sphingolipids.
- Acyl CoAs are transacylated to carnitine to form energy-equivalent acylcarnitines capable of being transported into the mitochondria where ß-oxidation occurs.
- Acyl CoAs are involved in the production of acetoacetate, a "ketone body" derived from fat metabolism when glucose is limiting.

Acyl-Carrier Protein

The acyl-carrier protein is a component of the multienzyme complex **fatty acid synthase**.[24] In ACP, the cofactor functions to transfer covalently bound intermediates between different active sites with successive cycles of condensations and reductions.[25] The nature of the fatty acid synthase complex varies considerably among different species; however, in each 4'-phosphopantetheine is the prosthetic group for the binding and transfer of the acyl units during this metabolism. The sulfhydryl group of the cofactor serves as the point of temporary covalent attachment of the growing fatty acid via a thiol linkage each time a malonic acid moiety is added by transfer to the cofactor. In this way, the cofactor appears to function as a swinging arm, allowing the growing fatty acid to reach the various catalytic sites of the enzyme.

Health Effects

Although pantothenic acid deficiency is exceeding rare, some benefits have been reported for the use of supplements of pantothenic acid and/or metabolites. These include:

- *Reduced serum cholesterol levels* High doses (500–1200 mg/day) of pantothine, the dimmer of pantetheine, has been shown to reduce serum total and low-density lipoprotein-associated cholesterol and triglycerides, and to increase high-density lipoprotein-associated cholesterol.[26]
- *Rheumatoid arthritis* A randomized control trial showed that high doses (up to 2 g/day) of calcium pantothenate reduced the duration of morning

---

[24] *Fatty acid synthase* is the name used to identify the multienzyme complex on which the several reactions of fatty acid synthesis (condensations and reductions) occur. The best studied complex is that of *Escherichia coli*; it consists of seven separate enzymes plus the small (10-kDa) protein ACP.

[25] The seven functional activities of the fatty acid synthase complex are *acetyltransferase, malonyltransferase, 3-ketoacyl synthase, 3-ketoacyl reductase, 3-hydroxyacyl dehydratase, enoyl reductase*, and *thioester hydrolase*.

[26] Binaghi, P., et al. (1990). *Minerva Med.* **81,** 475–479.

stiffness, the degree of disability, and the severity of pain for rheumatoid arthritis patients.[27]

- *Athelitic performance* Results have been inconsistent, some showing improved efficiency of oxygen utilization and reduced lactate acid accumulation,[28] others showing no benefits.[29]

VII. Pantothenic Acid Deficiency

Deficiencies Rare

Deprivation of pantothenic acid results in metabolic impairments, including reduced lipid synthesis and energy production. Signs and symptoms of pantothenic acid deficiency vary among different species; most frequently, they involve the skin, liver, adrenals, and nervous system. Owing to the wide distribution of the vitamin in nature, dietary deficiencies of pantothenic acid are rare; they are more common in circumstances of inadequate intake of basic foods and vitamins, and are often associated with (and mistakenly diagnosed as) deficiencies of other vitamins. Understanding of the presentation of pantothenic acid deficiency comes mostly from studies with experimental animals. These have shown a pattern of general deficiency signs (Table 15-2).

Antagonists

Pantothenic acid deficiency has been produced experimentally using purified diets free of the vitamin, or

by administering an antagonist. One antagonist is the analog **ω-methylpantothenic acid**, which has a methyl group in place of the hydroxymethyl group of the vitamin; this change prevents it from being phosphorylated and inhibits the action of pantothenic acid kinase. Other antagonists include desthio-CoA, in which the terminal sulfhydryl of the active metabolite is replaced with a hydroxyl group, and hopantenate, in which the three-carbon β-alanine moiety of the vitamin is replaced with the four-carbon γ-aminobutyric acid (GABA).

Deficiency Syndromes in Animals

Pantothenic acid deficiency in most species results in reduced growth and reduced efficiency of feed utilization. In rodents, the deficiency results in a scaly dermatitis, achromotrichia, alopecia, and adrenal necrosis. Congenital malformations of offspring of pantothenic acid-deficient dams have been reported. Excess amounts of porphyrins[30] are excreted in the tears of pantothenic acid-deficient rats, in a condition called *blood-caked whiskers*. Pantothenic acid-deficient chicks develop skin lesions at the corners of the mouth, swollen and encrusted eyelids, dermatitis of the entire foot (with hemorrhagic cracking),[31] poor feathering, fatty liver degeneration, thymic necrosis, and myelin degeneration of the spinal column with paralysis and lethargy. Chicks produced from deficient hens show high rates of embryonic and post-hatching mortality. Pantothenic acid-deficient dogs develop hepatic steatosis, irritability, cramps, ataxia, convulsions, alopecia, and death. Deficient pigs show similar nervous signs, develop hypertrophy and steatosis of the adrenals, liver, and heart, and show ovarian atrophy with impaired uterine development. Deficient fish show anorexia.

Marginal deficiency of pantothenic acid in the rat has been found to produce elevated serum levels of triglycerides and free fatty acids. The metabolic basis of this effect is not clear; however, it is possible that it involves a somewhat targeted reduction in cellular CoA concentrations, affecting the deposition of fatty acids in adipocytes (via impaired **acyl-CoA synthase**) but not the hepatic production of triglycerides.

Table 15-2. General signs of pantothenic acid deficiency

Organ system	Signs
General	
Appetite	Decrease
Growth	Decrease
Vital organs	Hepatic steatosis, thymic necrosis, adrenal hypertrophy
Dermatologic	Dermatitis, achromotrichia, alopecia
Muscular	Weakness
Gastrointestinal	Ulcers
Nervous	Ataxia, paralysis

---

[27] U.S. Practitioner Research Group (1980). *Practitioner* **224**, 208–211.

[28] Litoff, D., et al. (1985). *Med. Sci. Sports Excer.* **17** (Suppl.), 287.

[29] Nice, C., et al. (1984). *J. Sports Med. Phys. Fitness* **24**, 26–29.

[30] For example, protoporphyrin IX.

[31] This condition is often confused with that produced by biotin deficiency. Unlike the latter, in which lesions are limited to the foot pad, the lesions produced by pantothenic acid deficiency also involve the toes and superior aspect of the foot.

Deficiency Signs in Humans

Pantothenic acid deficiency in humans has been observed only in severely malnourished patients and in subjects treated with the antagonist ω-methylpantothenic acid. In cases of the former type, neurologic signs (paresthesia in the toes and sole of the feet) have been reported.[32] Subjects made deficient in pantothenic acid through the use of ω-methylpantothenic acid also developed burning sensations of the feet. In addition, they showed depression, fatigue, insomnia, vomiting, muscular weakness, and sleep and gastrointestinal disturbances. Changes in glucose tolerance, increased sensitivity to insulin, and decreased antibody production have also been reported.

Some evidence suggests that pantothenic acid intake may not be adequate for some people: Urinary pantothenic acid excretion has been found to be low for pregnant women, adolescents, and the elderly compared with the general population.

VIII. Pantothenic Acid Toxicity

Negligible Toxicity

The toxicity of pantothenic acid is negligible. No adverse reactions have been reported in any species following the ingestion of large doses of the vitamin. Massive doses (e.g., 10 g/day) administered to humans have not produced reactions more severe than mild intestinal distress and diarrhea. Similarly, no deleterious effects have been identified when the vitamin was administered parenterally or topically. It has been estimated that animals can tolerate without side effects doses of pantothenic acid as great as at least 100 times their respective nutritional requirements for the vitamin.

IX. Case Study

Instructions

Review the following experiment, paying special attention to the independent and dependent variables in the design. Then, answer the questions that follow.

Case

To evaluate the possible role of pantothenic acid and ascorbic acid in wound healing, a study was conducted on the effects of these vitamins on the growth of fibroblasts. Human fibroblasts were obtained from neonatal foreskin; they were cultured in a standard medium supplemented with 10% fetal calf serum and antibiotics.[33] The medium contained no ascorbic acid but contained 4 mg of pantothenic acid per liter. Cells were used between the third and ninth passages. Twenty-four hours before each experiment, the basal medium was replaced by medium supplemented with pantothenic acid (40 mg/l) or pantothenic acid (40 mg/l) plus ascorbic acid (60 mg/l). Cells (1.5×10^5) were plated in 3 ml of culture medium in 28-cm^2 plastic dishes. After incubation, they were collected by adding trypsin and then scraping; they were counted in a hemocytometer. The synthesis of DNA and protein was estimated by measuring the rates of incorporation of radiolabel from [^{3}H]thymidine and [^{14}C]proline, respectively. Total protein was measured in cells (lysed by sonication and solubilized in $0.5 N$ NaOH) and in the culture medium.

Results after 5 days of culture

Treatment	Cells ($\times 10^5$)	^{3}H (10^3 cpm)	^{14}C (10^3 cpm)	Cell protein (mg/dish)	Protein in medium (mg/ml)
Control	2.90 ± 0.16	11.6 ± 0.4	1.7 ± 1.0	10.0 ± 1.0	1.93 ± 0.01
Plus pantothenic acid	3.83 ± 0.14[a]	18.7 ± 0.5[a]	2.9 ± 0.1[a]	14.5 ± 0.9[a]	1.93 ± 0.02
Plus pantothenic acid and ascorbic acid	3.74 ± 0.19[a]	18.1 ± 0.8[a]	2.8 ± 0.1[a]	8.1 ± 0.9	2.11 ± 0.01[a]

[a]Significantly different from control value, $p < 0.05$.

---

[32] **Burning feet syndrome** was described during World War II in prisoners in Japan and the Philippines, who were generally malnourished. That large oral doses of calcium pantothenate provided some improvement suggested that the syndrome involved, at least in part, deficiency of pantothenic acid.

[33] Gentamicin and amphotericin B (Fungizone).

Case Questions

1. Why were thymidine and proline selected as carriers of the radiolabels in this experiment?
2. Why were fibroblasts selected (rather than some other cell type) for use in this study?
3. Assuming that the protein released into the culture medium is largely soluble procollagen, what can be concluded about the effects of pantothenic acid and/or ascorbic acid on collagen synthesis in this system?
4. What implications do these results have regarding wound healing?

Study Questions and Exercises

1. Diagram the areas of metabolism in which CoA and ACP (via fatty acid synthase) are involved.

2. Construct a decision tree for the diagnosis of pantothenic acid deficiency in humans or an animal species.

3. What key feature of the chemistry of pantothenic acid relates to its biochemical functions as a carrier of acyl groups?

4. What parameters might you measure to assess the pantothenic acid status of a human or animal?

Recommended Reading

Bender, D. A. (1999). Optimum nutrition: Thiamin, biotin and pantothenate. *Proc. Nutr. Soc.* **58,** 427–433.

Flodin, N. W. (1988). *Pharmacology of Micronutrients*, pp. 189–192. Alan R. Liss, New York.

Leonoardi, R., Zhang, Y. M., Rock, C. O., and Jackowski, S. (2005). Coenzyme A: Back in action. *Progr. Lipid Res.* **44,** 125–153.

Miller, J. W., Rogers, L. M., and Rucker, R. B. (2001). Pantothenic acid. Chapter 24 in *Present Knowledge in Nutrition*, 8th ed. (B. A. Bowman and R. M. Russell, eds.), pp. 253–260. ILSI Press, Washington, DC.

Plesofsky, N. S. (2001). Pantothenic acid, Chapter 9 in *Handbook of Vitamins*, 3rd ed. (R. B. Rucker, J. W. Suttie, D. B. McCormick, and L. J. Machlin, eds.), pp. 317–337. Marcel Dekker, New York.

Plesofsky-Vig, N., and Brambl, R. (1988). Pantothenic acid and coenzyme A in cellular modification of proteins. *Annu. Rev. Nutr.* **8,** 461–482.

Tahiliani, A. G., and Benlich, C. J. (1991). Pantothenic acid in health and disease. *Vit. Horm.* **46,** 165–228.

van den Berg, H. (1997). Bioavailability of pantothenic acid. *Eur. J. Clin. Nutr.* **51,** S62–S63.

Folate

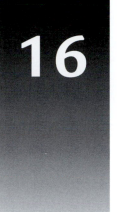

16

Using Streptococcus lactis *R as a test organism, we have obtained in a highly concentrated and probably nearly pure form an acid nutrilite with interesting physiological properties. Four tons of spinach have been extracted and carried through the first stages of concentration.... This acid, or one with similar chemical and physiological properties, occurs in a number of animal tissues of which liver and kidney are the best sources. ... It is especially abundant in green leaves of many kinds, including grass. Because of this fact, we suggest the name "folic acid" (Latin,* folium*—leaf). Many commercially canned greens are nearly lacking in the substance.*

—H. K. Mitchell, E. S. Snell, and R. J. Williams

I.	The Significance of Folate	356
II.	Sources of Folate	356
III.	Absorption of Folate	358
IV.	Transport of Folate	360
V.	Metabolism of Folate	362
VI.	Metabolic Functions of Folate	365
VII.	Folate Deficiency	375
VIII.	Pharmacologic Uses of Folate	377
IX.	Folate Toxicity	377
X.	Case Study	378
	Study Questions and Exercises	379
	Recommended Reading	379

Anchoring Concepts

1. Folate is the generic descriptor for folic acid (pteroylmonoglutamic acid) and related compounds exhibiting qualitatively the biological activity of folic acid. The term *folates* refers generally to the compounds in this group, including mono- and polyglutamates.
2. Folates are active as coenzymes in single-carbon metabolism.
3. Deficiencies of folate are manifested as anemia and dermatologic lesions.

Learning Objectives

1. To understand the chief natural sources of folates.
2. To understand the means of absorption and transport of the folates.
3. To understand the biochemical functions of the folates as coenzymes in single-carbon metabolism, and the relationship of that function to the physiological activities of the vitamin.
4. To understand the metabolic interrelationship of folate and vitamin B_{12} and its physiological implications.

Vocabulary

p-Acetaminobenzoylglutamate
Betaine
Cervical paralysis
7,8-Dihydrofolate reductase
Dihydrofolic acid (FH_2)
Folate
Folate-binding proteins (FBPs)
Folate receptor (FR)
Folate transporter
Folic acid
Folyl conjugase
Folyl polyglutamates
Folyl polyglutamate synthetase
5-Formimino-FH_4
5-Formyl-FH_4
10-Formyl-FH_4
Homocysteine
Homocysteinemia
Leukopenia
Macrocytic anemia
Megaloblasts
5,10-Methenyl-FH_4
Methionine synthase
Methionine synthetase
Methotrexate
5-Methyl-FH_4
5,10-Methylene-FH_4
5,10-Methylene-FH_4 dehydrogenase
5,10-Methylene-FH_4 reductase (MTHFR)
Methyl-folate trap
Methione synthase

Pernicious anemia
Pteridine
Pterin ring
Pteroylglutamic acid
Purines
S-adenosylmethionine (SAM)
Serine hydroxymethyltransferase
Single-carbon metabolism
Sulfa drugs
Tetrahydrofolate reductase
Tetrahydrofolic acid (FH_4)
Thymidylate
Thymidylate synthase
Vitamin B_{12}

I. The Significance of Folate

Folate is a vitamin that has only recently been appreciated for its importance beyond its essential role in normal metabolism, especially for its relevance to the etiologies of chronic diseases and birth defects. Widely distributed among foods, particularly those of plant foliar origin, this abundant vitamin is underconsumed by people whose food habits do not emphasize plant foods. Intimately related in function with vitamins B_{12} and B_6, its status at the level of subclinical deficiency can be difficult to assess and the full extent of its interrelationships with these vitamins and with amino acids remains incompletely elucidated.

Folate deficiency is an important problem in many parts of the world, particularly where there is poverty and malnutrition. It is an important cause of anemia, second only to nutritional iron deficiency. Evidence shows that marginal folate status can support apparently normal circulating folate levels while still limiting single-carbon metabolism. Thus, folate is emerging as having an important role in the etiology of homocysteinemia, which has been identified as a risk factor for occlusive vascular disease, cancer, and birth defects. It has been estimated that an increase in mean folate intake of $200\,\mu g$/day could reduce coronary artery disease deaths in the United States by 13,500 to 50,000. The finding of markedly reduced neural tube defects risk by periconceptional folate treatment has driven folate supplementation efforts in the United States and other countries. Still, there must be concern about the use of folate supple-

ments, particularly high-level supplements, as folate is known to mask the **macrocytic anemia** of vitamin B_{12} deficiency, which will lead to neuropathy if not corrected. For these several reasons, it is important to understand folate nutrition.

II. Sources of Folate

Distribution in Foods

Folates (**folyl polyglutamates**) occur in a wide variety of foods of both plant and animal origin (Table 16-1). Liver, mushrooms and green, leafy vegetables are rich sources of folate in human diets, while oilseed meals (e.g., soybean meal) and animal byproducts are important sources of folate in animal feeds. The folates in foods and feedstuffs are almost exclusively in reduced form as polyglutamyl derivatives of **tetrahydrofolic acid (FH_4)**. Very little free folate (folyl monoglutamate) is found in foods or feedstuffs.

Analyses of foods have revealed a wide distribution of general types of polyglutamyl folate derivatives, the predominant forms being **5-methyl-FH_4** and **10-formyl-FH_4**. The folates found in organ meats (e.g., liver and kidney) are about 40% methyl derivatives, whereas that in milk (and erythrocytes) is exclusively the methyl form. Some plant materials also contain mainly 5-methyl-FH_4 (e.g., lettuce, cabbage, orange juice), but others (e.g., soybean) contain relatively little of that form (~15%), the rest occurring as the 5- and 10-formyl derivatives. Most of the folates in cabbage are hexa- and heptaglutamates, whereas half of those in soybean are monoglutamates. More than a third of the folates in orange juice are present as monoglutamates, and nearly half are present as pentaglutamates. Liver and kidney contain mainly pentaglutamates, and ~60% of the folates in milk are monoglutamates (with only 4–8% each of di- to heptaglutamates).

Stability

Most folates in foods and feedstuffs (that is, folates other than **folic acid**[1] and **5-formyl-FH_4**) are easily oxidized and, therefore, are unstable to oxidation under aerobic conditions of storage and processing. Under such conditions (especially in the added presence of heat, light, and/or metal ions), FH_4

---

[1] Throughout this text, the term *folic acid* is used as the specific trivial name for the compound **pteroylglutamic acid**.

Table 16-1. Folate contents of foods

Food	Folate (μg/100 g)	Food	Folate (μg/100 g)
Dairy products		Other	
Milk	5–12	Eggs	70
Cheese	20	Brewers' yeast	1500
Meats		Vegetables	
Beef	5–18	Asparagus	70–175
Liver		Beans	70
Beef	140–1070	Broccoli	180
Chicken	1810	Brussels sprouts	90–175
Tuna	15	Cabbage	15–45
Cereals		Cauliflower	55–120
Barley	15	Peas	90
Corn	35	Soybeans	360
Rice		Spinach	50–190
Polished	15	Tomatoes	5–30
Unpolished	25	Fruits	
Wheat, whole	30–55	Apples	5
Wheat bran	80	Bananas	30
		Oranges	25

derivatives can readily be oxidized to the corresponding derivatives of **dihydrofolic acid (FH$_2$)** (partially oxidized) or folic acid (fully oxidized), some of which can react further to yield physiologically inactive compounds. For example, the two predominant folates in fresh foods, 5-methyl-FH$_4$ and 10-formyl-FH$_4$, are converted to 5-methyl-5,6-FH$_2$ and 10-formylfolic acid, respectively. For this reason, 5-methyl-5,6-FH$_2$ has been found to account for about half of the folate in most prepared foods. Although it can be reduced to the FH$_4$ form (e.g., by ascorbic acid), in the acidity of normal gastric juice, it isomerizes to yield 5-methyl-5,8-FH$_2$, which is completely inactive. Owing to their gastric anacidosis, this isomerization does not occur in pernicious anemia patients, who are thus able to utilize the partially oxidized form by absorbing it and subsequently activating it to 5-methyl-FH$_4$. Because some folate derivatives of the latter type can support the growth responses of test microorganisms used to measure folates,[2] some information in the available literature may overestimate the biologically useful folate contents of foods and/or feedstuffs. Substantial losses in the folate contents of food can occur as the result of leaching in cooking water when boiling (losses of total folates of 22% for asparagus and 84% for cauliflower have been observed), as well as oxidation, as described above. Due to such losses, green leafy vegetables can lose their value as sources of folates despite their relatively high natural contents of the vitamin.

Bioavailability

The biological availability of folates in foods has been difficult to assess quantitatively; estimates are variable among foods but generally indicate bioavailabilities less than half of folic acid. In general, folates appear to be less well utilized from plant-derived foods than from animal products

---

[2] *Lactobacillus casei, Streptococcus faecium* (formerly, *S. lactis* R. and *S. faecalis*, respectively), and *Pediococcus cerevisiae* (formerly, *Leuconostoc citrovorum*) have been used. Of these, *L. casei* responds to the widest spectrum of folates.

Table 16-2. Biologic availability to humans of folates in foods

Food/feedstuff	Bioavailability[a] (range of reported values, %)
Bananas	0–148
Cabbage	0–127
Eggs	35–137
Lima beans	0–181
Liver (goat)	9–135
Orange juice	29–40
Spinach	26–99
Tomatoes	24–71
Wheat germ	0–64
Brewers' yeast	10–100
Soybean meal	0–83

[a]Results expressed relative to folic acid.
Sources: Baker, H., Jaslow, S. P., and Frank, O. (1978). *J. Am. Geriatr. Soc.* **26,** 218–221; Baker, H., and Srikantia, S. G. (1976). *Am. J. Clin. Nutr.* **29,** 376–379; Tamura, T., and Stokstad, E. L. R. (1973). *Br. J. Haematol.* **25,** 513–532.

(Table 16-2). Several factors affect the biologic availability of food folates:

- *Antifolates in the diet* Folates can bind to the food matrices; many foods contain inhibitors of the intestinal brush border folate conjugase and/or folate transport.
- *Inherent characteristics of various folates* Folate vitamers vary in biopotency.
- *Nutritional status of the host* Deficiencies of iron and vitamin C status are associated with impaired utilization of dietary folate.[3]

Interactions of these factors complicate the task of predicting the bioavailability of dietary folates (Table 16-2). This problem is exacerbated by the methodological difficulties in evaluating folate utilization, which can be done through bioassays with animal models,[4] balance studies with humans, or isotopic methods to measure the appearance of folates in blood, excreta, and tissues.

III. Absorption of Folate

Hydrolysis of Folyl Polyglutamates

Under fasting conditions, folic acid, 5-methyl-FH$_4$, and 5-formyl-FH$_4$ are virtually completely absorbed, and most polyglutamyl folates are absorbed at efficiencies in the general range of 60–80%. Because the majority of food folates occur as reduced polyglutamates, they must be cleaved to the mono- or diglutamate forms for absorption. This is accomplished by the action of an exocarboxypeptidase folyl γ-glutamyl carboxypeptidase, more commonly called **folyl conjugase**.

Conjugase activity is widely distributed in the mucosa of the proximal small intestine, both intracellularly and in association with the brush border. These appear to be different enzymes: the 75 kDa intracellular enzyme is localized in the lysosomes and, has an optimum of pH 4.5–50, whereas the 700 kDa brush border enzyme has an optimum of pH 6.5–7.0 mw. Although the latter enzyme is present in lower amounts, it appears to be important for the hydrolysis of dietary folyl polyglutamates. Folyl conjugase activities have also been found in bile, pancreatic juice, kidney, liver, placenta, bone marrow, leukocytes, and plasma, although the physiological importance of the activity in these tissues is uncertain. In the uterus, conjugase activity is induced by estrogen. A genetic variant of the brush border enzyme has been identified in association with low serum folate concentrations and homocysteinemia, suggesting impaired utilization of dietary folates.

Loss of conjugase activity results in impaired folate absorption. Conjugase activity is reduced by nutritional zinc deficiency or by exposure to naturally occurring inhibitors in foods (Table 16-3). Studies with several animal models have demonstrated that chronic ethanol feeding can decrease intestinal hydrolysis of folyl polyglutamates and can impair the absorption, transport, cellular release, and metabolism of folates. Effects of this nature are thought to contribute to the folate deficiencies frequently

---

[3] Some anemic patients respond optimally to oral folate therapy only when they are also given iron. Patients with scurvy often have megaloblastic anemia, apparently owing to impaired utilization of folate. In some scorbutic patients, vitamin C has an antianemic effect; others require folate to correct the anemia.

[4] As with any application of information from studies with animal models, the validity of extrapolation is an issue important in assessing folate bioavailability. For example, the rat and many other species have little or no jejunal brush border conjugase activity, these species relying on the pancreatic conjugase for folate deconjugation. This contrasts with the pig and human, which deconjugate folates primarily by jejunal brush border activity, with activity of only secondary importance in the pancreatic juice.

Table 16-3. Inhibition of jejunal folate conjugase activities *in vitro* by components of selected foods

Food	Pig conjugase (% inhibition)	Human conjugase (% inhibition)
Red kidney beans	35.5	15.9
Pinto beans	35.1	33.2
Lima beans	35.6	35.2
Black-eyed peas	25.9	19.3
Yellow cornmeal	35.3	28.3
Wheat bran	−2.0	0
Tomato	8.1	14.2
Banana	45.9	46.0
Cauliflower	25.2	15.3
Spinach	21.1	13.9
Orange juice	80.0	73.4
Egg	11.5	5.3
Milk	13.7	–
Cabbage	12.1	–
Whole wheat flour	0.3	–
Medium rye flour	2.2	–

Source: Bhandari, S. D., and Gregory, J. F. (1990). *Am. J. Clin. Nutr.* **51**, 87–94.

observed among chronic alcoholics. However, there are other likely contributing factors, as enterocytes are known to be sensitive to ethanol toxicity, and many chronic alcoholics can have insufficient dietary intakes of the vitamin.

Natural conjugase inhibitors are contained in certain foods: cabbage, oranges, yeast, beans (red kidney, pinto, lima, navy, soy), lentils, and black-eyed peas.[5] The presence of conjugase inhibitors reduces folate bioavailability; this effect appears to be the basis for the low availability of the vitamin in orange juice. Folate absorption can also be reduced by certain drugs including cholestyramine (which binds folates), ethanol (which inhibits deconjugation), salicylazosulfapyridine,[6] diphenylhydantoin,[7] aspirin and other salicylates, and several nonsteroidal anti-inflammatory drugs.

Uptake

Dietary **folates** are absorbed as folic acid, 5-methyl-FH_4, and 5-formyl-FH_4 in most species, although some (e.g., dogs) appear also to absorb folyl polyglutamates. The overall efficiency of folate absorption appears to be ~50% (10–90%). Malabsorption of the vitamin occurs in diseases affecting the intestinal mucosa. A microclimate hypothesis has been proposed for the enteric absorption of folates. It holds that folate absorption is dependent on the pH of the proximal jejunum, with an optimum at pH 6.0–6.3. According to this hypothesis, the elevated absorption of folate in individuals with pancreatic exocrine insufficiency may be due to the low pancreatic excretion of bicarbonate in that condition. Loss of buffering capacity renders the intestinal lumenal milieu slightly more acidic, minimizing the charge on the folate molecule, thus facilitating its diffusion across the brush border membrane. Under more basic conditions (i.e., pH > 6.0), folate absorption falls off rapidly. Two jejunal brush border **folate-binding proteins (FBPs)**, thought to be involved in this process, have been isolated.

Three mechanisms are involved in folate absorption:

- *Folate transporter* Folic acid is actively transported across the jejunum, and perhaps the duodenum, by an Na^+-coupled, carrier-mediated process that is stimulated by glucose and shows a pH maximum at about pH 6. The transporter is a transmembrane protein with much greater affinities for folic acid than for reduced folates. The active transport process is maximal at lumenal folate concentrations of 10–20 μM. Its expression is suppressed by exposure to alcohol.[8] Hereditary folate malabsorption, apparently involving failure of transporter expression, has been reported.[9]

---

[5] The conjugase inhibitors in beans and peas reside in the seed coats and are heat labile.

[6] This drug, also called Azulfidine and sulfasalazine, is used to treat inflammatory bowel disorder.

[7] This drug, also called Dilantin, is an anticonvulsant.

[8] This effect appears to be the basis of substantial impairments in folate absorption in subjects consuming alcohol (Halsted, C. H., et al. [2002]. *J. Nutr.* **132**, 2367S–2372S).

[9] Hereditary folate malabsorption has been reported in some 30 patients, presenting at 2–6 months of age as megaloblastic anemia, mucositis, diarrhea, failure to thrive, recurrent infections, and seizures.

- *Folate receptor* A high-affinity, folate-binding protein, also called the **folate receptor (FR)**, has been identified in the intestine and other tissues. The intestine contains three isoforms, each of which is associated with the brush border. Two isoforms (α- and ß-) are glycosylphosphatidyl-inositol (GPI)-anchored to the membrane; one (β-) is a soluble protein. The GPI-anchored receptor FRα has been shown to cycle between intracellular and extracellular compartments while remaining bound to the membrane, thus effecting the high-affinity uptake of folate and nonmolar concentrations.

- *Diffusion* Folic acid can also be absorbed passively, apparently by diffusion. This nonsaturable process is linearly related to lumenal folate concentration and can account for 20–30% of folate absorption at high folate intakes.

Methylation

Folic acid taken up by the intestinal mucosal cell is reduced to FH_4, which can either be transferred without further metabolism to the portal circulation or alkylated (e.g., by methylation to 5-methyl-FH_4) before being transferred.

IV. Transport of Folate

Free in Plasma

In most species, folate is transported to the tissues mostly as monoglutamate derivatives in free solution in the plasma. The notable exception is the pig, in which FH_4 is the predominant circulating form of the vitamin. [10] The predominant form in portal plasma is the reduced form, tetrahydrofolic acid (FH_4). This is taken up by the liver, which releases it to the peripheral plasma after converting it primarily to 5-methyl-FH_4, but also to 10-formyl-FH_4. The concentration of 10-formyl-FH_4 is tightly regulated,[11] whereas that of 5-methyl-FH_4 is not; thus the latter varies in response to folate meals, and so on. Thus, folates of dietary origin are absorbed and transported to the liver as FH_4, which is converted to the methylated form and transported to the peripheral tissues.

Plasma folate concentrations in humans are typically in the range of 10–30 nM. Most circulates in free solution, but some is bound to low-affinity protein binders such as albumin, and others are bound to a soluble form of the high-affinity FBP. The latter is also found in high levels in milk. Erythrocytes contain greater concentrations of folate than, typically 50–100 nM. These stores are accumulated during erythropoiesis; the mature erythrocyte does not take up folate.

The folate levels of both plasma and erythrocytes are reduced by cigarette smoking; habitual smokers show plasma folate levels that are more than 40% less than those of nonsmokers.[12] While serum folates have been found to be normal among middle-class drinkers of moderate amounts of ethanol, more than 80% of impoverished chronic alcoholics show abnormally low serum levels and some 40% show low erythrocyte levels. This corresponds to a similar incidence (34–42%) of megaloblastosis of the bone marrow in alcoholic patients. These effects probably relate to the displacement of foods containing folates by alcoholic beverages, which are virtually devoid of the vitamin, as well as to direct metabolic effects: inhibition of intestinal folyl conjugase activity and decreased urinary recovery of the vitamin.

Cellular Uptake

The cellular uptake of folates occurs exclusively with monoglutamate derivatives found in the plasma, as the polyglutamates cannot cross biological membranes. The cellular uptake of folate involves the three processes outlined above for enteric absorption:

- *Folate transporter* The folate transporter is expressed in most tissues. It has affinities for various folates varying both between tissues and between the apical and basolateral membranes. Its affinities for folic acid are two orders of magnitude greater than those for reduced folates.

---

[10] The metabolic basis for this anomaly is not clear.

[11] In humans, the plasma level is held at about 80 ng/dl.

[12] These findings probably relate to the inactivation of cobalamins by factors (cyanides, hydrogen sulfide, nitrous oxide) in cigarette smoke (see Chapter 17).

- *Folate receptor*   A high-affinity FR is expressed in many tissues. Studies have shown that it mediates the uptake of folate in the kidney. Because the FR and transporter are localized on opposite aspects of polarized cells, it has been speculated that the FR may facilitate the movement of folate across the apical membrane into the cell, while the transporter, which shows a lower affinity for folate, facilitates the movement of the vitamin across the basolateral membrane and into the portal circulation.

Within cells, FH_4 is methylated to yield 5-methyl-FH_4, which is bound to intracellular macromolecules. As a result of methylation in the mammary gland, 5-methyl-FH_4 comprises three-quarters of the folates in breast milk. Folate is held in cells by conversion to folyl polyglutamates; polyglutamation traps folates inside cells at concentrations greater (by one to two orders of magnitude) than those of extracellular fluids.

Folate-Binding Proteins

Folate-binding proteins (FBPs) have been identified in plasma, milk, and several other tissues (e.g., erythrocytes, leukocytes, intestinal mucosa, kidney, liver, placenta, choroid plexus, and urine[13]). Each binds folates noncovalently with high affinity, such that the complex does not dissociate under physiological conditions.[14] Low concentrations (e.g., binding <10 ng of folic acid per deciliter) of FBPs have been found in sera of healthy humans; greater concentrations of FBPs have been found in folate-deficient subjects, pregnant women, human milk, and leukemic leukocytes. It is suggested that the FBPs found in plasma and milk are derived from cellular membranes in which they serve transport functions. This appears to be true of the FBPs in milk;[15] they have been shown to stimulate the enteric absorption of folate from that food. The liver contains two FBPs: one is the enzyme dimethylglycine dehydrogenase; the other is the enzyme sarcosine dehydrogenase. Each binds reduced folates with an affinity that is 100-fold greater than that for nonreduced forms (Table 16-4).

Table 16-4.   Differential binding of folate metabolites by folate-binding protein isoforms

Folate/metabolite	FBP isoform binding affinity
Folate	
5'-Methyl-FH_4	FBP-α > FBP-β by 50-fold
5'-Formyl-FH_4	FBP-α > FBP-β by 100-fold
Folate antagonist	
Methotrexate	FBP-α > FBP-β by 20-fold
Dideaza-FH_4	FBP-α > FBP-β by 10-fold

Source: Antony, A. C. (1996). *Annu. Rev. Nutr.* **16**, 501–521.

Isoforms of FBP cDNAs have been cloned: three from humans (FBP-σ, -β, and -γ) and two from murine L1210 cells. These have identical open reading frames and 3'-untranslated regions, but their 5'-untranslated regions differ in both sequence and length. Four human FBP genes have been located in chromosome 11q13.2→q13.5 within a 140-kilobase region;[16] their promoter lacks TATA or CAAT elements but has sequences recognized by transcription factors (*ets* oncogene-encoded transcription factor and SP1) that are thought to regulate FBP expression. The genes appear to have a single promoter located within an intron and containing a triplet of clustered SP1-binding sites and an initiator region. The regulation of FBP expression is not well understood, but it is clear that extracellular folate concentration plays an important role in that process, serving as an inverse stimulus to FBP expression.

The membrane FBPs appear to be anchored by glycosyl-phospholipids, probably via serinyl or asparaginyl residues. Because FBPs show different binding affinities for various folates (and folate antagonists), it is assumed that the transport of folates into cells depends on the relative expression of FBP isoforms. The best evidence for a transport role of the FBPs comes from studies of the maternal-to-fetal transfer of folate. That process has been shown to involve the concentration of 5'-methyl-FH_4 by placental FBPs on the maternally facing chorionic surface followed by the transfer of the vitamers to the fetal circulation down a descending concentration gradient. Folate

---

[13] Urinary FBP is presumed to be of plasma origin.

[14] Other proteins (e.g., albumin) bind folates nonspecifically, forming complexes that dissociate readily.

[15] There are two FBPs in milk. Each is a glycoprotein; one may be a degradation product of the other.

[16] FBP-α and FBP-β genes are found less than 23 kb apart in sequence, with two additional FBP-related genes located upstream of the FBP-α gene.

uptake in liver presumably occurs similarly; studies show the process to be electroneutral, involving the co-transport of H^+.

Tissue Distribution

In humans, the total body content of folate is 5–10 mg, about half of which resides in the liver in the form of tetra-, penta-, hexa- and heptaglutamates of 5-methyl-FH_4 and 10-formyl-FH_4.[17] The relative amounts of these single-carbon derivatives vary among tissues, depending on the rate of cell division. In tissues with rapid cell division (e.g., intestinal mucosa, regenerating liver, carcinoma), relatively low concentrations of 5-methyl-FH_4 are found, usually with concomitant elevations in 10-formyl-FH_4. In contrast, in tissues with low rates of cell division (e.g., normal liver), 5-methyl-FH_4 predominates. Brain folate (mostly 5-methyl-FH_4) levels tend to be very low, with a subcellular distribution (penta- and hexaglutamates mostly in the cytosol and polyglutamates mostly in the mitochondria) the opposite of that found in liver. That folate-deficient animals show relatively low hepatic concentrations of shorter chain-length folyl polyglutamates compared with longer chain-length folates suggests that the longer chain-length metabolites are better retained within cells. In the rat, uterine concentrations of folates show cyclic variations according to the menstrual cycle, with maxima coincident with peak estrogenic activity just before ovulation.[18] It has been suggested that tissue FBPs, which bind polyglutamate forms of the vitamin, may play important roles in stabilizing folates within cells, thus reducing their rates of metabolic turnover and increasing their intracellular retention.

V. Metabolism of Folate

There are three aspects of folate metabolism:

- *Reduction of the pteridine ring system* Reduction of the **pterin ring** from the two nonreduced states, folic acid and dihydrofolic acid (FH_2), to the fully reduced form tetrahydrofolic acid (FH_4) that is capable of accepting a single-carbon unit is accomplished by the cytosolic enzyme **7,8-dihydrofolate reductase** (Fig. 16-1).[19] This activity is found in high amounts in liver and kidney and in rapidly dividing cells (e.g., tumor).

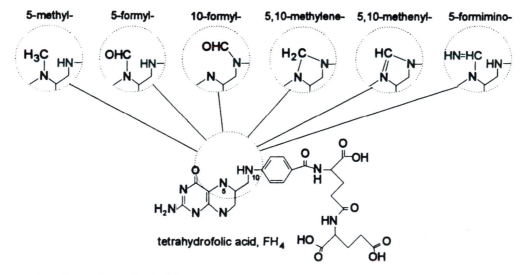

Fig. 16-1. Single-carbon units carried by folate.

---

[17] The hepatic reserve of folate should be sufficient to support normal plasma concentrations of the vitamin (>400 ng/dl) for at least 4 weeks. (Signs of megaloblastic anemia are usually not observed within 2–3 months of folate deprivation.) However, some evidence suggests that the release of folate from the liver is independent of nutritional folate status, resulting instead from the deaths of hepatocytes.

[18] On the basis of this type of observation, it has been suggested that estrogen enhancement of folate turnover in hormone-dependent tissues may be the basis of the effects of pregnancy and oral contraceptive steroids in potentiating low-folate status.

[19] Also called *tetrahydrofolate dehydrogenase*, this 65-kDa NADPH-dependent enzyme can reduce folic acid to FH_2 and, of greater importance, FH_2 to FH_4. The enzyme is potently inhibited by the drug methotrexate, a 4-aminofolic acid analogue.

The reductase is inhibited by several important drugs including the cancer chemotherapeutic drug **methotrexate**,[20,21] which appears to exert its antitumor action by inhibiting the reductase activity of tumor cells.

- *Reactions of the polyglutamyl side chain*   The folyl monoglutamates that are taken up by cells are trapped therein as polyglutamate derivatives that cannot cross cell membranes. Polyglutamate forms are also mobilized by side-chain hydrolysis to the monoglutamate. These conversions are catalyzed by two enzymes:

  - *Polyglutamation*   The conversion of 5-methyl-FH_4 to folyl polyglutamates is accomplished by the action of the ATP-dependent **folyl polyglutamate synthetase**,[22] which links glutamyl residues to the vitamin by peptide bonds involving the γ-carboxyl groups.[23] The enzyme requires prior reduction of folate to FH_4 or demethylation of the circulating 5-methyl-FH_4 (by vitamin B_{12}-dependent methionine synthetase). It is widely distributed at low concentrations in many tissues. That folyl polyglutamate synthetase is critical in converting the monoglutamyl transport forms of the vitamin to the metabolically active polyglutamyl forms was demonstrated by the discovery of a mutational loss of the synthetase activity, which produced lethal folate deficiency. In most tissues, the activity of the low-abundance enzyme is rate-limiting for folate accumulation and retention. Cells that lack the enzyme are unable to accumulate the vitamin.[24] Those lacking the mitochondrial enzyme cannot accumulate the vitamin in that subcellular compartment and, consequently, are deficient in mitochondrial single-carbon metabolism.

  - *Cellular conjugases*   Folyl polyglutamates are converted to derivatives of shorter chain length by lysosomal[25] γ-glutamyl carboxypeptidases, also referred to as cellular conjugases, some of which are zinc-metalloenzymes.

- *Acquisition of single-carbon moieties at certain positions (N-5 or N-10) on the pterin ring*   Folate is metabolically active as a variety of derivatives with single-carbon units at the oxidation levels of formate, formaldehyde, or methanol[26] substituted at the N-5 and/or N-10 positions of the pteridine ring system (Fig. 16-2). The main source of single-carbon fragments is **serine hydroxymethyltransferase** (Table 16-5), which uses the dispensable amino acid serine[27] as the single-carbon donor. Each folyl derivative is a donor of its single-carbon unit in metabolism;[28] thus, by cycling through the acquisition/loss of single-carbon units, each derivative delivers these species to a variety of metabolic uses. Most single-carbon folate derivatives in cells

---

[20] 4-Amino-10-methylfolic acid.

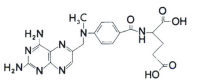

[21] Other inhibitors include the antimalarial drug pyrimethamine and the antibacterial drug trimethoprim.

[22] The mitochondrial and cytosolic forms of the enzyme are encoded by a single gene whose transcription has alternate start sites and the mRNA which has alternative translation sites.

[23] This enzyme also catalyzes the polyglutamation of the anticancer folate antagonist methotrexate, which enhances its cellular retention. Tumor cells, which have the greatest capacities to perform this side-chain elongation reaction, are particularly sensitive to the cytotoxic effects of the antagonist.

[24] Because polyglutamation is also necessary for the cellular accumulation and cytotoxic efficacy of antifolates such as methotrexate, decreased folyl polyglutamate synthase activity is associated with clinical resistance to those drugs.

[25] Lysosomes also contain a folate transporter, which is thought to be active in bringing folypolyglutamates into that vesicle.

[26] It should be noted that single carbons at the oxidation level of CO_2 cannot be transported by folates; such fully oxidized carbon is transported by biotin and thiamin pyrophosphate.

[27] Serine is biosynthesized from glucose in nonlimiting amounts in most cells.

[28] Although the route of its biosynthesis is unknown, eukaryotic cells contain significant amounts of 5-formyl-FH_4. That folyl derivative, also called *leucovorin, folinic acid,* and *citrovorum factor,* is used widely to reverse the toxicity of methotrexate and, more recently, to potentiate the cytotoxic effects of 5-fluorouracil.

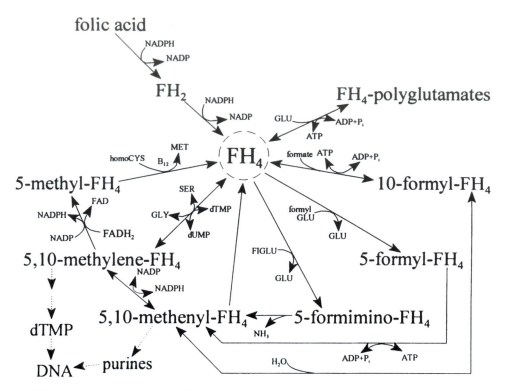

Fig. 16-2. Role of folate in single-carbon metabolism.

are bound to enzymes or FBPs; the concentrations of the free pools of folate coenzymes are therefore low, in the nanomolar range.

Catabolism

Tissue folates appear to turn over by the cleavage of the polyglutamates at the C-9 and N-10 bonds to liber-

ate the **pteridine** and p-aminobenzoylpolyglutamate moieties. This cleavage probably results from chemical oxidation of the cofactor in both the intestinal lumen (dietary and enterohepatically recycled folates) and the tissues. Once formed, p-aminobenzoylpolyglutamate is degraded, presumably by the action of folyl conjugase, and is acetylated to yield **p-acetaminobenzoylgluta- mate** and p-acetoaminobenzoate. The rate of folate

Table 16-5. Enzymes involved in the acquisition of single-carbon units by folates

Single-carbon unit	Folate derivative	Enzyme(s)
Methyl group	5-Methyl-FH$_4$	5,10-Methylene-FH$_4$ reductase
Methylene group	5,10-Methylene-FH$_4$	Serine hydroxymethyltransferase
		5,10-Methylene-FH$_4$ dehydrogenase
Methenyl group	5,10-Methenyl-FH$_4$	5,10-Methylene-FH$_4$ dehydrogenase
		5,10-Methenyl-FH$_4$ cyclohydrolase
		5-Formimino-FH$_4$ cyclohydrolase
		5-Formyl-FH$_4$ isomerase
Formimino group	5-Formimino-FH$_4$	FH$_4$:formiminotransferase
Formyl group	5-Formyl-FH$_4$	FH$_4$:glutamate transformylase
	10-Formyl-FH$_4$	5,10-Methenyl-FH$_4$ cyclohydrolase
		10-Formyl-FH$_4$ synthetase

catabolism appears to be related to the rate of intracellular folate utilization. Accordingly, urinary levels of *p*-acetoaminobenzoate are correlated with the total body folate pool. Folate breakdown is greatest under hyperplastic conditions (e.g., rapid growth, pregnancy[29]). Studies of the kinetics of folate turnover using isotopic labels have indicated at least two metabolic pools of the vitamin in nondeficient individuals: a larger, slow-turnover pool, and a smaller, rapid-turnover pool. At low to moderate intakes, 0.5–1% of total body folate appears to be catabolized and excreted per day (Table 16-6).

Excretion

Intact folates and the water-soluble side-chain metabolites *p*-acetaminobenzoylglutamate and *p*-acetaminobenzoate are excreted in the urine and bile. The total urinary excretion of folates and metabolites is small (e.g., ≤1% of total body stores per day). Folate conservation is effected by the reabsorption of 5-methyl-FH$_4$ by the renal proximal tubule; renal reabsorption appears to be mainly a nonspecific process, although an FBP-mediated process has also been demonstrated. Fecal concentrations of folates are usually rather high; however, they represent mainly folates of intestinal microfloral origin, as enterohepatically circulated folates appear to be absorbed quantitatively.

Table 16-6. Folate catabolic rates in humans

Folate intake (μg/day)	Estimated total body folate catabolic rate	
	(mg)	(% body pool/day)
200	28.5	0.47
300	31.5	0.61
400	32.2	0.82

Source: Gregory, J. F., et al. (1998). *J. Nutr.* **128,** 1896–1906.

VI. Metabolic Functions of Folate

Coenzymes in Single-Carbon Metabolism

The folates function as enzyme co-substrates in many reactions of the metabolism of amino acids and nucleotides, as well as the formation of the primary donor for biological methylations, **S-adenosylmethionine (SAM)**. In each of these functions, the fully reduced (tetrahydro-) form of each serves as an acceptor or donor of a single-carbon unit (Table 16-7). Collectively, these reactions are referred to as **single-carbon metabolism.**

Methionine and S-adenosylmethionine synthesis

As 5-methyl-FH$_4$, which is freely produced from 5,10-methenyl-FH$_4$, folate provides labile methyl groups for methionine synthesis from homocysteine.[30] Methionine is essential for the synthesis of proteins and polyamines, and is the precursor of SAM, which serves as a donor of "labile" methyl groups for more than 100 enzymatic reactions that have critical roles in metabolism.[31] *S*-Adenosylmethionine[32] also serves as a key regulator of the transsulfuration and remethylation pathways. This metabolism is catalyzed by two enzymes: **methylenetetrahydrofolate reductase (MTHFR)** and **methionine synthase.**[33] Methylenetetrahydrofolate reductase is necessary for the production of 5-methyl-FH$_4$, the obligate single-carbon donor for methionine synthesis.

Histidine catabolism

Cytosolic forminonotransferase catalyzes the final reaction in the catabolism of histidine by transferring the formimino group from formiminoglutamate (FIGLU) to FH$_4$.

---

[29] This effect may be an important contributor to the folate-responsive megaloblastic anemia common in pregnancies in parts of Asia, Africa, and Central and South America (where rates as high as 24% have been reported) as well as in the industrialized world (where rates of 2.5–5% have been reported).

[30] This is one of two pathways for the synthesis of methionine from homocysteine, the other using **betaine** as a methyl donor.

[31] By loss of the flux of methyl groups via 5-methyl-FH$_4$:homocysteine methyltransferase, folate deficiency causes a secondary hepatic choline deficiency.

[32] It is also an allosteric inhibitor of 5,10-methylene-FH$_4$ reductase and an activator of the pyridoxal phosphate-dependent enzyme cystathionine β-synthase, which catalyzes the condensation of homocysteine and serine to form cystathionine.

[33] Two genetic polymorphisms in methionine synthase have been identified. It is not clear whether either has functional significance.

Table 16-7. Metabolic roles of folate

Folate coenzyme	Enzyme	Metabolic role
5,10-Methylene-FH$_4$	Serine hydroxymethyltransferase	Receipt of a formaldehyde unit in serine catabolism (the mitochondrial enzyme important in glycine synthesis)
	Thymidylate synthetase	Transfers formaldehyde to C-5 of dUMP to form dTMP in pyrimidines
10-Formyl-FH$_4$	10-Formyl-FH$_4$ synthetase	Accepts formate from tryptophan catabolism
	Glycinamide ribonucleotide transformylase	Donates formate in purine synthesis
	5-Amino-4-imidazolecarboxamide transformylase	Donates formate in purine synthesis
	10-Formyl-FH$_4$ dehydrogenase	Transfers formate for oxidation to CO_2 in histidine catabolism
5-Methyl-FH$_4$	Methionine synthetase	Provides methyl group to convert homocysteine to methionine
	Glycine N-methyltransferase	Transfers methyl group from S-adenosylmethionine to glycine in the formation of homocysteine
5-Formimino-FH$_4$	Formiminotransferase	Accepts formimino group from histidine catabolism

Nucleotide metabolism

Though not required for the *de novo* synthesis of pyrimidines, folates are required for the synthesis of thymidylate, and they are also required for purine synthesis. Both roles are necessary for the *de novo* synthesis of DNA and thus for DNA replication and cell division. Accordingly, disruption of these functions impairs cell division and results in the macrocytic anemia of folate deficiency.

- *Thymidylate synthesis* Folates transport formaldehyde (as 5,10-methylene-FH$_4$) for **thymidylate** synthesis. The enzyme **thymidylate synthase**[34] catalyzes the conversion of deoxyuridine monophosphate (dUMP) to deoxythymidine monophosphate (dTMP), involving the transfer of formaldehyde from 5,10-methylene-FH$_4$ to dUMP. This step is rate-limiting to DNA replication, thus enabling the normal progression of the cell cycle. Thymidylate synthase is expressed only in replicating tissues;

the highest expression occurs during the S phase of the cell cycle.
- *Purine synthesis* Folates transport formate (as 10-formyl-FH$_4$, produced from 5,10-methylene-FH$_4$) in two steps in the synthesis of **purines** in the synthesis of adenine and guanine. In this way, formyl groups are used to provide the C-2 and C-8 positions of the purine ring, and FH$_4$ is regenerated. These reactions are catalyzed by aminoimidazolecarboxamide ribonucleotide tranformylase and glycinamide ribonucleotide tranformylase, respectively.

Single-Carbon Metabolism

Regulation

The regulation of single-carbon metabolism is effected by the interconversion of oxidation states of the folate intermediates. In mammalian tissues, the β-carbon of serine is the major source of single-carbon units for these aspects

---

[34] The antifolate 5-fluorodeoxyuridylate is active by forming a complex with the enzyme and its folate co-substrate.

of metabolism. That carbon fragment is accepted by FH_4 to form 5,10-methylene-FH_4 (by **serine hydroxymethyltransferase**), which has a central role in single-carbon metabolism. The latter derivative can be used directly for the synthesis of thymidylate (by thymidylate synthetase),[35] it can be oxidized to **5,10-methenyl-FH_4** (by **5,10-methylene-FH_4 dehydrogenase**) for use in the *de novo* synthesis of purines, or it can be reduced to 5-methyl-FH_4 (by MTHFR) for use in the biosynthesis of methionine. The result is the channeling of single-carbon units in several directions: to methionine, to thymidylate (for DNA synthesis), or to purine biosynthesis.

Because folyl polyglutamates have been found to inhibit a number of the enzymes of single-carbon metabolism, it has been suggested that variation in their polyglutamate chain lengths (observed under different physiological conditions) may play a role in the regulation of single-carbon metabolism.

The methyl-folate trap

The major cycle of single-carbon flux in mammalian tissues appears to be the serine hydroxymethyltransferase/5,10-methylene-FH_4 reductase/methionine synthetase cycle, in which the methionine synthetase reaction is rate limiting (Fig. 16-3). The committed step (5,10-methylene-FH_4 reductase) is feedback inhibited by S-adenosylmethionine and product inhibited by 5-methyl-FH_4. Methionine synthetase depends on the

transfer of labile methyl groups from 5-methyl-FH_4 to vitamin B_{12}, which, as methyl-B_{12}, serves as the immediate methyl donor for converting homocysteine to methionine. Without adequate vitamin B_{12} to accept methyl groups from 5-methyl-FH_4, that metabolite accumulates at the expense of the other metabolically active folate pools. This is known as the **methyl-folate trap**. The loss of FH_4 that results from this blockage in folate recycling blocks transfer of the histidine-formino group to folate (as **5-formimino-FH_4**) during the catabolism of that amino acid. This results in the accumulation of the intermediate formiminoglutamate (FIGLU). Thus, elevated urinary FIGLU levels after an oral histidine load are diagnostic of vitamin B_{12} deficiency.

Health Effects

Homocysteinemia

High circulating levels of homocysteine, which are estimated to occur in 5–7% of the U.S. population, have been associated with increased risks to cardiovascular disease, recurrent early pregnancy loss, and hip fracture. Accumulation of **homocysteine** can occur through elevated production of homocysteine from methionine and, probably to a lesser extent, through impaired disposal of homocysteine through transsulfuration to cystathionine. This results in **homocysteinemia**[36] and homocysteinuria.

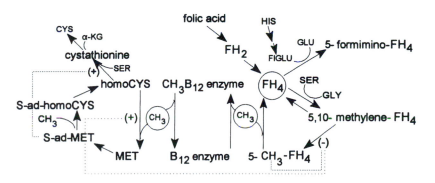

Fig. 16-3. Metabolic interrelationships of folate and vitamin B_{12}; basis of the "methyl folate trap." CYS, cysteine; α-KG, α-ketoglutarate; SER, serine; homoCYS, homocysteine; S-ad-homoCYS, S-adenosylhomocysteine; S-ad-MET, S-adenosylmethionine; MET, methionine.

---

[35] This is the sole *de novo* path of thymidylate synthesis. It is also the only folate-dependent reaction in which the cofactor serves as both a single-carbon donor and a reducing agent. Thymidylate synthase is the target of the anticancer drug 5-fluorouracil (5-FU). The enzyme converts the drug to 5-fluorodeoxyuridylate, which is incorporated into RNA and also is a suicide inhibitor of the synthetase. Inhibition of the synthetase results in the cellular accumulation of deoxyuridine triphosphate (dUTP), which is normally present at only very low concentrations, and the incorporation of deoxyuridine (dU) into DNA. DNA with this abnormal base is enzymatically cleaved at sites containing dU, leading to enhanced DNA breakage.

[36] Defined as a plasma concentration of homocysteine >14 μM.

Homocysteine can be converted to homocysteine thiolactone by methionyl tRNA synthetase, in an error-editing reaction that prevents its incorporation into the primary structure of proteins, but at high levels the thiolactone can react with protein lysyl residues. Protection against the damage to high-density lipoproteins that results from homocysteinylation is effected by a Ca^{++}-dependent homocysteine thiolactonase associated with those particles.[37]

Homocysteinemia can have congenital causes[38] and can also be related to nutritional status with respect to vitamin B_6, vitamin B_{12}, and folate.[39] It causes displacement of protein-bound cysteine, which results in changes in redox thiol status, probably via thiol–disulfide exchange and redox reactions. Such changes have also been observed in patients with cardiovascular disease, renal failure, or human immunodeficiency virus (HIV) infection, suggesting involvement of homocysteine-induced loss of extracellular antioxidant status in those disorders.

Experimental folate deprivation has been shown to cause elevated plasma homocysteine concentrations, and the use of folate-containing multivitamin supplements is associated with low mean plasma homocysteine levels. One prospective, community-based study found plasma homocysteine to be strongly inversely associated with plasma folate level (which was positively associated with the consumption of folate-containing breakfast cereals, fruits, and vegetables) and to be only weakly associated with plasma levels of vitamin B_{12} and pyridoxal phosphate (Table 16-8).[40] While early studies showed large regular doses of folate to reduce plasma homocysteine concentrations, more recent studies indicate that total folate (food + supplement) of 300–400 μg/day are necessary to support normal to low plasma homocysteine levels.

Homocysteinemia can respond to supplementation of folic acid. The relationship is linear up to daily folate intakes of about 0.4 mg. A meta-analysis of 25 randomized controlled trials showed that daily intakes of at least 0.8 mg folic acid are required to realize maximal reductions in plasma homocysteine levels (Table 16-9). The institution of population-wide folate supplementation has reduced homocysteine levels of Americans (Table 16-10). The MTHFR genotype can also affect plasma homocysteine levels: Individuals with the C677T T/T genotype have slightly lower levels of folate and slightly higher levels of homocysteine in comparison to other (C/C and C/T) genotypes (Table 16-11).

Table 16-8. Plasma homocysteine and vitamin levels in elderly subjects

Subject age (years)	Homocysteine		Folate (nM)	Vitamin B_{12} (pM)	Pyridoxal phosphate (nM)
	μM	Percent elevated			
			Men		
67–74	11.8	25.3	9.3	265	52.6
75–79	11.9	26.7	9.3	260	49.6
80+	14.1	48.3	10.0	255	47.6
Trend, p:	<0.001	<0.001	NS[a]	NS	NS
			Women		
67–74	10.7	19.5	10.4	302	59.9
75–79	11.9	28.9	10.2	289	52.2
80+	13.2	41.1	9.7	290	52.1
Trend, p:	<0.001	<0.001	NS	NS	NS

[a]NS, Not significant.

Source: Selhub, J., Jacques, P. F., Wilson, P. W., Rush, D., and Rosenberg, I. H. (1993). *J. Am. Med. Assoc.* **270**, 2693–2698.

---

[37] Jakubowski, H. (2000). *J. Nutr.* **130**, 377S–381S.

[38] Inherited deficiencies of cysteine β-synthase and 5,10-methylene FH_4 reductase have been identified in humans.

[39] Chronic alcoholics have been found to have mean serum homocysteine levels about half those of nonalcoholics. Chronic ethanol intake appears to interfere with single-carbon metabolism, and alcoholics are at risk of folate deficiency.

[40] Selhub, J., et al. (1996). *J. Nutr.* **126**, 1258S–1265S.

Table 16-9. Relationship of folic acid intake and plasma homocysteine reduction

Folic acid dose (mg/d)	% homocysteine reduction (95% CI)
0.8	13 (10–16)
0.9	20 (17–22)
0.10	23 (21–26)
2	23 (20–26)
5	25 (22–28)

Source: Homocysteine Lowering Trialists' Collaboration (2005). *Am. J. Clin. Nutr.* **82,** 806–812.

Cardiovascular disease

In 1969 Kilmer McCully pointed out a relationship between elevated plasma homocysteine levels and risk to occlusive vascular disease. Subsequently, epidemiologic studies have confirmed that relationship, demonstrating associations of moderate elevations in plasma homocysteine and risks of coronary, peripheral, and carotid arterial thrombosis and atherosclerosis, venous thrombosis, retinal vascular occlusion, carotid thickening, and hypertension (Table 16-12).[41] These observations are supported by studies in animal models that have shown folate deprivation to be thrombogenic. A meta-analysis of the results of 27 cross-sectional and case control studies[42] attributed 10% of total coronary artery disease to homocysteinemia. That analysis showed that a 5 μM increase in plasma homocysteine level increased the risk of coronary artery disease as much as a 0.5 mM (20 mg/dl) increase in total plasma cholesterol. More

recent considerations of available evidence suggest that homocysteinemia may not be a source of significant cardiovascular risk for healthy people, and prospective studies indicate that homocysteinemia is an important risk factor in high-risk subjects.

Cardiovascular end points have also been found to vary with plasma folate level independently of homocysteine. Furthermore, folate supplementation has been shown to reverse endothelial dysfunction independent of its effect in lowering plasma homocysteine level, and to reduce arterial pressure and increase coronary dilation. These effects likely involve the stimulation of nitric oxide production by 5-methylfolic acid, and perhaps also to inhibition of lipoprotein oxidation by folic acid.

Neural tube defects

Folate has an important role in normal embryogenesis, apparently involving its support of normal cell division. For some three decades, adequate folate status has been linked to reduced risks of abnormalities in early embryonic development and, specifically, to risk of malformations of the embryonic brain and/or spinal cord, collectively referred to as neural tube defects (NTDs).[43] These linkages have involved observations of high incidences of low-folate status among women with NTD birth compared to women with normal birth outcomes. Additional support came from the production of NTDs in animal models by the folate antagonist aminopterin. Seven clinical intervention trials have tested the hypothesis that supplemental folate can reduce NTD risk.

Table 16-10. Changes in plasma folate and homocysteine levels in the United States since the implementation of folate fortification of cereal foods

Survey year	Plasma folate		Plasma homocysteine	
	mean ± SE	% = 6.8 nmol/L	mean ± SE	% = 13 μmol/L
1988–1994	12.1 ± 0.3	18.4	8.7 ± 0.1	13.2
1999–2000	30.2 ± 0.7	0.8	7.0 ± 0.1	4.5
2001–2002	27.8 ± 0.5	0.2	7.3 ± 0.1	4.7

Source: Ganji, V., and Kafi, M. R. (2006). *J. Nutr.* **136,** 153–158.

---

[41] The low prevalence of coronary heart disease among South African blacks has been associated with their typically lower plasma homocysteine levels and their demonstrably more effective homocysteine clearance after methionine loading.

[42] Boushey, C. J., et al. (1995). *J. Am. Med. Assoc.* **274,** 1049–1057.

[43] Neural tube defects comprise the most common forms of congenital malformations, affecting 0.5–8 per 1000 live births. The term derives from the neural structures (brain, spinal cord, cranial bones, vertebral arches, meninges, overlying skin) formed from the embryonic neural tube in humans 20–28 days after fertilization. The most prominent neural tube defects are anencephaly and spina bifida. More than 95% of NTD pregnancies occur in families with no history of such defects; but women with one affected pregnancy or with spina bifida themselves face a risk of 3–4% of an NTD in a subsequent pregnancy.

Table 16-11. Relationship of MTHFR genotype to plasma folate and homocysteine levels

Genotype	N	Plasma folate (nmol/L)	Plasma homocysteine (μmol/L)
C/C	983	8.0 (3.4–22.2)[a]	12.9 (7.5–22.5)[a]
C/T	907	7.2 (2.5–20.9)	13.6 (8.1–33.4)
T/T	206	6.3 (2.6–26.6)	17.1 (8.1–67.1)

[a]Mean (95% CI).
Source: de Bree, A., et al. (2003). *Am. J. Clin. Nutr.* **77,** 687–693.

Table 16-12. Plasma homocysteine levels in myocardial infarction cases and controls

Parameter	Cases	Controls
Plasma homocysteine (nM)	11.1 ± 4.0	10.5 ± 2.8[a]
Cases ≥95th percentile in terms of homocysteine level	31	13
n (total number of cases)	271	271

[a]$p = 0.026$.
Source: Stamper, F. M. J., Malinow, M. R., Willett, W. C., Newcomer, L. M., Upson, B., Ullman, D., Tishler, P. V., and Hennekens, C. H. (1992). *J. Am. Med. Assoc.* **268,** 877–881.

One of these, a large, well-designed, multicentered trial conducted by the British Medical Research Council, found that a daily oral dose of 4 mg of folic acid reduced significantly the incidence of confirmed NTDs among the pregnancies of women at high risk for such disorders.[44]

The results of several studies (Table 16-13) show consistent protective effects of folates, indicating that periconceptual supplementation of the vitamin can reduce the risk of serious birth defects by as much as half. The largest controlled trial, conducted with some 250,000 subjects in China, showed that a daily supplement containing 400 μg folic acid, consumed with at least 80% compliance beginning before the periconceptual period, was associated with reductions in NTD risk of 85% in a high-prevalence area and 40% in a low-prevalence one.[45] Studies in the United States demonstrated the efficacy of folate supplements (400–4000 μg) in preventing second NTDs in women with prior NTD pregnancies.[46] A recent meta-analysis of four randomized, controlled trials concluded that periconceptional folate supplementation has a strong protective effect against NTDs.[47]

In consideration of this evidence, in 1992 the United States Public Health Service issued a recommendation that all women of childbearing age consume 0.4 mg folic acid daily to reduce their risks of an NTD pregnancy. In the following year, the United

Table 16-13. Results of placebo-controlled, clinical intervention trials of folate supplements in the prevention of neural tube defects

Study	Folate supplement	NTD rates, cases/total pregnancies		RR (95% CI)
		Placebo	Treatment	
Laurence et al. (1981)[a]	4 mg	4/51	2/60	0.42 (0.04–2.97)
Milunsky et al. (1989)[b]	4 mg ± multivitamins	21/602	6/593	0.34 (0.10–0.74)
Czeizel and Fritz (1992)[c]	0.8 mg + multivitamins	2/2104	0/2052	0.00 (0.00–0.85)

[a]Laurence, K. M., James, M., Miller, M. H., Tennant, G. B., and Campbell, H. (1981). *Br. Med. J.* **280,** 1509–1511 (women with NTD histories).
[b]Milunsky, A., Jick, H., Jick, S. S., Bruell, C. L., McLaughlin, D. S., Rothman, K. J., and Willett, W. (1989). *J. Am. Med. Assoc.* **262,** 2847–2852 (women with NTD histories).
[c]Czeizel, A. E., and Fritz, I. (1992). *J. Am. Med. Assoc.* **262,** 1634 (women without previous NTD births).

---

[44] The double-blind, randomized clinical trial involved 1817 women, each with a previous affected pregnancy, who were followed in 33 clinics in 7 countries. Each subject was randomly assigned to treatments consisting of a placebo or a multivitamin supplement (A, D, C, B_6, thiamin, riboflavin, and nicotinamide) and/or a placebo or folic acid (4 mg/day) in a complete factorial design, and the outcomes of their pregnancies were confirmed. Of a total of 1195 completed pregnancies, 27 had confirmed neural tube defects; these included 21 cases in both groups not receiving folate, but only 6 cases in both folate groups (relative risk, 0.28; 95% CI, 0.12–0.71). The multivitamin treatment did not significantly affect the incidence of NTDs (MRC Vitamin Research Group [1991]. *Lancet* **338,** 131–137).

[45] Berry, R. J., et al. (1999). *N. Eng. J. Med.* **341,** 1485–1490.

[46] Centers for Disease Control and Prevention (2000). *Morbid. Mortal. Weekly Rep.* **49,** 1–4; Stevenson, R. E., et al. (2000). *Pediatrics* **106,** 677–683.

[47] Lumley, J., et al. (2001). *Cochrane Database Syst. Rev.* CD001056.

States Food and Drug Administration ruled that all cereal grain products produced in that country be fortified with 140 µg folic acid per 100 g, and that additions of folic acid be allowed for breakfast cereals, infant formulas, medical and special dietary foods, and meal replacement products. Other countries have developed similar policies. Recent reviews[48] concluded that countries practicing folate fortification have experienced significant reductions in the incidence of NTDs as a result: United States, 19–31%; Costa Rica, 63–87%; Canada, 47–54%.

Although high levels of folate appear to reduce the risk of NTDs, the minimum effective dose has not been determined. Questions remain as to whether lower doses of the vitamin may also be effective, whether folate can reduce the incidence of NTDs among women without previous affected pregnancies, and whether such a high level of folate has significant side effects. Also, the mechanism of folate action in reducing the incidence of these birth defects remains unclear.

The metabolic basis of the protective effect of folate against teratogenic effects is not clear. It does not appear to involve differences in folate absorption, as women with histories of NTD births have been found to absorb the vitamin at rates comparable to those of women without NTD histories. Furthermore, severe, uncomplicated folate deficiency produces no neural tube changes in mice; and folic acid supplements have been shown to increase the incidence of brain and meningeal abnormalities and cleft palate in the fetuses of zinc-deficient rats.

Other serious pregnancy complications

Low-folate status has been associated with other congenital defects, including cleft lip and palate and defective development of limbs and the heart. Homocysteinemia has been associated with increased risks of hypertension, preeclampsia, and placental abruption.

Erythropoiesis

Folate is required for the production of new erythrocytes through its functions in the synthesis of purines and thymidylate required for DNA synthesis as well as through its function in regenerating methionine, the methyl donor for DNA methylation. The essen-

tiality of folate for the synthesis and repair of DNA is evidenced by the effects of folate deficiency: arrest of erythropoiesis prior to the late stages of differentiation, resulting in apoptotic reduction of cells surviving to postmitotic, terminal stages in the condition called megaloblastic anemia. That anemia can have folate-responsive components in subjects with apparently normal plasma folate levels, as indicated by the fact that addition of folate to iron supplements can improve the treatment of anemia pregnancy.

DNA methylation

Folate appears to have a role in the methylation of DNA by virtue of its function in single-carbon metabolism, as the methylation of cytosine is important in regulating gene transcription. Folate deprivation has been found to produce chromosomal breaks in megaloblastic bone marrow, reflecting DNA strand breaks and hypomethylation. The hypomethylation of DNA is believed to alter chromatin structure in ways that increase mutation rates. One study found hypomethylation within exons 5–8[49] of the *p53* gene; although genomewide hypomethylation was not observed, the deficiency was found to produce genomewide DNA strand breakage. Such results suggest that folate deficiency may affect carcinogenesis by creating fragile sites in the genome and potentially inducing proto-oncogene expression. A recent study showed that low-folate subjects with the T/T variant of MTHFR C677T polymorphism had relative hypomethylation of whole-blood DNA, compared to those with the C/C variant; those differences were not apparent among folate-adequate subjects of both genotypes.[50]

Cancer

Folate deprivation, by enhancing genomic instability and dysregulated gene transcription, appears to enhance predisposition to neoplastic transformation. Accordingly, low-folate status has been associated with increased risk of cancers of the colon, cervix, lung, oral and pharyngeal, head and neck, stomach and gastrointestinal tract, and brain. The best studied of these is colorectal cancer, for which ecological and case-control evidence suggests a protective effect of

---

[48] Yetley, E. A., and Rader, J. I. (2004). *Nutr. Rev.* **62,** S50–S59; Chen, L. T., and Rivera, M. A. (2004). *Nutr. Rev.* **62,** S40–S43; Mills, J. L., and Signore, C. (2004). *Birth Defects Res.* (Pt. A) **70,** 844–845.

[49] This region has been identified as one highly probable to undergo neoplastic transformation.

[50] Frisco, S., et al. (2002). *Proc. Nat. Acad. Sci.* **99,** 5606–5611.

the vitamin. These data also suggest that the protective effects of folate can be diminished by alcohol. Two large epidemiological studies have indicated that folate adequacy may reduce the effect of alcohol consumption in elevating breast cancer risk.[51] The results of a case-control study of women with mild to moderate cervical dysplasia support the hypothesis of a role of low-folate status as a risk factor: women infected with human papilloma virus showed a five-fold greater risk of dysplasia when they also had low serum folates compared with high levels.[52] Protective effects of folate against carcinogenesis have been indicated in animal tumor model studies, which have shown that folate deficiency serves as an effective co-carcinogen in colonic carcinogenesis.

Folate deprivation, by limiting cell proliferation, can impair the growth of established tumors. Accordingly, the MTHFR C677T T/T and the A1298C C/C genotypes are associated with moderate reductions in colorectal cancer risks.[53] It is thought that these genotypic effects relate to differences in relatively smaller associated thymidylate pools. Thus, the question has been raised as to whether populationwide folate fortification may have cancer-promoting effects.[54]

Immune function

That folate status may affect immune cell function is suggested by findings that folate deprivation of lymphocytes *in vitro* causes depletion of interleukin-2 and stimulates p53-independent apoptosis. Similar effects have not been observed *in vivo*. It has been noted that folate supplementation can stimulate natural killer (NK) cell cytotoxicity among subjects of low-folate status. Curiously, the opposite effect was observed among subjects consuming a high-folate diet, in whom NK cytotoxicity was inversely related to the plasma concentration of the nonmetabolized form of the vitamin, folic acid.[55]

Cognitive function

Folate is required to maintain homocysteine at low levels in the central nervous system. Hyperhomocysteinemia has been associated with increased risks to psychiactic and neurodegenerative disorders including depression, schizophrenia, Alzheimer's disease and Parkinson's disease. Studies have shown several ways homocysteine can be neurotoxic: through inhibition of methyltransferases involved in catecholamine methylation by the metabolite S-adenosylhomocysteine; through enhanced excitotoxicity leading to cell death by homocysteine oxidation products that act as agonists of the N-methyl-D-aspartate receptor; through oxidative stress resulting from the production of reactive oxygen species generated by the oxidation of homocysteine. Folate may also be directly involved in the regulation of neurotransmitter metabolism, as neuropsychiatric subjects with low erythrocyte folate levels and hyperhomocysteinemia have been found to show low cerebral spinal fluid levels of the serotonin metabolite 5-hydroxyindole acetic acid and reduced turnover of dopamine and noradrenaline. It has been suggested that folate may affect the metabolism of monamine neurotransmitters as a structural analog of tetrahydrobiopterin,[56] an essential cofactor in that metabolic pathway, and that the enzymes of folate metabolism, MTHFR, and dihydrofolate reductase may also function in tetrahydrobiopterin metabolism.

That cognitive impairment has been found to be correlated to plasma homocysteine level, but not to biomarkers of folate and/or vitamin B_{12} status, has raised questions about the clinical significance of those vitamins with respect to these outcomes. In fact, clinical studies of folate treatment have yielded mixed results. A systematic review of four randomized, controlled trials concluded that folic acid yielded no beneficial effects on measures of cognition or mood in older, healthy women;[57] but another review, of three randomized trials, suggested that folic acid may benefit the treatment of depression.[58]

---

[51] Zhang, S., et al. (1999). *J. Am. Med. Assoc.* **281**, 1632–1637; Rohan, T. E., et al. (2000). *J. Nat. Cancer Inst.* **92**, 266–269.

[52] Butterworth, C. E. J. et al. *J. Am. Med. Assoc.* **267**, 528–533; Liu, T., et al. (1993). *Cancer Epidemiol. Biomarkers Prev.* **2**, 525–530.

[53] Kono, S., and Chen, K. (2005). *Cancer Sci.* **96**, 535–542.

[54] Kim, Y. I. (2004). *Am. J. Clin. Nutr.* **80**, 1123–1128.

[55] Troen, A. M., et al. (2006). *J. Nutr.* **136**, 189–194.

[56] Both contain a pterin moiety.

[57] Malouf, M., et al. (2003). *Cochrande Database Syst. Rev.* CD004514.

[58] Taylor, M.J., et al (2004). *J. Psychopharmacol.* **18**, 251–256.

MTHFR polymorphisms

Genetic polymorphisms have been identified in the human MTHFR: a C/T substitution of base pair 677 (C677T); an A/C substitution of base pair 1298 (A1298C) (Table 16-14).

- *C677T* The C677T polymorphism is abundant in Caucasian and Asian populations, but is rare among African Americans. Individuals homozygous for the variant (T/T) have a form of MTHFR with lower specific activity, lower affinity for the flavin cofactor, and lower thermal stability[59] than the C/C form of the enzyme. They also show reduced plasma folate concentrations and mild homocysteinemia (Table 16-15). The distribution of cellular single-carbon units appears to be altered in T/T individuals: when fed a low-folate diet, individuals of the T/T genotype more frequently (44%) showed elevations in plasma homocysteine than did those of the C/T (20%) or C/C (15%) genotypes.[60] Individuals of the T/T genotype show the greatest homocysteine-lowering responses to folate supplements. These results suggest that substantial numbers of individuals may have elevated needs for folate.

- *A1298C* The allele frequencies of the A1298C polymorphism are similar to those of the C667T polymorphism. The A1298C polymorphism appears to be without significant physiological consequence unless combined with the C667T polymorphism; doubly heterozygous individuals have been found to have MTHFR specific activities of two-thirds those of doubly homozygous individuals.[61]

MTHFR polymorphisms have been related to various diseases.

- *Vascular disease* The T/T C677T MTHFR genotype has been identified as a risk factor for carotid intima-media thickening, a risk factor to vascular disease. One meta-analysis of 53 studies of MTHFR C677T genotype showed the T/T genotype to be associated with a 20% greater risk of venous thrombosis compared to the C/C genotype;[62] but another meta-analysis found the available evidence inconclusive.[63]

- *NTDs* The protective effect of folate supplementation against NTD risk may be limited to a subset of subjects with defective folate metabolism caused by MTHFR mutations. The T/T C677T genotype is associated with NTD risk, but the effect appears to be dependent on folate status. In

Table 16-14. Polymorphisms of proteins related to folate absorption and metabolism

Enzyme	Mutation	Wild-type	Genotype: frequency	
			Mutant homozygote	heterozygote
MTHFR	T6557C	C/C: 41%	T/T: 18%	C/T: 41%
	C1289A	A/A: 53%	C/C: 9%	A/C: 37%
brush border conjugase	T1561C	C/C: 92%	T/T: 0[a]	C/T: 8%
reduced folate transporter	G80A	A/A: 35%	G/G: 18%	A/G: 47%
methionine synthase	G2756A	A/A: 59%	G/G: 3%	A/G: 38%
methionine synthase reductase	G66A	A/A: 28%	G/G: 23%	A/G: 49%

[a]1 in 625 reported.
Source: Molloy, A. M. (2002). *J. Vit. Nutr. Res.* **72,** 46–52.

[59] For this reason the variant is frequently referred to as the "thermolabile enzyme."

[60] Kauwell, G. P. A., et al. (2000). *Metabolism* **49,** 1440–1443.

[61] Chango, A., et al. (2000). *Br. J. Nutr.* **83,** 593–596.

[62] Den Heijer, M., et al. (2005). *J. Thrombosis Haemostasis* **3,** 292–299.

[63] Lewis, S. J., et al. (2005). **doi,** 10.1136/bmj.e8611.658947.55

Table 16-15. Effect of 5,10-methylene-FH_4 reductase genotype on parameters of homocysteine, vitamin B_{12}, and folate status in humans

Metabolite	Genotype		
	−/−	+/−	+/+
Homocysteine (μM)	13.4 ± 3.4	13.2 ± 3.1	17.1 ± 11.5
Vitamin B_{12} (pM)	246 ± 130	271 ± 121	233 ± 94
Erythrocyte folate (nM)	541 ± 188	517 ± 182	643 ± 186
Plasma folate (nM)	12.8 ± 6.5	12.8 ± 6.7	9.5 ± 3.1

Source: van der Put, N. M., Stelgers-Theunissen, R. P., Frost, P., Trijbels, F. J., Estes, T. K., van Heuval, L. P., Mariman, E. C., den Heyer, M., Roger, R., and Bloom, H. J. (1995). *Lancet* **346,** 1070–1071.

a recent analysis, T/T homozygosity was associated with a fivefold increase in NTD risk for mothers not using multivitamin supplements, but was without effect for mothers using supplements.[64]

- *Down syndrome* Evidence suggests that T/T C677T genotype elevates risk in individuals also carrying a mutation in methionine synthase reductase; such individuals have also been found to have elevated risks of Down syndrome.[65]
- *Cognitive disorders* Studies have shown that individuals of the T/T C677T genotype have increased risks of depression and schizophrenia.
- *Cancer* Homozygosity for T/T C677T MTHFR has consistently been found to be associated with reduced risk for colorectal cancer.[66] The T/T genotype does not appear to affect risk for colorectal adenoma unless folate status is low, in which case it is related to increased risk. The T/T genotype has also been associated with increased risk for lymphocytic leukemia; these risks appear to be even greater in individuals with the combined C677T/A1298C heterozygous genotype.[67] Studies of the relationship of the MTHFR A1298C genotype on colorectal cancer have yielded variable results.
- *Methotrexate therapy* Individuals with the T/T C677T genotype have a higher risk of discontinuing methotrexate treatment for rheumatoid arthritis owing to adverse effects. In contrast,

individuals with the C/C A1298C genotype typically show improved efficacy of methotrexate therapy without increased side effects.

- *Bone mineral density* One study found that women of the T/T C677T genotype showed reduced bone mineral density if they had relatively low intakes of folate, vitamin B_{12}, and riboflavin.[68]

Masking vitamin B_{12} deficiency

High-level intakes of folate can interfere with the clinical diagnosis of vitamin B_{12} deficiency by preventing the common presenting sign, megaloblastic anemia. This phenomenon renders that sign as insufficient for diagnosing either deficiency without accompanying metabolic measurements of MMA (elevations of which indicate vitamin B_{12} deficiency) and FIGLU (elevations of which indicate folate deficiency). Folate supplementation does not mask the irreversible progression of neurological dysfunction and cognitive decline of vitamin B_{12} deficiency; but those signs develop over a longer timeline than does the anemia produced by the deficiency. Because vitamin B_{12} deficiency is estimated to affect 10–15% of the American population over 60 years. of age, the amount of folate for the fortification of wheat flour (140μg/100g flour) in the United States was chosen to provide an amount of added folate (100μg/person/day) sufficient for only a small proportion of the general

---

[64] Botto, L. D., et al. (1999). *Am. J. Epidemiol.* **150,** 323–324.

[65] Hobbs, C. A., et al. (2000). *Am. J. Hum. Genet.* **67,** 623–630.

[66] Kono, S., and Chen, K. (2005). *Cancer Sci.* **96,** 535–542.

[67] Skibola, C. F., et al. (1999). *Proc. Nat. Acad. Sci.* **96,** 12810–12834.

[68] Abrahamsen, B., et al. (2005). *Bone* **36,** 577–583.

population receiving a level (>1 mg/day) capable of masking vitamin B_{12} deficiency.

VII. Folate Deficiency

Contributing Factors to Folate Deficiency

The most important factor contributing to folate deficiency is insufficient dietary intake. Other factors can contribute, particularly when combined with low dietary intake of the vitamin. Those factors are shown in Table 16-16.

General Signs of Folate Deficiency

Deficiencies of folate result in impaired biosynthesis of DNA and RNA, and thus in reduced cell division, which is manifested clinically as anemia, dermatologic lesions, and poor growth in most species. The anemia of folate deficiency is characterized by the presence of large, nucleated erythrocyte-precursor cells, called macrocytes, and of hypersegmented[69] polymorphonuclear neutrophils, reflecting decreased DNA synthesis and delayed maturation of bone marrow.

Table 16-16. Contributing factors to folate deficiency

Poor dietary intake

Malabsorption

    Intestinal diseases: tropical sprue, celiac disease

    Gastric diseases: atrophic gastritis

    Drugs: alcohol, sulfasalazine, p-aminosalicylic acid, gastric acid-suppressants

    Genetic: hereditary folate malabsorption

Metabolic impairments

    Acquired: dihydrofolate reductase inhibitors (e.g., methotrexate); alcohol; sulfasalazine

    Genetic: methylenetetrahydrofolate reductase deficiency; glutamate formiminotransferase deficiency; methylenetetrahydrofolate reductase polymorphisms

Increased requirements: hemodialysis; prematurity; pregnancy; lactation

While clinical deficiency is usually detected as anemia, megaloblastic changes occur in other cells. These involve increased cellular DNA content, with defects characterized by DNA strand breakage and growth arrest in the G2 phase of the cell cycle just prior to mitosis. These defects are thought to result from the misincorporation of uracil into DNA in place of thymidylate—a potentially mutagenic situation.

Severely anemic individuals show weakness, fatigue, difficulty in concentrating, irritability, headache, palpitations, and shortness of breath. Folate deficiency also affects the intestinal epithelium, where impaired DNA synthesis causes megaloblastosis of enterocytes. This is manifested clinically as malabsorption and diarrhea, and is a contributor to the clinical picture of tropical sprue.

Signs and/or symptoms of folate deficiency are observed among individuals consuming inadequate dietary levels of the vitamin (Table 16-17). These effects are exacerbated by physiological conditions that increase folate needs (e.g., pregnancy, lactation, rapid growth), by drug treatments that reduce folate utilization, by aging, and by diseases of the intestinal mucosa.[70]

Methionine–Folate Linkage

Folate utilization is impaired by insufficient supplies of vitamin B_{12} and/or the indispensable amino acid methionine; therefore, dietary deficiencies of either of those nutrients can produce signs of folate deficiency. Patients with **pernicious anemia**[71] generally have impaired folate utilization and show signs of folate deficiency. The metabolic basis of this effect involves the **methionine synthetase** reaction, which is common to the functions of both folate and vitamin B_{12}. Methionine supplements cannot correct the low circulating folate levels caused by vitamin B_{12} deficiency. The amino acid appears to exert its action via S-adenosylmethionine, which inhibits 5,10-methylene-FH_4 reductase (thus reducing the *de novo* synthesis of 5-methyl-FH_4) and activates methionine synthetase.

---

[69] Neutrophil hypersegmentation is defined as >5% five-lobed or any six-lobed cells per 100 granulocytes.

[70] Examples include *tropical sprue* (inflammation of the mucous membranes of the alimentary tract) and other types of enteritis that involve malabsorption and, usually, diarrhea.

[71] Pernicious anemia is vitamin B_{12} deficiency resulting from the lack of the intrinsic factor required for the enteric absorption of that vitamin (see Chapter 17).

Table 16-17.   General signs of folate deficiency

Organ system	Signs
General	
Appetite	Decrease
Growth	Decrease
Dermatologic	Alopecia, achromotrichia, dermatitis
Muscular	Weakness
Gastrointestinal	Inflammation
Vascular	
Erythrocytes	Macrocytic anemia
Nervous	Depression, neuropathy, paralysis

Relationship with Zinc

Folate utilization can be impaired by depletion of zinc. Dietary zinc deficiency has been found in humans to reduce the absorption of folyl polyglutamates (*not* monoglutamates) and in animals to reduce liver folates. This is thought to indicate a need for zinc by the enzymes of folate metabolism. Studies have yielded inconsistent but mostly negative results concerning the effects of folate deficiency on zinc metabolism.

Deficiency Syndromes in Animals

Folate deficiency in animals is generally associated with poor growth, anemia, and dermatologic lesions involving skin and hair/feathers (Table 16-12). In chicks, severe anemia is one of the earliest signs of the deficiency. The anemia is of the macrocytic (megaloblastic) type, involving abnormally large erythrocyte size (the normal range in humans is 82–92 μm³) due to the presence of **megaloblasts**, which are also seen among the hyperplastic erythroid cells in the bone marrow. Anemia in folate deficiency is followed by **leukopenia** (abnormally low numbers of white

blood cells), poor growth, very poor feathering, perosis, lethargy, and reduced feed intake. Poultry with normally pigmented plumage[72] show achromotrichia due to the deficiency. Folate-deficient turkey poults show a spastic type of **cervical paralysis** in which the neck is held rigid.[73] Folate-deficient guinea pigs show leukopenia and depressed growth; pigs and monkeys show alopecia, dermatitis, leukopenia, anemia, and diarrhea; mink show ulcerative hemorrhagic gastritis, diarrhea, anorexia, and leukopenia. The deficiency is not easily produced in rodents unless a **sulfa drug**[74] or folate antagonist is fed, in which case leukopenia is the main sign.[75] Folate-responsive signs (reduced weight gain, macrocytic anemia) can be produced in catfish by feeding them succinylsulfathiazole. Folate deficiency in the rat has been shown to reduce exocrine function of the pancreas, in which single-carbon metabolism is important.[76]

Deficiency Signs in Humans

Folate deficiency in humans is characterized by a sequence of signs, starting with nuclear hypersegmentation of circulating polymorphonuclear leukocytes[77] within about two months of deprivation of the vitamin. This is followed by megaloblastic anemia and, then, general weakness, depression, and polyneuropathy. In pregnant women, the deficiency can lead to birth defects or spontaneous abortion. Elderly humans tend to have lower circulating levels of folate, indicating that they may be at increased risk of folate deficiency. Although the basis of this finding is not fully elucidated, it appears to involve age-related factors such as food habits that affect intake of the vitamin rather than its utilization.

That folate-responsive homocysteinemia can be demonstrated in apparently healthy free-living populations suggests the prevalence of undiagnosed suboptimal vitamin status. For example, twice-weekly treatments of elderly subjects with folate (1.1 mg) in combination with **vitamin B₁₂** (1 mg) and vitamin B₆

---

[72] Such breeds include the barred Plymouth Rock, the Rhode Island red, and the black Leghorn.

[73] Poults with cervical paralysis may not show anemia; the condition is fatal within a couple of days of onset, but responds dramatically (within 15 min) to parenteral administration of the vitamin.

[74] For example, sulfanilamide.

[75] Although leukopenia was manifested relatively soon after experimental folate depletion, rats kept alive with small doses of folate eventually also develop macrocytic anemia.

[76] Experimental pancreatitis can be produced in that species by treatment with ethionine, an inhibitor of cellular methylation reactions, or by feeding a diet deficient in choline.

[77] These cytological changes do not become manifest until well after circulating folate levels drop (by 6–8 weeks).

(5 mg) have been shown to reduce plasma concentrations of homocysteine by as much as half and also to reduce methylmalonic acid, 2-methylcitric acid, and cystathionine, despite the fact that their pretreatment plasma levels of those vitamins were not low.

Effects of Drugs

Several drugs can impair the absorption and metabolism of folates. These have proven to have clinical applications, ranging from the treatment of autoimmune diseases, to cancer and to malaria[78]—all instances in which cell proliferation can be suppressed through the inhibition of a folate-dependent step in single-carbon metabolism.

- *Methotrexate* Methotrexate, also called amethopterin, is an analog of folate, differing in two ways: the presence of an amino group replacing the 4-hydroxyl group on the pteridine ring and a methyl group at the N-10 position. These differences give methotrexate a greater affinity than the natural substrate for dihydrofolate reductase, resulting in its inhibition. Accordingly, the drug produces an effective folate deficiency, with reductions in thymidine synthesis and purines. This antiproliferative effect is the basis for the drug's role in the treatment of cancer, rheumatoid arthritis, psoriasis, asthma, and inflammatory bowel disease. Because side effects include those of folate deficiency, methotrexate is usually used with accompanying and carefully monitored folate supplementation to reduce the incidence of mucosal and gastrointestinal side effects.
- *5-Fluorouracil* The antineoplastic drug 5-fluorouracil is a substrate for thymidylate synthase, being incorporated into the nucleotide as 5-fluorodeoxyuridylate instead of dUMP. The abnormal product binds covalently with the enzyme to inhibit DNA synthesis.
- *Other drugs* Impairments in folate status/metabolism have been reported for anticonvulsants (diphenylhydantoin, phenobarbital), antiinflammatory drugs (sulfasalazine), glycemic control drugs (metformin), and alcohol.

VIII. Pharmacologic Uses of Folate

High doses of folate (e.g., 400 µg/day intramuscular; 5 mg/day oral) have been shown to correct the megaloblastic anemia of pernicious anemia patients. However, because folate does not affect the neurological lesions of pernicious anemia or vitamin B_{12} deficiency, it can, by correcting anemia, mask an underlying problem of vitamin B_{12} nutrition in its early (and more easily treated) stages.

Folate at treatment can also be effective in reducing elevated and normal plasma homocysteine levels. This effect may be realized with doses <1 mg; it appears to be greater when the vitamin is given in combination with vitamin B_{12}. High doses of 5-methylfolate have been found to benefit patients with acute psychiatric disorders.[79] Both depressed and schizophrenic patients responded to daily doses of 15 mg of 5-methylfolate with improved clinical and social outcomes compared with placebo controls.[80]

The U.S. Food and Drug Administration has recommended that women who have had a neural tube defect pregnancy should take 4 mg of folate daily. In addition, the agency has proposed adding folate to enriched breads, flours, corn meals, pastas, rice, and other grain products to achieve a target daily intake, for all women 15–44 years of age, of 0.4–1.0 mg of folate.

Individuals taking high-level folate supplements typically circulate significant amounts of nonmetabolized folic acid, which does not occur at nutritional doses of the vitamin.

IX. Folate Toxicity

No adverse effects of high oral doses of folate have been reported in animals, although parenteral administration of pharmacologic amounts (e.g., 250 mg/kg, which is about 1000 times the dietary requirement) has been shown to produce epileptic responses and

---

[78] Antifolates remain the first-line drug in the treatment of malaria worldwide. Unfortunately, the malarial parasite *Plasmodium falciparum* has developed resistance through mutations in dihydrofolate reductase (see Gregson, A., and Lpowe, C. G. [2005]. *Pharmacol. Rev.* **57,** 117–145).

[79] Nearly two-thirds of patients with megaloblastic anemia due to vitamin B_{12}/folate deficiency show neuropsychiatric complications.

[80] Godfrey, P. S., et al. (1990). *Lancet* **336,** 392–395.

renal hypertrophy in rats. Inconsistent results have been reported concerning the effects of high-folate levels (1- to 10-mg doses) on human epileptics. Some have indicated increases in the frequency or severity of seizures and reduced anticonvulsant effectiveness,[81] whereas others have shown no such effects. It has also been suggested that folate may form a nonabsorbable complex with zinc, thus antagonizing the utilization of that essential trace element at high intakes of the vitamin. Because studies with animal models have shown that folate treatment can exacerbate teratogenic effects of nutritional zinc deficiency, which is thought to be prevalent but is seldom detected in some areas and population groups, some have urged caution in recommending folate supplements to pregnant women.

X. Case Study

Instructions

Review the following case report, paying special attention to the diagnostic indicators on which the treatments were based. Then, answer the questions that follow.

Case

A 15-year-old girl was admitted to the hospital because of progressive withdrawal, hallucinations, anorexia, and tremor. Her early growth and development were normal, and she had done average schoolwork until she was 11 years old, when her family moved to a new area. The next year, she experienced considerable difficulty in concentrating and was found to have an IQ of 60. She was placed in a special education program, where she began to fight with other children and have temper tantrums; when punished, she became withdrawn and stopped eating. A year earlier, she had experienced an episode of severe abdominal pain for which no cause could be found, and she was referred to a mental health clinic. Her psychologic examination at that time had revealed inappropriate giggling, poor reality testing, and loss of contact with her surroundings. Her verbal and performance IQs were then 46 and 50, respectively. She was treated with thioridazine[82] and,

Laboratory findings

Parameter	Patient	Normal range
Electroencephalogram	Diffusely slow	
Spinal fluid		
Protein (mg/dl)	42	15–45
Cells	None	None
Urine		
Homocystine	Elevated	
Methionine	Normal	
Serum		
Homocystine	Elevated	
Methionine	Normal	
Folate (ng/ml)	3	5–21
Vitamin B_{12} (pg/ml)	800	150–900
Hematology		
Hemoglobin (g/dl)	12.1	11.5–14.5
Hematocrit (%)	39.5	37–45
Reticulocytes (%)	1	~1
Bone marrow	No megaloblastosis	

within 2 weeks, she ate and slept better and was helpful around the house. However, over the succeeding months, while she continued taking thioridazine, her functioning fluctuated and the diagnosis of catatonic schizophrenia was confirmed. Three months before the present admission, she had become progressively withdrawn and drowsy, and needed to be fed, bathed, and dressed. She also experienced visual hallucinations, feelings of persecution, and night terrors. On having a seizure, she was taken to the hospital.

Her physical examination on admission revealed a tall, thin girl with fixed stare and catatonic posturing, but no neurologic abnormalities. She was mute and withdrawn, incontinent, and appeared to have visual and auditory hallucinations. Her muscle tone varied from normal to diffusely rigid.

On the assumption that her homocysteinuria was due to cystathionase deficiency, she was treated with pyridoxine HCl (300 mg/day, orally) for 10 days. Her homocysteinuria did not respond; however, her mental status improved and, within 4 days, she was able to conduct some conversation and her hallucinations seemed to decrease. She developed new neurological

---

[81] High doses of folate appear to interfere with diphenylhydantoin absorption.

[82] An antischizophrenic drug.

signs: foot and wrist droop and gradual loss of reflexes. She was then given folate (20 mg/day orally) for 14 days because of her low serum folate level. This resulted in a marked decrease in her urinary homocystine and a progressive improvement in intellectual function over the next 3 months. She remained severely handicapped by her peripheral neuropathy, but she showed no psychotic symptoms. After 5 months of folate and pyridoxine treatment, she was tranquil and retarded, but showed no psychotic behavior; she left the hospital against medical advice and without medication.

The girl was readmitted to the hospital 7 months later (a year after her first admission), with a 2-month history of progressive withdrawal, hallucinations, delusions, and refusal to eat. The general examination was the same as on her first admission, with the exceptions that she had developed hyperreflexia and her peripheral neuropathy had improved slightly. Her mental functioning was at the 2-year-old level. She was incontinent, virtually mute, and had visual and auditory hallucinations. She was diagnosed as having simple schizophrenia of the childhood type. Folate and pyridoxine therapy was started again; it resulted in her decreased homocysteine excretion and gradual improvement in mental performance. After 2 months of therapy in the hospital, she was socializing, free of hallucinations, and able to feed herself and recognize her family. At that time, the activities of several enzymes involved in methionine metabolism were measured in her fibroblasts and liver tissue (obtained by biopsy).

Enzyme activities

| Enzyme | Tissue or cell type | Enzyme activity[a] | |
		Patient	Normal
Methionine adenyltransferase	Liver	20.6	4.3–14.5
Cystathionine-β-synthetase	Fibroblasts	25.9	3.7–65.0
Betaine:homocysteine methyltransferase	Liver	26.7	1.2–16.0
5-Methyl FH_4:homocysteine methyltransferase	Fibroblasts	3.5	2.9–7.3
5,10-Methylene FH_4 reductase	Fibroblasts	0.5	1.0–4.6

[a]Enzyme units.

Thereafter, she was maintained on oral folate (10 mg/day). She has been free of homocysteinuria and psychotic manifestations for several years.

Case Questions

1. On admission of this patient to the hospital, which of her symptoms were consistent with an impairment in a folate-dependent aspect of metabolism?

2. What finding appeared to counterindicate an impairment in folate metabolism in this case?

3. Propose a hypothesis for the metabolic basis of the observed efficacy of oral folate treatment in this case.

Study Questions and Exercises

1. Diagram the metabolic conversions involving folates in single-carbon metabolism.

2. Construct a decision tree for the diagnosis of folate deficiency in humans or an animal species. In particular, outline a way to distinguish folate and vitamin B_{12} deficiencies in patients with macrocytic anemia.

3. What key feature of the chemistry of folate relates to its biochemical function as a carrier of single-carbon units?

4. What parameters might you measure to assess folate status of a human or animal?

Recommended Reading

Bailey, L. B. (ed.). (1995). *Folate in Health and Disease*, 469 pp. Marcel Dekker, New York.

Bailey, L. B., Moyers, S., and Gregory, J. F. (2001). Folate. Chapter 21 in *Present Knowledge in Nutrition* 8th ed. (B. A. Bowman and R. M. Russell, eds.), pp. 214–229. ILSI Press, Washington, DC.

Bottiglieri, T. (2005). Homocysteine and folate metabolism in depression. *Prog. Neuro-Psychopharmacol.* **29,** 1103–1112.

Brody, T., and Shane, B. (2001). Folic acid, Chapter 12 in *Handbook of Vitamins*, 3rd ed. (R. B. Rucker, J. W. Suttie, D. B. McCormick, and L. J. Machlin, eds.), pp. 427–462. Marcel Dekker, New York.

Carmel, R. (2006). Folic acid, Chapter 28 in *Modern Nutrition in Health and Disease*, 10th ed. (M. E. Shils,

M. Shike, A. C. Ross, B. Cabellero, and R. J. Cousins, eds.), pp. 470–481. Lippincott, New York.

Cornel, M. C., de Smit, D. J., and de Jong-van den Berg, L. T. W. (2005). Folic acid—the scientific debate as a base for public policy. *Reprod. Toxicol.* **20,** 411–415.

de Bree, A., Vershuren, W. M. M., Kromhout, D., Kluijtmans, L. A. J., and Bloom, H. J. (2002). Homocysteine determinants and the evidence to what extent homocysteine determines the risk of coronary heart disease. *Pharmacol. Rev.* **54,** 599–618.

Eicholzer, M., Tönz, O., and Zimmermann, R. (2006). Folic acid: A public health challenge. *Lancet* **367,** 1352–1361.

Fenech, M. (2001). The role of folic acid and vitamin B_{12} in genomic stability of human cells. *Mutation Res.* **475,** 57–67.

Fingas, P. M., Wright, A. J. A., Wollfe, C. A., Hart, D. J., Wright, D. M. and Dainty, J. R. (2003). Is there more to folates than neural-tube defects? *Proc. Nutr. Soc.* **62,** 591–598.

Giovannucci, E. (2002). Epidemiological studies of folate and colorectal neoplasia: A review. *J. Nutr.* **132,** 2350S–2355S.

Gregory, J. F. (2001). Case study: Folate bioavailability. *J. Nutr.* **131,** 1376S–1382S.

Gregory, J. F., and Quinlivan, E. P. (2002). *In vivo* kinetics of folate metabolism. *Ann. Rev. Nutr.* **22,** 199–220.

Halsted, C. H., et al. (2002). Metabolic interactions of alcohol and folate. *J. Nutr.* **132,** 2367S–2372S.

Kaman, B. A., and Smith, A. K. (2004). A review of folate receptor alpha cycling and 5-methyltetrahydrofolate accumulation with an emphasis on cell models *in vitro*. *Adv. Drug Deliv. Rev.* **56,** 1085–1097.

Kim, Y. I. (2003). Role of folate in colon cancer development and progression. *J. Clin. Nutr.* **133,** 3731S–3739S.

Kono, S., and Chen, K. (2005). Genetic polymorphisms of methylenetetrahydrofolate reductase and colorectal cancer and adenoma. *Cancer Sci.* **96,** 535–542.

Koury, M. J., and Ponka, P. (2004). New insights into erythropoiesis: The roles of folate, vitamin B_{12}, and iron. *Ann. Rev. Nutr.* **24,** 105–131.

Lucock, M. (2000). Folic acid: Nutritional biochemistry, molecular biology and role in disease processes. *Mol. Genetics Metab.* **71,** 121–138.

Malinow, M. R. (1996). Plasma homocyst(e)ine: A risk factor for arterial occlusive diseases. *J. Nutr.* **126,** 1238S–1243S.

McNulty, H., and Pentieva, K. (2004). Folate bioavailability. *Proc. Nutr. Soc.* **63,** 529–526.

Mills, J. L., Scott, J. M., Kirke, P. N., McPartlin, J. M., Conley, M. R., Weir, D. G., Molloy, A. N., and Lee, Y. J. (1996). Homocysteine and neural tube defects. *J. Nutr.* **126,** 756S–760S.

Moat, S. J., Lang, D., McDowell, I. F. W., Clarke, Z. L., Madhavan, A. K., Lewis, M. J., and Goodfellow, J. (2004). Folate, homocysteine, endothelial function and cardiovascular disease. *J. Nutr. Biochem.* **15,** 64–79.

Molley, A. M. (2004). Folate and homocysteine interrelationships including genetics of the relevant enzymes. *Curr. Opin. Lipidol.* **15,** 49–57.

Quinlivan, E. P., Hanson, A. D., and Gregory, J. F. (2006). The analysis of folate and its metabolic precursors in biological samples. *Anal. Biochem.* **348,** 163–184.

Rampersand, G. C., Kauwell, G. P. A., and Bailey, L. P. (2003). Folate: A key to optimizing health and reducing disease risk in the elderly. *J. Am. Coll. Nutr.* **22,** 1–8.

Rush, D. (1994). Periconceptional folate and neural tube defect. *Am. J. Clin. Nutr.* **59,** 511S–516S.

Scott, J. M. (1999). Folate and vitamin B_{12}. *Proc. Nutr. Soc.* **58,** 441–448.

Sharp, L., and Little, J. (2003). Polymorphisms in genes in folate metabolism and colorectal neoplasia: A HuGE review. *Am. J. Epidemiol.* **159,** 423–442.

Stanger, O. (2002). Physiology of folic acid in health and disease. *Curr. Drug Metab.* **3,** 211–223.

Stover, P. J. (2004). Physiology of folate and vitamin B_{12} in Health and Disease. *Nutr. Rev.* **62,** S3–S12.

Tamura, T., and Picciano, M. F. (2006). Folate and human reproduction. *Am. J. Clin. Nutr.* **83,** 993–1016.

Ubbink, J. B. (1994). Vitamin nutrition status and homocysteine: An atherogenic risk factor. *Nutr. Rev.* **52,** 383–393.

van der Put, N. M., van Straaten, H. W., Trijbels, F. J., and Blom, H. J. (2001). Folate, homocysteine and neural tube defects: An overview. *Exp. Biol. Med.* **226,** 243–270.

Verhoef, P., and Stampfer, M. J. (1995). Prospective studies of homocysteine and cardiovascular disease. *Nutr. Rev.* **53,** 283–288.

Wagner, C. (1996). Symposium on the subcellular compartmentalization of folate metabolism. *J. Nutr.* **126,** 1228S–1234S.

Whittle, S. L. and Hughes, R. A. (2004). Folate supplementation and methotrexate treatment in rheumatoid arthritis: A review. *Rheumatol.* **43,** 267–271.

Vitamin B$_{12}$

17

Patients with Addisonian pernicious anemia have ... a "conditioned" defect of nutrition. The nutritional defect in such patients is apparently caused by a failure of a reaction that occurs in the normal individual between a substance in the food (extrinsic factor) and a substance in the normal gastric secretion (intrinsic factor).

— W. B. Castle and T. H. Hale

I.	The Significance of Vitamin B$_{12}$	382
II.	Sources of Vitamin B$_{12}$	382
III.	Absorption of Vitamin B$_{12}$	383
IV.	Transport of Vitamin B$_{12}$	385
V.	Metabolism of Vitamin B$_{12}$	386
VI.	Metabolic Functions of Vitamin B$_{12}$	387
VII.	Vitamin B$_{12}$ Deficiency	388
VIII.	Vitamin B$_{12}$ Toxicity	395
IX.	Case Study	395
	Study Questions and Exercises	397
	Recommended Reading	397

Anchoring Concepts

1. Vitamin B$_{12}$ is the generic descriptor for all *corrinoids* (compounds containing the cobalt-centered corrin nucleus) exhibiting qualitatively the biological activity of cyanocobalamin.
2. Deficiencies of vitamin B$_{12}$ are manifested as anemia and neurologic changes, and can be fatal.
3. The function of vitamin B$_{12}$ in single-carbon metabolism is interrelated with that of folate.

Learning Objectives

1. To understand the chief natural sources of vitamin B$_{12}$.
2. To understand the means of enteric absorption and transport of vitamin B$_{12}$.
3. To understand the biochemical functions of vitamin B$_{12}$ as a coenzyme in the metabolism of propionate and the biosynthesis of methionine.
4. To understand the metabolic interrelationship of vitamin B$_{12}$ and folate.
5. To understand the factors that can cause low vitamin B$_{12}$ status, and the physiological implications of that condition.

Vocabulary

Adenosylcobalamin
Anemia
Aquocobalamin
Cobalamins
Cobalt
Cyanocobalamin
Gastric parietal cell
Haptocorrin
Hypochlorhydria
Homocysteinemia
IF receptor
IF–vitamin B$_{12}$ complex
Intrinsic factor (IF)
Lipotrope
Megaloblastic anemia
Megaloblastic transformation
Methionine synthetase (also called methyl-FH$_4$ methyltransferase)
Methylcobalamin
Methylmalonyl-CoA mutase
Methylfolate trap
Methyl-FH$_4$ methyltransferase
5-Methyl-FH$_4$: homocysteine methyltransferase
Methylmalonic acid (MMA)
Methylmalonic acidemia
Methylmalonic aciduria
Methylmalonyl-CoA mutase
Ovolactovegetarian
Pepsin
Peripheral neuropathy
Pernicious anemia
R proteins
S-adenosylmethionine (SAM)
Schilling test
TC$_{II}$ receptor

Transcobalamin I (TC$_I$)
Transcobalamin II (TC$_{II}$)
Transcobalamin III (TC$_{III}$)
Vegan
Vitamin B$_{12}$ coenzyme synthetase

I. Significance of Vitamin B$_{12}$

Vitamin B$_{12}$ is synthesized by bacteria. It is found in the tissues of animals, which require the vitamin for critical functions in cellular division and growth; in fact, some animal tissues can store the vitamin in very appreciable amounts that are sufficient to meet the needs of the organism for long periods (even years) of deprivation. The vitamin is seldom found in foods derived from plants; therefore, animals and humans that consume strict vegetarian diets are very likely to have suboptimal intakes of vitamin B$_{12}$ that, if prolonged and uncorrected, will lead to **anemia** and, ultimately, to peripheral neuropathy. However, most vegetarians are either not strict **vegans** (who exclude all foods of animal origin) and many consume foods and/or supplements containing at least some vitamin B$_{12}$; for this reason, vitamin B$_{12}$ deficiency is not common. Nevertheless, the prevalence of low vitamin B$_{12}$ status is not uncommon, particularly among older people, and has been shown to be a factor in the prevalence of homocysteinemia, a risk factor for occlusive vascular disease.

II. Sources of Vitamin B$_{12}$

Distribution in Foods

Because the synthesis of vitamin B$_{12}$ is limited almost exclusively to bacteria, the vitamin is found only in foods that have been bacterially fermented and those derived from the tissues of animals that have obtained it from their ruminal or intestinal microflora, ingesting it either with their diet or coprophagously. Animal tissues that accumulate vitamin B$_{12}$ (e.g., liver[1]) are, therefore, excellent food sources of the vitamin (Table 17-1). The richest food sources of vitamin B$_{12}$ are dairy products, meats, eggs, fish, and shellfish. The principal vitamers in foods are methylcobalamin, deoxyadenosylcobalamin, and hydroxycobalamin. The richest sources of vitamin B$_{12}$ for animal feedstuffs are animal byproducts such as meat and bone meal, fish meal, and whey.

Human milk contains 260–300 pM vitamin B$_{12}$, almost exclusively bound to an R-protein, which declines to only half that level after the first 12 weeks of lactation. Breast milk vitamin B$_{12}$ levels of women consuming strict vegetarian diets are less than those of women consuming mixed diets, and tend to be inversely correlated with the length of time on the vegetarian diet. It has been observed that infant urinary methylmalonic acid levels increase, indicating

Table 17-1. Sources of vitamin B$_{12}$ in foods

Food	Vitamin B$_{12}$ (μg/100 g)	Food	Vitamin B$_{12}$ (μg/100 g)
Meats		Fish and sea food	
Beef	1.94–3.64	Herring	4.3
Beef brain	7.83	Salmon	3.2
Beef kidney	38.3	Trout	7.8
Beef liver	69–122	Tuna	2.8
Chicken	0.32	Clams	19.1
Chicken liver	24.1	Oysters	21.2
Ham	0.8	Lobster	1.28
Pork	0.55	Shrimp	1.9
Turkey	0.379	Other	
Dairy products		Eggs, whole	1.26
Milk	0.36	Egg whites	0.09
Cheeses	0.36–1.71	Egg yolk	9.26
Yogurt	0.06–0.62	Vegetables, grains, fruits	None contain vitamin B$_{12}$

---

[1] Vitamin B$_{12}$ was discovered as the antipernicious anemia factor in liver.

vitamin B$_{12}$ deficiency at maternal milk vitamin B$_{12}$ concentrations less than about 360 pM.

Some studies have indicated that, under certain conditions, some algae and other plants (e.g., peas, beans) may also be able to synthesize small amounts of vitamin B$_{12}$-like compounds.[2] However, foods derived from such sources have no value as sources of the vitamin. Contrary to popular belief, fermented soy or rice products do not contain significant amounts of vitamin B$_{12}$.

The microbial synthesis of vitamin B$_{12}$ by long-gutted animals depends on an adequate supply of cobalt, which must be ingested in the diet. If the supply of cobalt is sufficient, the rumen microbial synthesis of vitamin B$_{12}$ in ruminants is substantial. For that reason, not only do those species have no need for preformed vitamin B$_{12}$ in the diet, but their tissues tend to contain appreciably greater amounts of the vitamin than those of nonruminant species.

Stability

Vitamin B$_{12}$ is very stable in both crystalline form and aqueous solution. High levels of ascorbic acid have been shown to catalyze the oxidation of vitamin B$_{12}$ in the presence of iron to forms that are poorly utilized.

Bioavailability

It is very difficult to estimate the bioavailability of vitamin B$_{12}$, but its bioavailability in foods generally appears to be moderate. Studies have found that about 25–65% of the vitamin in eggs, meats, and fish is absorbed.[3] Bioavailability falls off rapidly at intakes (<2 mg/day) exceeding those sufficient to saturate the active transport mechanism for active transport across the gut, as incremental enteric absorption of the vitamin depends on diffusion, a process with no greater than 1% efficiency. Accordingly, about 1% of the vitamin is absorbed from vitamin B$_{12}$ supplements.[4]

III. Absorption of Vitamin B$_{12}$

Digestion

The naturally occurring vitamin B$_{12}$ in foods is bound in coenzyme form to proteins. The vitamin is released from such complexes on heating, gastric acidification, and/or proteolysis (especially by the action of **pepsin**). Thus, impaired **gastric parietal cell** function, as in achlorhydria, impairs vitamin B$_{12}$ utilization.

Protein Binding in the Gut

Free vitamin B$_{12}$ is bound to proteins secreted by the gastric mucosa:

- *R proteins*[5]   The binding of vitamin B$_{12}$ to these glycoproteins[6] may be adventitious. They are found in human gastric juice, intestinal contents, and several other bodily fluids. While R proteins have also been found in certain cells[7] in certain other species, they appear to be largely limited to humans. They show structural and immunologic similarities, their differences in electrophoretic mobility being due to differing carbohydrate contents. The **R proteins** in the intestine are not necessary for the enteric absorption of vitamin B$_{12}$, as they are normally digested proteolytically in the alkaline conditions of the small intestine, whereupon they release their ligands to be bound by **intrinsic factor (IF)**. However, because vitamin B$_{12}$ binds preferentially to R proteins rather than to IF under the acidic conditions of the stomach, they can interfere with the absorption of vitamin B$_{12}$. Patients with pancreatic exocrine insufficiency, and consequent deficiencies of proteolytic activities in the intestinal lumen, can achieve high concentrations of R proteins that render the vitamin poorly absorbed.
- *Intrinsic factor*   The intrinsic factor (IF) is synthesized and secreted, in most animals (including humans), by the gastric parietal cells in response to histamine, gastrin, pentagastrin, and the presence of food. Individuals

[2] Dagnelie, P. C., et al. (1991). *Am. J. Clin. Nutr.* **53,** 695–697.

[3] Heyssel, B. M., et al. (1966). *Am. J. Clin. Nutr.* **18,** 176–184; Doscherholmen, A., et al. (1975). *Proc. Soc. Exp. Biol. Med.* **149,** 987–990; Doscherholmen, A., et al. (1981). *Proc. Soc. Exp. Biol. Med.* **167,** 480–484.

[4] Berlin, H., et al. (1968). *Acta Med. Scand.* **184,** 247–258.

[5] These vitamin B$_{12}$-binding glycoproteins were named for their high electrophoretic mobilities, *rapid*.

[6] They contain sialic acid and fucose.

[7] For example, plasma, saliva, tears, bile, cerebrospinal fluid, amniotic fluid, leukocytes, erythrocytes, and milk.

with loss of gastric parietal cell function may be unable to use dietary vitamin B_{12}, as these cells produce both IF and acid, both of which are required for the enteric absorption of the vitamin.[8] For this reason, geriatric patients, many of whom are hypoacidic, may be at risk of low vitamin B_{12} status. A relatively small protein (the molecular masses of human and porcine IFs range from 44 to 63 kDa, and from 50 to 59 kDa, respectively, according to the carbohydrate moiety isolated with particular preparations), IF binds the four **cobalamins** (**methylcobalamin**, **adenosylcobalamin**, **cyanocobalamin**, and **aquocobalamin**) with comparable, high affinities under alkaline conditions. Intrinsic factor also binds a specific receptor in the ileal mucosal brush border. Cobalamin-binding appears to have an allosteric effect on the ileal receptor-binding center of IF, causing the protein complex to dimerize and increasing its binding to the receptor. Formation of the **IF–vitamin B_{12} complex** protects the vitamin from catabolism by intestinal bacteria, and protects IF from hydrolytic attack by pepsin and chymotrypsin. That some free IF has been found in the ileum indicates that absorption may occur for cobalamins synthesized by bacteria of that region of the small intestine.

Mechanisms of Absorption

Vitamin B_{12} is absorbed from the gut by two mechanisms:

- *Active transport*   The carrier-mediated absorption of vitamin B_{12} is highly efficient and quantitatively important at low doses (1–2 μg). Such doses appear in the blood within 3–4 hours of consumption. The active transport of vitamin B_{12} depends on the interactions of the IF-vitamin B_{12} complex with a specific receptor in the microvilli of the ileum. The ileal **IF receptor**, a glycoprotein, binds the IF–vitamin B_{12} complex, but little, if any, free IF or free vitamin B_{12}. Human and porcine IF receptors each consist of

two subunits: α subunits of 70 and 90 kDa, respectively (immunologically related to IF in each species); and hydrophobic β subunits of 130 or 140 kDa, respectively. In contrast, the canine IF receptor consists of a single 200-kDa unit. Receptor binding occurs at neutral pH and depends on Ca^{2+}, in the presence of which it forms a stable IF–vitamin B_{12}–IF receptor complex. The receptor is anchored to the brush border membrane and effects the enteric absorption of vitamin B_{12} through the endocytotic internalization of the receptor-bound complex. Biophysical studies of the canine IF receptor have revealed that most of it (83%) protrudes from the membrane, being anchored there by only about 17% of the protein structure. The absorption of vitamin B_{12} by the enterocyte involves the cellular uptake of the dissociated vitamin, with the release of the unbound IF to the intestinal lumen; It is not clear whether this uptake involves pinocytosis or movement of the receptor complex through the plasma membrane. Upon entering the enterocyte, the vitamin is bound to an intracellular protein that is immunologically similar to IF, and eventually transferred to the portal circulation bound to a specific carrier protein, **transcobalamin II (TC_{II})** (see below). Human patients who lack IF have very low abilities to absorb vitamin B_{12}, excreting in the feces 80–100% of oral doses (versus the 30–60% fecal excretion rates of individuals with adequate IF).

- *Simple diffusion*   Diffusion of the vitamin occurs with low efficiency (~1%) throughout the small intestine and becomes significant only at higher doses. Such doses appear in the blood within minutes of comsumption. This passive mechanism is utilized in therapy for pernicious anemia, in which patients are given high doses (>500 μg/day) of vitamin B_{12} *per os*. For such therapy, the vitamin must be given an hour before or after a meal to avoid competitive binding of the vitamin food.

---

[8] Individuals lacking IF are unable to absorb vitamin B_{12} by active transport. Such individuals can be given the vitamin by intramuscular injection (1 μg/day) or in high oral doses (25–2000 μg) to prevent deficiency. Randomized controlled trials have shown that an oral dose regimen of 1000 μg daily for a week, followed by the same dose weekly and, then, monthly can be as effective as intramuscular administration of the vitamin for controlling short-term hematological and neurological responses in deficient patients (Butler, C. C. [2006]. *Fam. Pract.* **23,** 279–285).

IV. Transport of Vitamin B$_{12}$

Transport Proteins

On absorption from the intestine, vitamin B$_{12}$ is initially transported in the plasma, most of which is bound as the adenosylcobalamin and methylcobalamin to an R protein called **transcobalamin I (TC$_I$)**. Most of the remainder is bound to another binding protein **transcobalamin II (TC$_{II}$)** synthesized in several tissues, including the intestinal mucosa, liever, seminal vesicles, fibroblasts, bone marrow, and macrophages. Three transcobalamins have been described:

- *Transcobalamin I (TC$_I$)* is a 60-kDa α-glycoprotein. This is an R protein, also referred to as **haptocorrin**. Vitamin B$_{12}$ bound to this protein appears to turn over very slowly (half-life, 9–10 days), becoming available for cellular uptake only over fairly long time frames. Because TC$_I$ occurs at very high concentrations in saliva, breast milk, and tears, and other secretions, it has been suggested that it may have antimicrobial activity through the sequestration of the vitamin.
- *Transcobalamin II (TC$_{II}$)* is smaller (38 kDa) and serves as the chief transport protein of the vitamin, binding it stoichiometrically in a 1:1 molar ratio.[9] While only 10–25% of plasma vitamin B$_{12}$ is bound to this transporter, the rapid turnover (half-life, 90 min.) of the protein-ligand complex renders TC$_{II}$ the only functional source of the vitamin for cellular uptake.
- *Transcobalamin III (TC$_{III}$)* is electrophoretically similar to TC$_I$ but antigenically similar to TC$_{II}$. Its metabolic role is less clear.

The movement of vitamin B$_{12}$ from the intestinal mucosal cells into the plasma appears to depend on the formation of the TC$_{II}$–vitamin B$_{12}$ complex (the vitamin is shuttled from IF to TC$_{II}$). This complex turns over rapidly; its half-life is about 6 min.[10] Within hours of absorption, however, much of the vitamin originally associated with TC$_{II}$ becomes bound to TC$_I$ and, in humans, to other plasma proteins (R proteins). Whereas deficiency of TC$_I$ does not appear to impair cobalamin metabolism, TC$_{II}$ is clearly necessary for normal cellular maturation of the hematopoietic system.[11] Because cobalamin is lost within days from TC$_{II}$, the amount bound to that protein can be a useful parameter of early-stage vitamin B$_{12}$ deficiency.

Transcobalamin Receptor

Membrane-bound receptor proteins for TC$_{II}$ occur in all cells. The **TC$_{II}$ receptor** is structurally similar to TC; it is a 50-kDa glycoprotein with a single binding site for the TC$_{II}$–vitamin B$_{12}$ complex. The binding is of high affinity and requires Ca^{2+}. It is thought that the cellular uptake of vitamin B$_{12}$ involves such TC$_{II}$ receptors mediating the pinocytotic entrance of the vitamin–TC$_{II}$ complex into the cell.

Role of R Proteins

In humans, most recently absorbed vitamin B$_{12}$ is transferred to the plasma R protein TC$_I$,[12] which bind approximately three-quarters of the circulating vitamin B$_{12}$ in that species. Owing to the specificity of the TC$_I$ for methylcobalamin, that vitamer predominates in the circulation of humans. Congenital deficiencies of this R protein results in low concentrations of vitamin B$_{12}$ in the plasma, but not in detectable losses in function, as cobalamins bound to TC$_I$ do not appear to be available for cellular uptake. Most other species lack R proteins; they transport the vitamin exclusively as the TC complex. Therefore, in species other than the human, the predominant circulating form is adenosylcobalamin.

Intracellular Protein Binding

After its cellular uptake, the TC$_{II}$–receptor complex is degraded in the lysosome to yield the free vitamin, which can be converted to methylcobalamin in the cytosol. Virtually all of the vitamin within the cell is bound to two vitamin B$_{12}$-dependent enzymes:

- **Methionine synthetase** (also called **methyl-FH$_4$ methyltransferase**) in the cytosol
- **Methylmalonyl-CoA mutase** in mitochondria

---

[9] About half of patients with acquired immunodeficiency syndrome (AIDS) have been found to have subnormal levels of holo-TC$_{II}$.

[10] Human plasma typically contains 500–1400 pmol of TC$_{II}$ per liter, with a vitamin B$_{12}$-binding capacity of about 800 pg/ml.

[11] A rare autosomal recessive deficiency in TC$_{II}$ has been described.

[12] Due to their affinity for R proteins, the TCs are grouped in a heterogeneous class of proteins called *R binders*.

Distribution in Tissues

Vitamin B$_{12}$ is the best stored of the vitamins. Under conditions of nonlimiting intake, the vitamin accumulates to very appreciable amounts in the body, mainly in the liver (about 60% of the total body store) and muscles (about 30% of the total). Body stores vary with the intake of the vitamin, but tend to be greater in older subjects. Hepatic concentrations approaching 2000 ng/g have been reported in humans; however, a total hepatic reserve of about 1.5 mg is typical. Mean total body stores of vitamin B$_{12}$ in humans are in the range of 2–5 mg. The greatest concentrations of vitamin B$_{12}$ occur in the pituitary gland; kidneys, heart, spleen, and brain also contain substantial amounts. In humans, these organs each contain 20–30 µg of vitamin B$_{12}$. The great storage and long biological half-life (350–400 days in humans) of the vitamin provide substantial protection against periods of deprivation. The low reserve of the human infant (~25 µg) is sufficient to meet physiological needs for about a year.

The predominant form in human plasma is methylcobalamin (60–80% of the total),[13] owing to the presence of TC$_I$ that selectively binds that vitamer (Table 17-2). However, the predominant vitamer in the plasma of other species, and in other tissues of all species, is adenosylcobalamin. (In humans, this form accounts for 60–70% of the total vitamin in liver and about 50% of that in other tissues.) Whereas methylcobalamin is the main form bound by TC$_I$ and TC$_{III}$, both it and adenosylcobalamin are bound in similar amounts by TC$_{II}$. Normal plasma vitamin B$_{12}$ concentrations vary widely among various mammalian species, from only hundreds (humans) to thousands (rabbits) of picomoles per liter.

The vitamin B$_{12}$ concentration of human milk varies widely (130–320 pg/ml) and is particularly great

Table 17-2. Cobalamins in normal human plasma

Cobalamin	Range (pmol/liter)
Total cobalamins	173–545
Methylcobalamin	135–427
Adenosylcobalamin	2–77
Cyanocobalamin	2–48
Aquacobalamin	5–67

(10-fold that of mature milk) in colostrum. Although those products contain TC$_{II}$, most of the vitamin (mainly methylcobalamin) is bound to R proteins, which they also contain in large amounts. In contrast, cow's milk, which does not contain R proteins, typically shows lower concentrations of the vitamin, present in that product mainly as adenosylcobalamin.

V. Metabolism of Vitamin B$_{12}$

Activation to Coenzyme Forms

Vitamin B$_{12}$ is delivered to cells in the oxidized form, hydroxycob(III)alamin, where it is reduced by thiol- and reduced flavin-dependent reduction of the cobalt center of the vitamin (to Co$^+$) to form cob(I)amin, also called vitamin B$_{12s}$. However, the vitamin is active in metabolism *only* as derivatives that have either a methyl group (methylcobalamin) or 5'-deoxyadenosinyl group (adenosylcobalamin) attached covalently to the **cobalt** atom. The conversion to these coenzyme forms involves two different enzymatic steps:

- *Generation of methylcobalamin* This step is catalyzed by the cytosolis enzyme **5-methyl-FH$_4$: homocysteine methyltransferase**. By producing methylcobalamin, it renders the vitamin a carrier for the single carbon unit in the regeneration of methionine from homocysteine.
- *Generation of adenosylcobalamin* The adenosylation of the vitamin occurs in the mitochondrial due to the action of **vitamin B$_{12}$ coenzyme synthetase**, which catalyzes the reaction of cob(II)amin with a deoxyadenosyl moiety derived from ATP. This step depends on the entry of hydroxycobalamin into the mitochondria and its subsequent reduction in sequential, one-electron steps involving NADH- and NADPH-linked aquacobalamin reductases[14] to yield cob(II)alamin.

Catabolism

Little, if any, metabolism of the corrinoid ring system is apparent in animals, and vitamin B$_{12}$ is excreted as the intact cobalamin. Apparently, only the free

---

[13] Methylcobalamin is lost preferentially, in comparison with the other forms of the vitamin, in pernicious anemia patients.

[14] These activities are derived from a cytochrome b_5/cytochrome b_5 reductase complex, and from a cytochrome P-450 reductase complex and an associated flavoprotein.

cobalamins (not the methylated or adenosylated forms) in the plasma are available for excretion.

Excretion

Vitamin B$_{12}$ is excreted via both renal and biliary routes at the daily rate of about 0.1–0.2% of total body reserves. (In humans this is 2–5 μg/day, thus constituting the daily requirement for the vitamin.) Although it is found in the urine, glomerular filtration of the vitamin is minimal (<0.25 μg/day in humans), and it is thought that urinary cobalamin is derived from the tubular epithelial cells and lymph. Urinary excretion of the vitamin after a small oral dose can be used to assess vitamin B$_{12}$ status; this is called the **Schilling test**. The biliary excretion of the vitamin is substantial, accounting in humans for the secretion into the intestine of 0.5–5 μg/day. Most (65–75%) of this amount is reabsorbed in the ileum by IF-mediated active transport. This enterohepatic circulation constitutes a highly efficient means of conservation, with biliary vitamin B$_{12}$ contributing only a small amount to the feces.

VI. Metabolic Functions of Vitamin B$_{12}$

Coenzyme Functions

Vitamin B$_{12}$ functions in metabolism in two coenzyme forms: adenosylcobalamin and methylcobalamin. Although several vitamin B$_{12}$-dependent metabolic reactions have been identified in microorganisms,[15] only two have been discovered in animals. These play key roles in the metabolism of propionate, amino acids, and single carbon. The reaction catalyzed by the adenosylcobalamin-dependent enzyme involves the splitting of a carbon-carbon bond of the coenzyme with the formation of a free radical on the coenzyme, which can be transferred through an amino acid residue on the enzyme to the substrate. The reaction catalyzed by the methylcobalamin-dependent enzyme is a simple transfer of the single carbon moiety.

The vitamin B$_{12}$-dependent enzymes of animals are as follows.

- *Methylmalonyl-CoA mutase* The adenosylcobalamin-dependent enzyme methylmalonyl-CoA mutase catalyzes the conversion of methylmalonyl-CoA to succinyl-CoA in the degradation of propionate formed from odd-chain fatty acids (and an important energy source for ruminants, in which it is produced by rumen microflora). That the propionic acid pathway is also important in nerve tissue per se is suggested by the delayed onset of the neurological signs of vitamin B$_{12}$ deficiency effected in animals by dietary supplements of direct (valine and isoleucine) or indirect (methionine) precursors of propionate. The mutase is a mitochondrial matrix enzyme, the dimmer of which binds two adenosylcobalamin molecules. In humans, methylmalonyl-CoA mutase is the first vitamin B$_{12}$-dependent enzyme to be affected by deprivation of the vitamin. Owing to loss of methylmalonyl-CoA mutase activity, vitamin B$_{12}$-deficient subjects show **methylmalonic aciduria**, especially after being fed odd-chain fatty acids. The accumulation of methylmalonic acid can disrupt normal glucose and glutamic acid metabolism, apparently by inhibiting the tricarboxylic acid (TCA) cycle. Vitamin B$_{12}$ deficiency can also cause a reversal of propionyl-CoA carboxylase activity, leading to the incorporation of the three-carbon propionyl-CoA in place of the two-carbon acetyl-CoA and resulting in the production of small amounts of odd-chain fatty acids. Increased methylmalonyl-CoA levels can also lead to its incorporation in place of malonyl-CoA, resulting in the synthesis of small amounts of methyl-branched chain fatty acids. It has been suggested that the neurological signs of vitamin B$_{12}$ deficiency may result, at least in part, from the production of these abnormal fatty acids in neural tissues.
- *Methionine synthase* Methionine synthetase catalyzes the methylation of homocysteine to regenerate methionine, serving as the methyl group carrier (via methylcobalamin) between the donor 5-methyltetrahydrofolate (5′-methyl-FH$_4$) and the acceptor homocysteine (Fig. 17-1).

---

[15] The following microbial enzymes require adenosylcobalamin: glutamate mutase, 2-methylene-glutarate mutase, L-β-lysine mutase, D-α-lysine mutase, D-α-ornithine mutase, leucine mutase, 1,2-dioldehydratase, glyceroldehydratase, ethanolamine deaminase, and ribonucleotide reductase; methylcobalamin is also required for the bacterial formation of methane and acetate.

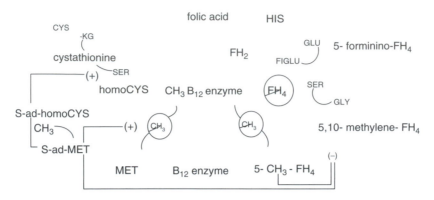

Fig. 17-1. Metabolic role of methycobalamin (CH$_3$B$_{12}$) and its relationship with folate in single-carbon metabolism. *Abbreviations:* CYS, cysteine; α-KG, α-ketoglutarate; SER, serine; homoCYS, homocysteine; S-ad-homoCys, S-adenosylhomocysteine; S-ad-MET, S-adenosylmethionine; MET, methionine.

Because of lost methionine synthetase activity, vitamin B$_{12}$-deficient subjects show reduced availability of methionine, the primary donor of methyl groups after its activation to **S-adenosylmethionine (SAM)**. Losses of SAM lead to impairments in the synthesis of creatine, phospholipids, and the neurotransmitter acetylcholine, all of which have broad impacts on physiological function. Thus, low vitamin B$_{12}$ status, results in the accumulation of both homocysteine and 5′-methyl-FH$_4$ (via the **methyl-folate trap**; see Chapter 16), the latter resulting in the loss of FH$_4$, the key functional form of folate. Methionine synthase can also catalyze the reduction of nitrous oxide to elemental nitrogen; in doing so it generates a free radical that inactivates the enzyme.

Other Effects

Cyanide metabolism

Cobalamins can bind cyanide to produce the nontoxic cyanocobalamin. For that reason hydroxocobalamin is a well-recognized cyanide antidote. Thus, it has been proposed that vitamin B$_{12}$ may have a role in the inactivation of the low levels of cyanide consumed in may fruits, beans, and nuts.

VII. Vitamin B$_{12}$ Deficiency

Contributors to Vitamin B$_{12}$ Deficiency

Deficiency of vitamin B$_{12}$ can be produced by several factors. Inadequate dietary intake is not the most common cause.

Vegetarian diets

Strict vegetarian diets, containing no meats, fish, animal products (e.g., milk, eggs), or vitamin B$_{12}$ supplements (e.g., multivitamin supplements, nutritional yeasts), contain practically no vitamin B$_{12}$ (Tables 17-3 and 17-4). Therefore, individuals consuming such diets typically show very low circulating levels of the vitamin; one study found 56% of vegetarian American women to have low serum concentrations (<148 pM) of vitamin B$_{12}$. Nevertheless, clinical signs among such individuals appear to be rare and may not become manifest for many years, although they are more common among breast-fed infants (Table 17-5). The vitamin B$_{12}$ content of breast milk has been found to vary inversely with the length of maternal vegetarian practice. Serum vitamin B$_{12}$ concentrations have also been found to vary inversely with the length of time of vegetarian practice, showing progressive declines through about 7 years (Fig. 17-2). This time compares very favorably with the estimated drawdown of hepatic stores of the vitamin.

Table 17-3. Vitamin B$_{12}$ and folate status of Thai vegetarians and mixed diet eaters

Group	Vitamin B$_{12}$ (pg/ml)	Folate (ng/ml)
Mixed diet		
Males	490	5.7
Females	500	6.8
Vegetarian		
Males	117[a]	12.0[a]
Females	153[a]	12.6[a]

[a] $p > 0.05$.
Source: Tungtrongchitr, V., *et al.* (1993). *Int. J. Vit. Nutr. Res.* **63,** 201–207.

Table 17-4. Plasma analytes (mean, 95% CI) indicative of vitamin B$_{12}$ status in vegetarians and nonvegetarians

Plasma analyte	Omnivorous subjects	Lacto- and lacto-ovo-vegetarians		Vegans	
		Vitamin users	Vitamin nonusers	Vitamin users	Vitamin nonusers
Vitamin B$_{12}$, pmol/L	287 (190–471)	303 (146–771)	179 (124–330)	192 (125–299)	126 (92–267)
Transcobalamin, pmol/L	54 (16–122)	26 (30–235)	23 (4–84)	14 (3–53)	4 (2–35)
Methylmalonic acid, nmol/L	161 (95–357)	230 (120–1344)	368 (141–2000)	708 (163–2651)	779 (222–3480)
Homocysteine, µmol/L	8.8 (5.5–16.1)	9.6 (5.5–19.4)	10.9 (6.4–27.7)	11.1 (5.3–25.9)	14.3 (6.5–52.1)
Folate, nmol/L	21.8 (14.5–51.5)	30 (14.8–119)	27.7 (16.0–76.9)	29.5 (18.8–71.8)	34.3 (20.7–72.7)

Source: Herrmann, W., et al. (2003). *Am. J. Clin. Nutr.* **78**, 131–136.

Table 17-5. Ranges of urinary methylmalonic acid excretion by breastfed infants of vegetarian and omnivorous mothers

Infant group	Methylmalonic acid range (µmol/mmol creatinine)
Vegetarian	2.6–790.9
Mixed-diet	1.7–21.4

Source: Specker, B. L., Miller, D., Norman, E. J., Greene, H., and Hayes, K. C. (1988). *Am. J. Clin. Nutr.* **47**, 89–92.

It should be remembered that not all vegetarians are strict vegans; many (called **ovolactovegetarians**) consume plant-based diets that also contain servings of dairy products, eggs, or fish to varying extents. Studies have shown that the occasional consumption of animal products (e.g., once per month) will support serum vitamin B$_{12}$ levels comparable to those of people eating traditional mixed diets (Table 17-6). In addition, such foods as *Nori* sp. and *Chlorella* sp. seaweeds, which may be eaten by vegetarians, appear to contain vitamin B$_{12}$.

Loss of gastric parietal cell function

One of the most common causes of vitamin B$_{12}$ deficiency is malabsorption of the vitamin owing to inadequate production of acid and/or IF by the gastric parietal cells.[16] Such conditions can be of two types:

- *Pernicious anemia* **Pernicious anemia** is the end result of autoimmune gastritis, also called

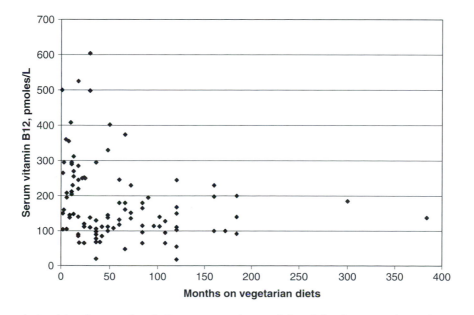

Fig. 17-2. Inverse relationship of serum vitamin B$_{12}$ concentrations and time following vegetarian eating practices in people in the northeastern United States. (*Adapted from:* Miller, D. R., et al. [1991]. *Am. J. Clin. Nutr.* **53**, 524–529.)

---

[16] Chronic atrophic gastritis can be a precancerous lesion, involving progressive metaplasia of the gastric mucosa leading to carcinoma.

Table 17-6. Impact of occasional consumption of animal products on vitamin B_{12} status of Americans in a macrobiotic community

Food	Consumed	Serum vitamin B_{12} (pM)	Urine methylmalonic acid (mmol/mol creatinine)
Dairy	Never	122	5.3
	≤1/week	183[a]	2.8[a]
	>1/week	179[a]	2.1[a]
Eggs	Never	139	4.8
	≤1/week	167	3.1
	>1/week	157	2.2
Sea foods[b]	Never	111	4.4
	≤1/week	145	5.3
	>1/week	161	2.6

[a]$p > 0.05$.
[b]Includes various sea vegetables (e.g., wakame, kombu, hijiki, arame, nori, dulse).
Source: Miller, D. R., Specker, B. L., Ho, M. L., and Norman, E. J. (1991). *Am. J. Clin. Nutr.* **53**, 524–529.

Type A chronic atrophic gastritis or gastric atrophy. It involves the destruction of the fundus and body of the stomach by antibodies to the membrane H^+/K^+-ATPase of the parietal cells. This causes progressive atrophy of parietal cells leading to **hypochlorhydria** and loss of IF production and resulting in severe vitamin B_{12} malabsorption. The condition presents as megaloblastic anemia within 2–7 years. Pernicious anemia is a disease of later life, with 90% of diagnosed cases being over 40 yrs of age. Reported prevalences vary from 50/100,000 to 4300/100,000, greater among women and among people of African descent. However, the disorder is likely to be widely underdiagnosed, as affected subjects may have neurological rather than hematological disease.

- *Atrophic gastritis due to* Helicobacter pylori *infection* Helicobacter pylori infection produces damage mostly to the stomach, referred to as Type B chronic atrophic gastritis, affecting an estimated 9–30% of Americans. The condition involves hypochlorhydria, which facilitates the proliferation of bacteria in the intestine. Both conditions limit and compete for the enteric absorption of vitamin B_{12}; however, reports of the effect of the condition on vitamin B_{12} status have been conflicting.

Pancreatic insufficiency

The loss of pancreatic exocrine function can impair the utilization of vitamin B_{12}. For example, about one-half of all human patients with pancreatic insufficiency show abnormally low enteric absorption of the vitamin. This effect can be corrected by pancreatic enzyme replacement therapy, using oral pancreas powder or pancreatic proteases. Thus, the lesion appears to involve specifically the loss of proteolytic activity, resulting in the failure to digest intestinal R proteins, which thus retain vitamin B_{12} bound in the stomach instead of freeing it for binding by IF.

Intestinal diseases

Tropical sprue[17] and ileitis involve damage to the ileal epithelium that can cause the loss of ileal IF receptors. Intestinal parasites such as the fish tapeworm *Diphyllobothrium latum* can effectively compete with the host for uptake of the vitamin. Explosively growing bacterial floras can do likewise. Protozoal infections such as *Giardia lamblia*, which cause chronic diarrhea, appear to cause vitamin B_{12} malabsorption in malnourished individuals.

Chemical factors

Several other factors can impair the utilization of vitamin B_{12}:

---

[17] Tropical sprue is endemic in south India, occurs epidemically in the Philippines and the Caribbean, and is frequently a source of vitamin B_{12} malabsorption experienced by tourists to those regions.

- *Certain xenobiotic agents* Biguanides,[18] alcohol, and smoking can damage the ileal epithelium to cause the loss of ileal IF receptors.
- *Nitrous oxide* Animal models of vitamin B$_{12}$ deficiency have been developed using exposure to nitrous oxide as the precipitating agent.[19] Nitrous oxide oxidizes the reduced form of cobalamin, cob(I)alamin, to the inactive form cob(II)alamin, causing rapid inactivation of the methylcobalamin-dependent enzyme and the excretion of the vitamin. Thus, repeated exposure to nitrous oxide results in the depletion of body cobalamin stores.
- *Oral contraceptive agents* The use of oral contraceptive agents (steroids) has been shown to cause a slight drop in plasma vitamin B$_{12}$ concentration; however, no signs of impaired function have been reported.

General Signs of Deficiency

Vitamin B$_{12}$ deficiency causes delay or failure of normal cell division, particularly in the bone marrow and intestinal mucosa. Because the biochemical lesion involves arrested synthesis of DNA precursors, the process depends on the availability of single carbon units. The vitamin B$_{12}$ deficiency-induced decreases in methionine biosynthesis, folate coenzymes (due to methylfolate "trapping"), and thymidylate synthesis all lead to a failure of DNA replication. This appears to be accompanied by uracil-misincorporation into DNA (due to the use of deoxyuridine instead of thymidine pyrophosphate by DNA polymerase), apparently resulting in double-stranded DNA damage and apoptosis. The reduced mitotic rate results in the formation of and abnormally large, cytoplasm-rich cells. This is called a **megaloblastic transformation**; it manifests itself as a characteristic type of anemia in which such enlarged cells are found (**megaloblastic anemia**).

Neurological abnormalities develop in most species. These appear to result from impaired methionine biosynthesis, but some investigators have proposed that neurological signs result instead from the loss of adenosylcobalamin. They are typically manifest with relatively late onset due to the effective storage and conservation of the vitamin. Neurological lesions of vitamin B$_{12}$ deficiency involve diffuse and progressive nerve demyelination, manifested as progressive neuropathy (often beginning in the peripheral nerves) and progressing eventually to the posterior and lateral columns of the spinal cord (Table 17-7).

Deficiency Syndromes in Animals

Vitamin B$_{12}$ deficiency in animals is characterized most frequently by reductions in rates of growth and feed intake and impairments in the efficiency of feed utilization. In a few species (e.g., swine) a mild anemia develops. In growing chicks and turkey poults, neurologic signs may appear. Vitamin B$_{12}$ deficiency has also been related to the etiology of perosis in poultry, but this effect seems to be secondary to those of methionine and choline, and related to the availability of labile methyl groups. Also related to limited methyl group availability (for the synthesis of phosphatidylcholine) in poultry is increased lipid deposition in the liver, heart, and kidneys. For this reason, vitamin B$_{12}$ is known as a **lipotrope** for poultry. Vitamin B$_{12}$ deficiency also causes embryonic death in the chicken, with embryos showing myopathies of the muscles of the leg, hemorrhage, myocardial hypertrophy, and perosis. Impaired utilization of dietary protein and testicular lesions (decreased numbers of seminiferous tubules showing spermatogenesis) have been observed in vitamin B$_{12}$-deficient rats.

Ruminants do not have dietary needs for vitamin B$_{12}$, relying instead on their rumen microorganisms

Table 17-7. Signs of vitamin B$_{12}$ deficiency

Organ system	Signs
General	
Growth	Decrease
Vital organs	Hepatic, cardiac, and renal steatosis
Fetus	Hemorrhage, myopathy, death
Circulatory	
Erythrocytes	Anemia
Nervous	Peripheral neuropathy

---

[18] Examples are guanylguanidine, amidinoguanidine, and diguanidine, the sulfates of which are used as reagents for the chemical determination of copper and nickel.

[19] Much of the toxicity of N$_2$O may actually be due to impaired vitamin B$_{12}$ function. Indeed, it is known that excessive dental use of *laughing gas* (which is N$_2$O) can lead to neurologic impairment.

to produce the vitamin in amounts adequate for their needs. Synthesis of the vitamin in the rumen is dependent on a continuous supply of dietary cobalt, as microbes can synthesize the organic portion of the corrin nucleus in the presence of cobalt to attach at the center. Sheep fed a diet containing less than about 70 μg of cobalt per kilogram of diet show signs of deficiency: inappetence, wasting, diarrhea, and watery lacrimation. Cobalt deficiency reduces hepatic cobalamin levels and increases plasma methylmalonyl-CoA levels but does not produce clinical signs; therefore, it is generally accepted that cattle are less susceptible than sheep to cobalt deficiency. Rumenal production of vitamin B$_{12}$ can also be affected by the composition of dietary roughage, the ratio of roughage to concentrate, and the level of dry matter intake. Most microbially produced vitamin B$_{12}$ appears to be bound to rumen microbes and is released for absorption only in the small intestine.

Deficiency Signs in Humans

Vitamin B$_{12}$ deficiency in humans is characterized by megaloblastic anemia and abnormalities of lipid metabolism. After prolonged periods, neurological signs affect approximately one-quarter of affected individuals. The neurological signs of vitamin B$_{12}$ deficiency in humans include **peripheral neuropathy**, which is characterized by numbness of the hands and feet, loss of proprioreception and vibration sense of the ankles and toes. Associated psychiatric signs can also be seen: memory loss, depression, irritability, psychosis, and dementia.

Distinguishing Deficiencies of Folate and Vitamin B$_{12}$

Some clinical signs (e.g., macrocytic anemia) can result from deficiencies of either vitamin B$_{12}$ or folate. The only metabolic process that is common to the two vitamins is the methyl group transfer from 5′-methyl-FH$_4$ to methylcobalamin for the subsequent methylation of homocysteine to yield methionine and the return of folate to its most important central metabolite, FH$_4$. Thus, deficiencies of either vitamin will reduce the FH$_4$ pool either directly by deprivation of folate or indirectly via the methylfolate trap, resulting from deprivation of vitamin B$_{12}$. In either case, the availability of FH$_4$ is reduced

and, consequently, its conversion ultimately to 5, 10-methylene-FH$_4$ is also reduced. This limits the production of thymidylate and thus of DNA, resulting in impaired mitosis, which manifests itself as macrocytosis and anemia. Similarly, the urinary excretion of the histidine metabolite formiminoglutamic acid (FIGLU) is elevated by deficiencies of either folate or vitamin B$_{12}$, as FH$_4$ is required to accept the formimino group, yielding 5′-formimino-FH$_4$. Studies have revealed that about half of subjects with either vitamin B$_{12}$ or folate deficiencies, and more than half of those with the combined deficiencies, show plasma methionine concentrations below normal.[20] Serum vitamin B$_{12}$ levels are highly correlated with those of methionine in vitamin B$_{12}$-deficient subjects.

While supplemental folate can mask the anemia or FIGLU excretion (especially after histidine loading) associated with vitamin B$_{12}$ deficiency by maintaining FH$_4$ in spite of the methylfolate trap, supplemental vitamin B$_{12}$ does not affect the anemia (or other signs) of folate deficiency. Although such signs as macrocytic anemia, urinary FIGLU, and subnormal circulating folate concentrations are, therefore, not diagnostic for either vitamin B$_{12}$ or folate deficiency (these deficiencies cannot be distinguished on the basis of these signs), the urinary excretion of **methylmalonic acid (MMA)** can be used for that purpose. Methylmalonic aciduria (especially after a meal of odd-chain fatty acids or a load of propionate) occurs only in vitamin B$_{12}$ deficiency (methylmalonyl-CoA mutase requires adenosylcobalamin). Therefore, patients with macrocytic anemia, increased urinary FIGLU, and low blood folate levels can be diagnosed as being vitamin B$_{12}$ deficient if their urinary MMA levels are elevated, but as being folate deficient if they are not (Table 17-8).

Subclinical Vitamin B$_{12}$ Deficiency

Marginal (subclinical) deficiencies of vitamin B$_{12}$ are estimated to be at least ten times more prevalent than the symptomatic deficiencies we have described. These are characterized by low vitamin B$_{12}$ status sufficient to produce metabolic abnormalities due to loss of vitamin B$_{12}$ coenzyme function characterized by elevated circulating levels of FIGLU, MMA, and homocysteine. A study of elderly Americans found that more than 4% showed elevations in urinary MMA levels; half also showed low serum vitamin

---

[20] Humans typically show plasma methionine concentrations in the range of 37–136 μM.

Table 17-8. Distinguishing vitamin B$_{12}$ and folate deficiencies

Deficiency	Urinary FIGLU[a]	Urinary MMA[b]	Serum homocysteine	Serum folate
Vitamin B$_{12}$	Elevated	Elevated	Increased	Decreased
Folate	Elevated	Normal	Increased	Decreased

[a]Formiminoglutamic acid.
[b]Methylmalonic acid.

B$_{12}$ levels.[21] Low cobalamin levels have been observed in 10–15% of apparently healthy, elderly Americans with apparently adequate vitamin B$_{12}$ intakes, and in 60–70% of those with low vitamin B$_{12}$ intakes.[22] The prevalence of low plasma vitamin B$_{12}$ concentrations in all Central American age groups was found to be 35–90%.[23] It would appear that poor absorption of the vitamin from foods generally accounts for a third of such cases.

Homocysteinemia

Owing to lost methionine synthetase activity, subclinical vitamin B$_{12}$ deficiency can result in a moderate to intermediate elevation of plasma homocysteine concentrations (see Fig. 17-1). This condition, called **homocysteinemia**, can also be produced by folate deficiency, which by the methyl-folate trap also limits methionine synthase activity. Vitamin B$_{12}$ deficiency may be the primary cause of homocysteinemia in many people; almost two-thirds of elderly subjects with homocysteinemia also show **methylmalonic acidemia**,

indicative of vitamin B$_{12}$ deficiency (Table 17-9). Moderately elevated plasma homocysteine concentrations are associated with arterial and venous thrombosis as well as atherosclerosis; the mechanisms for these effects appear to involve inhibition by homocysteine of anticoagulant mechanisms mediated by the vascular epithelium. Thus, homocysteinemia is a risk factor for coronary, cerebral, and peripheral arterial occlusive diseases as well as for carotid thickening. Still, less than a third of individuals with low circulating vitamin B$_{12}$ levels also show homocysteinemia.

Neurological function

The accumulation of methylmalonyl CoA under conditions of low vitamin B$_{12}$ status leads to the formation and incorporation of nonphysiologic fatty acids into neuronal lipids including those in myelin sheaths. Methylcobalamin is the obligate carrier of methyl groups for the synthesis of choline, the precursor of the neurotransmitter acetylcholine. These phenomena are thought to underlie the neurological

Table 17-9. Vitamin B$_{12}$ and folate status of elderly subjects showing homocysteinemia

Parameter	Serum homocysteine		Serum methylmalonic acid	
	>3 SD	≤3 SD	>3 SD	≤3 SD
Serum vitamin B$_{12}$ (pM)	197 ± 77[a]	325 ± 145	217 ± 83[a]	332 ± 146
Serum folate (nM)	12.7 ± 8.2[a]	22.9 ± 19.0	18.1 ± 12.5[a]	22.7 ± 19.5

[a]$p > 0.05$.
Abbreviation: SD, standard deviation.
Source: Lindenbaum, J., Rosenberg, I. H., Wilson, P. W. F., Stabler, S. P., and Allen, R. H. (1994). Prevalence of cobalamin deficiency in the Framingham elderly population. *Am. J. Clin. Nutr.* **60,** 2–11.

[21] Norman, E. J., et al. (1993). *Am. Med. J.* **94,** 589–594.
[22] Carmel, R., et al. (1999). *Am. J. Clin. Nutr.* **70,** 904–910; Carmel, R. (2000). *Ann. Rev. Med.* **51,** 357–375.
[23] Allen, L. H. (2004). *Nutr. Rev.* **62,** S29–S33.

lesions of vitamin B$_{12}$ deficiency and to be related specifically to the following conditions:

- *Cognition* Serum homocysteine levels have been found to be negatively correlated with neuropsychological tests scores. There is little evidence that vitamin B$_{12}$ treatment can improve cognitive function in most impaired patients, although a review of clinical experience in India suggested the value of the vitamin in improving frontal lobe and language function in patients.[24] Because low serum vitamin B$_{12}$ levels occur more frequently in patients with senile dementia of the Alzheimer's type than in the general population, some have suggested that the vitamin may have a role in that disorder. This hypothesis is supported by observations of inverse relationships of serum vitamin B$_{12}$ levels and platelet monoamine oxidase activities, and the finding that vitamin B$_{12}$ treatment reduced the latter.
- *Depression* Low plasma levels of vitamin B$_{12}$ (and folate) have been reported in nearly a third of patients with depression, who also tend to show homocysteinemia. A recent study[25] suggested that patients with high vitamin B$_{12}$ status may have better treatment outcomes, but randomized clinical trials of vitamin B$_{12}$ treatment have not been reported.
- *Schizophrenia* That patients with schizophrenia generally have elevated circulating levels of methionine, with many also having homocysteinemia, suggests perturbations in single-carbon metabolism that naturally suggests a role of vitamin B$_{12}$. Randomized clinical trials of vitamin B$_{12}$ treatment have not been reported.
- *Multiple sclerosis* It has been suggested that low vitamin B$_{12}$ status may exacerbate multiple sclerosis by enhancing the processes of inflammation and demyelination and by impairing those of myelin repair. Pertinent to this hypothesis are the results of a study that

found combination therapy with interferon-ß and vitamin B$_{12}$ to produce dramatic improvements in an experimental model of the disease.

Genomic stability

Vitamin B$_{12}$ and folic acid play critical roles in the prevention of chromosomal damage and hypomethylation of DNA. A cross-sectional study showed that the vitamin B$_{12}$ levels of buccal cells were significantly lower in smokers than in nonsmokers and that elevated levels of the vitamin were associated with reduced frequency of micronucleus formation.[26] Chromosomal aberrations have also been reported for some patients with pernicious anemia.[27]

Carcinogenesis

The finding that low, asymptomatic vitamin B$_{12}$ status produced aberrations in base substitution and methylation of colonic DNA in the rat model,[28] suggests that subclinical deficiencies of the vitamin may enhance carcinogenesis. This hypothesis is supported by the results of a prospective study that found significantly increased breast cancer risk among women ranking in the lowest quintile of plasma vitamin B$_{12}$ concentration,[29] and the finding of significantly different risks for esophageal squamous cell carcinoma and gastric cardia adenocarcinoma associated with polymorphisms of methylenetetrahydrofolate reductase,[30] which, because it catalyzes the production of 5′-methyl-FH$_4$, can limit the activity of the vitamin B$_{12}$-dependent enzyme methionine synthase.

Osteoporosis

That vitamin B$_{12}$ may affect bone health was suggested by the finding that osteoporosis was more prevalent among elderly Dutch women of marginal or deficient status with respect to the vitamin (Table 17-10).

[24] Rita, M., et al. (2004). *Neurol. (India)* **52,** 310–318.
[25] Levitt, A. J., et al. (1998). *Psychiat. Res.* **79,** 123–129.
[26] Piyathilke, C. J., et al. (1995). *Cancer Epid. Biomakers Prev.* **4,** 751–758.
[27] Jensen, M. K. (1977). *Mutat. Res.* **45,** 249–252.
[28] Choi, S. W., et al. (2004). *J. Nutr.* **134,** 750–755.
[29] Wu, K., et al. (1999) *Cancer Epidemiol. Biomarkers Prev.* **8,** 209–217.
[30] Stolzenber-Solomon, R. Z., et al. (2003). *Cancer Epidemiol. Biomarkers Prev.* **12,** 1222–1226.

Table 17-10. Relationship of vitamin B_{12} status and osteoporosis risk among elderly women

Plasma vitamin B_{12}, pmol/L	N	RR (95% CI)
>320	34	1.0
210–320	43	4.8 (1.0–23.9)
<210	35	9.5 (1.9–46.1)

Source: Dhonukshe-Rutten, R. A. M., et al. (2003). *J. Nutr.* **133**, 801–807.

Congenital Disorders of Vitamin B_{12} Metabolism

Several congenital deficiencies in proteins involved in vitamin B_{12} metabolism, each an autosomal recessive trait, have been reported in humans (Table 17-11). Most of these disorders result in signs alleviated by high parenteral doses of the vitamin. The exception is congenital R protein deficiency; the few documented cases have involved healthy individuals.

VIII. Vitamin B_{12} Toxicity

Vitamin B_{12} has no appreciable toxicity. Results of studies with mice indicate that it is innocuous when administered parenterally in very high doses. Localized, injection-site, sclerodermoid reaction[31] secondary to vitamin B_{12} injection has been reported. Dietary levels of at least several hundred times the nutritional requirements are safe. High plasma levels of the vitamin are indicative of disease,[32] rather than hypervitaminosis B_{12}.

IX. Case Study

Instructions

Review the following case report, paying special attention to the diagnostic indicators on which the treatment was based. Next, answer the questions that follow.

Case

A 6-month-old boy was admitted in comatose condition. He had been born at term, weighing 3 kg, the first child of an apparently healthy 26-year-old *vegan*.[33] The mother had knowingly eaten no animal products for eight years and took no supplemental vitamins. The infant was exclusively breastfed. He smiled at one–two months of age and appeared to be developing normally. At four months, his development began to regress; this was manifested by his loss of head control, decreased vocalization, lethargy, and increased irritability. Physical examination revealed a pale and flaccid infant who was completely unresponsive even to painful stimuli. His pulse was 136/min, respirations 22/min, and blood pressure 100 mmHg by palpation. His length was 65 cm (50th percentile for age) and his weight was 5.6 kg (<3rd percentile, and at the 50th percentile for 3 months of age).

Table 17-11. Congenital disorders of vitamin B_{12} metabolism

Condition	Missing/deficient factor	Signs/symptoms
Methylmalonic aciduria	Methylmalonyl-CoA mutase	Methylmalonic aciduria, homocysteinuria, lethargy, muscle cramps, vomiting, mental retardation
Lack of intrinsic factor	Intrinsic factor	Signs consistent with vitamin B_{12} deficiency
Imerslund-Gräsbeck syndrome	IF receptor	Specific malabsorption of vitamin B_{12}
Lack of transcobalamins	Transcobalamins	Severe (fatal) megaloblastic anemia appearing early in life
Lack of R proteins	R proteins	None

---

[31] Such reactions are not common, but have been reported for various drugs and for vitamin K.

[32] Elevated cobalamin levels are typical of myelogenous leukemia and promyelocytic leukemic, and are used as diagnostic criteria for polycythemia vera and hypereosinophilic syndrome. Several liver diseases (acute hepatitis, cirrhosis, hepatocellular carcinoma, and metastatic liver disease) can cause similar increases, which are due to increased levels of TC_I.

[33] A strict vegetarian.

His head circumference was 41 cm (3rd percentile). His optic disks[34] were pale. There were scattered ecchymoses[35] over his legs and buttocks. He had increased pigmentation over the dorsa of his hands and feet, most prominently over the knuckles. He had no head control and a poor grasp. He showed no deep tendon reflexes. His liver edge was palpable 2 cm below the right costal margin.

Laboratory results

Parameter	Patient	Normal range
Hemoglobin (g/dl)	5.4	10.0–15.0
Hematocrit (%)	17	36
Erythrocytes (×10^6/μl)	1.63	3.9–5.3
White blood cells (×10^3/μl)	3.8	6–17.5
Reticulocytes (%)	0.1	<1
Platelets (×10^3/μl)	45	200–480

A peripheral blood smear revealed mild macrocytosis[36] and some hypersegmentation of the neutrophils.[37] Bone marrow aspiration showed frank megaloblastic changes in both the myeloid[38] and the erythroid[39] series. Megakaryocytes[40] were decreased in number. The sedimentation rate, urinalysis, spinal fluid analysis, blood glucose, electrolytes, and tests of renal and liver function gave normal results. An electroencephalogram was markedly abnormal, as manifested by minimal background Θ activity and epileptiform transients in both temporal regions. Analysis of the urine obtained on admission demonstrated a markedly elevated excretion of methylmalonic acid, glycine, methylcitric acid, and homocysteine. Shortly after admission, respiratory distress developed, and 5 mg of folic acid was given, followed by transfusion of 10 ml of packed erythrocytes per kilogram body weight. Four days later, a repeat bone marrow examination showed partial reversal of the megaloblastic abnormalities.

Other laboratory results

Parameter	Patient	Normal range
Serum vitamin B$_{12}$ (pg/ml)	20	150–1000
Serum folates (ng/ml)	10	3–15
Serum iron (μg/dl)	165	65–175
Serum iron-binding capacity (μg/dl)	177	250–410

Cyanocobalamin (1 mg/day) was administered for 4 days. The patient began to respond to stimuli after the transfusion; however, the response to vitamin B$_{12}$ was dramatic. Four days after the initial dose he was alert, smiling, responding to visual stimuli, and maintaining his body temperature. As he responded, rhythmical twitching activity in the right hand and arm developed that persisted despite anticonvulsant therapy and despite a concomitant resolution of electroencephalographic abnormalities. The mother showed a completely normal hemogram. Her serum vitamin B$_{12}$ concentration was 160 pg/ml (normal, 150–1000 pg/ml), but she showed moderate methylmalonic aciduria. Her breast milk contained 75 pg of vitamin B$_{12}$/ml (normal, 1–3 ng/ml).

With vitamin B$_{12}$ therapy, the infant's plasma vitamin B$_{12}$ rose to 600 pg/ml, and he continued to improve clinically. The abnormal urinary acids and homocysteine disappeared by day 10; cystathionine persisted until day 20. On day 14, the Hb was 14.4 g/dl, hematocrit was 41%, and the WBC was 5700/ml. The platelet count became normal 20 days after admission. The unusual pigment on the extremities had improved considerably 2 weeks after he received the parenteral vitamin B$_{12}$ and disappeared gradually over the next month. The liver was no longer palpable. The twitching of the hands disappeared within a month of therapy. Developmental assessment at 9 months of age revealed him to be functioning at the 5-month age level. A month later, he was sitting

---

[34] Circular area of thinning of the sclera (the fibrous membrane forming the outer envelope of the eye) through which the fibers of the optic nerve pass.

[35] Purple patches caused by extravasation of blood into the skin, differing from petechiae only in size (the latter being very small).

[36] Occurrence of unusually large numbers of *macrocytes* (large erythrocytes) in the circulating blood; also called *megalocytosis*, *magalocythemia*, and *macrocythemia*.

[37] A type of mature white blood cell in the granulocyte series.

[38] Related to myocytes.

[39] Related to erythrocytes.

[40] An unusually large cell thought to be derived from the primitive mesenchymal tissue that differentiates from hematocytoblasts.

and taking steps with support. Head circumference had exhibited catch-up growth and at 44 cm was in the normal range for the first time since admission. His length was 70 cm (10th percentile) and weight 8.4 kg (10th percentile). By this time, the mother's serum vitamin B_{12} had dropped to only 100 pg/ml, and she began taking supplemental vitamin B_{12}.

Case Questions

1. Which clinical findings suggested that two important coenzyme forms of vitamin B_{12} were deficient or defective in this infant? How do the clinical findings relate specifically to each coenzyme?

2. What findings allow the distinction of vitamin B_{12} deficiency from a possible folic acid-related disorder in this patient?

3. Offer a reasonable explanation for the fact that the mother, who had avoided vitamin B_{12}-containing foods for 8 years before her pregnancy, did not show overt signs of vitamin B_{12} deficiency.

Study Questions and Exercises

1. Construct a decision tree for the diagnosis of vitamin B_{12} deficiency in humans or an animal species and, in particular, the distinction of this deficiency from that of folate..

2. What key feature of the chemistry of vitamin B_{12} relates to its coenzyme functions?

3. What parameters might you measure to assess the vitamin B_{12} status of a human or an animal?

4. What is the relationship of normal function of the stomach and pancreas to the utilization of dietary vitamin B_{12}?

Recommended Reading

Andrès, E., Loukili, N. H., Noel, E., Kaltenbach, G., Abdelgheni, M. B., Perrin, A. F., Noblet-Dick, M., Maloisel, F., Schlienger, J. L., and Blicklé, J. F. (2004). Vitamin B_{12} (cobalamin) deficiency in elderly patients. *Can. Med. Assoc. J.* **171**, 251–259.

Baik, H. W., and Russell, R. M. (1999). Vitamin B_{12} deficiency in the elderly. *Ann. Rev. Nutr.* **19**, 357–377.

Bailey, L. B. 2004. Folate and vitamin B_{12} recommended intakes and status in the United States. *Nutr. Rev.* **62**, S14–S20.

Banerjee, R., and Ragsdale, S. W. (2003). The many faces of vitamin B_{12}: Catalysis by cobalamin-dependent enzymes. *Ann. Rev. Biochem.* **72**, 209–247.

Beck, W. S. (2001). Cobalamin (Vitamin B_{12}), Chapter 13 in *Handbook of Vitamins*, 3rd ed. (R. B. Rucker, J. W. Suttie, D. B. McCormick, and Machlin L. J., eds.), pp. 463–512. Marcel Dekker, New York.

Bridden, A. (2003). Homocysteine in the context of cobalamin metabolism and deficiency states. *Amino Acids* **24**, 1–12.

Brown, K. L. (2005). Chemistry and enzymology of vitamin B_{12}. *Chem. Rev.* **105**, 2075–2149.

Carmel, R. (2006). Cobalamin (Vitamin B_{12}). Chapter, 29 in *Modern Nutrition in Health and Disease*, 10th ed. (M. E. Shils, M. Shike, A. C. Ross, B. Cabellero, and R. J. Cousins, eds.), pp. 482–497. Lippincott, New York.

Cooper, B. A., and Rosenblatt, D. S. (1987). Inherited defects of vitamin B_{12} metabolism. *Annu. Rev. Nutr.* **7**, 291–320.

Dwyer, J. T. (1991). Nutritional consequences of vegetarianism. *Ann. Rev. Nutr.* **11**, 61–91.

Ermens, A. A. M., Vlasveld, L. T., and Lindemans, J. (2003). Significance of elevated cobalamin (vitamin B_{12}) levels in blood. *Clin. Biochem.* **36**, 585–590.

Fenech, M. (2001). The role of folic acid and vitamin B_{12} in genomic stability of human cells. *Mutation Res.* **475**, 57–67.

Herrmann, W., and Geisel, J. (2002). Vegetarian lifestyle and monitoring of vitamin B-12 status. *Clin. Chim. Acta* **326**, 47–59.

Koury, M. J., and Ponka, P. (2004). New insights into erythropoiesis: The roles of folate, vitamin B_{12} and iron. *Ann. Rev. Nutr.* **24**, 105–131.

Kräutler, B. (2005). Vitamin B_{12}: Chemistry and biochemistry. *Biochem. Soc. Trans.* **33**, 806–810.

Marsh, E. N. G., and Drennan, C. L. (2001). Adenosylcobalamin-dependent isomerases: New insights into structure and mechanism. *Curr. Opin. Chem. Biol.* **5**, 499–505.

Metz, J. (1992). Cobalamin deficiency and the pathogenesis of nervous system disease. *Annu. Rev. Nutr.* **12**, 59–79.

Monsen, A. L. B., and Ueland, P. M. (2003). Homocysteine and methylmalonic acid in diagnosis and risk assessment from infancy to adolescence. *Am. J. Clin. Nutr.* **78,** 7–21.

Rita, M., Paola, T., Rodolfo, A, Tatiana, C., Giuseppe, C., and Antonio, B. (2004). Vitamin B$_{12}$ and folate depletion in cognition: A review. *Neurol. (India)* **52,** 310–318.

Sanders, T. A. B., and Reddy, S. (1994). Nutritional implications of a meatless diet. *Proc. Nutr. Soc.* **53,** 297–307.

Scott, J. M. (1997). Bioavailability of vitamin B$_{12}$. *Eur. J. Clin. Nutr.* **51,** S49–S53.

Scott, J. M. (1999). Folate and vitamin B$_{12}$. *Proc. Soc. Nutr. Soc.* **58,** 441–448.

Stabler, S. P. (2001). Vitamin B-12, Chapter 22 in *Present Knowledge in Nutrition,* 8th ed. (B. A. Bowman and R. M. Russell, eds.), pp. 230–240. ILSI Press, Washington, DC.

Stabler, S. P., and Allen, R. H. (2004). Vitamin B$_{12}$ deficiency as a worldwide problem. *Ann. Rev. Nutr.* **24,** 299–326.

Stover, P. J. (2004). Physiology of folate and vitamin B$_{12}$ in health and disease. *Nutr. Rev.* **62,** S3–S12.

Thorogood, M. (1995). The epidemiology of vegetarianism and health. *Nutr. Res. Rev.* **8,** 179–192.

Toh, B. H., van Driel, I. R., and Gleeson, P. A. (2006). Pernicious anemia. *N. Engl. J. Med.* **337,** 1441–1448.

Zetterberg, H. (2004). Methylenetetrahydrofolate reductase and transcobalamin genetic polymorphisms in human spontaneous abortion: Biological and clinical implications. *Reprod. Biol. Endocrinol.* **2,** 7–15.

Quasi-vitamins

18

Have all the vitamins been discovered? From all indications in the extensive recent and current publications in the scientific literature dealing with the purification and effects of "unidentified factors," the answer appears to be "no." It is from such studies that new vitamins may be recognized and characterized.

— A. F. Wagner and K. Folkers

I.	Is the List of Vitamins Complete?	400
II.	Choline	401
III.	Carnitine	406
IV.	*myo*-Inositol	413
V.	Pyrroloquinoline Quinone	418
VI.	Ubiquinones	420
VII.	Flavonoids	422
VIII.	Non-Provitamin A Carotenoids	425
IX.	Orotic Acid	428
X.	*p*-Aminobenzoic Acid	429
XI.	Lipoic Acid	429
XII.	Ineffective Factors	430
XIII.	Unidentified Growth Factors	431
	Study Questions and Exercises	431
	Recommended Reading	432

Anchoring Concepts

1. The designation "vitamin" is specific for animal species, stage of development or production, and/or particular conditions of the physical environment and diet.
2. Each of the presently recognized vitamins was initially called an accessory factor or an unidentified growth factor. These terms continue to be used to describe biologically active substances, particularly for species of lower orders.

Learning Objectives

1. To understand that the designation of a compound as a vitamin is biased in favor of dietary essentials for humans.
2. To understand that other substances have been proposed as vitamins.
3. To understand that choline and carnitine are vitamins for certain animal species.
4. To understand the metabolic functions of other conditionally essential nutrients: *myo*-inositol, pyrroloquinoline quinine, the ubiquinones, and orotic acid.
5. To understand why flavonoids, non-provitamin A carotenoids, *p*-aminobenzoic acid, and lipoic acid are not called vitamins.

Vocabulary

Acetylcholine
Acylcarnitine esters
Acylcarnitine translocase
p-Aminobenzoic acid
Arachidonic acid
Betaine
Betaine aldehyde dehydrogenase
Betaine:homocysteine methyltransferase
γ-Butyrobetaine hydroxylase
Ca^{2+} channel
Calcisomes
Carnitine
Carnitine acyltransferases I and II
Chelates
Choline
Choline acetyltransferase
Choline dehydrogenase
Choline kinase
Choline oxidase
Choline phosphotransferase
Coenzyme Q_{10} (CoQ_{10})
Cyanogenic glycoside
Cytidine diphosphorylcholine (CDP–choline)
Dimethylglycine
Eicosanoids
Flavanols
Flavonoids

Glycerylphosphorylcholine
Glycerylphosphorylcholine diesterase
myo-Inositol
Inositol 1,4,5-triphosphate (IP$_3$)
Intestinal lipodystrophy
Isoflavones
Labile methyl groups
Lecithin
Lipoic acid
Lipoamide
Lycopene
Lysolecithin
Lysyl oxidase
Lutein
Macular degeneration
Methionine
Orotic acid
Perosis
Phosphatidylcholine
Phosphatidylcholine glyceride
  choline transferase
Phosphatidylethanolamine
Phosphatidylethanolamine *N*-methyl
  transferase
Phosphatidylinositol (PI)
Phosphatidylinositol 4-phosphate (PIP)
Phospholipases A$_1$, A$_2$, B, C, and D
Phosphorylcholine
Phytic acid
Phytoestrogens
Pyrroloquinoline quinone (PQQ)
Quinoproteins
Second messenger
Sphingomyelin
Stearic acid
Trimethylamine
ε-*N*-Trimethyllysine
Ubiquinones
Vitamin B$_T$
Xanthophylls
Zeaxanthin

I. Is the List of Vitamins Complete?

Common Features in the Recognition of Vitamins

Reflection on the ways in which the traditional vitamins were recognized reveals a process of discovery involving both empirical and experimental phases (see Chapter 2). That is, initial associations between diet and health status were the sources of hypotheses that could be tested in controlled experiments. As is generally true in science, where hypotheses were clearly enunciated and adequate experimental approaches were available, insightful investigators were able to make remarkable progress in identifying these essential nutrients. Those endeavors, of course, also revealed that some unidentified factors were not new at all,[1] some identical or otherwise related to each other,[2] others biologically active but not essential in diets,[3] and still others to be without basis in fact.[4] The apparently irregular and often confusing array of informal names of the vitamins[5] reveals this history of discovery.

Limitations of Traditional Designations of Vitamins

The development of the vitamine theory was instrumental in conditioning thought such that the discovery of the vitamins could occur. Indeed, it provided the basis for the evolution of the operating definition that has been used to designate vitamin status for biologically active substances. However, after several decades of learning more and more about the metabolism and biochemical actions of the substances called vitamins, it has become clear that the traditional criteria for that designation[6] are, in several cases (e.g., vitamins D and C, niacin, and choline), inappropriate unless they are used with specific reference

---

[1] An example is vitamin T (also called "termitin," "penicin," "torutilin," "insectine," "hypomycin," "myocoine," or "sesame seed factor"). This extract from yeast, sesame seeds, or insects appeared to stimulate the growth of guppies, hamsters, baby pigs, chicks, mice, and insects: promoted wound healing in mice; and improved certain human skin lesions. It was found to be a varied mixture containing folate, vitamin B$_{12}$, and amino acids.

[2] For example, vitamins M, B$_c$, B$_{10}$, T, and B$_x$ were found to be various forms of folate.

[3] For example, the ubiquinones.

[4] For example, pangamic acid (vitamin B$_{15}$), laetrile (vitamin B$_{17}$), orotic acid (vitamin B$_{13}$), and vitamins H$_3$ and U.

[5] See Appendix A.

[6] See Chapter 1.

to animal species, stage of development, diet or nutritional status, and physical environment. However, because it is often more convenient to consider nutrients by general group without such referents, the designation of vitamin status has become a bit arbitrary as well as anthropocentric in that the traditional designation of the vitamins reflects, to a large extent, the nutritional needs of humans and, to a lesser extent, those of domestic animals. For example, although it is now very clear that 1,25-dihydroxycholecalciferol [1,25-(OH)$_2$-cholecalciferol] is actually a hormone produced endogenously by all species exposed to sunlight, the parent compound cholecalciferol continues to be called vitamin D$_3$ in recognition of its importance to the health of many people whose minimal sunlight exposure renders them in need of it in their diets.

Other species may have obligate dietary needs for substances that are biosynthesized by humans and/or higher animals. Such substances can be considered to be vitamins in the most proper sense of the word. Available evidence indicates this to be true for at least three substances, and some reports have suggested this for others.

It is also the case that specific physiological states resulting from specific genetics, disease, or dietary conditions may place an individual incapable of synthesizing a metabolite, resulting in a need for the preformed nutrient from exogenous sources such as the diet. Several such conditionally essential nutrients have characteristics of vitamins for affected individuals.

Finally, as more is learned, it is certainly possible that more vitamins may be discovered.

Quasi-vitamins

It is useful to recognize the other factors that appear to satisfy the criteria of vitamin status for only a few species or under only certain conditions and to do so without according them the full status of a vitamin. This is done using the term *quasi-vitamin*. The list of quasi-vitamins includes:

- Factors required for some species
  - *Choline*—required in the diets of young growing poultry for optimal growth and freedom of leg disorders
  - *Carnitine*—required for growth of certain insects

  - *Myo-inositol*—clearly required for optimal growth of fishes and to prevent intestinal lesions in gerbils
- Factors for which evidence of nutritional essentiality is less compelling
  - *Pyrroloquinoline quinine*
  - *Ubiquinones*
  - *Flavonoids*
  - *Some non-provitamin A carotenoids*
  - *Orotic acid*
  - *p-Aminobenzoic acid*
  - *Lipoic acid*

In addition, the biologically active properties of certain natural products (unidentified growth factors, or UGFs) are worthy of consideration in as much as at most of the consensus vitamins were initially recognized as UGFs. Also included in this chapter are discussions of ineffective factors often confused with vitamins.

The quasi-vitamins:

Choline	Pyrroloquinoline quinone	Bioflavonoids
Carnitine	Ubiquinones	p-Aminobenzoic acid
myo-Inositol	Orotic acid	Lipoic acid

II. Choline

A Known Metabolite Acting Like a Vitamin

The discovery of insulin by Banting and Best in the mid-1920s led to studies of the metabolism of depancreatized dogs that showed dietary lecithin (phosphatidylcholine) to be effective in mobilizing the excess lipids in the livers of insulin-deprived animals. Best and Huntsman showed that choline was the active component of lecithin in mediating this effect. Choline had been isolated by Strecker in 1862, and its structure had been determined by Bayer shortly after that. Yet, it was the findings revealing choline as a lipotropic factor that stimulated interest in its nutritional role.

Poultry Have Special Needs for Choline

In 1940, Jukes showed that choline is required for normal growth and the prevention of the leg disorder called **perosis**[7] in turkeys; he found that the amount required to prevent perosis is greater than that required to support normal growth. Further studies by Jukes and by Norris's group at Cornell showed that **betaine**, the metabolic precursor to choline, was not always effective in preventing choline-responsive perosis in turkeys and chicks. These findings stimulated further interest in the metabolic roles and nutritional needs for choline, as it was clear that its function was more than simply that of a lipotrope.

Chemical Nature

Choline is the trivial designation for the compound 2-hydroxy-N,N,N-trimethylethanaminium [also, (β-hydroxyethyl)trimethylammonium]. It is freely soluble in water and ethanol, but insoluble in organic solvents. It is a strong base and decomposes in alkaline solution with the release of trimethylamine. The prominent feature of its chemical structure is its triplet of methyl groups, which enables it to serve as a methyl donor.

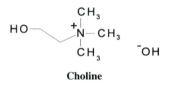

Choline

Distribution in Foods and Feedstuffs

All natural fats contain some choline; therefore, the vitamin is widely distributed in foods and feedstuffs (Table 18-1). The factor occurs naturally mostly in the form of **phosphatidylcholine** (also called **lecithin**), which, because it is a good emulsifying agent, is used as an ingredient or additive in many processed foods and food supplements. Some dietary choline (< 10%) is present as the free base and **sphingomyelin** (phosphatidylcholine analogs containing, instead of a fatty acid, sphingosine [2-amino-4-octadecene-1,3-diol] at the glycerol α-carbon). Choline is added (as choline chloride and choline bitartrate) to infant formulas as a means of fortification. The richest sources in human diets[8] are egg yolk, glandular meats (e.g., liver, kidney, brain), soybean products, wheat germ, and peanuts. The best sources of choline for animal feeding

Table 18-1. Choline contents of common foods

Food	Choline (mg/g)	Food	Choline (mg/g)
Meats		Vegetables	
Beef brain	410	Asparagus	128
Beef liver	630	Cabbage	46
Beef kidney	333	Carrots	10
Ham	120	Cauliflower	78
Trout	84	Lettuce	18
Cereals		Soybeans	237
Barley	139	Peanuts	145
Oats	151	Dairy and egg products	
Rice, polished	126	Milk	10
Wheat germ	423	Egg yolk	1713

are the germs of cereals, legumes, and oilseed meals (e.g., soybean meal). Corn is notably low in choline (half the levels found in barley, oats, and wheat). Wheat is rich in the choline-sparing factor betaine; therefore, the choline needs of livestock fed diets based on wheat are much lower than those of animals fed diets based on corn. Little is known about the bioavailability of choline in foods and feedstuffs. Naturally occurring choline, as well as the choline salts used as supplements to human diets and animal feeds, have good stability.

Absorption

Choline is released from phosphatidylcholine by hydrolysis in the intestinal lumen. This is accomplished enzymatically through the action of phospholipases produced by the pancreas (**phospholipase A$_2$**, which cleaves the β-ester bond) and the intestinal mucosa (**phospholipases A$_1$ and B**, both of which cleave the α-ester bond to yield **glycerylphosphorylcholine**). The mucosal enzymes are much less efficient than the pancreatic enzyme. Therefore, most of the phosphatidylcholine that is ingested is absorbed as **lysolecithin** (deacylated only in the α position), which is reacylated to yield phosphati-

---

[7] Perosis occurs in rapidly growing, heavy-bodied poultry, and involves the misalignment of the tibiotarsus and consequent slippage of the Achilles tendon. This impairs ambulation and can reduce feeding, consequently impairing growth. Perosis can also be caused by dietary deficiencies of niacin or manganese.

[8] Choline intakes of Americans have been estimated to be 443 ± 88 mg/day for women and 631 ± 157 mg/day for men (Fischer, L. M., et al. [2005]. *J. Nutr.* **135,** 826–829).

dylcholine. This reaction involves the dismutation of two molecules of lysolecithin to yield one molecule of glycerylphosphorylcholine and one molecule of phosphatidylcholine. Analogous reactions occur with sphingomyelin, which, unlike phosphatidylcholine, is not degraded in the intestinal lumen, but is taken up intact by the intestinal mucosa. When free choline or one of its salts is consumed, a large amount (e.g., nearly two-thirds) is catabolized by intestinal microorganisms to the end product **trimethylamine**,[9] much of which is absorbed and excreted in the urine. The remaining portion is absorbed intact. Phosphatidylcholine is not subject to such extensive microbial metabolism and, therefore, produces less urinary trimethylamine.

Choline is absorbed in the upper portion of the small intestine by a saturable, carrier-mediated process involving a carrier localized in the brush border, and efficient at low lumenal concentrations ($<4\,\mathrm{m}M$). At high lumenal concentrations, it is also absorbed by passive diffusion.

Uptake and Transport

Recently absorbed choline is transported into the lymphatic circulation (or the portal circulation in birds, fishes, and reptiles) primarily in the form of phosphatidylcholine bound to chylomicra, which are subject to clearance to the lipoproteins that circulate to the peripheral tissues. Thus, choline is transported to the tissues predominantly as phospholipids associated with the plasma lipoproteins (Table 18-2).

Table 18-2. Distribution of phospholipids in plasma lipoproteins

Lipoprotein class	Phospholipid content (% total weight)
High-density lipoproteins (HDLs)	~30
Low-density lipoproteins (LDLs)	~22
Very low-density lipoproteins (VLDLs)	10–25
Chylomicra	3–15

Choline is taken up into cells by three transport systems:[10]

- By a high-affinity, Na^+-dependent transporter (CHT1) that provides choline for the synthesis of acetylcholine in cholinergic neurons
- By low-affinity, Na^+-independent transporters of the family of organic cation transporters (OCTs)
- By passive diffusion

Choline is present in all tissues as an essential component of phospholipids in membranes of all types. It is stored in the greatest concentrations in the essential organs (e.g., brain, liver, kidney) in the forms of phosphatidylcholine and sphingomyelins. Placental tissues are unique in that they accumulate large amounts of acetylcholine, presumably to meet fetal needs, which is otherwise present only in the parasympathetic nervous system.

Biosynthesis

There are three means of phosphatidylcholine biosynthesis: methylation of ethanolamine, reaction of cytidine diphosphate, and phospholipid base exchange (e.g., substitution of choline for serine, ethanolamine, or inositol in endogenous phospholipids). Of these, only the methylation pathway involves the *de novo* synthesis of choline. Most species can synthesize choline, as phosphatidylcholine, by the sequential methylation of **phosphatidylethanolamine** by **phosphatidylethanolamine N-methyltransferase** (Fig. 18-1). This activity is actually due to two enzymes: a cell inner membrane enzyme adds the first methyl group; a cell outer membrane enzyme adds the second and third methyl groups. Each enzyme uses *S*-adenosylmethionine as the methyl donor. The first is rate limiting to choline synthesis. Owing to developmental deficiencies of this methylating enzyme, which is low in male rats and absent from chicks until about 13 weeks of age, animals can require dietary sources of preformed choline. The chick has an absolute need, while the rat requires choline only if this methylation pathway is limited by the low availability of methyl groups, in which case the feeding of methyl donors

---

[9] The characteristic fishy odor of this product is identifiable after consumption of a choline supplement.

[10] It has also been suggested that choline-specific tansporter-like proteins (CHTLs) may participate in the cellular uptake of choline.

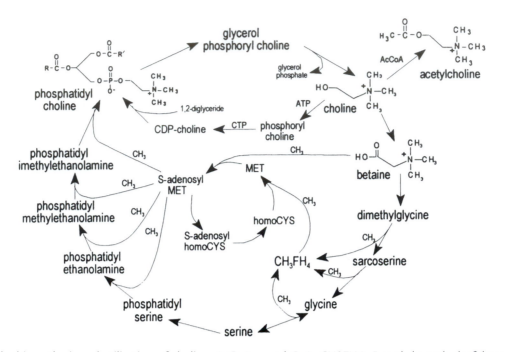

Fig. 18-1. The biosynthesis and utilization of choline. AcCoA, acetyl-CoA; CH3FH4, 5-methyl tetrahydrofolate; CTP, cytidine triphosphate; homoCYS, homocysteine; MET, methionine.

(methionine, betaine) spares the need for choline. Phosphatidylethanolamine *N*-methyltransferase activity is greatest in liver, but is also found in many other tissues. It accounts for the synthesis of 15–40% of the phosphatidylcholine in the liver most of the balance being derived from the cytidine diphosphate (CDP)–choline pathway.

Metabolism

Choline is released in free form in the tissues by the actions of **phospholipase C**, which cleaves the circulating form (phosphatidylcholine) to yield a diglyceride and **phosphorylcholine**. The latter species is converted to free choline by alkaline phosphatase. In addition, peripheral tissues also contain phospholipase B activity and can therefore produce glyceryl-phosphorylcholine from the circulating form of the vitamin. That product can then be cleaved by **glyceryl-phosphorylcholine diesterase** to yield free choline. The brain also contains **phospholipase D**, which cleaves free choline directly from the circulating form (also yielding glycerylphosphate).

Free choline can be oxidized by the mitochondrial enzyme **choline dehydrogenase** to yield betaine alde-

hyde, which is then converted by the cytosolic enzyme **betaine aldehyde dehydrogenase** to betaine.[11] This dual enzyme system is called **choline oxidase**; it is found is several tissues (e.g., liver and kidney), but is notably absent from brain, muscle, and blood. It is induced by dietary choline. Choline is oxidized to betaine at a rate that is an order of magnitude greater than that of its incorporation into phosphorylcholine. Betaine cannot be reduced back to form choline, but it can donate its methyl groups to homocysteine to produce **dimethylglycine** and **methionine** by the action of the enzyme **betaine:homocysteine methyltransferase**. Therefore, while the choline oxidase pathway removes free choline from the body, it also serves as a source of **labile methyl groups**.

Free choline is phosphorylated by the cytosolic enzyme **choline phosphotransferase** (also called **choline kinase**), using ATP as the phosphate donor. This step occurs in many tissues and constitutes the first step in the generation of **cytidine diphosphorylcholine (CDP–choline)**, which combines with diacylglycerol (by the action of **phosphatidylcholine glyceride transferase**) in the synthesis of phosphatidylcholine.

Only a small fraction of choline is acetylated, but that amount provides the important neurotransmitter

[11] 1-Carboxy-*N,N,N*-trimethylmethanaminium hydroxide inner salt.

acetylcholine. This step involves the reaction of choline with acetyl-CoA and is catalyzed by an enzyme **choline acetyltransferase** localized in cholinergic nerve terminals, as well as in certain other nonnervous tissues (e.g., placenta). Because brain choline acetyltransferase does not appear to be saturated with either substrate, it is likely that the availability of choline (as well as that of acetyl-CoA) may determine the rate of synthesis of acetylcholine.

Metabolic Functions

Choline has five essential functions in metabolism:

- *As phosphatidylcholine*
  ○ A structural element of biological membranes
  ○ A precursor to ceramide,[12] the basic structure of sphingolipids, which play roles in transmembrane signal transduction[13]
  ○ A promoter of lipid transport (as a lipotrope)
- *As acetylcholine*, it is a neurotransmitter, occurring primarily in the parasympathetic nervous system.
- *As a component of platelet-activating factor* (1-*O*-alkyl-2-acetyl-*sn*-glycero-3-phosphocholine), it is important in clotting, inflammation,[14] uterine ovum implantation, fetal maturation, and induction of labor.
- *As a component of plasmalogen*, it has a role in myocardial function.[15]
- *As a source of labile methyl groups*, after its irreversible oxidation to betaine, it is a source of labile methyl groups for transmethylation reactions in the formation of methionine from homocysteine, or of creatine from guanidoacetic acid. This function links choline to folate metabolism: Because the biosynthesis of methionine by the methylation of homocysteine by 5-methyltetrahydrofolate cannot meet all of the intracellular demands for S-adenosylmethionine, choline constitutes an important dietary source of labile methyl groups for homocysteine transmethylation.

Conditions of Need

Choline deprivation can produce signs in young poultry (e.g., chicks less than about 13 weeks of age) and in older poultry and other animals fed diets deficient in methyl groups (methionine-deficient diets). Choline deprivation in other animal species can cause signs if the intake of methionine is also limited. Those signs include depressed growth, hepatic steatosis, and hemorrhagic renal degeneration. The fatty infiltration of the liver that occurs in choline-deficient animals is presumed to be due to the need for phosphatidylcholine for hepatic lipoprotein (mainly very low-density lipoprotein, VLDL) synthesis, which in turn is necessary for the export of triglycerides. Poultry also show perosis, but this disorder is thought to be a secondary lesion related to impaired lipid transport.

Clear needs for dietary choline have also been demonstrated for fish.[16] The signs of deficiency include impaired weight gain and efficiency of feed utilization and hepatic steatosis. It is generally assumed that most fishes cannot synthesize choline at levels sufficient to meet their physiological needs.

Rats fed a choline-deficient diet or treated with methotrexate show 30–40% reductions in hepatic and brain levels of folate, resulting in a shift toward longer polyglutamate metabolites and in the undermethylation of DNA. Pregnancy and lactation result in significant decreases in hepatic choline levels.

Choline deficiency have not been reported in humans, but this may only reflect the adequacy of other methyl donors in the types of subjects frequently studied. One study, in which healthy adults were fed a diet adequate (but not excessive) in methionine and folacin, showed that deprivation of choline produced signs of hepatic dysfunction (increased serum transaminase activities) that were corrected by feeding choline. Furthermore, some evidence supports benefits of choline in the treatment of diseases involving hepatic steatosis and of liver dysfunction associated with total parenteral feeding of low-choline fluids.

---

[12] Ceramide is formed by adding a fatty acid to the amino group of sphingosine. Among the biological activities of ceramide are the stimulation of *apoptosis* (i.e., programmed cell death).

[13] Phospholipid-mediated signal transduction involves membrane phospholipases that trigger the generation of inositol-1,4,5-triphosphate, which acts to release Ca^{2+} from stores in the endoplasmic reticulum.

[14] Overproduction of platelet-activating factor has been shown to produce a hyperresponsive condition, as occurs in asthma.

[15] High levels of plasmalogen are found in the sarcolemma. It is thought that the adverse effects of myocardial ischemia may involve the breakdown of plasmalogen.

[16] For example, red drum (*Sciaenops ocellutus*) and striped bass (*Morone* spp.).

Role in Carcinogenesis

Choline deficiency in animal models has been found to increase the incidence of spontaneous hepatocarcinomas in the absence of any known carcinogen and to enhance hepatocarcinogenesis induced chemically. These effects have been shown to involve both the initiation and promotion phases of carcinogenesis. They would appear to result from metabolic responses to choline deprivation, in particular, decreases in tissue levels of S-adenosylmethionine resulting in hypomethylation of DNA and the consequent changes in gene transcription, including modified expression of p53 protein. They may also be related to the progressive increase in hepatocyte proliferation that occurs after parenchymal cell death in the regenerating choline-deficient liver. Similar results have been found in mice (but not rats) treated with the choline precursor diethanolamine.

Health Effects

The intake of choline can affect the concentrations of the neurotransmitter acetylcholine in the brain, suggesting that choline loading may be beneficial to patients with diseases involving deficiencies of cholinergic neurotransmission. Indeed, studies with animal models have shown choline supplementation during development to enhance cognitive performance, particularly on more difficult tasks; to increase electrophysiological responsiveness; and to provide some protection against alcohol and other neurotoxic agents.

In humans, large doses (multiple-gram quantities) of choline have been used to increase brain choline concentrations above normal levels, thereby stimulating the synthesis of acetylcholine in nerve terminals. Such supplementation has been found to help in the treatment of tardive dyskinesia, a movement disorder involving inadequate neurotransmission at striatal cholinergic interneurons.[17] Choline supplements have also been used with some success to improve free memory in subjects without dementia[18] and to diminish short-term memory losses associated with Alzheimer's disease,[19] a disorder involving deficiency of hippocampal cholinergic neurons. In fact, it has been suggested that auto-cannibalism of membrane phosphatidylcholine may be an underlying defect in that disease. This is supported by the fact that patients treated with anticholinergic drugs develop short-term memory deficits resembling those associated with hippocampal lesions.

Phosphatidylcholine has been reported to reduce manic episodes in patients, suggesting that it can be centrally active; however, such treatment has been found to exacerbate depression among tardive dyskinesia patients.

Toxicity

The toxicity of choline appears to be very low. However, deleterious effects have been reported for the salt choline chloride; these have included growth depression, impaired utilization of vitamin B_6, and increased mortality. The cause of these effects is not clear, however; the apparent toxicity of that form of the vitamin may actually have been due to the perturbation of acid–base balance caused by the high level of chloride administered with large doses of the salt. In humans, high doses (e.g., 20 g) have produced dizziness, nausea, and diarrhea.

III. Carnitine

Insect Growth Factor

In the 1950s, a group of entomologists at the University of Illinois, Fraenkel and colleagues, found that the successful growth of the yellow mealworm *Tenebrio molitor* in culture required the feeding of a natural substance that they found to be present in milk, yeast, and many animal tissues. They purified the growth factor, which they named **vitamin B_T**, from whey solids and identified it as **carnitine**,[20] a known metabolite isolated at the turn of the century from extracts of mammalian muscle. Although this finding established carnitine as a biologically active substance, the first

---

[17] Tardive dyskinesia is prevalent among patients treated with neuroleptic drugs (drugs affecting the autonomic nervous system) and is characterized by choreoathetotic movements [involuntary movements resembling both *chorea* (irregular and spasmodic) and *athetosis* (slow and writhing)] of the face, the extremities, and, usually, the trunk.

[18] Spiers, P., et al. (1996). *Arch. Neurol.* **53,** 441–448; Ladd, S. L., et al. (1993). *Clin. Neuropharmacol.* **16,** 540–549; Sitram, N., et al. (1978). *Life Sci.* **22,** 1555–1560.

[19] Alvarez, X. A., et al. (1997). *Methods Find. Exp. Clin. Pharmacol.* **19,** 201–210.

[20] Carter, H. E., Bhattacharyya, P. K., Weidman, K. R., and Fraenkel, G. (1952). *Arch. Biochem. Biophys.* **38,** 405–426.

indication of its metabolic role came a decade later when Fritz at the University of Michigan found that it stimulated the *in vitro* oxidation of long-chain fatty acids by subcellular fractions of heart muscle. More recently, research interest in carnitine has increased dramatically, stimulated by the finding of Broquist and colleagues at Vanderbilt University that carnitine is biosynthesized by mammals from the amino acid lysine, which is limiting in the diets of many Third World populations, and by the description by Engel and colleagues of clinical syndromes (of apparently genetic origin) associated with carnitine deficiency.

Chemical Nature

Carnitine is the generic term for a number of compounds including L-carnitine (β[-]-β-hydroxy-γ-[*N,N,N*-trimethylaminobutyrate][21]) and its acetyl and propionyl esters. Only the L-isomer is biologically active.

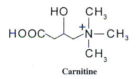

Carnitine

Biosynthesis

Carnitine is synthesized in mammals from two indispensable amino acids—lysine and methionine—which provide the methyl groups. Carnitine biosynthesis has been investigated most extensively in the rat; available evidence indicates that the biosynthetic pathways in humans, and probably other mammals, are identical. The process (see Fig. 18-2) commences with the enzymatic trimethylation of a peptide-bound lysine residue to form **ε-*N*-trimethyllysine,** using *S*-adenosylmethionine as the methyl donor. The ε-*N*-trimethyllysine, released as the protein turns over, is converted to L-carnitine through a sequence of enzymatic reactions involving two Fe^{2+}- and ascorbate-dependent hydroxylases and one NAD^+-dependent dehydrogenase. Carnitine biosynthesis can be stimulated by the catabolic state (e.g., fasting), thyroid hormone, and the peroxisome proliferator clofibrate.[22] That tissue carnitine concentrations are depressed in vitamin B_6 deficiency suggests that the vitamin may be required for carnitine biosynthesis; serine hydroxymethyltranferase, a pyridoxal 5'-phosphate-dependent enzyme, has the capacity to cleave 3-hydroxy-6-*N*-trimethyllysine.

The enzymes that catalyze the conversion of ε-*N*-trimethyllysine to γ-butyrobetaine appear to occur in all tissues. In contrast, the last enzyme in the biosynthetic pathway, **γ-butyrobetaine hydroxylase**, is present only in liver, kidney, and brain. In human liver and kidney, it is present as multiple isoenzymes; the activity increases during development,[23] reaching maximum in the mid-teens. Little direct evidence is available concerning the quantitative aspects of carnitine biosynthesis relative to physiological needs in humans. That healthy adults can

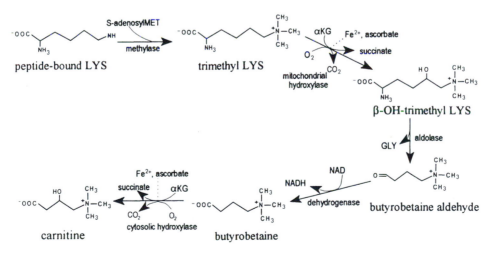

Fig. 18-2. The biosynthesis of carnitine. αKG, α-ketoglutarate; LYS, lysine; GLY, glycine.

---

[21] Molecular weight = 161.2.

[22] This effect appears to involve the receptor peroxisome proliferator-activated nuclear receptor α (PPARα).

[23] For example, the hepatic γ-butyrobetaine hydroxylase activities of three infants and a 2.5-year-old boy were 12 and 30%, respectively, of the mean adult activity.

synthesize carnitine at rates sufficient for their needs is indicated by findings that subjects in Southeast Asia, whose cereal-based diets provide very little preformed carnitine, show plasma carnitine concentrations[24] comparable to those of subjects in Western nations, whose diets tend to have abundant amounts of the factor. Similarly, attempts to produce carnitine deficiency in experimental animals by restricting carnitine in the diet have proved unsuccessful, apparently owing to their capacities to biosynthesize the factor. However, because neonates of several species, including humans, have been found to have low tissue carnitine levels when fed low-carnitine diets, it is likely that the total carnitine biosynthetic capacity may be immature in newborns, thus rendering them dependent on their diets for preformed carnitine. That the milks of various species contain appreciable amounts of carnitine supports this view. For example, human milk contains 28–95 nmol of carnitine per milliliter, and cow's milk contains 190–270 nmol of carnitine per milliliter.

Dietary Sources

The available data concerning the carnitine contents of foods are scant and must be considered suspect, owing to the use of nonstandard analytical methods.

Nevertheless, it is apparent that materials of plant origin tend to be low in carnitine, whereas those derived from animals tend to be rich in the factor (Table 18-3). Red meats and dairy products are particularly rich sources.

Absorption

Carnitine appears to be absorbed across the gut by an active process dependent on Na^+ co-transport, as well as by a passive, diffusional process that may be important for the absorption of large doses of the factor. The efficiency of absorption appears to be high, ca. 54–87%. High doses are absorbed at lower efficiencies (1–18%), with <1% appearing in the urine and very little appearing in the feces. The uptake of carnitine from the intestinal lumen into the mucosa is rapid, and about half of that taken up is acetylated in that tissue.

Transport

Carnitine is released slowly from tissues (e.g., erythrocytes) into the plasma in both the free and acetylated forms, which are found there in simple solution. Plasma total carnitine concentrations in healthy adults are 30–89 μM, with men typically showing slightly greater (by ~15%) concentrations

Table 18-3. Approximate amounts of total carnitine in selected foods and feedstuffs

Food/feedstuff	Carnitine (μg/100 g)	Food/feedstuff	Carnitine (μg/100 g)
		Plant origin	
Avocado	1.25	Alfalfa	2.00
Cabbage	—[a]	Barley	—[a]
Cauliflower	0.13	Casein, vit.	1.5
Orange juice	—[a]	Casein, acid washed	0.4
Peanut	0.76	Corn	—[a]
Spinach	—[a]	Wheat	0.35–1.22
Bread	0.24	Torula yeast	1.60–3.29
		Animal origin	
Beef	59.8–67.4	Beef liver	2.6
Beef kidney	1.8	Beef heart	19.3
Chicken	4.6–9.1	Lamb, muscle	78.0
Cow's milk	0.53–3.91	Egg	—[a]

[a]—, None detected.
Source: Mitchell, M. (1978). *Am. J. Clin. Nutr.* **31,** 293–306.

---

[24] Mean ± SD: men, 59 ± 12 μM (n = 40); women, 52 ± 12 μM (n = 45).

than women. Carnitine is taken up, against concentration gradients, by peripheral tissues, most of which can also synthesize it. Tissue uptake is effected by high-affinity, Na^+-dependent transporters[25] related to the organic cation transporters. Carnitine is located principally in the skeletal muscle, which contains some 95% of the body's carnitine. The carnitine concentrations of skeletal muscles are typically 70-fold that of plasma; somewhat smaller differences have been reported between other tissues and extracellular fluids. Skeletal muscle carnitine concentrations in healthy adults are 11–52 nmol/mg noncollagen protein, with men and women showing comparable concentrations.

Excretion

The turnover of carnitine in muscle is relatively slow; however, it is increased substantially by exercise, which reduces muscle carnitine concentrations. The turnover times for carnitine in human tissues have been estimated to be ~8 days in skeletal muscle and heart, 11.6 hr in liver and kidney, and 68 min in extracellular fluid. Whole-body turnover time has been estimated to be 66 days, indicating significant reutilization of carnitine among the various tissues of the body. Exercise appears to produce a preferential mobilization of free carnitine, thus resulting in an apparent shift toward fatty acid esters of carnitine in the muscle. Carnitine is highly conserved by the human kidney, which reabsorbs more than 90% of filtered carnitine, thus playing a dominant role in the regulation of plasma carnitine concentration. Renal excretion of carnitine adapts to the level of carnitine intake. A small amount of carnitine is normally found in the urine, even in subjects with low plasma carnitine concentrations; some of this may come from the renal secretion of carnitine either in free form or as short-chain **acylcarnitine esters**. Short-chain acyl-CoAs are normally utilized as rapidly as they are generated, and little acylcarnitine accumulates. Some conditions, however, lead to the accumulation and, thus, excretion of acylcarnitine: propionic aciduria (propionyl-CoA carboxylase deficiency) and methylmalonic aciduria (methylmalonyl-CoA mutase deficiency), owing either to hereditary abnormali-

ties or dietary deficiencies (of biotin and vitamin B_{12}, respectively); and supplemental dietary choline.

Metabolic Function

Carnitine functions in the transport of long-chain fatty acids (fatty acyl-CoA) from the cytosol into the mitochondrial matrix for oxidation as sources of energy (Fig. 18-3). The mitochondrial inner membrane is impermeable to long-chain fatty acids and their CoA derivatives, which are therefore dependent on activation as carnitine esters for entry into that organelle. This transport process, referred to as the carnitine transport shuttle, is effected by two transesterifications involving fatty acyl esters of CoA and carnitine and the action of three mitochondrial enzymes: **carnitine acyltransferases I and II**, and **carnitine translocase.**

Carnitine acyltransferase I resides on the outer side of the inner mitochondrial membrane, while carnitine acyltransferase II is located on the matrix side and **acylcarnitine translocase** spans the inner membrane. The acyltransferases catalyze the formation and hydrolysis of fatty acylcarnitine esters.[26] The translocase catalyzes the exchange of carnitine and acylcarnitines (produced by carnitine acyltransferase I) across the membrane. The result of the concerted action of these enzymes is that long-chain fatty acids are brought into the mitochondrion by being esterified to carnitine and transported as fatty acylcarnitine

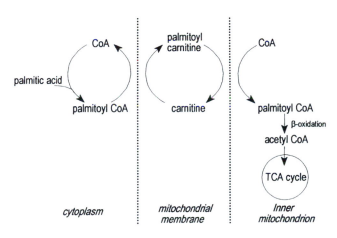

Fig. 18-3.   The carnitine transport shuttle.

---

[25] At least five carnitine transporters have been cloned.

[26] The carnitine acyltransferases are actually a family of related enzymes. Six carnitine acyltransferases with different but overlapping chain-length specificities have been isolated from mitochondria (three each from the inner and outer sides of the inner membrane).

esters, after which carnitine is released and returned to the outer side of the membrane, thus rendering the free fatty acid available for β-oxidation within the mitochrondrion. It has been suggested that the carnitine transport shuttle may also function in the reverse direction by transporting acetyl groups back to the cytoplasm for fatty acid synthesis.[27] Under normal metabolic conditions, it appears that short-chain acyl-CoAs are generated at rates comparable to their use rates such that acylcarnitine does not accumulate. However, under conditions of propionic acidemia or methylmalonic acidemia and aciduria, which occur in vitamin B_{12} deficiency, the urinary excretion of acylcarnitine is enhanced owing to the increased formation of short-chain acylcarnitines.

The activity of the carnitine transport shuttle is typically low at birth but increases dramatically after birth. For example, the carnitine palmitoyl transferase I activity in rat liver increases nearly fivefold within 24 hr of birth, peaking within 2–3 days. Similar increases in the hepatic activities of carnitine acetyltransferase I and carnitine palmitoyl transferase I have been observed in human infants. These increases correspond to the parallel development of fatty acid oxidation in the heart, liver, and adipose tissue and suggest that the carnitine transport shuttle is rate limiting to that process. While the mechanism of the postpartum increase in carnitine transport shuttle activity remains poorly understood, it is clear that one factor influencing it is carnitine status.

Carnitine appears also to have biological actions similar to those of glucocorticoids. Evidence suggests that carnitine can bind the glucocorticoid receptor and effect the receptor-mediated release of cytokines.

Conditions of Need

Essential nutrient for insects

Carnitine is an essential nutrient for some insect species, including beetles of the family *Tenebrionidei*,[28]

the beetle *Oryzaephilus surinamensis*, and the fly *Drosophila melanogaster*. It is presumed that carnitine plays the same essential role in the metabolism of fatty acids in insects that it does in mammals, and that their special requirement for the factor as an essential nutrient is due to their inability to synthesize it from endogenous sources. For these species, carnitine clearly is a vitamin.[29]

Conditional needs of mammals

Needs for preformed carnitine have also been demonstrated in mammals. Neonatal rabbits fed a carnitine-free colostrum replacer or a carnitine-free weaning diet showed abnormally low tissue and urinary carnitine levels, decreased plasma total and VLDL–cholesterol, and increased apolipoprotein levels. Carnitine needs have been demonstrated in rats under conditions in which carnitine biosynthesis is impaired by nutritional deprivation of the amino acids lysine or methionine. It is estimated that about 0.1% of the lysine required by the rat may be consigned to carnitine biosynthesis; rats fed lysine-deficient diets have been shown to develop mild depressions in tissue carnitine concentrations and to suffer growth depression and fatty liver, both of which are at least partially alleviated by feeding carnitine.[30]

Carnitine deficiencies can also result from genetic disorders of carnitine metabolism that affect its tissue utilization. Disorders in which carnitine metabolism is specifically affected are of two types:

- *Primary muscle carnitine deficiency* This is thought to involve defective transport of carnitine into skeletal muscle due to deficiency of carnitine palmitoyltransferase II or acylcarnitine translocase. The major clinical features include mild to severe muscular weakness and, frequently, excessive lipid accumulation in skeletal muscle fibers.

---

[27] Even if such a reverse shuttle were to function, its contribution to fatty acid synthesis would be insignificant in comparison with that of the citrate shuttle, which transports acetyl-CoA to the cytoplasm by the action of a citrate cleavage enzyme.

[28] A family of mealworms.

[29] Carnitine is an amino acid, but because it has no role in protein synthesis it meets the criteria of vitamin status (an organic compound that is distinct from fats, carbohydrates, and proteins; see Chapter 1).

[30] The feeding of a lysine-deficient diet to rats produced a severe depression in growth, but only marginal depressions in the carnitine concentrations of some tissues (e.g., the carnitine concentrations of skeletal muscle and heart were each about 70% of normal). In addition, the carnitine concentration in the liver rose. Despite that increase, hepatic steatosis occurred unless L-carnitine was fed. Experiments have shown that such mild carnitine deficiency produced in lysine-deficient rats can, indeed, reduce palmitic acid oxidation in homogenates of those tissues. Other experiments showed that rats fed low-protein diets limiting in methionine had reduced growth and developed fatty livers. Supplementation of that diet with 0.2% L-carnitine overcame part of the growth depression and markedly reduced the hepatic signs.

- *Primary systemic carnitine deficiency* This has a much more heterogeneous clinical picture, including such features as multiple episodes of metabolic encephalopathy, cardiomyopathy, hypoglycemia, hypoprothrombinemia, hyperammonemia, and hepatic steatosis. The etiology of this syndrome is thought to be heterogeneous; carnitine biosynthesis is thought to be normal, but, in at least some cases, renal carnitine reabsorption is impaired.

Carnitine deficiency has also been recognized as a secondary feature of a variety of other genetic disorders (e.g., organic acidurias[31] and Fanconi syndrome[32]) in which the renal tubular loss of total carnitine and of acylcarnitine esters in particular are elevated. It is thought that, in these abnormal metabolic conditions, carnitine may function to remove excess organic acids. If true, this would be a new physiological role for carnitine.

Table 18-4. Apparent carnitine deficiency in protein-malnourished children

Group	Plasma carnitine (µmol/dl)	Plasma albumin (g/dl)
Healthy controls	$9.0 \pm 0.6(8)^a$	$3.5 \pm 0.1(8)$
Undernourished patients	$6.4 \pm 0.9(10)$	$2.7 \pm 0.2(5)$
Patients with marasmus	$3.7 \pm 0.5(12)$	$2.7 \pm 0.2(8)$
Patients with Kwashiorkor	$2.6 \pm 0.5(13)$	$1.7 \pm 0.1(9)$

^{a}Mean $\pm$ SD for (n) children.
Source: Khan, L., and Bamji, M. S. (1977). *Clin. Chim. Acta* **75**, 163–169.

Health Effects

Carnitine supplementation of the diets of pregnant and lactating sows has been shown to improve the growth and nursing of piglets,[33] indicating suboptimal endogenous carnitine biosynthesis in the gestating and neonatal periods of that species.

Low plasma or tissue carnitine levels have been associated with several conditions. Carnitine-deficient individuals, diagnosed by low muscle and/or plasma carnitine levels, typically show lipid accumulation in muscle with high risk of encephalopathy, progressive muscular weakness, and cardiomyopathy.

Infants and children

Abnormally low circulating carnitine levels have been found in humans with severe protein malnutrition (Table 18-4). Low plasma carnitine concentrations, which responded to nutritional therapy, have also been found in children with schistosomiasis and associated signs of anemia and protein malnutrition (low serum albumin) in the Middle East. Two steps in the biosynthesis of carnitine require Fe^{2+} (the mitochondrial ε-N-trimethyllysine hydroxylase and the cytosolic γ-butyrobetaine hydroxylase). Therefore, it is possible that both the iron deficiency (manifested as anemia) and the protein deficiency (manifested as a low serum albumin concentration) of these patients may have reduced their abilities to synthesize carnitine.

Neonates appear to have compromised endogenous carnitine synthesis (i.e., very low hepatic γ-butyrobetaine hydroxylase activities); their carnitine status is dependent on that of the mother, on the placental transfer of carnitine *in utero*, and on the availability of exogenous sources[34] after birth. Accordingly, infants fed soy-based formulas (which contain little or no carnitine) have been found to be unable to maintain normal plasma carnitine levels, whereas intravenous administration of L-carnitine allows them to do so. Preterm infants can be at special risk in this regard. Although their plasma carnitine levels tend to be nearly normal, they can be depleted rapidly during the course of intravenous feeding with solutions that have not been supplemented with carnitine. One

---

[31] Examples include isovaleric, glutaric, propionic, and methylmalonic acidemias, which result from long- and medium-chain acyl-CoA dehydrogenase deficiencies.

[32] Fanconi syndrome is a renal disease characterized by the excessive renal excretion of a number of metabolites that are normally reabsorbed (e.g., amino acids).

[33] Ramanau, A. (2005). *Br. J. Nutr.* **93**, 717–721.

[34] Examples are mother's milk, prepared infant formulas, and milk replacers. It has been suggested that natural selection has resulted in mother's milk containing carnitine in proportion to the needs of the infant. In fact, the greatest concentrations of carnitine in human milk occur during the first 2–3 days of suckling. During the first 3 weeks of lactation, the carnitine content of human milk varies from 50 to 70 nmol/ml; after that time, it declines to abut 35 nmol/ml by 6–8 weeks. Most milk-based infant formulas contain comparable or slightly greater amounts of carnitine. However, formulas based on soybean protein or casein and casein hydrolysate contain little or no carnitine. Lipid emulsions also contain no appreciable carnitine.

study found the plasma carnitine concentrations of preterm infants (gestational age < 36 weeks) to drop from 29 to $13\,\mu M$ during total parenteral feeding.

The consequences of suboptimal carnitine status would appear to be great for the infant, who at birth changes from a pattern of energy metabolism based on glucose as the major fuel to one based on the utilization of fats.[35] Thus, for the newborn, free fatty acids appear to be the preferred metabolic fuels, especially for the heart and skeletal muscle (tissues depending on the oxidation of fatty acids for more than half of their total energy metabolism), when glucose availability is limited. Accordingly, carnitine is an important cofactor for neonatal energy metabolism.

Carnitine deficiency in human infants has been found to produce several subclinical biochemical changes. Infants fed soy-based formula diets for as long as 2 weeks after birth have shown reduced hepatic carnitine concentrations with associated reductions in hepatic fatty acid oxidation and ketogenesis. Hypertriglyceridemia has also been reported in infants fed soy-based diets not supplemented with carnitine. However, the long-term physiological consequences of these reductions are unknown and no clinical symptoms of carnitine deficiency in infants have been described.

Hepatic function

Hypocarnitinemia (plasma concentrations $< 55\,\mu M$) and tissue carnitine depletion appear to be common in patients with advanced cirrhosis, who not only tend to have marginal intakes of carnitine and its precursors, but also have loss of hepatic function, including the capacity to synthesize carnitine. Carnitine supplementation has been found to protect against ammonia-induced encephalopathy in cirrhotics.[36]

Renal function

Patients with renal disease managed with chronic hemodialysis can be depleted of carnitine[37] owing to the loss of carnitine in the dialysate, which greatly exceeds the amount normally lost in the urine.[38] Tissue depletion of carnitine has been related to the complications attendant to hemodialysis: hyperlipidemia, cardiomyopathy, skeletal muscle asthenia, and cramps. Although randomized, controlled trials have not been conducted, clinical experience and the results of small, open-label studies have suggested that carnitine administration to dialysis patients can increase hematocrit, allow a lower erythropoietin dose, and reduce intradialytic hypotension and fatigue.[39]

Diabetes

Reduction in the carnitine-dependent transport of fatty acids into the mitochondria, resulting in cytosolic triglyceride accumulation, has been implicated in the pathogenesis of insulin resistance. Studies have also shown that carnitine can stimulate the insulin-mediated disposal of glucose. These findings suggested that carnitine status affects the control of glycolysis and/or gluconeogenesis. A clinical trial found carnitine to reduce fasting plasma glucose levels and to increase fasting triglycerides in type II diabetics.[40]

Cardiovascular function

Studies have shown that carnitine supplementation can benefit cardiac function.[41] Supplementation of rats with carnitine has been shown to produce effects on prostaglandins that are associated with cardioprotection (i.e., lowering of the ratios of 6-keto-prostaglandin $F_{1\alpha}$ to thromboxane B_2 and leukotriene B_4 [LTB_4]), and to reduce myocardial

---

[35] At birth, plasma free fatty acids and β-hydroxybutyrate concentrations are rapidly elevated owing to the mobilization of fat from adipose tissue. These elevated levels are maintained by the utilization of high-fat diets such as human milk and many infant formulas, which typically contain more than 40% of total calories as lipid.

[36] Malaguarnera, M., et al. (2003). *World J. Gastroenterol.* **11**, 7197–7202.

[37] In one study, the muscle carnitine concentrations of eight patients after hemodialysis was only 10% of that of healthy controls. It is of interest, however, that not all hemodialysis patients experience carnitine depletion. Some show chronic hypocarnitinemia, whereas others show a return of plasma carnitine concentrations to normal or higher than normal within about 6 hr after dialysis. The recovery of the latter group is hastened (to about 2 hr) if each patient is given 3 g of D,L-carnitine orally at the end of the dialysis period.

[38] This can be prevented by adding carnitine to the dialysate (e.g., 65 nmol/ml).

[39] Handleman, G. J. (2006). *Blood Purif.* **24**, 140–142.

[40] Rahbar, A. R., et al. (2005). *Eur. J. Clin. Nutr.* **59**, 592–596.

[41] Ferrari, R., et al. (2004). *Ann. N.Y. Acad. Sci.* **1033**, 79–91.

injury after ischemia and reperfusion. Randomized, controlled trials with cardiac patients have shown carnitine treatment to reduce left ventrical dilatation and prevent ventricular remodeling. Long-term studies with chronic heart failure patients showed that carnitine supplementation improved exercise capability.

Neurologic function

Because animal studies have shown that acetylcarnitine treatment can induce the release of acetylcholine in the striatum and hippocampus, a multicenter, randomized, clinical intervention trial with Alzheimer's disease patients found attenuated progression for several parameters of behavior, disability, and cognitive performance.[42] One study found carnitine supplementation to reduce attention problems and aggressive behavior in boys with attention-deficit hyperactivity disorder.[43]

Male reproductive function

Epididymal tissue and spermatozoa typically contain high concentrations of carnitine. Studies in rodent models as well as humans indicate that carnitine levels are related to sperm count, motility, and maturation, and that carnitine supplementation can improve sperm quality.[44]

Thyroid function

Carnitine appears to be a peripheral agonist of thyroid hormone action. A randomized, controlled trial found administration of carnitine to be effective in reversing symptoms of hyperthyroidism.[45]

Athletic performance

Although it has been suggested that oral carnitine supplementation may attenuate the deleterious effects of hypoxic training and thus hasten recovery from strenuous exercise, a recent review of the published literature concluded that there is no evidence that carnitine supplements can improve athletic performance.[46]

IV. *myo*-Inositol

Antialopecia Factor

Although ***myo*-inositol** had been discovered in extracts of animal tissues almost 100 years earlier, interest in its potential nutritional role was first stimulated in the 1940s when Wolley reported it to be a new vitamin required for normal growth and for the maintenance of normal hair and skin of the mouse (the "mouse antialopecia factor"). Subsequently, that original report was questioned regarding the adequacy of the diet with respect to other known vitamins. Nevertheless, several groups found that dietary supplements of *myo*-inositol stimulated growth of chicks, turkeys, rats, and mice in ways that appeared to depend on other factors such as biotin and folate. Whether the observed effects were actually responses to a missing nutrient was debated owing to the observation by Needham that the daily urinary excretion of *myo*-inositol by the rat exceeds the amount ingested, which led to the conclusion that the factor was synthesized by that species. However, *myo*-inositol was found to be essential for the growth of most cells in culture. More recently, it has been found that deprivation of *myo*-inositol can render the hepatic triglyceride accumulation by the rat susceptible to influence by the fatty acid composition of dietary fat, indicating a function resembling that of an essential nutrient. Furthermore, Hegsted and colleagues at Harvard found that the female Mongolian gerbil[47] develops **intestinal lipodystrophy** when depleted of the factor. In fact, that group demonstrated a dietary requirement for *myo*-inositol to prevent that disorder in the gerbil fed a diet containing adequate levels of all other known nutrients.

Chemical Nature

Myo-inositol is a water-soluble, hydroxylated, cyclic six-carbon compound (*cis*-1,2,3,5-*trans*-4,6-cyclohexanehexol). It is the only one of the nine possible stereoisomeric forms of cyclohexitol with biological activity.

[42] Spagnoli A., et al. (1991). *Neurology* **41,** 1726–1732.

[43] Van Oudheusden, L. J., and Scholte, H. R. (2002). *Prostaglandins Leukotrienes Essent. Fatty Acids* **67,** 33–38.

[44] Ng, C. M., et al. (2004). *Ann. N.Y. Acad. Sci.* **1033,** 177–188.

[45] Benvenga, S., et al. (2004). *Ann. N.Y. Acad. Sci.* **1033,** 158–167.

[46] Brass, E. P. (2004). *Ann. N.Y. Acad. Sci.* **1033,** 67–78.

[47] *Meriones unguiculatus*.

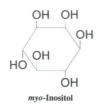

myo-Inositol

Biosynthesis from Glucose

It appears that most, if not all, mammals can synthesize *myo*-inositol *de novo* ultimately from glucose; biosynthetic capacity has been found in the liver, kidney, brain, and testis of rats and rabbits, and in the kidney[48] and other tissues in humans. The biosynthesis involves the cyclization of glucose 6-phosphate to inositol 1-phosphate by inositol-1-phosphate synthase, followed by a dephosphorylation by inositol-1-phosphatase.

Dietary Sources

myo-Inositol occurs in foods and feedstuffs in three forms: free *myo*-inositol, **phytic acid**,[49] and inositol-containing phospholipids. The richest sources of *myo*-inositol are the seeds of plants (e.g., beans, grains, and nuts) (Table 18-5). However, the predominant form occurring in plant materials is phytic acid (which can comprise most of the total phosphorus present in materials such as cereal grains[50]). Because most mammals have little or no intestinal phytase activity, phytic acid is poorly utilized as a source of either *myo*-inositol or phosphorus.[51,52] In animal products, *myo*-inositol occurs in free form as well as in inositol-containing phospholipids (primarily **phosphatidylinositol—PI**); free *myo*-inositol predominates in brain and kidney, whereas phospholipid inositol predominates in skeletal muscle, heart, liver, and pancreas. The richest animal sources of inositol are organ meats. Human milk is relatively rich in *myo*-inositol (colostrum, 200–500 mg/liter; mature milk, 100–200 mg/liter) in comparison with cow's milk (30–80 mg/liter). A disaccharide form of *myo*-inositol, 6-β-galactinol (6-*O*-β-D-galactopyranosyl-*myo*-inositol), comprises about one-sixth of the nonlipid *myo*-inositol in that material.

---

[48] Renal synthesis of *myo*-inositol has been found to be about 4 g/day (~2 g/kidney/day).

[49] Inositol hexaphosphate:

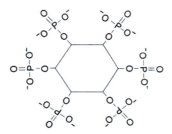

[50] Of the total phosphorus present, phytic acid phosphorus comprises 48–73% for cereal grains (corn, barley, rye, wheat, rice, sorghum), 48–79% for brans (rice, wheat), 27–41% for legume seeds (soybeans, peas, broad beans), and 40–65% for oilseed meals (soybean meal, cottonseed meal, rapeseed meal).

[51] The bioavailability of phosphorus from most plant sources is relatively good (>50%) for ruminants, which benefit from the phytase activities of their rumen microflora. Nonruminants, however, lack their own intestinal phytase and thus generally derive much less phosphorus from plant phytic acid, depending on the phytase contributions of their intestinal microflora. For pigs and rats, such contributions appear to be significant, giving them moderate abilities (about 37 and 44%, respectively) to utilize phytic acid phosphorus. In contrast, the chick, which has a short gut and rapid intestinal transit time and, thus, has only a sparse intestinal microflora, can use little (about 8%) phytic acid phosphorus.

[52] Phytic acid can also form a very stable chelation complex with zinc (Zn^{2+} is held by the negative charges on adjacent pyrophosphate groups), thus reducing its nutritional availability. For this reason, the bioavailability of zinc in such plant-derived foods as soybean is very low.

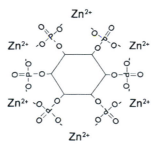

Table 18-5.   Total *myo*-inositol contents of selected foods

Food	*myo*-Inositol (mg/g)	Food	*myo*-Inositol (mg/g)
Vegetables		Fruits	
Asparagus	0.29–0.68	Apple	0.10–0.24
Beans		Cantaloupe	3.55
Green	0.55–1.93	Grape	0.07–0.16
White	2.83–4.40	Grapefruit	1.17–1.99
Red	2.49	Orange	3.07
Broccoli	0.11–0.30	Peach	0.19–0.58
Cabbage	0.18–0.70	Pear	0.46–0.73
Carrot	0.52	Strawberry	0.13
Cauliflower	0.15–0.18	Watermelon	0.48
Celery	0.05	Cereals	
Okra	0.28–1.17		
Pea	1.16–2.35	Rice	0.15–0.30
Potato	0.97	Wheat	1.42–11.5
Spinach	0.06–0.25	Meats	
Squash, yellow	0.25–0.32	Beef	0.09–0.37
Tomato	0.34–0.41	Chicken	0.30–0.39
Dairy products, eggs		Lamb	0.37
Milk	0.04	Pork	0.14–0.42
Ice cream	0.09	Turkey	0.08–0.23
Cheese	0.01–0.09	Liver	
Egg		Beef	0.64
Whole	0.09	Chicken	1.31
Yolk	0.34	Pork	0.17
Nuts		Tuna	0.11–0.15
Almond	2.78	Trout	0.11
Peanut	1.33–3.04		

Source: Clements, R. S., Jr., and Darnell, B. (1980). *Am. J. Clin. Nutr.* **33,** 1954–1962.

The U.S. Food and Drug Administration classifies *myo*-inositol among the substances generally recognized as safe and, therefore, can be used in the formulation of foods without the demonstrations of safety and efficacy required by the Food, Drug and Cosmetic Act. It is added to many prepared infant formulas (at about 0.1%). It is estimated that typical American diets provide adults with about 900 mg of *myo*-inositol per day, slightly over half of which is in phospholipid form.

Absorption

The enteric absorption of free *myo*-inositol occurs by active transport; the uptake of *myo*-inositol from the small intestine is virtually complete. The enteric absorption of phytic acid, however, depends on the ability to digest that form and on the amounts of divalent cations in the diet/meal. Most animal species lack intestinal phytase activities and are, therefore, dependent on the presence of a gut microflora that produces those enzymes. For species that harbor such microfloral populations (e.g., ruminants and long-gutted nonruminants), phytate is digestible, thus constituting a useful dietary source of *myo*-inositol. Dietary cations (particularly Ca^{2+}) can reduce the utilization of phytate by forming insoluble (and, thus, nondigestible and nonabsorbable) phytate **chelates**. Because a large portion of the total *myo*-inositol in mixed diets typically is in the form of phytic acid, the utilization of *myo*-inositol from high-calcium diets can be less than half of that from diets containing low to moderate amounts of the mineral.[53] Little information is available concerning the mechanism of absorption of phospholipid *myo*-inositol; it is probable that it is analogous to that of phosphatidylcholine.[54]

Transport

myo-Inositol is transported in the blood predominantly in the free form; the normal circulating concentration of *myo*-inositol in humans is about 30 μM. A small but significant amount of phosphatidylinositol (PI) is found in association with the circulating lipoproteins. Free *myo*-inositol appears to be taken up by an active transport process in some tissues (kidney, brain) and by carrier-mediated diffusion in others (liver). The active process requires Na^+ and energy, and is inhibited by high levels of glucose. Apparently, because of this antagonism, untreated diabetics show impaired tissue uptake and impaired urinary excretion of *myo*-inositol.

Metabolism

Free *myo*-inositol is converted to PI within cells either by *de novo* synthesis by reacting with the liponucleotide cytidine diphosphate (CDP)-diacylglycerol,[55] or by an exchange with endogenous PI.[56] Phosphatidylinositol can, in turn, be sequentially phosphorylated to the monophosphate (**phosphatidylinositol 4-phosphate**, **PIP**) and diphosphate (phosphatidylinositol 4,5-diphosphate, PIP_2) forms by membrane kinases.[57] Thus, in tissues, *myo*-inositol is found as the free form, as PI, PIP, and PIP_2.[58] The *myo*-inositol-containing phospholipids tend to be enriched in **stearic acid** (predominantly at the 1-position) and **arachidonic acid** (predominantly at the 2-position) in comparison with the fatty acid compositions of other phospholipids. For example, the *myo*-inositol-containing phospholipids on the plasma membrane from human platelets contain about 42 mol% stearic acid and about 44 mol% arachidonic

acid. The greatest concentrations of *myo*-inositol are found in neural and renal tissues.

The turnover of the *myo*-inositol phospholipids is accomplished intracellularly. Phosphatidylinositol phosphates can be catabolized by cellular phosphomonoesterases (phosphatases), ultimately to yield PI. In the presence of cytidine monophosphate, PI synthetase functions (in the reverse direction) to break down that form to yield CDP-diacylglycerol and *myo*-inositol. The kidney appears to perform most of the further catabolism of *myo*-inositol, first clearing it from the plasma and converting it to glucose and, then, oxidizing it to CO_2 via the pentose phosphate shunt. The metabolism of *myo*-inositol appears to be relatively rapid; the rat can oxidize half of an ingested dose in 48 hr.

Metabolic Functions

The metabolically active form of *myo*-inositol appears to be phosphatidylinositol, which is thought to have several physiologically important roles:

- As an effecter of the structure and function of membranes
- As a source of arachidonic acid for eicosanoid production
- As a mediator of cellular responses to external stimuli

Phosphatidylinositol has been proposed to be active in the regulation of membrane-associated enzymes and transport processes. For example, phosphatidylinositol is an endogenous activator of a microsomal Na^+,K^+-ATPase, an essential constituent of acetyl-CoA carboxylase, a stimulator of tyrosine hydroxylase, a factor bound to alkaline phosphatase and 5′-nucleotidase, and a membrane anchor for acetylcholinesterase. It has been suggested that such effects involve the special membrane-active properties conferred on the phospholipid by its unique fatty acid composition. For example, its polar head group and highly nonpolar fatty acyl

---

[53] For the same reason, the bioavailability of calcium is also low for high-phytate diets. This effect also occurs for the nutritionally important divalent cations Mn^{2+} and Zn^{2+}; the bioavailability of each is reduced by the presence of phytic acid in the diet.

[54] This would involve hydrolysis by pancreatic phospholipase A in the intestinal lumen to produce a lysophosphatidylinositol, which, on uptake by the enterocyte, would be reacylated by an acyltransferase or hydrolyzed further to yield glycerylphosphorylinositol.

[55] This step is catalyzed by the microsomal enzyme CDP diacylglycerol–inositol 3-phosphatidyltransferase (also called PI synthetase).

[56] This reaction is stimulated by Mn^{2+}; like phosphatidylinositol synthetase, it is localized in the microsomal fraction of the cell.

[57] These are ATP:phosphatidylinositol 4-phosphotransferase and ATP:phosphatidylinositol-4-phosphate 5-phosphotransferase, respectively. They are located on the cytosolic surface of the erythrocyte membrane. There is no evidence that *myo*-inositol can be isomerized or phosphorylated to the hexaphosphate level; however, such prospects would be of interest, as the isomer D-*chiro*-inositol has been shown to promote insulin function, and inositol hexaphosphate (phytic acid) has been found to be anticarcinogenic in a variety of animal models.

[58] The disaccharide 6-β-galactinol appears to be a unique mammary metabolite.

chains may facilitate specific electrostatic interactions, while providing a hydrophobic microenvironment for enzyme proteins on or in membranes. Such properties may render phosphatidylinositol an effective anchor for the hydrophobic attachment of proteins to membranes. Phosphatidylinositol also serves as a source of releasable arachidonic acid for the formation of the **eicosanoids**[59] by the cellular activities of cyclooxygenase and/or lipoxygenase. Although phosphatidylinositol is less abundant in cells than the other phospholipids (phosphatidylcholine, phosphatidylethanolamine, and phosphatidylserine), its enrichment in arachidonic acid renders it an effective source of that eicosanoid precursor.

That the metabolism of phosphatidylinositol is activated in target tissues by stimuli producing rapid (e.g., cholinergic or α-adrenergic agonists) or medium-term (e.g., mitogens) physiological responses suggests a mediating role of such responses. It is thought that this role involves the conversion of the less abundant species, phosphatidylinositol diphosphate (PIP_2), to the water-soluble metabolite **inositol 1,4,5-triphosphate (IP_3)**, which serves as a **second messenger** to activate the release of Ca^{2+} from intracellular stores.[60]

Inositol phosphate receptors on the cell surface have been shown to effect primary control over the hydrolysis of PIP_2 by regulating the activity of phospholipase C (phosphodiesterase) on the plasma membrane. Thus, receptor occupancy activates the hydrolysis of PIP_2, which is favored at low intracellular concentrations of Ca^{2+}, to produce IP_3 and, perhaps, other inositol polyphosphates. The IP_3 that is produced signals the release of Ca^{2+} from discrete organelles called **calcisomes**, as well as the entry of Ca^{2+} into the cell across the plasma membrane.[61] This process involves a specific IP_3 receptor on the calcisomal membrane; the binding of IP_3 to this receptor opens a **Ca^{2+} channel** closely associated with the receptor.

It is thought that the IP_3-stimulated entry of Ca^{2+} into the cell involves an increase in the permeability to Ca^{2+} of the plasma membrane that is signaled by the emptying of the IP_3-sensitive intracellular pool.

The mechanism whereby the IP_3-sensitive pool and the plasma membrane communicate to effect this response is not understood. There is also some evidence to suggest that 1,2-diacylglycerol, which is formed from the receptor-stimulated metabolism of the *myo*-inositol-containing phospholipids, may also serve a second messenger function in activating protein kinase C for the phosphorylation of various proteins important to cell function. According to this hypothesis, 1,2-diacylglycerol functions with Ca^{2+} and phosphatidylserine, both of which are known to be involved in the activation of protein kinase C.

Conditions of Need

Although early reports indicated dietary needs for *myo*-inositol to prevent alopecia in rodents, fatty liver in rats, and growth retardation in chicks, guinea pigs, and hamsters, more recent studies with more complete diets have failed to confirm such needs. Hence, it has been concluded that most, if not all, of those lesions actually involved deficiencies of other nutrients (e.g., biotin, choline, and vitamin E). Because *myo*-inositol appears to be synthesized by most, if not all, species, it has been suggested that the observed responses to dietary supplements of *myo*-inositol may have involved favorable effects of the compound on the intestinal microflora. This hypothesis would suggest that the addition of *myo*-inositol to diets would be beneficial when those diets contain marginal amounts of such factors as choline and biotin, the gut synthesis of which can be important. Accordingly, it has been shown that supplements of *myo*-inositol reduced hepatic lipid accumulation in rats fed a choline-deficient diet, improved growth in rats fed a diet deficient in several vitamins, and reduced the incidence of fatty liver in and improved the growth of chicks fed a biotin-deficient diet containing an antibiotic. Thus it appears that, under certain conditions, animals can have needs for preformed *myo*-inositol. Such conditions are not well

---

[59] The eicosanoids include prostaglandins, thromboxanes, and leukotrienes. The prostaglandins are hormone-like substances secreted for short-range action on neighboring tissues; they are involved in inflammation, in the regulation of blood pressure, in headaches, and in the induction of labor. The functions of the leukotrienes and thromboxanes are less well understood; they are thought to be involved in regulation of blood pressure and in the pathogenesis of some types of disease.

[60] There is some controversy concerning whether other inositol phosphates [e.g., inositol 1,3,4,5-tetraphosphate (IP_4), which is a product of a 3-kinase acting on IP_3] can also signal Ca^{2+} mobilization. Evidence suggests that, in at least some cells, IP_3 and IP_4 may have cooperative roles in Ca^{2+} signaling.

[61] The Ca^{2+}-mobilizing activity of IP_3 is terminated by its dephosphorylation (via a 5-phosphatase) to the inactive inositol-1,4-bisphosphate, or by its phosphorylation (via a 3-kinase) to a product of uncertain activity, IP_4.

defined, but it has been suggested that they include such situations as disturbed intestinal microflora,[62] diets containing high levels of fat,[63] and a physical environment creating physiological stress.

For a few species, however, overt dietary needs for *myo*-inositol have been demonstrated. These include several fishes and the gerbil. Studies with fishes have shown dietary deprivation of *myo*-inositol to result in anorexia, fin degeneration, edema, anemia, decreased gastric emptying rate, reduced growth, and impaired efficiency of feed utilization. Studies with gerbils have shown *myo*-inositol deprivation to result in intestinal lipodystrophy, with associated hypocholesterolemia and reduced survival. Interestingly by, these effects are observed only in female gerbils; males appear to have a sufficient testicular synthesis of *myo*-inositol. For at least these species, *myo*-inositol must be considered a dietary essential.

Health Effects

Inositol supplementation has been found to be beneficial in certain situations:

- *Preterm infants* Three randomized, clinical trials have found inositol supplementation to improve survival and reduce retinopathy of prematurity, bronchial dysplasia, and intraventricular hemorrhage.[64]
- *Psoriasis* A small, randomized clinical trial with psoriasis patients found supplementation with inositol to reduce the severity of symptoms.[65]
- *Psychiatric disorders* Because mood stabilizers such as lithium, valproate, and carbamazepine function by the stabilization of inositol signaling, it has been suggested that inositol may have value in the treatment of depression and other psychiatric disorders. While inositol supplementation has been reported to be helpful in treating bipolar depression and bulimia nervosa with binge eating, the limited findings in this area to date do not indicate clear benefits.

V. Pyrroloquinoline Quinone

Newly Discovered Coenzyme

In the late 1970s, studies of specialized bacteria, the methylotrophs,[66] resulted in the discovery of a new enzyme cofactor, **pyrroloquinoline quinone (PQQ)**. That cofactor was found in several different bacterial oxidoreductases. Subsequently, PQQ has been identified in several other important enzymes (now collectively called **quinoproteins**) in yeasts, plants, and animals. In 1989, Killgore and colleagues at the University of California demonstrated the beneficial effects of PQQ in preventing skin lesions in mice fed a diet containing low concentrations of that factor.

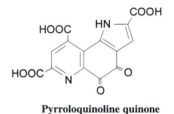

Pyrroloquinoline quinone

Chemical Nature

Pyrroloquinoline quinone, sometimes called methoxatin, is a tricarboxylic acid with a fused heterocyclic (o-quinone) ring system.[67] Its C-5 carbonyl group is very reactive toward nucleophiles,[68] leading to adduct formation.

Dietary Sources

Little quantitative information is available concerning the distribution of PQQ in foods and feedstuffs. Some reports indicate PQQ to be present in egg yolk, adrenal tissue, and many citrus fruits in the range of 500–20,000 ppb and in casein, starch, and isolated soy protein in the range of 10–100 ppb.

Metabolic Function

In bacterial quinoproteins, PQQ is covalently bound to the apoprotein, probably by an amide or ester

---

[62] For example, antibiotics can reduce the number of microorganisms that normally produce *myo*-inositol as well as other required nutrients.

[63] High-fat diets may increase the needs for *myo*-inositol for lipid transport.

[64] Howlett, A., and Ohlsson, A. (2003). *Cochrane Database Syst. Rev.*, CD000366.

[65] Allan, S. J. R., et al. (2004). *Br. J. Dermatol.* **150,** 966–969.

[66] The methylotrophs dissimilate single-carbon compounds (e.g., methane, methanol, and methylamine).

[67] 4,5-Dihydro-4,5-dioxo-1*H*-pyrrolo[2,3-*f*]quinoline-2,7,9-tricarboxylic acid.

[68] For example, amino groups, thiol groups.

bond via its carboxylic acid group(s). The redox behavior of PQQ involves its ability to form adducts that facilitate both one- and two-electron transfers. In dehydrogenases its function appears to involve electron transfers of both types (substrate oxidation by a two-electron transfer to PQQ, followed by single-electron transfer to such acceptors as copper-containing proteins and cytochromes). Accordingly, two forms of the cofactor, the semiquinone $PQQH\bullet$ and the catechol $PQQH_2$, have been found in the bacterial quinoproteins.

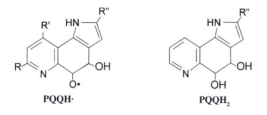

The role of PQQ in eukaryotes is less clear. Although several animal quinoproteins have been proposed, more recent investigations using sensitive physical methods have failed to confirm earlier claims of covalent binding of PQQ or derivatives at the active centers of those enzymes. One important enzyme that has been proposed to be a quinoprotein is **lysyl oxidase**, which plays a key role in the cross-linking of collagen and elastin by catalyzing the oxidative deamination of peptidyllysine to peptidyl-α-aminoadipic-δ-semialdehyde. Studies indicate that the needs of this and related enzymes may not be for PQQ at all, but rather for a tyrosine derivative, peptide-bound trihydroxyphenylalanine (6-hydroxydopa).[69] In fact, the apparent quinone requirement of plasma monoamine oxidase, after which other putative animal quinoproteins have been modeled, has been found to be satisfied by 6-hydroxydopa.

Conditions of Need

Killgore and colleagues fed mice for 10 weeks a chemically defined diet that contained <30 ppb PQQ.

It was supplemented with vitamins[70] at five times the required levels, and special precautions were taken to minimize the potential for exposure of mice to PQQ from microbial sources.[71] The positive control group was treated in like manner, but was fed the basal diet supplemented with 800 ppb PQQ. The results showed a clear difference in rate of growth in favor of the PQQ-supplemented mice. Furthermore, about one-quarter of the PQQ-deprived animals showed friable skin, mild alopecia, and a hunched posture. About one-fifth of the PQQ-deprived mice died by 8 weeks of feeding, with aortic aneurysms or abdominal hemorrhages. The most frequent sign, friable skin, was taken to suggest an abnormality of collagen metabolism; subsequent study revealed increased collagen solubility (indicating reduced cross-linking) and abnormally low activities of lysyl oxidase in PQQ-deprived animals. Attempts to breed PQQ-deprived mice were unsuccessful; mice fed the low-PQQ diet for 8–9 weeks produced either no litters or litters in which the pups were immediately cannibalized at birth. Subsequent work by the same group has shown deprivation of PQQ to have immunopathologic effects in mice: altered mitogenic responses and reduced interleukin 2 levels. More recent results from the same laboratory have shown that PQQ-deprivation of growing mice elevated the plasma levels of glucose, alanine, glycine, and serine, and reduced the amounts and function of hepatic mitochondria.[72]

These results show physiologic impairment due to PQQ deprivation. Still, the absence of a clear enzyme cofactor function renders the metabolic significance of these effects difficult to assess. It has been proposed that PQQ and/or PQQ-derived factors may not function as specific enzyme cofactors at all, acting instead as oxidant radical scavengers. Nevertheless, a PQQ reductase activity has been identified in bovine erythrocytes.[73] There is still much to be learned about the metabolism, distribution, and biochemical functions of PQQ. At present, while it is clear that PQQ and/or related factors can have nutritional significance, available evidence is insufficient to support designating PQQ as a vitamin.

---

[69] 6-Hydroxydopa is also called *topa quinone*.

[70] Thiamin, pyridoxine, vitamin A, vitamin E, vitamin B_{12}, folate, vitamin K_2, and biotin.

[71] An antibiotic (2% succinylsulfathiazole) was added to the diet; the major dietary ingredients were autoclaved; drinking water was distilled and ultrafiltered; and the mice were housed in a laminar flow cage unit with air filtered to prevent the passage of microbes.

[72] Stites, T., et al. (2006). *J. Nutr.* **136**, 390–396.

[73] This activity has been called a flavin reductase or NADPH-dependent methemoglobin reductase; however, it shows a much lower K_m value for PQQ ($2\mu M$) than for flavins (about $30\mu M$).

VI. Ubiquinones

Chemical Nature

The **ubiquinones** are a group of tetra-substituted 1,4-benzoquinone derivatives with isoprenoid side chains of variable length. Originally isolated from the unsaponifiable fractions of the hepatic lipids from vitamin A-deficient rats, the principal species of the group (ubiquinone[50][74]) was subsequently identified as an essential component (**coenzyme Q$_{10}$ or CoQ$_{10}$**) of the mitochondrial electron transport chains of most prokaryotic and all eukaryotic cells. In the four decades since that recognition, the term *coenzyme Q* has come to be used to describe generally this family of compounds, all of which are synthesized from precursors in the inner mitochondrial membrane. The structure of the 6-chromanol portion of the CoQ group is remarkably similar to the oxidized form of vitamin E, tocopherylquinone, the difference being the two methoxyl groups on the CoQ$_{10}$ ring in place of two methyl groups on the tocopherylquinone ring.

Metabolic Function

Mitochondrial respiratory chain component

The ubiquinones function as electron acceptors for complexes I and II of mitochondrial electron transport chains. They pass electrons from flavoproteins (e.g., NADH or succinic dehydrogenases) to the cytochromes via cytochrome b_5. They perform this function by undergoing reversible reduction/oxidation to cycle between the 1,4-quinone (oxidized) and 1,4-dihydroxybenzene (reduced) species (Fig. 18-4).

Antioxidant

Its redox capacity allows CoQ$_{10}$ to function beyond the nonelectron transport chain as a membrane-bound antioxidant that protects and thus spares α-tocopherol in subcellular membranes. Along with α-tocopherol, β-carotene, and selenium, CoQ$_{10}$ has been shown to provide significant protection from lipid peroxidation in animal models. In some tissues (e.g., liver) its effect appears to be greater than those of the other antioxidant nutrients.[75] Administration of CoQ$_{10}$ has been found to protect against myocardial damage mediated by free-radical mechanisms (ischemia, drug toxicities) in animal models. It has been proposed that CoQ$_{10}$ plays a major role in the determination of membrane potentials of subcellular membrane systems.

Biosynthesis

Coenzyme Q$_{10}$ is synthesized in most tissues. The biosynthetic process derives the isoprenyl side chain from mevalonate, the ring system from tyrosine, the hydroxyl groups from molecular oxygen, and the methyl groups from *S*-adenosylmethionine to produce a 50-carbon polyiosoprene chain (i.e., containing 10 isoprene units). Because endogenous tissue biosynthesis appears sufficient to support membrane saturation levels, supplementation increases tissue levels above normal in only liver and spleen. That older animals show lower CoQ levels suggest that the biosynthetic rate may decline with age.

Dietary Sources

Few empirical data for the ubiquinone contents of foods are available, however, the localization of

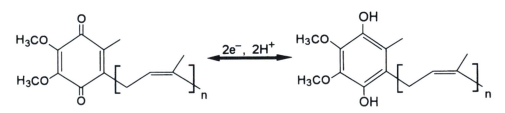

Fig. 18-4. Redox function of ubiquinones.

---

[74] The conventions of nomenclature for the ubiquinone/CoQ group are similar to those for the vitamin K group. For the ubiquinones, the number of side-chain carbons is indicated parenthetically; for the CoQ designation, the number of side-chain isoprenyl units is indicated in subscript.

[75] Leibovitz, B., et al. (1990). *J. Nutr.* **120,** 97–104.

coenzyme Q_{10} in the mitochondrial electron transport chain and in other cellular membranes would predict that the most important food sources would be tissues of high cellularity and those rich in mitochrondria such as heart and muscle.

Absorption and Tissue Distribution

It is assumed that the ubiquinones are absorbed, transported and taken up into cells by mechanisms analogous to those of the tocopherols. Coenzyme Q_{10} is distributed in all membranes in the cell. Relatively great concentrations of CoQ_{10} are found in the liver, heart, spleen, kidney, pancreas, and adrenals.[76] The total CoQ_{10} pool size in the human adult is estimated to be 0.5–1.5 g. Tissue ubiquinone levels increase under the influence of oxidative stress, cold acclimation, and thyroid hormone treatment, and appear to decrease with cardiomyopathy, other muscle diseases, and aging.

Conditions of Need

Metabolic needs for CoQ are linked to vitamin E status. Although CoQ_{10} itself does not spare vitamin E for preventing gestation-resorption syndrome in the rat, the oxidized form, that is, the 6-chromanol moiety of hexahydro-CoQ_4, has been found to prevent the syndrome in vitamin E-deficient rats and to produce significant reductions (but not full protection) in both the anemia and the myopathy of vitamin E-deficient rhesus monkeys. In fact, the responses (e.g., increased reticulocyte count, reduced creatinine excretion, reduced dystrophic signs) were more rapid than have been observed in therapy with α-tocopherol. Thus, it appears that dietary ubiquinones may be important as potential sources of antioxidant protection, but that they share that role with other antioxidant nutrients, several of which are likely to be more potent in this regard. For this reason, and because of the lack of evidence of specifically impaired physiological function due to deprivation of coenzyme Q, these compounds are be considered vitamins.

Health Effects

Studies with animal models[77] have shown that supplemental CoQ_{10} can help maintain the integrity of cardiac muscle under cardiomyopathic conditions.

Clinical trials with humans have indicated benefits of supplemental CoQ_{10} of several types:

- *Neurologic conditions*   Modest improvements in symptoms were reported from a small, randomized, controlled trial with Parkinson's disease patients.[78]
- *Migraine*   A small, open-label trial reported CoQ_{10} to reduce headache frequency.[79]
- *Congestive heart failure*   A meta-analysis of randomized, controlled trials showed CoQ_{10} supplements to reduce dyspnea, edema, and the frequency of hospitalization.[80]
- *Hypertension*   A systematic review of eight randomized, controlled trials suggested that CoQ^{10} supplementation to decrease systolic pressure by an average of 16 mm Hg, and diastolic pressure by an average of 10 mm Hg.[81]
- *Atherosclerosis*   A randomized, controlled trial found CoQ_{10} supplementation after myocardial infarction to reduce subsequent myocardial events and cardiac deaths.[82]
- *Endothelial dysfunction*   A randomized, controlled trial found CoQ_{10} supplementation to improve endothelial function of peripheral arteries of dyslipidemic patients with type II diabetes.[83]
- *Tolerance to cancer chemotherapy*   A systematic review of six randomized, controlled trials suggested that CoQ_{10} supplementation provided some protection against cardiac or hepatic toxicity.[84]

---

[76] The contributions of foods and feedstuffs, many of which are now known to contain appreciable concentrations of ubiquinones, to these high tissue levels are unknown.

[77] For example, cardiomyopathy induced in the rat by feeding a fructose-based, copper-deficient diet.

[78] Muller, T., et al. (2003). *Neurosci. Lett.* **341,** 201–204.

[79] Sandor, P. S., et al. (2005). *Neurol.* **64,** 713–715.

[80] Soja, A. M., et al. (1997). *Mol. Aspects Med.* **18,** S159–S168.

[81] Rosenfeldt, F., et al. (2003). *Biofactors* **18,** 91–100.

[82] Singh, R. B., et al. (2003). *Mol. Cell. Biochem.* **246,** 75–82.

[83] Watts, G. F., et al. (2002). *Diabetologia* **45,** 420–426.

[84] Roffe, L., et al. (2004). *J. Clin. Oncol.* **22,** 4418–4424.

VII. Flavonoids

Synergists of Vitamin C

The group of compounds now referred to as the **flavonoids** was discovered by Szent-Györgyi as the factor in lemon juice or red peppers that potentiated in the guinea pig the antiscorbutic activity of the ascorbic acid contained in those foods. The factor was variously called citrin, vitamin P,[85] and vitamin C_2, but was ultimately found to be a mixture of phenolic derivatives of 2-phenyl-1,4-benzopyrane, the flavane nucleus.

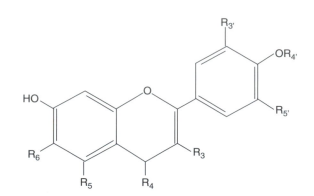

Fig. 18-5. General structure of flavonoids.

Ubiquitous Plant Metabolites

Flavonoids are ubiquitous in foods and feedstuffs of plant origin; more than 6000 different flavonoids have been identified, each a secondary metabolite of shikimic acid. Flavonoids have a wide variety of functions in plant tissues: natural antiobiotics,[86] predator feeding deterrents, photosensitizers, UV-screening agents, metabolic and physiologic modulators. They represent the major sources of red, blue, and yellow pigments other than the carotenoids. Flavonoids are polyphenolic compounds containing two aromatic rings linked by an oxygen-containing, heterocyclic ring (Fig. 18-5).

There are seven general classes of flavonoids, classified by their common ring substituents:

- *Flavonols* These derivatives (R_3 hydroxy, R_4 keto) include quercetin, kaempferol, isorhamnetic, and myricetin, the most abundant flavonoids in human diets. Flavonols are found in a variety of fruits and vegetables, often as glycosides. Relatively high amounts (15–40 mg/ 100 g) are found in broccoli, kale, leeks, and onions; flavanols are also found in red wine, tea, and fruit juices.
- *Flavanols* These derivatives (R_3 hydroxy) include catechin, epicatechin, epigallocatechin and their gallate derivatives. They are found in apples, apricots, and red grapes (2–20 mg/100 g); green tea and dark chocolate are rich in catechins (40–65 mg/100 g).

- *Flavones* This group of some 300 compounds retains the basic flavane nucleus structure. It includes apigenin and luteolin in very high concentrations (>600 mg/100 g) in parsley, and in lower but significant amounts in cereal grains, celery and citrus rinds (which contain polymethoxylated forms).
- *Proanthocyanidins* These derivatives are polymeric flavanols, also called condensed tannins. They are present in all plants. These polyphenols have strong antioxidant properties in *vitro*.
- *Anthocyanins* These derivatives (R_3 and R_4 reduced) exist as glycosides, their aglycone chromophores being referred to as anthocyanidins. There are several hundred anthocyanidins, the most common of which are cyanidin, delphinidin, malvinidin, pelargonidin, peonidin, petunidin, and malvidin. Most are red or blue pigments. The richest sources (up to 600 mg/100 g) are raspberries, black berries, and blue berries; cherries, radishes, red cabbage, red skinned potato, red onions, and red wine are also good sources (50–150 mg/100 g). Anthocyanins have antioxidant properties. Unlike other flavonoids, anthocyanins are relatively unstable to cooking and high-temperature food processing.
- *Flavanones* These derivatives (R_4 keto, "C" ring otherwise reduced) are found primarily in citrus fruit (15–50 mg/100 g) where they are also present as *O*- and *C*-glycosides and methoxylated derivatives. They include eriocitrin, neoericitrin, hesperidin, neohesperidin, naringin, narirutin, didymin, and poncirin.

---

[85] The letter *P* indicated the permeability vitamin because it improved capillary permeability.

[86] That is, as phytoalexins.

- *Isoflavones* These derivatives ("B" aromatic ring liked at R_3) are contained only in legumes mostly as glycosides; **isoflavones** include daidzein, genistein, and glycitein, which are also referred to as **phytoestrogens** due to the affinities of their 7- and 4′-hydroxyl groups to binding mammalian estrogen receptors. Soy products can contain 25–200 mg/100 g).

Flavonoids in Foods

The consumption of flavonols, flavones, and flavanols has been estimated to average 50 mg/day in the United States,[87] with the intake proanthocyanidins being comparable. The greatest contributors of flavonoids in human diets are fruits and vegetables, fruit juices being the richest sources and apples the prime source in most Western diets (Table 18-6). Most flavonoids tend to be concentrated in the outer layers of fruit and vegetable tissues (e.g., skin, peel). In general, the flavonoid contents of leafy vegetables are high, whereas those of root vegetables (with the notable exception of onions with colored skins) are low. The average daily intake of flavonoids from a typical American diet has been estimated to be ~1 g.

Flavonoid Utilization

The hydroxyl groups of these polyphenols enable them to form glycosidic linkages with sugars, and most flavonoids occur naturally as glycosides.

Flavonoid glycosides appear to be hydrolyzed by glycosidases in saliva, the brush border of the intestines, and the intestinal microflora. Hindgut bacteria can also degrade the flavanoid by cleaving the heterocyclic ring, leading to the formation of various phenolic acids and their lactones, some of which may be absorbed from the colon. Upon absorption, flavonoids are conjugated as glucuronides or sulfates in the liver and are degraded to a variety of phenolic compounds that are rapidly excreted.

Health Effects of Flavonoids

Antioxidant activity

Flavonoids are able to chelate divalent metal cations (e.g., Cu^{2+}, Fe^{2+}), thus serving antioxidant functions by removing those catalysts of lipid peroxidation reactions. For example, the flavonol quercetin, which has multiple phenolic hydroxyl groups, a carbonyl group at C-4, and free C-3 and C-5 hydroxyl groups, can scavenge superoxide radical ions, hydroxyl radicals, and fatty acyl peroxyl radicals. Flavonols and some proanthocyanins have been shown to inhibit macrophage-mediated LDL oxidation *in vitro*, probably by protecting LDL–α-tocopherol from oxidation or by reacting with the tocopheroxyl radical to regenerate α-tocopherol. This would appear to be the basis of the observed effects of flavonoids in reducing capillary fragility and/or permeability. This antioxidant potential can contribute to chemical measurements

Table 18-6. Flavonoid contents of selected foods

Food	Quercetin (mg/kg)	Kaempferol (mg/kg)	Myricetin (mg/kg)	Luteolin (mg/kg)
Lettuce	7–30	<2	<1	<1
Onion	284–486	<2	<1	<1
Endive	<1	15–95	<1	<1
Red pepper	<1	<2	<0.5	7–14
Broad beans	20	<2	26	<1
Apples	21–72	<2	<1	<1
Strawberries	8–10	8–10	<1	<1
Black tea	17–25	13–17	3–5	<1
Red wine	4–16	<1	7–9	<1
Apple juice	3	<1	<0.5	<1

Source: Hertog, M. G. L. (1996). *Proc. Nutr. Soc.* **55**, 385–397.

[87] Similar estimates have been made for northern European diets.

of "total antioxidant capacity" in foods. Studies with animal models have found flavanols in tea to reduce oxidative DNA damage and other biomarkers of oxidative damage.

Enzyme modulation

Flavonoids have been found to interact with all classes of enzymes and to selectively affect the activities of some. This includes induction of phase II enzymes (e.g., epoxide reductase, UDP-glucoronosyltansferase, glutathione-S-transferase, NAD(P)H: quinone oxidoreductase) by affecting their transcription through binding to promoter regions of their respective genes; and inhibition of other enzymes (e.g., aldose reductase, phosphodiesterase, *O*-methyltransferase, and several serine- and threonine-kinases) by direct binding to the respective protein. For example, studies have found tea flavanols to inhibit redox-sensitive transcription factors (NFκB, AP-1), inhibit prooxidative enzymes (lipooxygenases, cyclooxygenases, nitric oxide synthase, xanthine oxidase), induce phase II enzymes, and induce antioxidant enzymes (glutathione *S*-transferases, superoxide dismutases). Such effects have been cited as the basis of the prospective anti-inflammatory roles of flavonoids.[88] Flavanones have been shown to induce phase II enzymes and to exert anti-inflammatory effects; naringin, in particular, has been implicated in the effect of grapefruit juice in inhibiting cytochrome P450-dependent drug metabolism.[89]

Chronic disease

Some epidemiologic studies have demonstrated associations of diets high in flavonoids (mainly quercetin) with reduced risks of cardiovascular diseases (high-flavonoid diets have been associated with 21 to 53% reductions in prevalence[90]) and cancers of the lung and rectum (diets high in catechins from fruit have been associated with 44–47% reductions in prevalence[91,92]). Because such diets are typically rich in fruits and vegetables, these studies do not indicate whether the protective factor(s) are flavonoids or some other phytochemicals, vitamins, or minerals (e.g., β-carotene, ascorbic acid, fiber) also provided by those foods.

Cardioprotective effects have been attributed to vasodilatory effects and blood pressure reduction, antioxidant protection of LDLs against lipid peroxidation, inhibition of platelet aggregation, and reduced inflammation. Quercetin has been found to inhibit the activation of *c*-Jun N-terminal kinase in the modulation of angiotensin-induced hypertrophy of vascular smooth muscle cells. Various proanthocyanins have been shown to inhibit platelet activation; to inhibit the expression of interleukin-2; and to lower serum levels of glucose, triglyceride, and cholesterol.

Various flavones have been found to inhibit cell proliferation and angiogenesis *in vitro* and to inhibit phorbol ester-induced skin cancer in the mouse model. These effects may involve inhibition of protein kinase C, stimulation of DNA repair mechanisms, and altered carcinogen metabolism. Some proanthocyanins have been shown to induce apoptosis.

Antiestrogenic effects of soy isoflavones

That soy isoflavones can be antiestrogenic was demonstrated by a study of Asian women in which the intake of soy products was found to be inversely associated with circulating levels of estrogen.[93] This effect relates to the binding of isoflavones to estrogen receptors α and ß, thus affecting the estrogen-synthetic activity of 17ß-steroid oxidoreductase, as well as estrogen-dependent signal transduction pathways. This is believed to underlie epidemiological observations of inverse associations of soy products and symptoms of menopause or premenstrual syndrome. Some, but not all, clinical trials have found the consumption of soy products to reduce menopausal symptoms by as much as 50–60%,[94] and a recent study found soy consumption effective in reducing

---

[88] Middleton, E., Jr., et al. (2000). *Pharmacol. Rev.* **52,** 673–751.

[89] This effect, which involves inhibition of the CYP3A4 isoform, may also involve other flavanones present in grapefruit juice. The potency of this effect is evidenced by the fact that a single glass of grapefruit juice can affect the biological activity of drugs metabolized by this enzyme system, increasing the activities of some and decreasing the activities of others.

[90] Arts, I. C. W., and Hollman, P. C. H. (2005). *Am. J. Clin. Nutr.* **81,** 317S–325S.

[91] Knekt, P., et al. (2002). *Am. J. Clin. Nutr.* **76,** 560–568.

[92] Arts, I. C., et al. (2002). *Cancer Causes Control.* **13,** 373–382.

[93] Nagata, C., et al. (1998). *J. Nat. Cancer Inst.* **90,** 1830–1835.

[94] Albertazzi, P., et al. (1998). *Obstet. Gynecol.* **91,** 6–11; Upmalis, D. H., et al. (2000). *Menopause* **7,** 236–242.

premenstrual syndrome symptoms.[95] As their estrogenic character might suggest, the consumption of soy isoflavones has been associated with higher bone mineral density in a limited number of epidemiological studies. Clinical trials conducted to test the hypothesis that soy isoflavones may be useful in improving bone mineralization for the prevention of osteoporosis have yielded inconsistent results.[96]

Other effects

It has been suggested that health benefits attributed to traditional, herbal medicaments may be due to bioactive flavonoids. Evidence supporting such a hypothesis includes the findings that bilberry anthocyanins reduce retinal hemorrhage in type 2 diabetics, and that certain proanthocyanins can inhibit bacterial adherence to uroepithelial cell surfaces, suggesting a role in reducing urogenital tract infections.

Despite these provocative findings, the paucity of clinical trial data makes the clinical value of flavonoids unclear. Although flavonoid supplementation may be beneficial under some circumstances, their effects would appear to be pharmacologic ones, and there is no firm evidence of unique nutritional roles. On this basis the flavonoids are not considered vitamins.

VIII. Non-Provitamin A Carotenoids

The carotenoids are polyisoprenoid compounds produced by plants for the purposes of harvesting light for photosynthesis and quench free radicals, thereby protecting against oxidative stress. Both functions are possible due to the capabilities of the conjugated double bond systems of these compounds, which enable them to accept unpaired electrons by delocalizing that electronegativity across multiple carbons. Accordingly, carotenoids have potent antioxidant capabilities. This property allows some carotenoids to function in vision; however, those without the ß-ionone head group necessary for that and other vitamin A functions (see Chapter 5), lack pro-vitamin A activity. These include some carotenes and oxygen-

ated analogs called xanthophylls. The most common non-provitamin A carotenoids in human diets are lycopene, lutein, zeaxanthin, and canthoxanthin (see Fig. 18-6).

Non-Provitamin A Carotenoids in Foods

Most non-provitamin A carotenoids are pigments occurring in red, yellow, and orange-colored plant tissues (see Fig. 18-7). The dominant form in U.S. diets is lycopene, the nonaromatic, polyisoprenoid precursor to the biosynthesis of ß-carotene in plants.[97] It is found in significant amounts in such red-colored foods as tomatoes, watermelon, pink grapefruit, and guava. It is estimated that Americans consume an average of 3.3 to 10.5 mg lycopene daily; estimates from European studies have been similar. The xanthophyll lutein is present in significant concentrations in spinach, kale, corn, broccoli, collards, and eggs; lutein and zeaxanthin in corn represent major sources of pigmentation for poultry diets.[98] The xanthophyll astaxathin is the source of pink coloration of salmon.

Utilization of Non-Provitamin A Carotenoids

Non-provitamin A carotenoids in foods are utilized by the same processes as those by which their provitamin A counterparts are utilized (see Chapter 5). Their

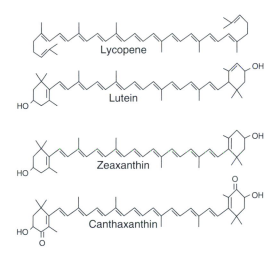

Fig. 18-6. Structures of major non-provitamin A carotenoids.

---

[95] Bryant, M. (2005). *Br. J. Nutr.* **93,** 731–739.

[96] Messina, M., et al. (2004). *Curr. Opin. Clin. Nutr. Metab. Care* **7,** 649–658.

[97] Plants convert lycopene to ß-carotene by forming to ß-rings at its ends through the action of lycopene cyclase.

[98] That is, to promote desirable colorations of egg yolks and broiler skin.

Table 18-7. Non-provitamin A carotenoids in fruits and vegetables

Food	Lycopene (µg/100 g)	Lutein and zeaxanthin (µg/100 g)	Cryptoxanthin (µg/100 g)
Apple, raw	0	45	0
Apricot, canned	65	2	0
Asparagus, raw	0	640	0
Avocado, raw	0	320	0
Broccoli, cooked	0	1,800	0
Beans, green	0	7,400	0
Brussels sprouts	0	1,300	0
Cabbage, red	0	26	0
Carrot, raw/cooked	0	260	0
Celery	0	3,600	0
Collards	0	16,300	0
Corn	0	780	0
Endive	0	4,000	0
Grapefruit, pink	3,360	0	0
Kale	0	21,900	0
Kiwi fruit	0	180	0
Leek, raw	0	1,900	0
Lettuce, leaf	0	1,400	0
Lettuce, romaine	0	1,800	0
Mango	0	0	54
Mustard greens	0	9,900	0
Nectarine	0	15	43
Okra, raw	0	6,800	0
Onion, yellow, raw	0	16	0
Orange	0	14	149
Papaya	0	0	470
Peach, canned	0	28	47
Pear, raw	0	110	0
Peas, green	0	1,700	0
Pepper, green, raw	0	700	0
Pumpkin	0	1,500	0
Spinach, cooked	0	12,600	0
Squash, summer	0	1,200	0
Swiss chard, raw	0	11,000	0
Tangerine	0	20	106
Tomato juice, canned	8,580	330	0
Tomato paste, canned	6,500	190	0
Tomato, raw	3,100	100	0
Watermelon, raw	4,100	14	0

Source: Nangles, A. R., et al. (1993). *J. Am. Diet. Assoc.* **93,** 284–296.

enteric absorption is effected by micelle-dependent diffusion and are subject to the antagonistic effects of binding to heat-labile food proteins.

Health Effects

It has been suggested that non-provitamin A carotenoids may account for the apparently protective associations of diets high in fruits and vegetables against cancer and other chronic diseases. This hypothesis has been tested in studies that have assessed carotenoid status on the basis of serum/plasma concentrations, or that have imputed carotenoid intakes from estimates of food intake and standard food carotenoid contents.

Lycopene

That **lycopene** may have an anticarcinogenic role has been suggested by the results of epidemiological studies.[99] A recent review of epidemiological findings indicated some evidence for a protective association of lycopene intake and lung cancer.[100] One study found patients with the precancerous lesion, oral leukoplakia, to respond in a dose-dependent manner to lycopene supplementation.[101]

More evidence is available for cancer of the prostate. A meta-analysis of 11 case-control studies and 10 cohort or nested case-control studies found prostate cancer risk to be inversely related to serum concentration of lycopene,[102] suggesting risk reduction of 25–30%. The same analysis, however, detected no significant associations of disease risk and the frequency of consumption of tomatoes, tomato products, or food lycopene, although some studies in which tomato consumption was high did report protective effects. The few intervention studies conducted to date have found lycopene supplementation to reduce cancer biomarkers: oxidative DNA damage in leukocytes and prostate tissues.[103] Studies with prostate cancer

cells in culture have shown them to be sensitive to lycopene, which causes cell cycle arrest and apoptosis. Lycopene exposure has been found to upregulate the expression of a gene affecting intercellular gap junction communication increases which are associated with decreased cell proliferation.[104] Still, supporting studies using animal models of carcinogenesis have been very limited, and their results varied. Thus, the practical importance of lycopene as a determinant of cancer risk reduction remains unclear.

Other health effects of lycopene are possible. A recent clinical intervention study found that oral lycopene treatment significantly reduced the incidence of preeclampsia (by 47%), disastolic pressure (by 5.5 mm Hg), and interuterine growth retardation (by 41%) in primigravida women.[105]

Lutein and zeaxanthin

These xanthophylls are present in high concentrations in the normal primate retina in an area originally named the "macula lutea" or "yellow spot" for its color. The human retina contains 25–200 ng of these pigments, **zeaxanthin** being concentrated in the center and **lutein** being distributed about the periphery. Other mammals lack maculae; however, carotenoid-rich oil droplets have been found in birds, reptiles, amphibians, and fish.[106] Because carotenoids are not synthesized by the host, the carotenoid content of the macula is dependent on dietary intake. Studies have revealed that the average macular pigments of populations are low.[107] While the function of macular carotenoids is not clear, it has been suggested that they serve to protect the macula from the damaging effects of blue-wavelength photons (they absorb in the range of 420–480 nm, reducing by as much as 90% the incoming energy in this range from reaching macular photoreceptors) and scavenge reactive oxygen species formed in photoreceptors, thus to improve visual acuity. That the autofluorescent

---

[99] Giovannucci, E. (2005). *J. Nutr.* **135,** 2030S–2031S.

[100] Arab, L., et al. (2002). *Exp. Biol. Med.* **227,** 894–899.

[101] Singh, M., et al. (2004). *Oral Oncol.* **40,** 591–596.

[102] Entinan, M., et al. (2004). *Cancer Epidemiol. Biomarkers Prev.* **13,** 340–345.

[103] Stacewicz-Sapuntzakis, M., and Bowen, P. E. (2005). *Biochim. Biophys. Acta* **1740,** 202–205.

[104] That is, connexin 43; Heber, D., and Lu, Q. Y. (2002). *Exp. Biol. Med.* **227,** 920–923.

[105] Sharma, J. B., et al. (2003). *Internat. J. Gynecol. Obstet.* **81,** 257–262.

[106] It has thus been speculated that the development of the macula was an evolutionary step associated with the development of color vision.

[107] Hammond, B. R., Jr., et al. (2002). *Invest. Ophthalmol. Vis. Sci.* **43,** 47–50; Snodderly, D. M., et al. (2004). *Invest. Ophthalmol. Vis. Sci.* **45,** 531–538.

pigment lipofuscin[108] accumulates in the retina with age, suggests oxidative stress as part of the etiology of the disease.

For these reasons, it has been suggested that lutein and zeaxanthin may protect against age-related **macular degeneration**, a leading cause of severe vision loss in industrialized countries.[109] Some epidemiological studies have supported this hypothesis, finding that people who consume diets rich in these xanthophylls tend to show lower rates of this disorder.[110] A recent randomized, controlled, clinical trial using lutein plus antioxidants as the intervention agent in patients with progressive atrophic macular degeneration reported improvements in several aspects of visual acuity;[111] otherwise there have been no empirical tests of this attractive hypothesis. That **xanthophylls** may be effective in supporting vision is supported by findings from another trial that lutein supplements improved visual acuity in cataract patients[112] and visual field in patients with retinitis pigmentosa.[113]

IX. Orotic Acid

Intermediate in Pyrimidine Biosynthesis

Orotic acid was isolated in the late 1940s from distillers' dried solubles[114] and was called, for a while, vitamin B_{13}. It is a substituted pyrimidine (1,2,3,6-tetrahydro-2,6-dioxo-4-pyrimidinecarboxylic acid).

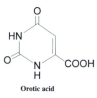

Orotic acid

Dietary Sources

Orotic acid is found in root vegetables (beets, carrots) and is associated with the whey fraction of milk. Notably, human milk lacks orotic acid.

Metabolic Function

Orotic acid is biosynthesized from N-carbamylphosphate by dehydration (via dihydroorotase), which is oxidized (via orotate reductase) to orotate. It is an important intermediate in the biosynthesis of pyrimidines.

When studies failed to confirm vitamin-like activity, that designation of this normal metabolite was dropped. In fact, orotic acid supplements (0.1%) to the diets of rats have been found to induce hepatic steatosis and hepatomegaly, and to increase hepatic levels of uracil nucleotides, presumably by increasing the flux through the pyrimidine pathway. These adverse effects have not been observed in other species (monkeys, guinea pigs, hamsters, mice, or pigs). On the basis of present understanding, orotic acid cannot be considered a vitamin.

Health Effects

Recent interest in orotic acid has concerned its hypocholesterolemic effect, an apparent consequence of its inhibition of hepatic cholesterol synthesis at the level of 3-hydroxy-3-methylglutaryl-CoA reductase. Studies have also found magnesium orotate to improve ventricular function and exercise tolerance in cardiac patients, but this effect would appear to be due to treatment of magnesium depletion and not the orotate moiety per se. Orotic acid has been used therapeutically for neonatal jaundice, hyperproteinemia, gout, and degenerative retinal disease.

---

[108] This appears to result from the condensation of two molecules of all-*trans*-retinal with one of the phosphatidylethanolamines, a complex that is taken up by the retinal pigment epithelium and converted to a stable pyridinium bisretinoid that is cytotoxic and causes apoptosis and, hence, macular degeneration.

[109] With an estimated prevalence of nearly 1.5%, age-related macular degeneration affects some 1.75 million Americans. The NIH-sponsored Age-Related Eye Disease Study [AREDS] found that 25% of patients with early signs did not develop severe vision loss when given a supplement containing zinc, ß-carotene, and vitamins E and C over a 5-year period (Age-Related Eye Disease Study Group [2001]. *Arch. Ophthamol.* **122**, 883–892).

[110] Seddon, J. M., et al. (1994). *J. Am. Med. Assoc.* **272**, 1413–1419.

[111] Richer, S., et al. (2004). *Opthalmol.* **75**, 216–230.

[112] Olmedilla, B., et al. (2003). *Nutrition* **19**, 21–24.

[113] Bahrami, H., et al. (2006). *Ophthalmol.* **6**, 23–25.

[114] This feedstuff consists of the dried aqueous residue from the distillation of fermented corn. It is used mainly as a component of mixed diets for poultry, swine, and dairy calves. It is rich in several B vitamins and has been valued as a source of unidentified growth factors, particularly for growing chicks and turkey poults.

X. *p*-Aminobenzoic Acid

Precursor to Folate in Bacteria

p-**Aminobenzoic acid** is an essential growth factor for many species of bacteria, which use it as a precursor for the biosynthesis of folate. Some early studies showed responses of chicks (increased growth) and rats (enhanced lactation) to *p*-aminobenzoic acid-supplemented diets containing marginal concentrations of folate. For a time *p*-aminobenzoic acid was called vitamin B_x. Such responses, however, were shown to be due to the use by the intestinal microflora of *p*-aminobenzoic acid for the synthesis of folate made available to the host either directly in the gut or indirectly via the feces. Because animals lack the enzymes of the folate synthetic pathway, they cannot convert this bacterial precursor to the actual vitamin. Therefore, *p*-aminobenzoic acid is not a vitamin.

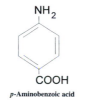

p-Aminobenzoic acid

Still, *p*-aminobenzoic acid can be biologically active. It can antagonize the bacteriostatic effects of sulfonamide drugs owing to similarities in chemical structure. It has a very high absorbance in the ultraviolet (UV) range and is used as a UV-screening agent in sun-blocking preparations. In a randomized, controlled trial,[115] it was found to inhibit fibroblast proliferation and to promote the reduction of fibrous plaques that cause penile deformation in patients with Peyronie's disease.[116]

Because its metabolism is limited, *p*-aminobenzoic acid can be used in clinical situations as a marker of the completeness of 24-hour urine collections, 70–85% appearing in the urine after a single oral dose.[117] Its glutamyl ester, *p*-aminobenzoylglutamate, is the primary catabolite of folate, produced by cleavage of the C9-N10 bond (see Chapter 16). Excreted in the urine as *p*-acetamidobenzoylglutamate, urinary levels

reflect the total body folate pool and can thus serve as an indicator of long-term folate status.[118]

XI. Lipoic Acid

Metabolic Functions

Coenzyme

Lipoic acid (6-thiocytic acid) is an essential cofactor for the oxidative decarboxylations of α-keto acids where, linked to the ε-amino group of a lysine residue of the enzyme dihydrolipoyl transacetylase, it is one of several prosthetic groups in the multienzyme, lactate dehydrogenase complex. In that catalysis, the amide form, **lipoamide**, undergoes reversible acylation/deacylation to transfer acyl groups to CoA as well as reversible redox ring opening/closing, which is coupled with the oxidation of the α-keto acid.[119] Thus, lipoic acid, occupies a critical position in energy metabolism, regulating the flow of carbon into the tricarboxylic acid cycle.

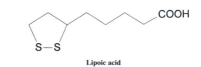

Lipoic acid

Antioxidant

The ability to undergo interconversion between disulfide (lipoic acid) and sulfhydryl (dihydrolipoic acid) forms enables this metabolite to function as a metabolic antioxidant, quenching reactive oxygen species and other free radicals and chelating prooxidant metal ions. Its function in this regard is related to those of other metabolic antioxidants in the network of protection against oxidative stress.

Dietary Sources

Lipoic acid is present in a wide variety of foods but generally at low levels. The best sources are tissues rich in mitochrondia (e.g., heart, kidney) or chloroplasts (i.e., dark green leafy vegetables such as spinach).[120] In these foods, most of the factor appears to occur bound to lysyl residues in proteins. Although the

---

[115] Weidner, W., et al. (2005). *Eur. Urol.* **47**, 530–535.

[116] Peyronie's disease is a benign condition of the penis characterized by the formation of fibrous plaques within the tunica albuginea, usually resulting in penile deformity with some degree of erectile dysfunction.

[117] Jakobsen, J., et al. (2003). *Eur. J. Clin. Nutr.* **57**, 138–142.

[118] Wolfe, J. M., et al. (2003). *Am. J. Clin. Nutr.* **77**, 919–923.

[119] That is, the conversion of pyruvate to acetyl CoA and α-ketoglutarate to succinyl CoA.

[120] Lodge, J. K., et al. (1997). *J. Appl. Nutr.* **49**, 3–11.

bioavailability of food forms of lipoyllysine have not been determined, it is likely that they are relatively low, as studies with purified lipoic acid have indicated efficiencies of enteric absorption of 20–38%.

Conditions of Need

Some species of bacteria (e.g., *Streptococcus faecalis, Lactobacillus casei*) and protozoa (e.g., *Tetrahymena geleii*) have clear needs for exogenous sources of lipoic. However, no deficiency signs have been reported, and lipoic acid supplements to chicks, rats, and turkey poults fed low-lipoic acid, purified diets have been without effect. Animals synthesize lipoic acid from octanoic acid by the introduction of sulfur atoms at two positions. This process, not fully elucidated, occurs in the mitochrondia. Therefore, lipoic acid is not considered a vitamin.

Health Effects

That lipoic acid can function as an antioxidant suggests that its metabolic effects, like those of other antioxidants, may be related to general antioxidant status and prooxidant "tone." Accordingly, lipoic acid has been found to reduce signs of vitamin C and vitamin E deficiency in rodent models, and to increase tissue levels of reduced glutathione. On the basis of such results, it has been proposed that lipoic acid may have value in the prevention and/or treatment of other chronic diseases associated with oxidative stress. Recent interest has centered on the prospective benefits of lipoic acid in diabetes and neurodegenerative diseases:

- *Diabetes* Studies with experimental animals have shown that supplemental lipoic acid can reduce lipid peroxidation induced by exercise, and increase the rate of glucose disposal, reduce cataract formation, and improve motor neuron conductivity in models of diabetes. Clinical trials with type II diabetic subjects have found lipoic acid treatment to increase glucose clearance[121] and to reduce blood glucose levels and lipid peroxidation products[122] as well as the severity of cardiovascular neuropathy.[123]

- *Multiple sclerosis* A trial with patients with multiple sclerosis indicated that lipoic acid may be useful in treatment by reducing serum matrix metalloproteinase-9 and reducing T-cell migration into the central nervous system.[124]

XII. Ineffective Factors

The term *vitamin* has been used from time to time in association with factors with no apparent metabolic activity that would justify that designation. Furthermore, opportunities afforded by patent law permitted a substance to be trade-named a vitamin in the 1940s, a situation bound to mislead the uninformed.

Vitamin B₁₅

A substance isolated from apricot kernels and other natural sources was trade-named "vitamin B_{15}" and was also called pangamic acid by its discoverers;[125] it was patented with a claim of therapeutic efficacy against a wide range of diseases of the skin, respiratory tract, nerves, and joints—despite the fact that no data were presented in the patent application. Whereas pangamic acid was originally described as *d*-gluconodimethylamino acetic acid (the ester of *d*-gluconic acid and dimethylglycine), the term now appears to be used indiscriminately; products also containing *N,N*-diisopropylammonium dichloroacetate, sodium gluconolactone, *N,N*-dimethylglycine, calcium gluconate, and/or glycine in various proportions also go by the names pangamic acid, pangamate, aangamik 15, and vitamin B_{15}. Thus, vitamin B_{15} is not a definable chemical entity; in fact, the substance originally called pangamic acid has frequently been absent from such preparations. Of the compounds likely to be present, *N,N*-diisopropylammonium dichloroacetate is known to be hypotensive, hypothermic, and potentially toxic, and dichloroacetate is a weak mutagen. Despite intermittent popular interest in these preparations,[126] the only information that would appear to support positive clinical results comes from anecdotal sources and the undocumented claims by vendors of these preparations. No substantive data appear to have ever been presented to support any beneficial biological effects of the so-called

---

[121] Jacob, S., et al. (1996). *Exp. Clin. Endcrinol. Diabetes* **104**, 284–288.

[122] Ziegler, D., et al. (1995). *Diabetol.* **38**, 1425–1433.

[123] Tankova, T., et al. (2004). *Rom. J. Intern. Med.* **42**, 457–464.

[124] Yadav, V., et al. (2005). *Mult. Scler.* **11**, 159–165.

[125] Ernst Krebs, Sr., and Ernst Krebs, Jr.—not to be confused with the great biochemist Sir Hans Krebs.

[126] For example, in its March 13, 1978, cover story, *New York* Magazine presented vitamin B_{15} as a possible cure for everything short of a transit strike.

vitamin B$_{15}$, and there is no evidence that deprivation of the factor(s) caused any physiological impairment.

Gerovital

As its name implies, Gerovital was promoted as a nutritional substance that alleviated age-related degenerative diseases. Also called vitamin H$_3$ and vitamin GH3, it is actually a buffered solution of procaine HCl, the dental anesthetic Novocain.[127] Its health claims are unsubstantiated.

Laetrile

Sometimes called vitamin B$_{17}$, laetrile was first isolated from apricot kernels. It is a discrete chemical entity, the **cyanogenic glycoside** 1-mandelonitrile-β-glucuronic acid. The term *laetrile* is often used interchangeably with the related cyanogenic glycoside amygdalin, which occurs naturally in the seeds of most fruits. These compounds have been claimed effective in cancer treatment, owing either to the cyanide they provide as being selectively toxic to tumor cells, or to the disease itself being a result of an unsatisfied metabolic need for laetrile. The contention that either compound provides a source of cyanide ignores the fact that animals, lacking β-glucosidases, cannot degrade the mandelonitrile moiety. In fact, laetrile and amygdalin are each nontoxic to animals and humans for that reason. Apricot kernels and other fruit seeds, however, contain β-glucosidases; if these are liberated (e.g., by crushing) before eating such seeds, then cyanide poisoning can occur.[128] Extensive animal tumor model studies and clinical trials have tested the putative antitumor effects of laetrile; these have yielded consistently negative results.

XIII. Unidentified Growth Factors

Since the discovery of vitamin B$_{12}$, experimental nutritionists have observed many instances of stimulated growth by the addition of natural materials to purified diets. Many such responses have been found to involve interrelationships of known nutrients.[129] Some have involved diet palatability and thus the rate of food intake of experimental animals. Some have resulted in the discovery of new essential nutrients (e.g., selenium). Other responses remain to be understood. For young monogastrics (particularly poultry) several feedstuffs are popularly regarded as having UGF activity:

- Condensed fish solubles
- Fish meal
- Dried whey
- Brewers' dried yeast
- Corn distillers' dried solubles
- Other fermentation residues

Elucidating the nature of these UGFs has been complicated by the fact that the growth responses are small and, often, poorly reproducible. This suggests that other interacting effects of environment, gut microfloral, diet, and so on, may be involved. As has happened in the past, perhaps the next vitamins will be discovered through studies of these or other UGFs.

Study Questions and Exercises

1. List the questions that must be answered in determining the eligibility of a substance for vitamin status.

2. For each of the substances discussed in this chapter, list the available information that would support its designation as a vitamin, and that which would refute such a designation.

3. Outline the general approaches one would need to take in order to characterize the UGF activity of a natural material such as fish meal for the chick.

4. Prepare a concept map of the relationships of micronutrients and physiological function, including the specific relationships of the traditional vitamins, the quasi-vitamins, and ineffective factors.

---

[127] Procain hydrochloride, that is, 4-aminobenzoic acid 2-(diethylamino)-ethyl ester hydrochloride.

[128] Normally, cyanide poisoning is not a problem for animals that eat apricot or peach kernels, as those seeds generally pass intact through the gut.

[129] An example is the enhancement, by the natural chelating activity in corn distillers' dried solubles, of the utilization of zinc by chicks fed a soybean meal-based diet.

Recommended Reading

Carnitine

Atkins, J., and Clandinin, M. T. (1990). Nutritional significance of factors affecting carnitine dependent transport of fatty acids in neonates: A review. *Nutr. Res.* **10,** 117–128.

Calabrese, V., Stella, A. M. G., Calvani, M., and Allan, D. (2005). Acetylcholine and cellular response: Roles in nutritional redox homeostasis and regulation of longevity genes. *J. Nutr. Biochem.* **17,** 73–88.

Engel, A. G., Banker, B. Q., and Eiben, R. M. (1997). Carnitine deficiency: Clinical, morphological, and biochemical observations in a fatal case. *J. Neurol. Neurosurg. Psychiatry* **40,** 313–322.

Ferrari, R., Merli, E., Cicchitelli, G., Mele, D., Fucili, A., and Ceconi, C. (2004). Therapeutic effects of L-carnitine and propionyl-L-carnitine on cardiovascular diseases: A review. *Ann. N.Y. Acad. Sci.* **1033,** 79–91.

Foster, D. W. (2004). The role of the carnitine system in human metabolism. *Ann. N.Y. Acad. Sci.* **1033,** 1–16.

Garrow, T. A. (2001). Choline and carnitine, Chapter 25 in *Present Knowledge in Nutrition*, 8th ed. (B. A. Bowman and R. M., Russell, eds.), pp. 261–270. ILSI Press, Washington, DC.

Mingrove, G. (2004). Carnitine in type 2 diabetes. *Ann. N.Y. Acad. Sci.* **1033,** 99–107.

Natecz, K. A., Miecz, D., Berezowski, V., and Cecchelli, R. (2004). Carnitine: Transport and physiological functions in the brain. *Mol. Aspects Med.* **25,** 551–567.

Rebouche, C. J. (2006). Carnitine, Chapter 33 in *Modern Nutrition in Health and Disease* (M. E. Shils, M. Shike, A. C. Ross, B. Caballero, and R. J. Cousins, eds.), pp. 537–544. Lippincott, New York.

Stanley, C. A. (2004). Carnitine deficiency disorders in children. *Ann. N.Y. Acad. Sci.* **1033,** 42–51.

Vaz, F. M., and Wanders, R. J. A. (2002). Carnitine biosynthesis in mammals. *Biochem. J.* **361,** 417–429.

Winter, S. C. (2003). Treatment of carnitine deficiency. *J. Inherit. Metab. Dis.* **26,** 171–180.

Wolf, G. (2006). The discovery of a vitamin role for carnitine: The first 50 years. *J. Nutr.* **136,** 2131–2134.

Choline

Chan, M. M. (1991). Choline, in *Handbook of Vitamins* (L. J. Machlin, ed.), 2nd ed., pp. 537–556. Marcel Dekker, New York.

Garrow, T. A. (2001). Choline and carnitine, Chapter 25 in *Present Knowledge in Nutrition,* 8th ed. (B. A. Bowman and R. M. Russell, eds.), pp. 261–270. ILSI Press, Washington, DC.

Newborne, P. M. (2002). Choline deficiency associated with diethanolamine carcinogenicity. *Toxicol. Sci.* **67,** 1–3.

Zeisel, S. H., and Niculescu, M. D. (2006). Choline and phosphatidylcholine, Chapter 32 in *Modern Nutrition in Health and Disease* (M. E. Shils, M. Shike, A. C. Ross, B. Caballero, and R. J. Cousins, eds.), pp. 525–536. Lippincott, New York.

Flavonoids

Blumberg, J. B., and Milbury, P. E. (2006). Dietary flavonoids, Chapter 28 in *Present Knowledge in Nutrition*, 9th ed., vol. I (B. A. Bowman and R. M. Russell, eds.), pp. 361–370. ILSI Press, Washington, DC.

Engler, M. B., and Engler, M. M. (2006). The emerging role of flavonoid-rich cocoa and chocolate in cardiovascular health and disease. *Nutr. Rev.* **64,** 109–118.

Hertog, M. G. (1996). Epidemiological evidence on potential health properties of flavonoids. *Proc. Nutr. Soc.* **55,** 385–397.

Hollman, P. C. H. (1997). Bioavailability of flavonoids. *Eur. J. Clin. Nutr.* **51,** S66–S69.

Knekt, P., Kumpulainen, J., Järvinen, R., Rissanen, H., Heliövaara, M., Reunanen, A., Hakulinen, T., and Aromaa, A. (2002). Flavonoid intake and risk of chronic disease. *Am. J. Clin. Nutr.* **76,** 560–568.

Nijveldt, R. J., van Nood, E., van Hoorn, D. E. C., Boelens, P. G., van Norren, K., and Leeuwen, P. A. M. (2001). Flavonoids: A review of probable mechanisms of action and potential applications. *Am. J. Clin. Nutr.* **74,** 418–425.

Peluso, M. R. (2006). Flavonoids attenuate cardiovascular disease, inhibit phosphodiesterase, and modulate lipid homeostasis in adipose tissue and liver. *Proc. Soc. Exp. Biol. Med.* **231,** 1287–1299.

Rice-Evans, C. A., and Packer, L., eds. (2003). *Flavonoids in Health and Disease*, Marcel Dekker, New York, 467 pp.

Ross, J. A., and Kasum, C. M. (2002). Dietary flavonoids: Bioavailability, metabolic effects, and safety. *Ann. Rev. Nutr.* **22,** 19–34.

myo-Inositol

Bennett, M., Onnebo, S. M. N., Azevedo, C., and Saiardi, A. (2006). Inositol pyrophosphates: Metabolism and signaling. *Cell Mol. Life Sci.* **63,** 552–564.

Downes, C. P., Gray, A., and Lucocq, J. M. (2006). Probing phosphoinositide functions in signaling and membrane trafficking. *Trends Cell Biol.* **15,** 259–268.

Shamsuddin, A. (1999). Metabolism and cellular functions of IP_6: A review. *Anticancer Res.* **19,** 3733–3736.

York, J. D. (2006). Regulation of nuclear processes by inositol polyphosphates. *Biochim. Biophys. Acta* **1761,** 552–559.

Lipoic Acid

Bilska, A., and Wlodek, L. (2005). Lipoic acid—the drug of the future. *Pharmacol. Rep.* **57,** 570–577.

Marquet, A., Bui, B. T. S., and Florentin, D. (2001). Biosynthesis of biotin and lipoic acid. *Vitamins Hormones* **61,** 51–101.

Packer, L., Kramer, K., and Rimbach, G. (2001). Molecular aspects of lipoic acid in the prevention of diabetes complications. *Nutr.* **17,** 888–895.

Packer, L., Witt, E. H., and Tritschler, H. J. (1995). Alpha-lipoic acid as a biological antioxidant. *Free Radic. Biol. Med.* **19,** 227–250.

Non-Provitamin A Carotenoids

Bartlett, H., and Eperjesi, F. (2003). Age-related macular degeneration and nutritional supplementation: A review of randomized controlled trials. *Ophthal. Physiol. Opt.* **23,** 383–399.

Clinton, S. K. (2005). Tomatoes or lycopene: A role in prostate carcinogenesis. *J. Nutr.* **135,** 2057S–2059S.

Cooper, D. A., Eldridge, A. L., and Peters, J. S. (1999). Dietary carotenoids and certain cancers, heart disease and age-related macular degeneration: A review of recent research. *Nutr. Rev.* **57,** 201–214.

Giovannucci, E. (2002). A review of epidemiologic studies of tomatoes, lycopene and prostate cancer. *Proc. Soc. Exp. Biol. Med.* **227,** 852–859.

Granado, F., Olmedilla, B., and Blanco, I. (2003). Nutritional and clinical relevance of lutein in human health. *Br. J. Nutr.* **90,** 487–502.

Handelman, G. J. (2001). The evolving role of carotenoids in human biochemistry. *Nutr.* **17,** 818–822.

Heber, D., and Lu, Q. Y. (2002). Overview of mechanisms of action of lycopene. *Exp. Biol. Med.* **227,** 920–923.

Krinsky, N. I., Landrum, J. T., and Bone, R. A. (2003). Biological mechanisms of the protective role of lutein and zeaxanthin in the eye. *Ann. Rev. Nutr.* **23,** 171–201.

Mares-Perlman, J. A., Millen, A. E., Ficek, T. L., and Hankinson, S. E. (2002). The body of evidence to support a protective role for lutein and zeaxanthin in delaying chronic disease. *Overview. J. Nutr.* **132,** 518S–524S.

Stringham, J. M., and Hammond, B. R., Jr. (2005). Dietary lutein and zeaxanthin: Possible effects on visual function. *Nutr. Rev.* **63,** 59–64.

Orotic Acid

Salerno, C., and Crifo, C. (2002). Diagnostic value of urinary orotic acid levels: Applicable separation methods. *J. Chromatog.* **781,** 57–71.

Pyrroloquinoline Quinone

Christensen, H. N. (1994). Is PQQ a significant nutrient in addition to its role as a therapeutic agent in the higher animal? *Nutr. Rev.* **52,** 24–25.

Duine, J. A., van de Meer, R. A., and Green, B. (1990). The cofactor pyrroloquinoline quinone. *Annu. Rev. Nutr.* **10,** 297–318.

Harris, E. D. (1992). The pyrroloquinoline quinone (PQQ) coenzymes: A case of mistaken identity. *Nutr. Rev.* **50,** 263–274.

Killgore, J., Smidt, C., Duich, L., Romero-Chapman, N., Tinker, D., Reiser, K., Melko, M., Hyde, D., and Rucker, R. B. (1989). Nutritional importance of pyrroloquinoline quinone. *Science* **245,** 850–852.

Smidt, C. R., Steinberg, F. M., and Rucker, R. B. (1991). Physiologic importance of pyrroloquinoline quinone. *Proc. Soc. Exp. Biol. Med.* **197,** 19–26.

Ubiquinones

Bonakdar, R. A., and Guardneri, E. (2005). Coenzyme Q10. *Compl. Altern. Med.* **72,** 1065–1070.

Crane, F. L. (2001). Biochemical functions of coenzyme Q_{10}. *Ann. N.Y. Acad. Sci.* **20,** 591–598.

Folkers, K., and Langsjoen, P. (1993). Nutrition and cardiac health: A deficiency of coenzyme Q_{10} is a dominant molecular cause of heart failure. *J. Optimal Nutr.* **2,** 24–274.

Linnance, A.W., et al. (2002). Human aging and global function of coenzyme Q_{10}. *Ann. N.Y. Acad. Sci.* **959,** 396–411.

Olson, R. E., and Rudney, H. (1983). Biosynthesis of ubiquinone. *Vitamins Hormones* **40,** 1–43.

USING CURRENT KNOWLEDGE OF THE VITAMINS

III

Sources of the Vitamins

19

The intakes of vitamins into the body calculated from standard tables are rarely accurate.

—J. Marks

I.	Vitamins in Foods	437
II.	Vitamin Contents of Feedstuffs	441
III.	Predicting Vitamin Contents	441
IV.	Vitamin Bioavailability	448
V.	Vitamin Losses	449
VI.	Vitamin Supplementation and Fortification of Foods	451
VII.	Vitamins in Human Diets	454
VIII.	Vitamin Supplements	457
IX.	Vitamin Labeling of Foods	459
X.	Vitamins in Livestock Feeds	461
	Study Questions and Exercises	466
	Recommended Reading	467

Anchoring Concepts

1. Estimates of the vitamin contents of many foods and feedstuffs are available.
2. For some vitamins, only a portion of the total present in certain foods or feedstuffs is biologically available.
3. The total vitamin intake of an individual is the sum of the amounts of bioavailable vitamins in the various foods, feedstuffs, and supplements consumed.

Learning Objectives

1. To understand the sources of error in estimates of the vitamin contents of foods and feedstuffs.
2. To understand the concept of a core food and to know the core foods for each vitamin.
3. To understand the sources of potential losses of the vitamins from foods and feedstuffs.
4. To understand which of the vitamins are most likely to be in insufficient supply in the diets of humans and livestock.

5. To understand the means available for the supplementation of individual foods and total diets with vitamins.

Vocabulary

Bioavailability
Core foods
National Nutrient Database
Nutrition Labeling and Education Act (NLEA)
Vitamin premix
Vitamin–mineral premix

I. Vitamins in Foods

Tabulated Vitamin Content Data

The formal compilation of food composition data was initiated by the U.S. Department of Agriculture (USDA) food chemist W. O. Atwater in 1896. Since that time, developing information on the nutrient composition of foods has been an ongoing program of the USDA in cooperation with Land Grant colleges and universities and, in more recent times, with the private sector, being in the interest of corporate feed producers to have reliable data for content in the feedstuffs of those nutrients that most directly affect the cost of their formulations. Nutrient composition data for foods are available in many forms (e.g., books, wall charts, tables, and appendices of books, computer tapes, and diskettes); however, most compilations derive from the USDA **National Nutrient Database**. These data are available as the *USDA Nutrient Database for Standard Reference*, release 19, and can be accessed via the Internet.[1] Other data relevant to the vitamin status and intakes of

---

[1] http://www.ars.usda.gov/main/site_main.htm?modecode=12354500

Americans can be found in other public access databases:

- *What We Eat in America:*[2] Results from US National Health and Nutrition Examination Surveys (NHANES) 2001–2002 and 2003–2004.
- *USDA Food Surveys, 1965–1998:*[3] Results from the *USDA Continuing Surveys of Food Intakes by Individuals (CSFII)* 1985–1986 and 1989–1991; *Portion Size Report,* 1989–1991; *Diet, Health and Knowledge Surveys (DHKS),* 1994–1996 and 1998; *Nationwide Food Surveys,* 1977–1978 and 1987–1988.
- *Nutrient Content of the Food Supply Report, 1909–2000:*[4] Historical data on the amounts of nutrients available per capita per day in food available for consumption in the United States.
- *USDA U.S. Food Supply Series:*[5] Annual estimates of amounts of about 350 foods that disappear into civilian food consumption at or before retail distribution
- *FDA Total Diet Studies:*[6] Conducted yearly to assess the levels of various nutritional elements, pesticide residues, and contaminants in the U.S. food supplement and in representative diets of selected age–sex groups

Similar, but less extensive, databases have been developed in some other countries,[7] and efforts are being made to standardize the collection, compilation, and reporting of food nutrient composition data on a wordwide basis.[8]

The nutrient composition of feedstuffs has, with few exceptions,[9] been developed less systematically and extensively. Data sets presently in the public domain have been compiled largely from original reports in the scientific literature. Therefore, the effects of uncontrolled sampling, multiple and often old analytical methods, multiple analysts, unreported analytical precision, unreported sample variance, and so on are likely to be far greater for the nutrient databases for feedstuffs than for the corresponding databases for foods.

Use of any database for estimating vitamin intake is limited for reasons concerning the accuracy and completeness of the data. Although the USDA National Nutrient Database (see Table 19-1, Appendix D) is much more complete than most feed tables with respect to data for vitamins, it is only reasonably complete with respect to thiamin, riboflavin, and niacin; data for vitamins D and E are particularly scant.[10] In addition, accurate and robust[11] analytical methods are available only for vitamin E, thiamin, riboflavin, niacin, and pyridoxine. For the other vitamins, this means that the quality of available analytical data can render them unacceptable for inclusion in the database or be low enough to raise serious questions concerning reliability.

Core Foods for Vitamins

Foods are the most important sources of vitamins in the daily diets of humans. However, the vitamins are unevenly distributed among the various foods that comprise human diets (Table 19-2). Therefore, the evaluation of the degree of vitamin adequacy of total diets is served by knowing which foods are likely to

---

[2] http://www.ars.usda.gov/Services/docs.htm?docid=14018

[3] http://www.ars.usda.gov/Services/docs.htm?docid=7787

[4] http://www.usda.gov/cnpp/nutrient_content.html

[5] http://209.48.219.50/Query.htm

[6] http://www.cfsan.fda.gov/~comm/tds-toc.html

[7] For example, the Swiss food composition database (http://food.ethz.ch:2000/swifd/) and the Mexican food composition database (MEXFOODS) (http://pobox.com/~mexfoods).

[8] This is the purpose of the INFOODS project of the United Nations University Food and Nutrition Program (http://www.crop.cr.inz/foodinfo/infoods/admin/0admin.html).

[9] The notable exception in the public domain was the program at the University of Maryland, which involved the ongoing analysis of feedstuffs commonly used in feeding poultry in the United States. That program focused on macronutrients. It was discontinued in the late 1970s; the last version of the data (i.e., *1979 Maryland Feed Composition Data*) was published as a supplement in the Proceedings of the Maryland Nutrition Conference in that year. Other widely used feed tables [e.g., Scott, M. L., Nesheim, M. C., and Young, R. J. (1982). "Nutrition of the Chicken," pp. 482–489. Scott Assoc., Ithaca, NY] were derived in part from this source.

[10] In 1987, Hepburn (Human Nutrition Information Service Report No. Adm-382, pp. 68–74) estimated that the USDA National Nutrient Data Bank contained vitamin values for the following percentages of entries: 83% for vitamin C, 64% for pyridoxine and vitamin B_{12}, 61% for retinol equivalents, 56% for folate, and 28% for vitamin E. In computer-based diet analysis programs, missing data can cause underestimates of the amounts of nutrients present or consumed; programs that fail to identify missing data will therefore underrepresent the uncertainty associated with the estimates they produce.

[11] Accuracy is minimally influenced by such factors as unusual technical skill of the analyst or particular instrumental conditions.

Table 19-1.   Adequacy of the USDA national nutrient database vitamin contents of foods

Food	A	D	E	K	C	Thiamin	Riboflavin	Niacin	B$_6$	Pantothenic acid	Folate	B$_{12}$
Baby foods	●		•	○	●	●	●	●	•	○	•	•
Baked foods												
Breads	○		•	○		●	●	●	●	•	•	○
Sweet goods	•		•			●	●	●	•	•	•	•
Cookies and crackers	•		•			●	●	●	●	•	•	•
Beverages	•			•	•	•	•	•	•	•	•	
Breakfast cereals	•	○	•	○	•	•	•	•	•	•	•	•
Candies	•		○		•	○	•	•	•	•	•	○
Cereal grains												
Whole	•		•	•		●	●	●	●	●	●	
Flour			•	○		●	●	●	●	●	●	
Pasta			○	○		●	●	●	●	●	●	
Dairy products	●	●	•	•	●	●	●	●	●	●	•	●
Eggs and egg products	•	•	•	•	○	●	●	●	●	●	•	●
Fast foods	●	○	•	○	•	●	●	●	•	•	○	•
Fats and oils	•	•	•	•								
Fish, shellfish												
Raw	•	•	•	○		•	•	•	•	•	•	•
Cooked	○	●	•	○		○	○	○	○	•	•	○
Fruits												
Raw	●	○	•	●	●	●	●	●	●	•	•	
Cooked	•	○	○	•	•	•	•	•	•	•	•	
Frozen, canned	●	○	○	•	●	●	○	●	•	•	•	
Legumes												
Raw	•		●	•		●	●	●	•	●	●	
Cooked	○		●	○		●	●	●	•	●	●	
Meat												
Beef	●	•	•	•		●	●	●	●	•	•	●
Lamb	•	•	•	○		●	●	●	•	•	•	●
Pork	•	•	•	○		●	●	●	●	•	•	●
Sausage	•	•	○	○	●	●	●	●	●	•	•	●
Veal	•	•	•	○		●	●	●	●	•	●	●
Poultry	•	•	•	○		●	●	●	•	•	•	•
Nuts, seeds	•	•	•	○	•	•	•	•	•	•	○	
Snack foods	•	•	•	○	○	•	●	●	•	•	•	○
Soups	●	○	○	●	●	●	●	●	•	○	○	•
Vegetables												
Raw	●	•	•	●	●	●	●	●	•	○	•	
Cooked	•	•	○	•	•	•	•	•	•	○	•	
Frozen	●	○	○	●	●	●	●	●	○	•	•	
Canned	●	○	○	●	●	●	●	●	○	•	•	

Key: (○) Few or no data; (•) inadequate data; (●) substantial data.

Source: Beecher, G. R., and Matthews, R. H. (1990). Nutrient composition of foods. In *Present Knowledge in Nutrition* (M. Brown, ed.), 6th ed., pp. 430–439. International Life Science Institute-Nutritional Foundation, Washington, DC.

Table 19-2.   Core foods for the vitamins

Vitamin A	Vitamin D	Vitamin E	Vitamin K
As retinol:	Milk[a]	Vegetable oils	Broccoli
Milk (breast, animal[a])	Ghee		Asparagus
Butter, ghee, margarine[a]	Margarine[a]		Lettuce
Liver	Cheese		Cauliflower
Eggs	Chicken (skin)		Cabbage
Small fish (eaten whole)	Liver		Brussels sprouts
As carotene:	Fatty fish (cod, herring)		Turnip greens
Red palm oil	Cod liver oil		Liver
Dark/medium-green leaves (spinach, kale, amaranthus, beans, cassava, cowpea, sweet potato)	Egg yolk		Spinach
Yellow/orange vegetables (carrot, pumpkin, sweet potato, cassava)			
Yellow/orange fruits (mango, pawpaw)			
Yellow maize			

Vitamin C	Thiamin	Riboflavin	Niacin
Tomatoes	Meats	Eggs	Meats
Potatoes	Potatoes	Liver	Eggs
Peppers	Liver	Meats	Fish
Pumpkins	Whole grains	Some fish	Whole grains
Citrus fruits (oranges)	Some fish	Asparagus	Legumes
Other fruits (guavas, berries, plantains, bananas)	Legumes	Milk	Milk
Yams	Oilseeds	Whole grains	Liver
Cassava	Milk	Green leaves	Peanuts
Milk (breast, animal)	Eggs	Legumes	

Vitamin B$_6$	Biotin	Pantothenic acid	Folate	Vitamin B$_{12}$
Meats	Liver	Liver	Tomatoes	Liver
Cabbage	Egg yolk	Milk	Beets	Fish
Potatoes	Cauliflower	Meats	Potatoes	Eggs
Liver	Kidney	Eggs	Wheat germ	Milk
Beans	Peanuts	Fish	Cabbage	
Whole grains	Soybeans	Whole grains	Eggs	
Peanuts	Wheat germ	Legumes	Meats	
Soybeans	Oatmeal		Spinach	
Some fish	Carrots		Asparagus	
Milk			Liver, kidney	
			Beans	
			Peanuts	
			Whole grains	
			Milk	

[a]The high vitamin content is due to fortification.

contribute significantly to the total intake of each particular vitamin, by virtue both of the frequency and the amount of the food consumed as well as the probable concentration of the vitamin in that food. Identifying such **core foods** is difficult because both the voluntary intakes of foods by free-living people and the concentrations of vitamins in those foods are extremely difficult to estimate quantitatively with acceptable certainty. Nevertheless, attempts to do that have indicated a manageable number of core foods for each of the vitamins. For example, for Americans it has been estimated that 80% of the total intakes of several vitamins are provided by 50 to 200 foods.[12]

II. Vitamin Contents of Feedstuffs

Vitamins in Feedstuffs

Several feedstuffs commonly used in the formulation of livestock diets contain nutritionally significant concentrations of vitamins (Table 19-3). However, a core feedstuffs concept (analogous to the core food concept) for vitamins is less useful in the practice of animal nutrition than it is in human nutrition because, unlike the ways in which people are fed or chose to feed themselves, the economic considerations in feeding livestock generally dictate the use of a relatively small number of feedstuffs with few (if any) day-to-day changes in diet formulation.[13] In livestock production, the continued use of the same or very similar diets has resulted in the empirical development of knowledge about the vitamin contents of feedstuffs.

III. Predicting Vitamin Contents

Sources of Inaccuracy

The availability of data for the vitamin contents of foods and feedstuffs can be extremely useful in making judgments concerning the adequacy of food supplies and feedstuff inventories; however, estimates of the nutrient intakes of individuals as determined on the basis of these data are seldom accurate, owing to the variety of factors that may alter the nutrient composition of a food or feedstuff before it is actually ingested. The errors associated with such estimates are particularly great for vitamins.

The sources of error in estimating vitamins in foods and feedstuffs are as follows:

- *Analytical errors*   Errors in the sampling of and actual analysis of foods and feedstuffs for vitamins can be an important contributor to the inaccuracy of predicted values.[14] Analytical errors are less likely to be problematic for vitamin E, thiamin, riboflavin, niacin, and pyridoxine, for which robust analytical techniques (i.e., not prone to analyst effects) are available.

- *Natural variation in vitamin contents*   The concentrations of vitamins in individual foods and feedstuffs can vary widely. The vitamin contents of materials of animal origin can be affected by the conditions imposed in feeding the source animal, which can be highly variable according to country of origin, season of the year, size of the farm, age at slaughter, the composition of the diets used, and so on. For example, the vitamin E content of poultry meat is greater from chickens fed supplements of the vitamin than from those that are not.[15]

- *Genetic sources of variation*   For foods and feedstuffs of plant origin, vitamin contents may vary among different cultivars of the same species (Fig. 19-1) and according to local agronomic factors and weather conditions that affect growth rate and yield (Table 19-4A and B). Between-cultivar differences of as much as several orders of magnitude have been reported for most vitamins. In some cases, these differences correspond to other, readily identified characteristics of the plant. For example, the ascorbic acid contents of lettuce, cabbage, and asparagus tend to be relatively high

---

[12] Using data from the 1976 Nationwide Food Consumption Survey and the Continuing Survey of Food Intakes by Individuals, USDA nutritionists have estimated that, on a national basis, Americans obtain 80% of their total intakes of the following vitamins from the following numbers of foods: vitamin A, 60; vitamin E, 100; thiamin, 168; riboflavin, 165; niacin, 159; pyridoxine, 175; folate, 129; vitamin B$_{12}$, 58.

[13] For example, starting broiler chicks are typically fed the same diet from hatching to 3 weeks of age, and laying hens in some management systems may be fed the same diet for 20 weeks before the formula is changed.

[14] For this reason, most nutrient analytical methods have been standardized by the Association of Official Analytical Chemists.

[15] A practical example of this comparison is the intensively managed commercial poultry flock fed formulated feeds in the United States versus the small courtyard flock largely subsisting on table scraps, insects, and grasses in China and much of the developing world.

Table 19-3. Feedstuffs containing significant amounts of vitamins

Vitamin A	Vitamin D	Vitamin E
None[a]	None[a]	Dehydrated alfalfa meal
		Sun-cured alfalfa meal
		Wheat germ meal
		Corn germ meal
		Stabilized vegetable oils

Vitamin K	Vitamin C	Thiamin
Dehydrated alfalfa meal	None[a,b]	None[a]
Sun-cured alfalfa meal		

Riboflavin	Niacin	Vitamin B_6
Dried skim milk	Barley	Sunflower seed meal
Peanut meal	Cottonseed meal	Sesame meal
Brewers' yeast	Dried fish solubles	Meat and bone meal
Dried buttermilk	Rice bran, polishings	
Dried whey	Wheat bran	
Torula yeast	Corn gluten feed	
Corn distillers' solubles	Fish meals	
Liver and glandular meal	Peanut meal	
	Torula yeast	
	Corn gluten meal	
	Corn distillers' solubles	
	Liver and glandular meal	
	Sunflower seed meal	
	Brewers' yeast	

Biotin	Pantothenic acid	Folate
Corn germ meal	Molasses	Dried brewers' grains
Brewers' yeast	Rice polishings	Dehydrated alfalfa meal
Molasses	Sunflower seed meal	Brewers' yeast
Torula yeast	Peanut meal	Soybean meal
Hydrolyzed feathers	Torula yeast	Torula yeast
Safflower meal	Liver and glandular meal	Meat and bone meal
	Brewers' yeast	Corn distillers' solubles
		Sun-cured alfalfa meal

Vitamin B_{12}	Choline	
Dried fish solubles	Liver and glandular meal	
Liver and glandular meal	Dried fish solubles	
Hydrolyzed feathers	Soybean meal	
Fish meals	Corn distillers' solubles	
Crab meal		
Dried skim milk		
Dried butter milk		
Meat and bone meal		

[a]Instability of the vitamin in most feedstuffs renders few, if any, predictable sources of appreciable amounts of it.
[b]Not required by livestock species.

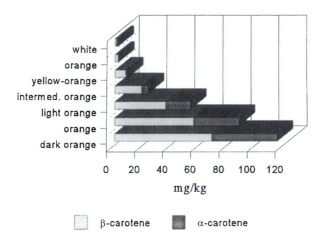

white
orange
yellow-orange
intermed. orange
light orange
orange
dark orange

0   20   40   60   80   100   120

mg/kg

▨ β-carotene   ▉ α-carotene

Fig. 19-1. Variation in carotene contents among carrot cultivars. (*From* Leferriere, W., and Gabelman, F. S. [1968]. *Proc. Am. Soc. Hortic. Sci.* **93,** 408–416.)

in the colored and darker green varieties, and darker orange varieties of carrot tend to have greater pro-vitamin A contents than do lighter-colored carrots. However, vitamin contents are not necessarily related to such physical traits or to each other.

The substantial variation in reported values for vitamins in many plant foods suggests that it may be possible to breed plants for higher vitamin contents. This notion is not new; however, contents of vitamins or other micronutrients have yet to be widely included in the breeding strategies of plant breeders, whose efforts are driven primarily by agronomic issues and considerations of consumer acceptance (i.e., market demand). Unfortunately, many of the latter considerations, notably appearance and "freshness," have little relation to vitamin content. In a world where greater access to vitamin A would be important to some 250 million children who are at risk of that deficiency, and where greater access to ascorbic acid would reduce the anemia that affects 4 of every 10 women, the possibility of improving the vitamin and other micronutrient contents of plants (particularly the staples that feed the poor) through genetic modification cannot be ignored. Even in the industrialized world, where diet-related chronic diseases are growing problems, underexploited opportunities exist to develop vitamin/mineral-rich fruits and

vegetables and to use these aspects of specific, good nutrition as marketing "hooks."

- *Environmental effects* For many plants, growing conditions that favor the production of lush vegetation will result in increased concentrations of several vitamins. Such environmental factors as day length, light intensity and quality, and temperature strongly affect the concentrations of vitamins, especially carotenes and ascorbic acid. Tomatoes, for example, show very strong effects of light, with shaded fruits having less ascorbic acid than those exposed to light.[16] Low temperatures have been shown to increase the ascorbic acid contents of beans and potatoes, the thiamin contents of broccoli and cabbage, the riboflavin contents of spinach, wheat, broccoli, and cabbage, and the niacin contents of spinach and wheat. However, low temperatures decrease thiamin in beans and tomatoes, riboflavin in beans, niacin in tomatoes, and carotenoids in carrots, sweet potatoes, and papayas. Conditions at harvest can also affect the vitamin content of some crops; for example, the vitamin E content of fungus-infected corn grain can be less than half that of nonblighted corn. Legumes such as alfalfa and soybeans contain the enzyme lipoxygenase, which, if not inactivated (by drying) soon after harvest, catalyzes lipid oxidation reactions, resulting in massive destruction of carotenoids and vitamin E. Accordingly, the vitamin contents of plant foods can be markedly different in different parts of the world and can show marked seasonal and annual changes. These fluctuations can be as great as 8-fold for the α-tocopherol content of alfalfa hay within a single season and 11-fold for the ascorbic acid content of apples produced in different years.

- *Effects of agronomic practices* Soil and crop management practices can affect the vitamin contents of edible plant tissues. These relationships are extremely complex, varying according to the soil type, plant species, and vitamin in question. In general, mineral fertilization can increase plant contents of ascorbic acid (P, K, Mn, B, Mo, Cu, Zn, Co),

---

[16] This effect has been documented in response to a cloudy day and to the difference between exposed and shaded sides of the same fruit.

Table 19-4A. Fold variations in reported vitamin contents of fruit and vegetable cultivars: β-carotene, ascorbic acid, α-tocopherol, thiamin, and riboflavin

Plant	β-Carotene	Ascorbic acid	α-Tocopherol	Thiamin	Riboflavin
Apple		29		3.0	10
Apricot	2.9			1.5	1.3
Banana		9			
Barley				2.3	
Bean	2.3	2.9		2.7	3.7
Blueberry	17	3.0		1.3	1.8
Cabbage		3.8		2.5	2.8
Carrot	80	1.4		6.9	5.5
Cassava	113	1.9			
Cauliflower		1.7		1.4	1.4
Cherry	3.5	4.2		2.0	1.5
Collard	1.4	1.6			2.1
Cowpea				2.9	3.0
Grape		3.0		7.5	3.4
Grapefruit	9.3	1.3			
Guava		11			
Lemon		1.2			
Maize	24		2.0	1.8	
Mango	3.8	91			2.0
Muskmelon		20			
Nectarine	4.8	4.7		1.0	1.3
Oat				1.8	
Orange	6.8	1.5			
Palm, oil	5.1				
Papaya	5.7	2.7		1.3	1.5
Pea	4.3	3.4		5.2	1.7
Peach	6.0	4.2		2.0	1.7
Peanut				1.4	1.9
Pear		16		7.0	5.0
Pepper, green	1.3	1.8	18		
Pepper, chili	46	10			
Plum	3.2	1.5			1.2
Potato		5.1		2.5	6.2
Rapeseed, oil			3.4		
Raspberry		2.3			
Soybean		2.4	1.2		
Spinach		1.6			
Squash					
Summer		9.4			
Winter		3.5			
Strawberry		4.3			

Table 19-4A. Fold variations in reported vitamin contents of fruit and vegetable cultivars: β-carotene, ascorbic acid, α-tocopherol, thiamin, and riboflavin—Cont'd

Plant	β-Carotene	Ascorbic acid	α-Tocopherol	Thiamin	Riboflavin
Sunflower			2.7		
Sweet potato	89	3.1		2.9	3.1
Taro		3.2		4.9	2.5
Tomato	20	15		1.6	
Turnip, greens		1.1			
Watermelon	15				
Wheat			29	7.9	5.2
Yam		1.9		3.0	3.9

Source: Mozafar, A. (1994). *Plant Vitamins: Agronomic, Physiological and Nutritional Aspects*, pp. 43–87. CRC Press, Boca Raton, Fl.

Table 19-4B. Fold variations in reported vitamin contents of fruit and vegetable cultivars: niacin, pyridoxine, biotin, pantothenic acid, and folate

Plant	Niacin	Pyridoxine	Biotin	Pantothenic acid	Folate
Apple	2.0		1.1	4.0	
Apricot	1.3				
Avocado	1.5	1.6		13	
Barley	1.1			1.2	
Bean	3.8	2.2			4.6
Blueberry	1.7				
Cherry	1.5				
Cowpea	2.2	1.5	1.5	1.3	
Grape	2.4				
Maize	5.5			1.3	
Mango	18				
Nectarine	1.3				
Oat	1.4				
Papaya	2.3				
Pea	1.2	1.3			2.2
Peach	1.2				
Peanut	1.5				
Pear	4.0		1.1	2.5	
Pepper, green	1.2				
Plum	4.5				
Potato	2.7	3.2			
Rye	1.3				
Strawberry	1.3				
Sweet potato	3.4			2.2	
Taro	4.9				
Wheat	5.0	8.6		2.6	
Yam	2.7				

Source: Mozafar, A. (1994). *Plant Vitamins: Agronomic, Physiological and Nutritional Aspects*, pp. 43–87. CRC Press, New York.

carotenes (N, Mg, Mn, Cu, Zn, B), thiamin (N, P, B), and riboflavin (N). However, nitrogen fertilization tends to decrease ascorbic acid concentrations despite increased yields. Organic fertilizers appear to increase the concentrations of some vitamins, in particular thiamin and vitamin B_{12}. Some of these effects may be due to the lower nitrate contents in organic fertilizers compared with inorganic ones; but organic fertilizers tend also to contain those vitamins that plant roots have recently been found able to absorb.

Practices that affect light exposure and plant growth rate can also affect plant vitamin contents. For example, ascorbic acid, the biosynthesis of which is related to plant carbohydrate metabolism, has been shown to be greater in field-grown versus greenhouse-grown tomatoes;[17] in peas, grapes, and tomatoes grown at lower planting densities; in lower yielding or smaller apples; and in field-ripened versus artificially ripened[18] apples.

- *Tissue variation*   Another source of variation in food vitamin contents comes from the fact that most vitamins are not distributed uniformly among the various edible tissues of plants (Figs. 19-2, 19-3, and 19-4). In fact, the gradients of several nutrients are found in plants, corresponding to the anatomical distribution of the phloem and xylem vascular network. Thus, relatively higher concentrations have been observed for ascorbic acid in the stem end of oranges and pears, the top ends of pineapples, the apical ends of potatoes, the tuber end of sweet potatoes, both the lower and upper portions of carrots, the top ends of turnips, and the stem tips of asparagus, bamboo shoots, and cucumbers. In general, exposed tissues (i.e., skin/peel and outer leaves) tend to contain greater concentrations of vitamins, particularly ascorbic acid, which is largely distributed in chloroplasts in tissues exposed to light.[19] In cereal grains, thiamin and niacin tend to be concentrated in tissues[20] that are removed in milling; therefore, breads made

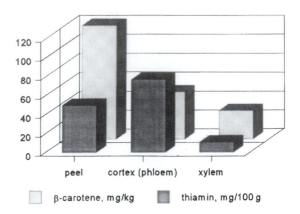

β-carotene, mg/kg   thiamin, mg/100 g

Fig. 19-2.   Tissue distribution of vitamins in carrots. (*From* Yamaguchi et al. [1952]. *Proc. Am. Soc. Hortic. Sci.* **60,** 351–358.)

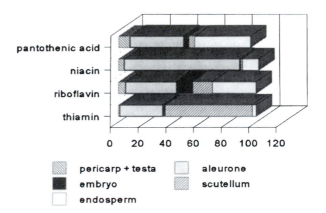

pericarp + testa   aleurone

embryo   scutellum

endosperm

Fig. 19-3.   Tissue distribution of vitamins in wheat. (*From* Hinto et al. [1953]. *Nature* (London) **173,** 993–997.)

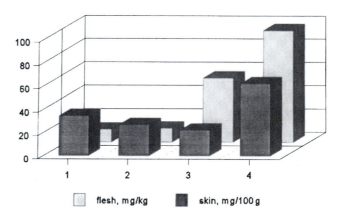

flesh, mg/kg   skin, mg/100 g

Fig. 19-4.   Tissue distribution of ascorbic acid in four apple cultivars. (*From* Gross, E. [1943]. *Garterbauwissenschaften* **17,** 500–507.)

---

[17] This difference can be as great as twofold.

[18] By exposure to ethylene either in storage or in transit to market.

[19] As much as 35–40% of the ascorbic acid in green plants may be present in chloroplasts, where its concentration can be as great as 50 m*M.* In the case of citrus fruits, three-quarters of the ascorbic acid is located in the peel.

[20] That is, the scutellum and aleurone layer.

from refined wheat flour tend to be much lower in those vitamins than are products made from maize, which is not milled. Mobilization of seed vitamin stores and, in some cases, biosynthesis of vitamins occur during germination such that young seedlings (sprouts) tend to have relatively high vitamin contents.

Potential of Biotechnology to Increase Vitamin Contents of Foods

Agricultural biotechnologies can increase the available vitamin contents of foods. Increasing vitamin content has not been an explicit goal in crop improvement, which has centered on economically important traits such those related to yield and disease resistance. However, the "hidden hunger" of micronutrient malnutrition, wihch emerged in the wake of remarkable increases in staple grain productivity due to the concerted plant breeding efforts of the "green revolution," drew attention to the needs for vitamin A, iron, iodine, and other micronutrients that are limiting in the diets of the poor of many countries. Consequently, the international agricultural biotechnology community has responded, demonstrating the potential for increasing vitamin contents of food using both traditional plant breeding techniques and those of genetic engineering.

- *Plant breeding*   Many crops show variations in vitamin contents of their edible tissues. Such variation between plants offers the possibility of breeding for increased amounts. An example is the case of maize (corn), various lines of which

vary from nondetectable to very large amounts of carotenoids, including those that can yield vitamin A metabolically (Table 19-5).

- *Genetic engineering*   That genetic engineering can be used to increase the vitamin contents of foods was demonstrated by Potrynkus and colleagues, who succeeded in producing a transgenic rice capable of biosynthesizing vitamin A.[21] This work, which spanned a decade and cost some $100 million, involved the introduction of the entire β-carotene biosynthetic pathway into rice endosperm, using genes from daffodil (*Narcissus pseudonarcissus*) and a bacterium (*Erwina uredovora*). The result is a line of rice that contains an appreciable amount of β-carotene, which they named *Golden*Rice™ (Table 19-6). It has been noted that *Golden*Rice™ does not contain enough provitamin A activity to have a major impact on prevalent vitamin A deficiency in poor, rice-eating countries.[22] However, its real value resides in its proof of the concept that vitamin contents of staple foods can be increased through genetic technologies.

Accommodating Variation in Vitamin Contents of Foods and Feedstuffs

To accommodate these sources of potential error, estimates of the vitamin contents of foods and feedstuffs have generally been made by analyzing multiple representative samples of each material. For the nutrient contents of feedstuffs it is a common practice to discount the average analytical value by 10–25% as a hedge against overestimating nutrient content. For

Table 19-5. Variation in carotenoid contents of lines of maize (corn)

Line	Carotenoid concentrations, µg/g				
	β-Carotene	**α-Carotene**	**Lutein**	**Zeaxanthin**	**β-Cryptoxanthin**
White	0.05 ± 0.002	Not detected	0.10 ± 0.01	0.09 ± 0.01	Not detected
Yellow	0.77 ± 0.14	0.44 ± 0.04	16.8 ± 0.6	5.4 ± 0.5	2.6 ± 0.4
Orange	5.6 ± 0.1	0.58 ± 0.02	15.7 ± 0.3	11.6 ± 0.03	5.4 ± 0.0
Dark orange	13.9 ± 0.7	1.53 ± 0.04	19.1 ± 4.5	11.8 ± 0.7	5.3 ± 0.7

Source: Howe, J. and Tanumihardjo, S.A. (2006). *J. Nutr.* **136**, 2562–2567.

---

[21] Ye et al. (2000). *Science* **287**, 303–305.

[22] Accounting for degradation (25%) during storage, *Golden*Rice™ should provide some 18% of the RDA for a 4-year-old child, an important increment.

Table 19-6. Use of recombinant DNA technologies to produce provitamin A containing rice

Line	β-Carotene content, (μg/g)
Normal rice	Not detected
GoldenRice™[a]	1.6

[a]Ye et al. (2000). *Science* **287,** 303–305.

both foods and feedstuffs, nutrient content databases typically include only a single value, the mean of all analyses, without indicating the variance around that mean. The practical necessity of using databases so constructed means that the nutritionist is faced with the dilemma of estimating vitamin intake through the use of data that are likely to be inaccurate to an uncertain and unascertainable degree. Thus, if an average value of 150 mg/kg is used to represent the ascorbic acid concentration of potatoes, as is frequently the case, then it must be recognized that half of all samples will exceed that value (thus yielding an underestimate), while half will contain less than that value (thus, yielding an overestimate). In constructing databases for use in meal planning or feed formulation, a better way to accommodate such natural variation is to enter into the database values discounted by a multiple of the standard deviation that would yield an acceptably low probability of overestimating actual nutrient amounts.[23] That approach, however, requires a fairly extensive body of data from which to generate mean-ingful estimates of variance. Few, if any sets of food/feedstuff vitamin composition data are that extensive.

IV. Vitamin Bioavailability

Bioavailability

Apart from considerations of analytical accuracy and natural variation associated with estimates of the vitamin contents of foods and feedstuffs, chemical analyses of vitamin contents may not provide useful information regarding the amounts of vitamin that are biologically available (Table 19-7). The concept of **bioavailability** (see Chapter 3) relates to the proportion of an ingested nutrient that is absorbed, retained, and metabolized through normal pathways to exert normal physiological function. Many vitamins can be present in foods and feedstuffs in forms that are not readily absorbed by humans or animals. The chemical analyses of such vitamins will yield measures of the total vitamin contents, which will be overestimates of the biologically relevant amounts. In the cases of niacin, biotin, pyridoxine, vitamin B_{12}, and choline, which in certain foods and feedstuffs can be poorly utilized, only the biologically available amounts have nutritional relevance. For those in particular, it would be useful to have methods for assessing vitamin bioavailability. An *in vitro* method has been developed to measure niacin bioavailability;[24] but for most vitamins bioavailability must be determined experimentally using appropriate animal models.

Table 19-7. Foods and feedstuffs with low vitamin bioavailabilities

Vitamin	Form	Food/feedstuff
Vitamin A	Provitamins A	Corn
Vitamin E	Nontocopherols	Corn oil, soybean oil
Ascorbic acid	Ascorbinogen	Cabbage
Niacin	Niacytin	Corn, potatoes, rice, sorghum grain, wheat
Pyridoxine	Pyridoxine 5′-β-glucoside	Corn, rice bran, unpolished rice, peanuts, soybeans, soybean meal, wheat bran, whole wheat
Biotin	Biocytin	Barley, fish meal, oats, sorghum grain, wheat
Choline	Phospholipids	Soybean meal

---

[23] This approach was originated in the 1950s by G. F. Combs, Sr. (the author's father) at the University of Maryland when he developed the Maryland Feed Composition Table. The data included in that table were based on replicate analyses from multiple samples of each feedstuff and were expressed as the mean –0.9 SD units. That adjustment was selected to allow a likelihood of overestimating actual nutrient concentration of $p = 0.20$, a level that was acceptable in his judgment.

[24] This method, developed by Prof. Kenneth Carpenter, involves the comparison of the amounts of niacin determined chemically before (free niacin) and after (total niacin) alkaline hydrolysis. The free niacin thus determined correlates with the available niacin determined using the growth response of niacin-deficient rats fed a low-tyrosine diet.

Vitamin bioavailabilities can be affected by several extrinsic and intrinsic factors:

- *Extrinsic factors*
  - *Concentration*—effects on solubility and absorption kinetics
  - *Physical form*—effects of physical interactions with other food components and/or of coatings, emulsifiers, etc., vitamin supplements
  - *Food/diet composition*—effects on intestinal transit time, digestion, vitamin emulsification, vitamin absorption, and/or intestinal microflora
  - *Nonfood agonists*—cholestyramine, alcohol, and other drugs that may impair vitamin absorption or metabolism
- *Intrinsic factors*
  - *Age*—age-related differences in gastrointestinal function
  - *Health status*—effects on gastrointestinal function

V. Vitamin Losses

The vitamins contained in foods can be lost in several ways (Table 19-8).

- *Storage losses*   The storage of untreated foods can result in considerable losses due to postharvest oxidation and enzymatic decomposition. The ascorbic acid contents of cold-stored apples and potatoes can drop by two-thirds and one-third, respectively, within 1–2 months. Those of some green vegetables can drop to 20–78% of original levels after a few days of storage at room temperature. Such losses can vary according to specific techniques of food processing and preservation.
- *Losses in milling grain*   The milling of grain to produce flour involves the removal of large amounts of the bran and germ portions of the native product. Because those portions are typically rich in vitamin E and many of the water-soluble vitamins, highly refined flours[25] are low in these vitamins (Figs. 19-5 and 19-6).
- *Losses in thermal processing*   Vitamins are subjected to destructive forces during thermal processing in the preservation of foods. *Blanching*, which is a mild heat treatment used to inactivate potentially deleterious enzymes, reduce microbial numbers, and decrease interstitial

Table 19-8.   Effects of food preservation techniques on vitamin contents of foods

Technique	Main effects	Vitamins destroyed[a]
Blanching	Partial removal of oxygen	Vitamin C (10–60%)[b,c]
	Partial heat inactivation of enzymes	Thiamin (2–30%), riboflavin (5–40%), niacin (15–50%), carotene (<5%)[c]
Pasteurization	Removal of oxygen[d]	Thiamin (10–15%)
	Inactivation of enzymes	Minor losses (1–5%) of niacin, vitamin B$_6$, riboflavin, and pantothenic acid
Canning	Exclusion of oxygen	Highly variable losses[e,f]
Freezing[g]	Inhibition of enzyme activity[h]	Very slight losses of most vitamins
Frozen storage[g]		Substantial losses of vitamin C and pantothenic acid; moderate losses of thiamin and riboflavin
Freeze drying	Removal of water	Very slight losses of most vitamins
Hot air drying	Removal of water	10–15% losses of vitamin C and thiamin
γ Irradiation	Inactivation of enzymes	Some losses (about 10%) of vitamins C, E, K, and thiamin

[a]Actual losses are variable, depending on exact conditions of time, temperature, etc.
[b]Loss of vitamin C is due to both oxidation and leaching.
[c]Losses of oxidizable vitamins can be reduced by rapid cooling after blanching.
[d]Vitamin losses are usually small, owing to the exclusion of oxygen during this process.
[e]Losses in addition to those associated with heat sterilization before canning.
[f]For example, 15% loss of vitamin C after 2 years at 10°C.
[g]Thawing losses are associated with vitamin leaching into the syrup.
[h]While enzymatic decomposition is completely inhibited in frozen vegetables, reactivation occurs during thawing such that significant vitamin losses can occur. This is avoided by rapidly blanching before freezing.

[25] Such flours consist mainly of the starchy endosperm.

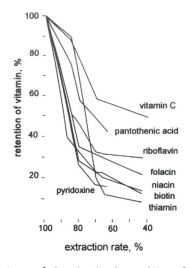

Fig. 19-5. Loss of vitamins in the making of flour. (*From* Moran, T. [1959]. *Nutr. Abstr. Rev.* **29,** 1.)

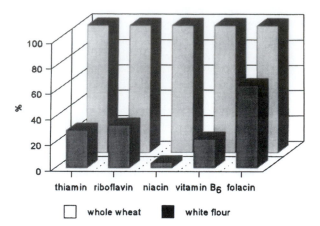

Fig. 19-6. Vitamin contents of whole wheat versus white flour.

gases, usually is minimally destructive, although it can result in the leaching of water-soluble vitamins from foods blanched in hot water. Otherwise, blanching usually improves vitamin stability. In contrast, canning and other forms of high-temperature treatment can accelerate reactions of vitamin degradation, depending on the chemical nature of the food (i.e., its pH, dissolved oxygen and moisture contents, presence of transition metals and/or other reactive compounds) (Table 19-9). Canning can, therefore, result in major losses of vitamins.

- *Other processing losses*   Freezing and drying usually result in only minor losses of most vitamins. Losses associated with ionizing (γ) irradiation vary according to the energy dose but are generally low (less than 10%).
- *Cooking losses*   Cooking can introduce further losses of vitamins from native food materials. However, methods used for cooking vary widely between different cultures and among different individuals, making vitamin losses associated with cooking highly variable. The washing of vegetables in water before cooking can result in the extraction of water-soluble vitamins,

Table 19-9.   Typical losses of vitamins through canning

Food	Vitamin A	Vitamin C	Thiamin	Riboflavin	Niacin	Vitamin B_6	Biotin	Pantothenic acid	Folate
Asparagus	43	54	67	55	47	64	0		75
Lima bean	55	76	83	67	64	47		72	62
Green bean	52	79	62	64	40	50		60	57
Beet	50	70	67	60	75	9		33	80
Carrot	9	75	67	60	33	80	40	54	59
Corn	32	58	80	58	47	0	63	59	72
Mushroom		33	80	46	52		54	54	84
Green pea	30	67	74	64	69	69	78	80	59
Spinach	32	72	80	50	50	75	67	78	35
Tomato	0	26	17	25	0		55	30	54

Source: Lund, D. (1988). "Nutritional Evaluation of Food Processing" (E. Karmas and R. S. Harris, eds.), 3rd ed., pp. 319–354. Van Nostrand Reinhold, New York.

particularly if they are soaked for long periods of time. The peeling of vegetables can remove vitamins associated with the outer tissues.[26] Vitamin losses associated with cooking processes are also highly variable but generally amount to about 50% for the less stable vitamins. The greatest losses are associated with long cooking times under conditions of exposure to air. Vitamin losses are less when food is cooked rapidly, as in a pressure cooker or a microwave oven, or by high-temperature stir frying. The baking of bread can reduce the thiamin content of flour by about 25% without affecting its contents of niacin or riboflavin.

handling foods through each of these steps is so great that the only way to estimate vitamin intakes of people is to analyze the vitamin contents of foods as they are eaten.

Vitamin losses from foods can be minimized by:

- Using fresh food instead of stored food
- Using minimum amounts of water in food preparation and cooking
- Using minimum cooking (where necessary, using high temperatures for short periods of time)
- Avoiding the storage of cooked food before it is eaten

Cumulative Losses of Vitamins from Foods

The losses of vitamins from foods are cumulative. Every step in the postharvest storage, processing, and cooking of a food can contribute to the loss of its vitamin contents (Table 19-10). In theory, these losses can be modeled and thus predicted. However, in practice, the variation in the actual conditions of

VI. Vitamin Supplementation and Fortification of Foods

Availability of Purified Vitamins

All of the vitamins are produced commercially in pure forms. Most are produced by chemical synthesis, but some are also isolated from natural sources

Table 19-10. General stabilities of vitamins to food processing and cooking

Vitamin	Conditions that enhance loss
Vitamin A	Highly variable but significant losses during storage and preparation
Vitamin D	(Stable to normal household procedures)
Vitamin E	Frying can result in losses of 70–90%; bleaching of flour destroys 100%; other losses in preparation or baking are small
Vitamin K	(Losses not significant due to synthesis by intestinal microflora)
Vitamin C	Readily lost by oxidation and/or extraction in many steps of food preparation, heat sterilization, drying, and cooking
Thiamin	Readily lost by leaching, by removal of thiamin-rich fractions from native foods (e.g., flour milling) and by heating; losses as great as 75% may occur in meats, and 25–33% in breads
Riboflavin	Readily lost on exposure to light (90% in milk exposed to sunlight for 2 hr, 30% from milk exposed to room light for 1 day), but very stable when stored in dark; small losses (12–25%) on heating during cooking
Niacin	Leached during blanching of vegetables ($\leq$40%), but very stable to cooking
Pyridoxine	Leached during food preparation; pasteurization causes losses of 67%; roasting of beef causes losses of about 50%
Biotin	(Apparently very stable; limited data)
Pantothenic acid	Losses of 60% by milling of flour and of about 30% by cooking of meat; small losses in vegetable preparation
Folate	(Data not available)
Vitamin B$_{12}$	Only small losses on irradiation of milk by visible or ultraviolet light

---

[26] For example, the peeling of potatoes can substantially reduce the ascorbic acid content of that food.

(e.g., the fat-soluble vitamins)[27] and some are produced microbiologically (e.g., thiamin, riboflavin, folate, pyridoxine, biotin, pantothenic acid, and vitamin B_{12}[28]). Before their commercial synthesis became feasible, which began only in the 1940s, vitamins were extracted from such natural sources as fish oils and rose hip syrup. Today, the production of vitamins is based predominantly on their chemical synthesis and/or microbiological production, the latter having been greatly impacted by the emergence of new techniques in biotechnology.[29] With the notable exception of the tocopherols,[30] there is no basis to the notion that biopotencies of vitamins prepared by chemical/microbiological synthesis are at least as great as those of vitamins isolated from natural sources. In some cases, synthetic vitamins may be appreciably more bioavailable than the vitamin from natural sources (e.g., purified niacin versus protein-bound niacytin; purified biotin versus protein-bound biocytin).

The use of purified vitamins offers obvious advantages for purposes of ensuring vitamin potency in a wide variety of formulated products, including fortificants and additives for foods and feeds, nutritional supplements, pharmaceuticals, and ingredients in cosmetics. The annual world production of vitamins is estimated to exceed 20,000 metric tons.[31] Vitamins are produced by at least 30 firms in some 17 countries; but 6 companies[32] presently dominate the world market.

Addition of Vitamins to Foods

The addition of vitamins to certain foods is a common practice in most countries. In some cases, vitamins are added to selected, widely used foods (e.g., bread,[33] milk,[34] margarine[34]) for the purpose of ensuring vitamin adequacy of populations; this is called *fortification*.[35] In other cases, vitamins are added to restore the vitamin content to that originally present before processing (*revitaminization*, e.g., white flour), to increase the amounts of vitamins already present (*enrichment*), or to make foods carriers of vitamins not normally present (*vitaminization*, e.g., many breakfast cereals). Vitamins are also added to a variety of formula foods: infant formulas, liquid nutrient supplements, enteral formulas used for tube feeding, and parenteral formulas used for intravenous feeding.

In the United States, the addition of nutrients to foods is regulated by the Food and Drug Administration (FDA), which has identified as candidates for addition to foods 22 nutrients including 12 vitamins (Table 19-11).[36] Since 1966 the USDA and USAID[37] have also routinely fortified or enriched foods provided as foreign aid under Public Law 480 (Table 19-12).[38] In addition, many antixerophthalmia programs have used vitamin A fortification of such foods as dried milk, wheat flour, sugar, tea, margarine, and MSG.[39]

---

[27] Examples include the following: vitamin A from fish liver, vitamin D_3 from liver oil or irradiated yeast, vitamin E from soybean or corn oils, and vitamin K from fish meal.

[28] The commercial production of vitamin B_{12} is strictly from microorganisms.

[29] The industrial production of the vitamins has been nicely reviewed: O'Leary, M. J. (1993). Industrial production, in *The Technology of Vitamins in Food* (P. B. Ottaway, ed.), pp. 63–89. Chapman & Hall, London.

[30] There is evidence that several vitamers E produced by chemical synthesis vary in biopotency (see Chapters 3 and 7). This is due to both the positions and numbers of their ring-methyl groups, the most biopotent being the trimethylated (α) form, as well as the stereochemical form of the isoprenoid side chain. The most potent vitamer is the one that occurs naturally, *RRR*-α-tocopherol.

[31] The growth of commercial vitamin production has been steady since the discovery of vitamin B_{12}. For example, in 1950 annual world vitamin production was estimated to be only 1567 metric tons.

[32] BASF, Daiichi, Hoffmann-La Roche, Merck, Rhône-Poulenc, and Takeda.

[33] In the United States, thiamin, riboflavin, niacin, and iron are added to white flour.

[34] In most Western countries, both vitamin A and vitamin D are added.

[35] The term *fortification* has come to be used to describe all types of additions of vitamins to foods.

[36] In addition to these vitamins, the following nutrients are approved: protein, calcium, phosphorus, magnesium, potassium, manganese, iron, copper, zinc, and iodine.

[37] United States Agency for International Development.

[38] The cost of this fortification is very low relative to the total value of the commodities. In 1993, the U.S. government provided through its P.L. 480 programs a total of 7.78 million metric tons of food assistance valued at $2.28 billion. The ingredients (vitamins and minerals) used to enrich the processed and soy-fortified commodities cost less than 2.5% of the value of the product; those used to enrich the more expensive blended food supplements cost less than 5% of the product value.

[39] That is, monosodium glutamate, used as a seasoning.

Table 19-11. Vitamins approved by the FDA for addition to foods

Vitamin	Recommended level of addition (per 100 kcal)
Vitamin A	250 IU
Vitamin D	20 IU
Vitamin E	1.5 IU
Vitamin C	3 mg
Thiamin	75 μg
Riboflavin	85 μg
Niacin	1.0 mg
Vitamin B$_6$	0.1 mg
Biotin	15 μg
Pantothenic acid	0.5 mg
Folate[a]	20 μg
Vitamin B$_{12}$	0.3 μg

[a]Effective 1998, the FDA required adding 140 μg/100 g of most enriched flour, breads, corn meals, rice, noodles, macaroni, and other grain products.

Stabilities of Vitamins in Fortified Foods

The stabilities and bioavailabilities of vitamins added to foods depend on the form of vitamin used, the composition of the food to which it is added, and the absorption status of the individual ingesting that food. The less stable vitamins can be lost from foods during storage, depending on the conditions (time, temperature, and moisture) of that storage (Fig. 19-7).

The chemical stabilities of some vitamins can be improved by using a more stable chemical form or formulation. For example, the calcium salt of pantothenic acid is more stable than the free acid form, and esters of vitamins A and E (retinyl acetate, tocopheryl acetate) are much more resistant to oxidation

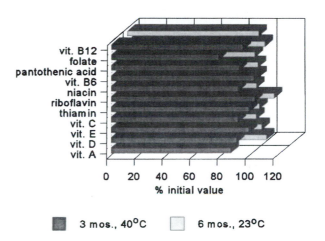

Fig. 19-7. Stabilities of vitamins added to a breakfast cereal. (*From* Anderson et al. [1976]. *Food Technol.* **30,** 110–114.)

Table 19-12. Vitamins added to P.L. 480 Title II commodities

Vitamin	Amount added per 100 g[a]				
	Processed blended foods		Soy-fortified cereals	Nonfat dry milk	Others
	Wheat–soy	Corn–soy			
Vitamin A (IU)	2314	2314	2204–2645	5000–7000	2204–2645
Vitamin D (IU)	198	198			
Vitamin E[b] (IU)	7.5	7.5			
Vitamin C (mg)	40.1	40.1			
Thiamin[c] (mg)	0.28	0.28	0.44–0.66		0.44–0.66
Riboflavin (mg)	0.39	0.39	0.26–0.40		0.26–0.40
Niacin (mg)	5.9	5.9	3.5–5.3		3.5–5.3
Pyridoxine[d] (mg)	0.165	0.165			
Pantothenic acid (mg)	2.75	2.75			
Folate (μg)	198	198			
Vitamin B$_{12}$ (μg)	3.97	3.97			

[a]The processed blended foods are also fortified with calcium, phosphorus, iron, zinc, iodine, and sodium; the soy-fortified cereals and other processed foods are fortified with calcium and iron.
[b]Added as all-*rac*-α-tocopheryl acetate.
[c]Added as thiamin mononitrate.
[d]Added as pyridoxine hydrochloride.

than the free alcohol forms. Vitamin preparations can also be coated or encapsulated[40] in ways that exclude oxygen and/or moisture, thus rendering them more stable. They are often spray-dried, spray-congealed, or prepared as adsorbates to improve their handling characteristics. Owing to such approaches, purified vitamins added to foods have been found to be as stable and bioavailable, if not more so, than the forms of the vitamins intrinsic to foods.

Efficacy of Vitamin Fortification

Fortified foods constitute important sources of vitamins for millions of people. Fortification of wheat flour with niacin was the basis for eliminating pellagra in the United States (Fig. 19-8). Today, fortified cereals and dairy products provide the average American 2–3 μg of vitamin D each day—nearly a third of total vitamin D intakes.[41] Other foods, such as orange juice, are now also being fortified with vitamin D. Countries with prevalent vitamin A deficiency have investigated the utility of vitamin A fortification. Guatemala instituted the fortification of table sugar with vitamin A (15 μg/g) in the 1970s;

the practice reduced the incidence of vitamin A deficiency among preschool children by an estimated 50%. Vitamin A-fortification of other foods, including table salt, monosodium glutamate, fish sauce, instant noodles, cereal grains, tea, and yogurt, have also proven efficacious to varying degrees. The folate status of Americans has been significantly increased through the mandatory fortification of cereal products instituted in 1996. This program, designed to increase folate intakes by an average of 100 μg/person/day, appears to have resulted in increases of twice that target, so that the folate intakes of most Americans meet or exceed the adult RDA (400 μg/day) (Fig. 19-9).

VII. Vitamins in Human Diets

Foods of both plant and animal origin provide vitamins in mixed diets for humans (Table 19-13; Fig. 19-10):[42]

- *Meats and meat products*   Generally excellent sources of thiamin, riboflavin, niacin, pyridoxine, and vitamin B_{12}. Liver (including that from poultry or fish) is a very good source of vitamins

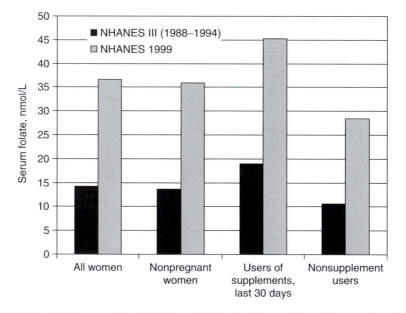

Fig. 19-8. Efficacy of niacin-fortification on pellagra incidence in the United States. (*After* Miller, D. F. [1978]. *Food Prod. Dev.* **12,** 30–37.)

---

[40] Gelatin, edible fats, starches, and sugars are used for this purpose.

[41] Calvo et al. (2004). *Am. J. Clin. Nutr.* **80,** 1710S–1716S.

[42] Variations on the pyramid approach have been produced. These include a modified food guide pyramid for lactovegetarians and vegans (Venti, C. A., and Johnson, C. A. [2002]. *J. Nutr.* **132,** 1050–1054); a Mediterrean diet temple food guide. (Fidanza, F., and Alberti, A. [2005]. *Nutr. Today* **40,** 71–78); a Brazilian food pyramid (Philippi, S. T. [2005]. *Nutr. Today* **40,** 79–83); and the Harvard healthy eating guide (Willett, W. C. [2005]. *Eat, Drink, and Be Healthy*, Simon & Schuster, New York, 299 pp.

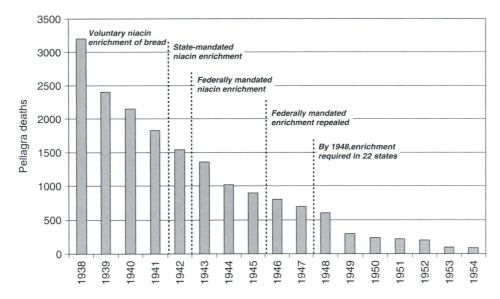

Fig. 19-9.   Efficacy of folate fortification in the United States. (*After* Bailey, L. B. [2004]. *Nutr. Rev.* **62**, S14–S20.)

A, D, E, and B$_{12}$, as well as folacin. Egg is a good source of biotin. Animal products, however, are generally not good sources of vitamin C or K (the exception being pork liver) or folate.

- *Beans, peas, and lentils*   Generally good sources of thiamin, riboflavin, niacin, vitamin B$_6$, biotin, pantothenic acid, and folate.
- *Milk products*   Important sources of vitamins A and C, thiamin, riboflavin,[43] pyridoxine, and

vitamin B$_{12}$. Because milk is widely enriched with irradiated ergosterol (vitamin D$_2$), it is also an important source of vitamin D.[44]

- *Vegetables*   Generally good sources of vitamins A, K, and C, and pyridoxine.
- *Fruits*   Generally good sources of vitamin C; some (e.g., mangoes) are also good sources of vitamin A grain products; generally good sources of thiamin, riboflavin, and niacin.

Table 19-13.   Percentage of vitamins provided by major food groups in western-type diets

Food	Vitamin A	Vitamin C	Thiamin	Riboflavin	Niacin	Vitamin B$_6$	Vitamin B$_{12}$
Vegetables	39.4	51.8	11.7	6.9	12.0	22.2	—
Legumes	—	—	5.4	—	8.2	5.4	—
Fruits	8.0	39.0	4.4	2.2	2.5	8.2	—
Grain products	—	—	41.2	22.1	27.4	10.2	1.6
Meats	22.5	2.0	27.1	22.2	45.0	40.0	69.2
Milk products	13.2	3.7	8.1	39.1	1.4	11.6	20.7
Eggs	5.8	—	2.0	4.9	—	2.1	8.5
Fats and oils	8.2	—	—	—	—	—	—
Other	2.7	3.4	—	—	3.3	—	—

Source: Sauberlich, H. E., Kretsch, M. J., Johnson, M. L., and Nelson, R. A. (1982). In *Animal Products in Human Nutrition* (D. C. Beitz and R. G. Hansen, eds.), p. 339. Academic Press, New York.

---

[43] In the United States, milk products supply an estimated 40% of the required riboflavin.
[44] This practice has practically eliminated rickets in countries that use it.

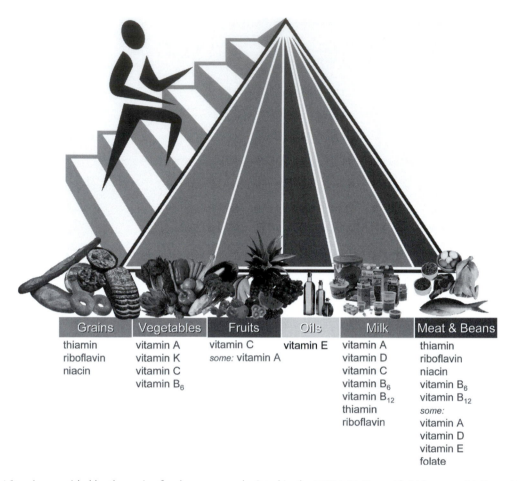

Fig. 19-10. Vitamins provided by the major food groups, as depicted in the USDA MyPyramid. (*After* www.MyPyramid.gov).

Vitamins in Breast Milk and Formula Foods

The vitamin contents of foods that are intended for use as the main or sole components of diets (e.g., human milk, infant formulas, parenteral feeding solutions) are particularly important determinants of the vitamin status of individuals consuming them. Studies of the vitamin contents of human milk have yielded variable results, particularly for the fat-soluble vitamins. In general, it has been observed that the concentrations of all vitamins (except vitamin B_{12}) in human milk tend to increase during lactation. In comparison with cow's milk, human milk contains more of vitamins A, E, C, and niacin, but less vitamin K, thiamin, riboflavin, and pyridoxine (Table 19-14).

Because infant formulas and parenteral feeding solutions are carefully prepared and quality-controlled products, each is formulated largely from purified or partially refined ingredients to contain known amounts of the vitamins. For parenteral feeding

Table 19-14. Vitamin contents of human and cow's milk

Vitamin	Human milk	Cow's milk
Vitamin A (retinol) (mg/liter)	0.60	0.31
Vitamin D_3 (μg/liter)	0.3	0.2
Vitamin E (mg/liter)	3.5	0.9
Vitamin K (mg/liter)	0.15	0.6
Ascorbic acid (mg/liter)	38	20
Thiamin (mg/liter)	0.16	0.40
Riboflavin (mg/liter)	0.30	1.90
Niacin (mg/liter)	2.3	0.8
Pyridoxine (mg/liter)	0.06	0.40
Biotin (μg/liter)	7.6	20
Pantothenic acid (mg/liter)	0.26	0.36
Folate (mg/liter)	0.05	0.05
Vitamin B_{12} (g/liter)	<0.1	3

Source: Porter, J. W. G. (1978). *Proc. Nutr. Soc.* **37**, 225.

solutions, however, some problems related to vitamin nutrition have occurred. One problem involved biotin, which was not added to such solutions before 1981 in the belief that intestinal synthesis of the vitamin was adequate for all patients except children with inborn metabolic errors or individuals ingesting large amounts of raw egg white. When it was found that children supported by total parenteral nutrition (TPN) frequently suffered from gastrointestinal abnormalities that responded to biotin,[45] the vitamin was added to TPN solutions.[46] Another problem with parenteral feeding solutions has been the loss of fat-soluble vitamins and riboflavin either by absorption to the plastic bags and tubing most frequently used, or by decomposition on exposure to light. Such effects can reduce the delivery of vitamins A, D, and E to the patient by two-thirds and to result in the loss of one-third of the riboflavin.

VIII. Vitamin Supplements

A common sight on the shelves of American supermarkets, grocery, drug, and health food stores is the wide variety of individual and multivitamin supplements that is available. Many multivitamin preparations also contain trace minerals. The use of vitamin supplements among peoples in developed countries is great enough to make this means a significant contributor to the vitamin nutriture of those populations. Several surveys have found that about half of the U.S. population takes oral vitamin supplements at least occasionally, and that about one-quarter do so daily.[47] Whether individuals take vitamin supplements appears to be affected by strong socioeconomic influences. For example, results of the 1987 U.S. National Health Interview Survey indicated that vitamin supplement use was greatest among individuals who believe that diet affects disease (vs. those who do not), nondrinkers and lighter drinkers of alcohol (vs. heavy drinkers), former smokers and individuals who never smoked (vs. current smokers), and individuals in the lowest three quartiles of body mass index (kg/m^2). Vitamin supplement use appears to be higher in certain subgroups (Table 19-15), for example, health professionals, vegetarians, the elderly, and readers of health-focused magazines. The median levels of supplement use by Americans are one to two times the RDAs for vitamins A, D, and B_6, niacin, pantothenic acid, and folate, and greater than

Table 19-15. Prevalence of vitamin supplement use by Americans

| Population | Percentage who are daily users of supplements | | | | |
	Any	Multitype	Vitamin A	Vitamin C	Vitamin E
Total	23.2	17.4	1.2	7.6	4.1
Sex					
Men	19.2	14.9	1.2	6.9	3.6
Women	26.8[a]	15.6	1.3	8.3[a]	4.6[a]
Race					
White	24.8[a]	18.5[a]	1.3	4.5[a]	7.1[a]
Black	15.9	12.2	4.5[a]	2.4	1.7
Hispanic	18.6	14.0	5.5	3.0	3.3[a]
Other	17.2	13.5	5.8	2.1	5.0[a]

[a]Significantly differen t from rate of lowest percentile group.
Source: Subar, A. F., and Block, G. (1990). *Am. J. Epidemiol.* **132,** 1091-1101.

---

[45] These patients appeared to have had altered gut microflora secondary to antibiotic treatment.

[46] Although there are no recommended dietary allowances (RDAs) for biotin, it has been suggested that biotin supplements be given to individuals being fed parenterally (infants, 30 μg/kg/day; adults, 5 μg/kg/day). These levels are consistent with the adequate intakes (infants, 5–6 μg/day; children, 8–25 μg/day; adults, 30 μg/day) of the Food Nutrition Board of the Institute of Medicine (1998).

[47] The prevalence of daily vitamin supplement use has been estimated at 21.4% [National Health and Examination Survey (NHANES), 1971–1974], 22.8% (NHANES-II, 1976–1980), 39.9% (FDA, 1983), 36.4% [National Health Interview Survey (NHIS), 1986], and 23.1 (NHIS, 1987).

Table 19-16. Average daily intakes of vitamin supplements by Americans

Vitamin	Total population, percentile			Daily supplement users, percentile			
	50th	75th	90th	25th	50th	75th	90th
Vitamin A (IU)	0	2,466	5,000	1,699	5,000	5,000	10,010
Vitamin D (IU)	0	148	400	136	395	400	400
Vitamin E (IU)	0	20	30	12	30	30	230
Vitamin C (mg)	0	60	368	39	60	307	629
Thiamin/riboflavin (mg)	0	0.8	1.5	0.6	1.5	1.5	7.6

Source: Subar, A. F., and Block, G. (1990). *Am. J. Epidemiol.* **132,** 1091–1101.

twice the RDAs for vitamins E, C, and B_{12}, thiamin, and riboflavin (Tables 19-16 and 19-17).

Studies have shown that nutritional supplement users tend to be more health conscious and have better diets, more education, and higher incomes than the general population. Many consumers report concern over the vitamin adequacy of their diets; most report concern for their health/wellness and that of their families. Two-thirds of American consumers consider nutritional supplements as helpful in preventing or treating such ailments as cancer, memory deficits, lack of energy, osteoporosis, colds and flu, arthritis, depression, stress, heartburn, high cholesterol level, and hypertension.

The most popular vitamin supplements purchased by American consumers are vitamins E and C; antioxidant mixtures containing both of those vitamins;[48] folic acid; and vitamin B complex containing folic acid and vitamins B_6 and B_{12}. The combined retail sales of vitamin and mineral supplements in the United States is estimated to be about $3 billion, some 40% of which is composed of multivitamin sales. Drug stores, supermarkets, and health food stores account for most (over 70%) of these sales. In the United States dietary supplements are regulated by the FDA under the Dietary Supplement Health and Education Act of 1994.[49]

Efficacy of Vitamin Supplements

Some studies have shown benefits of vitamin supplementation in populations with access to diverse diets. Folate supplements were shown to reduce the risk of hip fractures;[50] vitamin D supplements were found to increase the efficacy of supplemental calcium in reducing risk to nonvertebral fractures;[51] and a multivitamin supplement was found to protect against wasting in HIV-infected women.[52] Nevertheless, most randomized, controlled trials with vitamins A, C, E, B_6, and B_{12}, and folate have not shown consistent efficacy in reducing cardiovascular risk[53] or progression of atherosclerosis.[54] Furthermore, it has been suggested that intervention with vitamin E may actually increase all-cause mortality,[55] and an intervention with β-carotene increased lung cancer incidence in male smokers.[56]

---

[48] Such antioxidant mixtures typically also contain β-carotene and selenium.

[49] This legislation charges the FDA to establish a framework for assuring safety, outline guidelines for literature displayed where supplements are sold, provide for use of claims and nutritional support statements, require ingredient and nutritional labeling, and establish good manufacturing practice regulations. The law changes previous legislation in that dietary supplements are no longer subject to the premarket safety evaluations required of other food ingredients.

[50] Sato et al. (2005). *J. Am. Med. Assoc.* **293,** 1082–1088.

[51] Bischoff-Ferrari et al. (2005). *J. Am. Med. Assoc.* **293,** 2257–2264.

[52] Villamor et al. (2005). *Am. J. Clin. Nutr.* **82,** 857–865.

[53] Morris, C. D., and Carson, S. (2003). *Ann. Intern. Med.* **139,** 56–70; Davey-Smith, G., and Ebrahim, S. (2005). *Lancet* **366,** 1679–1681; Barclay, L., and Vega, C. (2006). www.medscape.com/viewarticle/527591 (accessed July 20, 2006).

[54] Bleys et al. (2006). *Am. J. Clin. Nutr.* **84,** 880–887.

[55] Miller et al. (2005). *Ann. Intern. Med.* **142,** 37–46.

[56] Albanes et al. (1996). *J. Nat. Cancer Inst.* **88,** 1560–1570.

Table 19-17. Effects of supplement use on vitamin intakes of Americans

Vitamin	Total population		Supplement users	
	Mean	% CV[a]	Mean	% CV[a]
Vitamin A (IU)	7419	67	8673	49
Vitamin C (mg)	277	110	422	84
Thiamin (mg)	7.5	231	13.0	172
Riboflavin (mg)	7.3	220	12.4	168
Niacin (mg)	35.4	98	50.3	84

[a]Coefficient of variation.
Source: Bowering, J., Subar, A. F., and Clancy, K. L. (1988). *Nutr. Res.* **8,** 1073–1077.

Guidelines for the Use of Vitamin Supplements

Healthy individuals can and should obtain adequate amounts of all nutrients, including vitamins, from a well-balanced diet based on a variety of foods of good quality. Such an approach minimizes the risks of deficiencies as well as excesses of all nutrients. It also acknowledges that foods can provide health benefits that have yet to be fully elucidated.

Nevertheless, certain circumstances may warrant the use of vitamin supplements:

- Folate for women who may conceive, are pregnant, or are lactating[57]
- Several vitamins for individuals with very low caloric intakes (such that their consumption of total food is insufficient to provide all nutrients)
- Vitamin B_{12} for vegetarians[58] and all persons over 50
- A single dose of vitamin K for newborn infants to prevent abnormal bleeding
- Certain vitamins for patients with diseases or medications that may interfere with vitamin utilization

For other persons with varied, balanced diets, the actual benefit of taking vitamin supplements is doubtful.

IX. Vitamin Labeling of Foods

Labeling Food Nutrients

The labeling of nutrient contents of foods is a relatively new practice, having been instituted in the United States in 1972. The U.S. regulations were respecified by the **Nutrition Labeling and Education Act (NLEA)** of 1990, the purpose of which was to provide, through a consistent food label format, useful information to consumers about the foods they eat in the context of their daily diets. The nutrition labeling of foods has the potential to influence consumer food use choices to the extent that the label information is accessible and can be acquired, processed, and used (Fig. 19-11).[59]

This U.S. program involves compulsory labeling for most prepared and packaged foods.[60] It

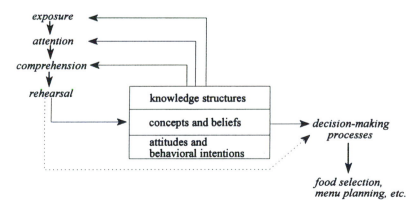

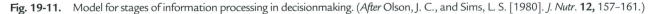

Fig. 19-11. Model for stages of information processing in decisionmaking. (*After* Olson, J. C., and Sims, L. S. [1980]. *J. Nutr.* **12,** 157–161.)

---

[57] Pregnant and lactating women may also need supplements of iron and calcium.

[58] Some vegetarians may also not receive adequate amounts of calcium, iron, and zinc.

[59] It is thought that individuals experience a sequence of interactions with new information before adopting a new behavior.

[60] The act excludes foods containing few nutrients, such as plain coffee, tea, spices; foods produced by small businesses; and foods prepared and served by the same establishment.

encourages voluntary labeling, either for individual products or at the point of purchase, for the most frequently consumed fresh fruits,[61] vegetables,[62] or seafood[63] and at the point of purchase for fresh poultry and meats, and for prepared foods served in restaurants. In addition to information about the name of the product and its manufacturer and the measure/count of food contents, the act requires the food label to carry information about the ingredients, serving size and number of servings, and quantities of specified food components and nutrients (Fig. 19-12). Vitamin and mineral content information must be presented in comparison with a standard, the Reference Daily Intakes (RDIs) (Table 19-18).[64] For the information they present, nutrition labels

Table 19-18. Reference daily intakes used in food labeling[a]

Nutrient	Amount
Protein[a]	50 g
Minerals	
Calcium	1000 mg
Iron	18 mg
Iodine	150 µg
Copper	2 mg
Vitamins	
Vitamin A	5000 IU
Vitamin D	400 IU
Vitamin E	30 IU
Vitamin C	60 mg
Thiamin	1.5 mg
Riboflavin	1.7 mg
Niacin	20 mg
Vitamin B$_6$	2 mg
Pantothenic acid	10 mg
Biotin	300 µg
Folate	400 µg

[a]RDI varies according to target group.

draw on the USDA National Nutrient Data Bank, or an alternative data bank developed by the Produce Marketing Association.

Labeling Vitamins

The NLEA requires that information about vitamin A and vitamin C be carried on all food labels (Fig. 19-12). The law makes optional the disclosure of contents of other nutrients including vitamins for which RDAs have been established. In all cases, information must be presented according to the specified format, known as the Nutrition Facts Label.[65] Other countries have adopted similar food labels (Fig. 19-13).

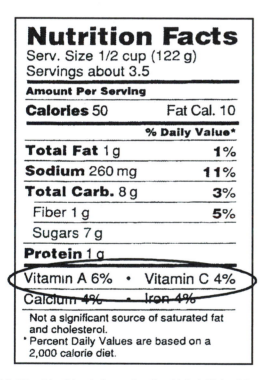

Fig. 19-12. Nutrition information food label, United States.

---

[61] Bananas, apples, watermelons, oranges, cantaloupe, grapes, grapefruits, strawberries, peaches, pears, nectarines, honeydew melons, plums, avocados, lemons, pineapples, tangerines, cherries, kiwi fruits, and limes.

[62] Potatoes, iceberg lettuce, tomatoes, onions, carrots, celery, corn, broccoli, cucumbers, bell peppers, leaf lettuce, sweet potatoes, mushrooms, green onions, green beans, summer squash, and asparagus.

[63] Shrimp, cod, pollack, catfish, scallops, salmon, flounder, sole, oysters, orange roughy, mackerel, ocean perch, rockfish, whiting, clams, haddock, blue crabs, rainbow trout, halibut, and lobster.

[64] RDI values are based on the respective Recommended Dietary Allowances (RDAs) and are compared to Daily Reference Values (DRVs). The RDIs replaced (largely in name only) the U.S. RDA values, which are based on the 1968 RDAs, used before 1990. Most labels use the RDIs developed for adults and children 4 years of age or older; foods targeted to a certain age group must use the RDI developed for that group.

[65] A good overview of the U.S. Nutrition Food Label is available at the U.S. Food and Drug Administration Center for Food Safety and Applied Nutrition Web site: http://www.cfsan.fda.gov/~dms/foodlab.html

```
INGREDIENTS: WHOLE WHEAT,
WHEAT BRAN, SUGAR, SALT, MALT,
THIAMIN HYDROCHLORIDE,
PYRIDOXINE HYDROCHLORIDE,
FOLIC ACID, REDUCED IRON, BHT.

         NUTRITION INFORMATION
                  PER 30 g
             SERVING CEREAL
             (175 mL, ¾ CUP)

ENERGY            Cal     100
                  kJ      420
PROTEIN           g       3.0
FAT               g       0.6
CARBOHYDRATE              24.0
SUGARS            g       4.4
STARCH            g       16.6
FIBRE             g       3.0
SODIUM            mg      265
POTASSIUM         mg      168

          PERCENTAGE OF
           RECOMMENDED
           DAILY INTAKE

THIAMIN           %       46
NIACIN            %       6
VITAMIN B₆        %       10
FOLACIN           %       8
IRON              %       28
```

Fig. 19-13. Nutrition information food label, Canada.

X. Vitamins in Livestock Feeds

Vitamins in Animal Feeds

Unlike human diets, formulated diets for livestock generally do not provide adequate amounts of vitamins unless they are supplemented with either certain vitamin-rich feedstuffs or purified vitamins. In general, the relative vitamin adequacy of unsupplemented animal feeds depends on the relative complexity (the number of feedstuffs used in the mixture) of the diet. The vitamin contents of simple rations tend to be less than those of complex ones (Table 19-20). For example, complex diets such as those used for feeding poultry or swine in the 1950s[66] would be expected to contain in their constituent feedstuffs more than an adequate amount of vitamin B_{12}, and adequate (or nearly so) amounts of vitamin K, vitamin E, thiamin, riboflavin, niacin, pyridoxine,

pantothenic acid, folate, and choline. In contrast, the simpler rations (based almost exclusively on corn and soybean meal) that are used today contain lower amounts, if any, of the more costly vitamin-rich feedstuffs previously used. Such simple rations can be expected to contain in constituent feedstuffs adequate levels only of vitamin E, thiamin, pyridoxine, and biotin. The availability of stable, biologically available, and economical vitamins facilitated this change in complexity of animal feeds by replacing with inexpensive mixtures of vitamins the more costly vitamin-rich feedstuffs used previously.

Losses of Vitamins from Feedstuffs and Finished Feeds

The vitamin contents of feedstuffs and finished feeds[67] are subject to destruction in ways very similar to those of foods (Table 19-19). The storage losses that can occur in particular feedstuffs are dependent on the conditions of temperature and moisture during storage; heat and humidity enhance oxidation reactions of several of the vitamins (vitamins A and E, thiamin, riboflavin, biotin). Vitamin losses are, therefore, minimized by drying feedstuffs quickly and storing them dry in weather-proof bins. Where the drying of a feedstuff is slow[68] or incomplete,[69] or where leaky bins are used for its storage, vitamin losses are greatest.

Table 19-19. Vitamins most likely to be limiting in human diets and nonruminant livestock feeds

Humans	Livestock
Vitamin A	Vitamin A
Vitamin E	Vitamin E
Vitamin C	Niacin
Riboflavin	Riboflavin
Folate	Pantothenic acid
Vitamin D, if house-bound	Vitamin D, if raised indoors
Vitamin B_{12}, if strict vegetarian	Vitamin K, if raised on slatted or raised wire floors
	Vitamin B_{12}, if raised on slatted or raised wire floors
	Choline, chicks only

---

[66] Those complex diets contained, in addition to a major grain and soybean meal, small amounts of the following: alfalfa meal, corn distillers' dried solubles, fish meal, meat, and bone meal.

[67] Complete, blended, ready-to-feed rations.

[68] For example, sun drying enhances the destruction of vitamin E in corn (although sun curing of cut hay is essential to provide vitamin D activity).

[69] Where moisture is not reduced to less than about 15%.

Vitamin losses from finished feeds are usually greater than those of individual feedstuffs. Finished feeds are supplemented with essential trace elements, some of which (Cu^{2+}, Fe^{3+}) can act as catalytic centers of oxidation reactions leading to vitamin destruction. Such effects are particularly important in high-energy feeds (e.g., broiler diets), which generally contain significant amounts of polyunsaturated fats. It is a common practice in many countries to compress many of these (and other) feeds into pellet form[70] by processes involving steam, heat, and pressure. Evidence suggests that pelleting can enhance the bioavailability of niacin and biotin, which occur in feedstuffs in bound forms; but it generally results in the destruction of vitamins A, D, E, K_3, C, and thiamin.

Vitamin Supplements Simplify Feed Formulations

As purified sources of the vitamins have become available at low cost, it has become possible to use fewer feedstuffs in less complicated blends to produce diets of high quality that will support efficient and predictable animal performance (Table 19-20). Thus, many feedstuffs formerly valuable as sources of vitamins (e.g., brewers' yeast, dried buttermilk, *green feeds*[71]) are no longer economical to use in intensive animal management systems.[72]

The use of purified vitamins as supplements to animal feeds has increased the economy of animal feeding by obviating the need to include relatively expensive vitamin-rich feedstuffs in favor of lower-priced feedstuffs that are lower in vitamin content but provide useful energy and protein (Table 19-21). In modern practice, the addition of vitamins to animal feeds is accomplished by preparing a mixture of the specific vitamins required with a suitable carrier[73] to ensure homogeneous distribution in the feed as it is mixed. Such a preparation is referred to as **vitamin premix** (Tables 19-22 and 19-23) and is handled in much the same way as other feedstuffs in the blending of animal feeds. Typically, vitamin premixes are formulated to be blended into diets at rates of 0.5–1.0%.[74]

Premixes generally also contain synthetic antioxidants [e.g., ethoxyquin, butylated hydroxytoluene (BHT)] to enhance vitamin stability during storage.[75] In many cases, trace minerals are included in **vitamin–mineral premixes**.[76] It is standard practice in the formulation of vitamin premixes to use amounts of vitamins that, when added to the expected amounts intrinsic to the component feedstuffs, will provide a comfortable excess above those levels found experimentally to be required to prevent overt deficiency signs. This is done in view of the many potential causes of increased vitamin needs; owing to the low cost of vitamin supplementation, this approach is considered a kind of low-cost[77] nutrition insurance.

---

[70] There are many reasons for pelleting finished feeds. Pelleting prevents demixing of the feed during handling and transit. It can improve the economy of feed handling owing to the associated increase in bulk density. For the same reason, it can improve the consumption of bulky, low-density feeds. It can also improve the efficiency of feed utilization by reducing wastage at the feeder. It is thought that the metabolizable energy values of some feedstuffs may be improved by the steam treatment used in pelleting (e.g., soybean meal with significant residual antitryptic activity). Pelleting also improves the handling of feeds that are very dusty.

[71] For example, fresh cabbage and grass.

[72] This phenomenon is most true in the economically developed parts of the world. In the developing world, such factors as the shortage of hard currency may make purified sources of vitamins too expensive to use in animal diets, thus making natural sources of the vitamins more valuable. Under such circumstances, it is prudent to exploit a wide variety of local feedstuffs, food wastes, and food byproducts in the formulation of animal feeds that are adequate in terms of vitamins as well as all other known nutrients.

[73] Examples include soybean meal, finely ground corn or wheat, corn gluten meal, and wheat middlings.

[74] The cost of the vitamin premix typically represents less than 2% of the total cost of most finished feeds. Of that amount, approximately two-thirds of the vitamin cost is accounted for by vitamin E, niacin, vitamin A, and riboflavin (roughly in that order).

[75] Studies have shown that the loss of vitamin A from poultry feeds stored at moderate temperatures (about 15% in 30 days) was slightly reduced (to about 10%) by the addition of any of several synthetic antioxidants. Under conditions of high temperature and high humidity, vitamin A losses from finished feeds can be much greater (e.g., 80–95%). Maximal protection by antioxidants is expected under conditions in which vitamin oxidation is moderate (e.g., short-term feed storage in hot, humid environments).

[76] Owing to the presence of mineral catalysts in oxidative reactions, the stabilities of oxidant-sensitive vitamins in compound premixes can be expected to be less than in premixes of the vitamins alone.

[77] Vitamin premixes usually account for only 1–2% of the total cost of feeds for nonruminant livestock.

Table 19-20.   Vitamins provided by constituent feedstuffs in two chick starter diets

Ingredient	Percentage in:	
	1936 diet[a] (complex)	Contemporary diet (simple)
Cornmeal	27.5	69.61
Oats	10.0	
Wheat bran	20.0	
Wheat middlings	10.0	
Soybean meal, 49% protein	10.0	19.08
Meat and bone meal	10.0	4.78
Poultry by-product meal		7.00
Dried whey	5.0	
Dehydrated alfalfa meal	5.0	
Blended fat		3.18
Limestone	2.0	
Salt	0.5	0.25
D,L-Methionine (98%)		0.10
Trace minerals	+[b]	+[c]
Vitamins	+[d]	+[e]
Vitamins provided by feedstuffs: per kilogram of diet		
Vitamin A (IU)	6000 (400)[f]	1360 (91)[f,g]
Vitamin E (IU)	27 (270)	20.5 (205)[g]
Vitamin K (mg)	0.73 (146)	0 (0)[g]
Thiamin (mg)	4.7 (261)	3.1 (172)
Riboflavin (mg)	5.4 (150)	2.3 (64)[g]
Niacin (mg)	69.9 (259)	28.3 (105)[g]
Pyridoxine (mg)	5.7 (190)	5.3 (177)
Biotin (g)	208 (139)	141 (94)
Pantothenic acid (mg)	15.7 (157)	7.4 (74)[g]
Folate (mg)	0.81 (145)	0.32 (58)
Vitamin B_{12} (g)	6.5 (72)	21.0 (233)[g]
Choline (mg)	1115 (86)	1395 (107)[g]

[a]This was a state-of-the-art diet for starting chicks at Cornell University in 1942.
[b]$MnSO_4$, 125 mg/kg.
[c]Provides per kilogram of diet: ZnO, 66 mg; $MnSO_4$, 220 mg; Na_2SeO_3, 220 g.
[d]Vitamin D_3, 790 IU/kg.
[e]Provides per kilogram of diet: vitamin A, 4400 IU; vitamin D_3, 2200 IU; vitamin E, 5.5 IU; vitamin K_3, 2 mg; riboflavin, 4 mg; nicotinic acid, 33 mg; pantothenic acid, 11 mg; vitamin B_{12}, 1 g; choline, 220 mg.
[f]Numbers in parentheses give amounts of each vitamin as a percentage of current (1984) recommendations of the U.S. National Research Council.
[g]Included in the vitamin–mineral premix.

Table 19-21. Insufficient amounts of vitamins in turkey starter diet feedstuffs

Vitamin	Level from feedstuffs, NRC requirement %	
	Simple feed[a]	Complex feed[b]
Vitamin A	20	40
Vitamin E	130	130
Thiamin	170	160
Riboflavin	60	90
Niacin	30	60
Vitamin B_6	130	100
Pantothenic acid	90	110
Biotin	120	140
Folate	50	50
Vitamin B_{12}	0	74
Choline	90	100

[a]Corn, 40.5%; soybean meal, 51.2%; animal fat, 4%; $CaHPO_4$, 3%; limestone, 0.8%; salt, 0.3%; methionine, 0.15%; trace minerals, 0.05%.
[b]Milo, 20.5%; wheat, 20%; soybean meal, 33.9%; poultry meal, 6%; animal fat, 5%; meat and bone meal, 5%; fish meal, 4%; alfalfa meal, 2%; distillers' grains and solubles, 2%; limestone, 0.7%; $CaHPO_4$, 0.5%; salt, 0.3%; methionine, 0.13%; trace minerals, 0.05%.
Source: Anonymous. (1989). *Vitamin Nutrition for Poultry*, pp. 13–14. Hoffman-La Roche, Inc., Nutley, NJ.

Table 19-22. Vitamins generally included in vitamin premixes for livestock diets

Vitamin	Poultry	Piglets	Hogs	Calves	Cattle
Vitamin A	+	+	+	+	+
Vitamin D_3	+	+	+	+	+
Vitamin E	+	+	+	+	+[a]
Vitamin K	+	+	+[a]		
Ascorbic acid	+[b]	+		+	
Thiamin		+[a]		+[a]	
Riboflavin		+	+	+	+[a]
Niacin	+	+			
Pyridoxine	+[a]	+	+[a]	+[a]	
Pantothenic acid		+	+	+	+[a]
Biotin	+[a]	+[a]	+[a]		
Folate					
Vitamin B_{12}	+	+		+[a]	
Choline	+	+			

[a]Sometimes added.
[b]Added in situations of stress.

Stabilities of Vitamins in Finished Feeds

It should be remembered, however, that purified vitamins may not always be cheap, particularly in developing countries. Under those circumstances, the appropriate way to assess the value of using vitamin supplements is to compare their market prices with the estimated loss of production realized by not supplementing feeds that can be economically produced using locally available feedstuffs.

Stabilities of Vitamins in Finished Feeds

Vitamins tend to be less stable in vitamin–mineral premixes used for livestock feeds owing to the redox reactions catalyzed by trace elements and physical abrasion of protective coatings (Table 19-24). Vitamin premixes that contain choline chloride typically show accelerated losses of vitamin B_6, which reacts with choline. During the storage of finished feeds, the migration of moisture to the shady, relatively cool side of a feed bin can result in the development of pockets of relatively high moisture, which can both enhance the chemical degradation of vitamins and support the growth of vitamin-consuming fungi. Feeds that are pelleted or extruded are also exposed to friction, pressure, heat, and humidity, all of which enhance vitamin loss.

Table 19-23.   Examples of vitamin premixes for animal feeds

Vitamin	Units/1000 kg diet		
	Practical diet[a] for chicks[c]	**Semipurified diet[b] for chicks[d]**	**Semipurified diet[b] for rats[e]**
Vitamin (IU) A[f]	8,800,000	50,000	40,000,000
Vitamin D_3 (IU)	2,200,000	4,500,000	1,000,000
Vitamin E (IU)[g]	5,500	50,000	50,000
Menadione $NaHSO_3$ (g)	2.2	1.5	50
Thiamin HCl (g)	15	6	
Riboflavin (g)	4.4	15	6
Niacin (g)	33	50	30
Pyridoxine HCl (g)	6	7	
d-Calcium pantothenate (g)	11	20	16
Biotin (mg)	0.6	0.2	
Folic acid (g)	6	2	
Vitamin B_{12} (mg)	10	20	10
Choline chloride (g)	220	2,000	+[h]
Minerals	+[i]	+[j]	+[j]
Other ingredients			
Antioxidant[k] (g)	125	100	100
Carrier (g)	To weight[l]	To weight[m]	To weight[m]

[a]Composed of nonpurified natural feedstuffs (e.g., corn, soybean meal).
[b]Composed of purified/partially purified ingredients (e.g., isolated soy protein, casein, sucrose, starch).
[c]From Scott et al. (1982). *Nutrition of the Chicken*, 3rd ed., p. 494. M. L. Scott and Associates, Ithaca, NY.
[d]Ibid., p. 546.
[e]AIN-76 diet, American Society for Nutritional Sciences (formerly, American Institute of Nutrition).
[f]As all-*trans*-retinyl palmitate.
[g]As all-*rac*-tocopheryl acetate.
[h]Added as 0.2% choline bitartrate.
[i]Includes 66 g of ZnO, 220 g of $MnSO_4$, and 220 mg of Na_2SeO_3.
[j]Includes $CaHPO_4•2H_2O$, $CaCO_3$, KH_2PO_4, $NaHCO_3$, $KHCO_3$, KCl, NaCl, $MnSO_4•H_2O$, $FeSO_4•7H_2O$, $MgCO_3$, $MgSO_4$, KIO_3, $CuO_4•5H_2O$, $ZnCO_3$, $CoCl_2$, $NaMoO_4•2H_2O$, and/or Na_2SeO_3 in amounts appropriate for the composition of the particular diet.
[k]For example, ethoxyquin, BHT.
[l]Corn meal.
[m]Sucrose.

Table 19-24. Typical stabilities of vitamins in a broiler feed

Vitamin	Percentage retention of activity			
	Premix storage (2 months)	Pelleting and conditioning (93°C, 1 min)	Feed storage (2 weeks)	Cumulative retention
Vitamin A[a]	98	90	92	81
Vitamin D$_3$	98	93	93	85
Vitamin E[b]	99	97	98	94
Vitamin K[c]	92	65	85	51
Thiamin[d]	99	89	98	86
Riboflavin	99	89	97	85
Niacin	99	90	93	83
Vitamin B$_6$[e]	99	87	95	82
Biotin	99	89	95	84
Pantothenic acid[f]	99	89	98	86
Folate	99	89	98	86
Vitamin B$_{12}$	100	96	98	86

[a]All-*trans*-retinyl acetate.
[b]All-*rac*-α-tocopheryl acetate.
[c]Menadione sodium bisulfite complex.
[d]Thiamin mononitrate.
[e]Pyridoxine hydrochloride.
[f]Calcium pantothenate.
Source: BASF. (1992). *Keeping Current*. Publication No. 9138. BASF, Ludwigshafen, Germany.

Study Questions and Exercises

1. For a core food for any particular vitamin, construct a flow diagram showing all of the processes, from the growing of the food to the eating of it by a human, that might reduce the useful amount of that vitamin in the food.

2. In consideration of the core foods for the vitamins and your personal food habits, which vitamin(s) might you expect to have the lowest intakes from your diet? Which might you expect to be low in the typical American diet? Which might you expect to be low in vegetarian and low-meat diets?

3. Use a concept map to show the relationships of vitamin supplementation of animal feeds to the concepts of chemical stability, bioavailability, and physiological utilization.

4. Prepare a flow diagram to show the means by which you might first evaluate the dietary vitamin status of a specific population (e.g., in an institutional setting), and then improve it, if necessary.

5. What principles should be used in planning diets to ensure adequacy with respect to the vitamins (and other nutrients)?

Recommended Reading

Ball, G. F. M. (1998). *Bioavailability and Analysis of Vitamins in Foods.* Chapman & Hall, New York, 569 pp.

Beecher, G. R., and Matthews, R. H. (1990). Nutrient composition of foods in *Present Knowledge in Nutrition* (M. Brown, ed.), pp. 430–443. International Life Science Institute-Nutritional Foundation, Washington, DC.

Eitenmiller, R. R., and Landen, W. O., Jr. (1999). *Vitamin Analysis of the Health and Food Sciences.* CRC Press, New York, 518 pp.

Holden, J. M., Harnly, J. M., and Beecher, G. R. (2006). Food Composition, Chapter 57 in *Present Knowledge in Nutrition* 9th ed. (B. A. Bowman and R. M. Russell, eds.), vol. II, pp. 781–794. ILSI Press, Washington, DC.

Mozafar, A. (1994). *Plant Vitamins: Agronomic, Physiological and Nutritional Aspects.* CRC Press, Boca Raton, FL.

Ottaway, P. B. (ed.) (1999). *The Technology of Vitamins in Foods.* Chapman & Hall, London, 270 pp.

Porter, D. V., and Earle, R. O. (eds.). (1990). *Nutrition Labeling: Issues and Directions for the 1990s.* National Academy Press, Washington, DC.

West, C. E., and Poortvliet, E. J. (1993). *The Carotenoid Content of Foods with Special Reference to Developing Countries.* International Science and Technology Institute, Arlington, VA, 210 pp.

Assessing Vitamin Status

20

[T]he old idea, that the state of nutrition of a child could be at once established by mere cursory inspection by the doctor, has to be abandoned.... [Such methods] gave us very little information about the occurrence of the milder degrees of deficiency, or of the earlier stages of their development.

—L. J. Harris

I.	General Aspects of Nutritional Assessment	469
II.	Assessment of Vitamin Status	471
III.	Vitamin Status of Human Populations	474
	Study Questions and Exercises	483
	Recommended Reading	484

Clinical evaluation
Dietary evaluation
Hidden hunger
Nutritional assessment
Sociologic evaluation

Anchoring Concepts

1. Detection of suboptimal vitamin status at early stages (before manifestation of overt deficiency disease) is desirable for the reason that vitamin deficiencies are most easily correctable in their early stages.
2. Vitamin status can be estimated by evaluating diets and food habits, but these methods are not precise.
3. Vitamin status can be determined by measuring the concentrations of vitamins and metabolites, and the activities of vitamin-dependent enzymes, in samples of tissues and urine.
4. Suboptimal status is more probable for some vitamins than for others.

Learning Objectives

1. To understand the requirements of valid methods for assessing vitamin status.
2. To understand the methods available for assessing the vitamin status of humans and animals.
3. To be familiar with available information regarding the vitamin status of human populations.

Vocabulary

Anthropometric evaluation
Biochemical evaluation

I. General Aspects of Nutritional Assessment

Nutritional assessment, in any application, has three general purposes:

- To detect deficiency states.
- To evaluate the nutritional qualities of diets, food habits, and/or food supplies.
- To predict health effects.

The need to understand and describe the health status of individuals, a basic tenet of medicine, spawned the development of methods to assess nutrition status as appreciation grew for the important relationship between nutrition and health. The first applications of nutritional assessment were in investigations of feed-related health and production problems of livestock and, later, in examinations of human populations in developing countries. Activities involving human populations, consisting mainly of organized nutrition surveys, resulted in the first efforts to standardize both the methods employed to collect such data and the ways in which the results are interpreted.[1] More recently,

---

[1] In 1955, the U.S. government organized the Interdepartmental Committee on Nutrition for National Defense (ICNND) to assist developing countries in assessing the nutritional status of their peoples, identifying problems of malnutrition, and developing practical ways of solving their nutrition-related problems. The ICNND teams conducted nutrition surveys in 24 countries. In 1963, the ICNND published the first comprehensive manual [ICNND. (1963). *Manual for Nutrition Surveys*, 2nd ed. U.S. Government Printing Office, Washington, DC] in which analytical methods were described and interpretive guidelines were presented.

nutritional assessment has also become an essential part of the nutritional care of hospitalized patients, and has become an increasingly important means of evaluating the impact of public nutrition intervention programs.

Systems of Nutritional Assessment

Three types of nutritional assessment systems have been employed in both population-based studies and the care of hospitalized patients:

- *Nutrition surveys*   Cross-sectional evaluations of selected population groups; conducted to generate baseline nutritional data, to learn overall nutrition status, and to identify subgroups at nutritional risk
- *Nutrition surveillance*   Continuous monitoring of the nutritional status of selected population groups (e.g., at-risk groups) for an extended period of time; conducted to identify possible causes of malnutrition
- *Nutrition screening*   Comparison of individuals' parameters of nutritional status with predetermined standards; conducted to identify malnourished individuals requiring nutritional intervention

Methods of Nutritional Assessment

Systems of **nutritional assessment** can employ a wide variety of specific methods. In general, however, these methods fall into five categories:

- *Dietary evaluation*   Estimation of nutrient intakes from evaluations of diets, food availability, and food habits (using such instruments as food frequency questionnaires, food recall procedures, diet histories, and food records)

- *Anthropometric evaluation*   Estimation of nutritional status on the basis of measurements of the physical dimensions and gross composition of an individual's body
- *Clinical evaluation*   Estimation of nutritional status on the basis of recording a medical history and conducting a physical examination to detect *signs* (observations made by a qualified observer) and symptoms (manifestations reported by the patient) associated with malnutrition
- *Biochemical evaluation*   Estimation of nutritional status on the basis of measurements of nutrient stores, functional forms, excreted forms, and/or metabolic functions
- *Sociologic evaluation*   Collection of information on nonnutrient-related variables known to affect or be related to nutritional status (e.g., socioeconomic status, food habits and beliefs, food prices and availability, food storage and cooking practices, drinking water quality, immunization records, incidence of low birth weight infants, breastfeeding and weaning practices, age- and cause-specific mortality rates, birth order, family structure).

Typically, nutritional assessment systems employ many or all of these types of methods for the complete evaluation of nutritional status. Some of these approaches, however, are more informative than others with respect to specific nutrients and particularly to early stages of vitamin deficiencies (Table 20-1).

Risk Factors for Vitamin Deficiency

The risk of suboptimal vitamin status is determined largely by factors that limit access to a diet that provides these nutrients and/or limit the body's ability to utilize them on ingestion. Therefore, many factors can

Table 20-1.   Relevance of assessment methods to the stages of vitamin deficiency

	Most informative methods				
Stage of deficiency	Dietary	Biochemical	Anthropometric	Clinical	Sociologic
1. Depletion of vitamin stores	+	+			
2. Cellular metabolic changes		+	+	+	
3. Clinical defects		+	+	+	
4. Morphological changes			+	+	
5. Behavioral					+

affect vitamin adequacy/inadequacy, but several are dominant in determining risk to vitamin deficiency:

- *Monotonous diet*   A diet with little food variety,[2] particularly one based primarily on milled cereal grains
- *Low-caloric intake*   A low intake of total food
- *Enteric malabsorption*   The existence of any acquired or innate problem limiting the absorption of nutrients across the gut
- *Impaired vitamin retention/utilization*   The existence of any acquired or innate problem of hepatic or renal metabolism

II. Assessment of Vitamin Status

Approaches

The assessment of vitamin status is best achieved by the application of biochemical methods, clinical evaluation, and, to a lesser extent, dietary methods. Anthropometric evaluation can be informative regarding energy and protein status, but yields no information relevant to vitamin status. Clinical evaluation can be effective in the diagnosis of late-stage vitamin deficiencies, that is, those involving physiologic dysfunction and/or morphological changes. However, overt vitamin deficiency syndromes are relatively rare compared with the incidence of suboptimal vitamin status, about which clinical evaluation is informative. Diets and food habits that are likely to provide insufficient amounts of available vitamins can be identified by dietary evaluation. However, as discussed in Chapter 19, these methods are almost always imprecise with respect to vitamins, and the parameters they measure usually have greater inherent variability than those for other nutrients. The detection of early-stage vitamin deficiencies is, therefore, best achieved using the various biochemical methods that are available.

Requirements of Useful Biochemical Methods

Many biochemical parameters of vitamin status can be identified. However, in order to be useful for the purposes of assessment of vitamin status, a parameter must satisfy several requirements:

- Correlate with the rate of vitamin intake, at least within the nutritionally significant range, and respond to deprivation of the vitamin.
- Relate to a meaningful period of time.
- Relate to normal physiologic function.
- Be measurable in an accessible specimen.
- Be technically feasible, reproducible, and affordable.
- Have an available base of normative data.

Available Biochemical Methods for Assessing Vitamin Status

The ideal parameter of vitamin status would be a measure of actual metabolic function of the vitamin. In some cases this is possible;[3] however, in most cases, direct measurement of vitamin metabolic function is not possible owing to the absence of a discrete functional parameter,[4] the existence of more than one metabolic function with different sensitivities to vitamin supply,[5] the function of the vitamin in a loosely bound fashion, which is unstable to the methods of tissue preparation,[6] among several reasons. Therefore, other parameters are useful for assessing vitamin status. These include measurements of the vitamin in accessible tissues (Tables 20-2, 20-3, and 20-4) or in urine, certain metabolites, or other enzymes related to the metabolic function of the vitamin.

---

[2] This may include a strict vegetarian diet that does not include some source of vitamin B_{12}.

[3] Examples include the measurement of prothrombin time to assess vitamin K status, and the measurement of stimulation coefficients of erythrocyte transketolase and glutathione reductase to assess thiamin and riboflavin status, respectively.

[4] For example, vitamin E appears to function as a biological lipid antioxidant. Measuring that function, however, is not possible with any physiological relevance because all of the known products of lipid peroxidation (e.g., malonaldehyde, alkanes) are known to be metabolized. This makes such measurements difficult to interpret with respect simply to vitamin E status.

[5] For example, pyridoxal phosphate is a cofactor for each of two enzymes involved in the metabolic conversion of tryptophan to niacin: kynureninase and transaminase. Although the cofactor is essential for the activity of each enzyme, kynureninase has a much greater affinity for pyridoxal phosphate ($K_m = 10^{-3}\ M$) than does the transaminase ($K_m = 10^{-8}\ M$). Therefore, under conditions of pyridoxine deprivation, the transaminase activity can be reduced even though kynureninase activity is unaffected.

[6] For example, the metabolically active forms of niacin, NAD(P)H, function as the cosubstrates of many redox enzymes. These enzyme–cosubstrate complexes are only transiently associated; therefore, dilution of biological specimens results in their dissociation and usually in the oxidation of the cosubstrate.

Table 20-2. Tissues accessible for biochemical assessment of vitamin status

Tissue or cell type	Relevance
Blood	
Plasma/serum	Contains newly absorbed nutrients as well as vitamins being transported to other tissues and, therefore, tends to reflect recent nutrient intake; this effect can be reduced by collecting blood after a fast
Erythrocytes	With a half-life of about 120 days, they tend to reflect chronic nutrient status; analyses can be technically difficult
Leukocytes	Have relatively short half-lives and, therefore, can be used to monitor short-term changes in nutrient status; isolation of these cells can present technical difficulties
Tissue	
Liver, adipose, bone marrow, muscle	Sampling is invasive, requiring research or clinical settings
Hair, nails	Easily collected and stored specimens offer advantages, particularly for population studies of trace element status; not useful for assessing vitamin status

Table 20-3. Limitations of some biochemical methods of assessing vitamin status

Vitamin	Parameter	Limitation(s)
Vitamin A	Plasma[a] retinol	Reflects body vitamin A stores only at severely depleted or excessive levels; confounding effects of protein and zinc deficiencies and renal dysfunction
Vitamin D	Plasma[a] alkaline phosphatase	Affected by other disease states
Vitamin E	Plasma[a] tocopherol	Affected by blood lipid transport capacity
Thiamin	Plasma[a] thiamin	Low sensitivity to changes in thiamin intake
Riboflavin	Plasma[a] riboflavin	Low sensitivity to changes in riboflavin intake
Vitamin B_6	RBC glutamic-pyruvic transaminase	Genetic polymorphism
Folate	RBC folates	Also reduced in vitamin B_{12} deficiency
	Urinary FIGLU[b]	Also increased in vitamin B_{12} deficiency
Vitamin B_{12}	Urinary FIGLU[b]	Also increased in folate deficiency

[a]Or serum.
[b]FIGLU, Formiminoglutamic acid.

Interpreting Results of Biochemical Tests of Vitamin Status

The guidelines originally developed by the ICNND are generally used for interpreting the results of biochemical parameters of vitamin status. It is important to note, however, that those interpretive guidelines were originally developed for use in surveys of populations. Their relevance to the assessment of the vitamin status of individuals is not straightforward, owing to issues of intraindividual variation and confounding effects, which may be quantitatively more significant for individuals than for populations. For example, intraindividual (within-person) variation is frequently noted in serum analytes. Therefore, a measurement of a single blood sample may not be appropriate for estimating the usual circulating level of the analyte of an individual, even though it may be useful in estimating the mean level of a population. Several factors can confound the interpretation of parameters of vitamin status: those affecting the response parameters directly, drugs that can increase vitamin

Table 20-4. Biochemical methods for assessing vitamin status

Vitamin	Functional parameters	Tissue levels	Urinary excretion
Vitamin A		Serum retinol[a]	
		Change in serum retinol with oral vitamin A dose[b]	
		Liver retinyl esters	
Vitamin D		Serum 25-$(OH)_2$-vitamin D_3[a]	
		Serum vitamin D_3	
		Serum 1,25-$(OH)_2$-D_3	
		Serum alkaline phosphatase	
Vitamin E	Erythrocyte hemolysis	Serum tocopherols[a]	
		Serum malondialdehyde	
		Serum 1,4-isoprostanes	
		Breath alkanes	
Vitamin K	Clotting time		
	Prothrombin time[a]		
Vitamin C		Serum ascorbic acid	Ascorbic acid
		Leukocyte ascorbic acid[a]	Ascorbic acid after load[c]
Thiamin	Erythrocyte transketolase stimulation[a]	Blood thiamin	Thiamin (thiochrome)
		Blood pyruvate	Thiamin after load[c]
Niacin		RBC NAD[a]	1-Methylnicotinamide
		RBC NAD:NADP ratio	1-Methyl-6-pyridone-3-carboxamide
		Plasma tryptophan	
Riboflavin	RBC glutathione reductase stimulation[a]	Blood riboflavin	Riboflavin
			Riboflavin after load[c]
Vitamin B_6	RBC transaminase	Plasma pyridoxal phosphate	Xanthurenic acid after tryptophan load[a,c]
		RBC transaminase stimulation	
		RBC pyridoxal phosphate	Quinolinic acid
		Plasma pyridoxal	4-Pyridoxic acid
Biotin		Blood biotin[a]	Biotin
Pantothenic acid	RBC sulfanilamide acetylase	Serum pantothenic acid	Pantothenic acid
		RBC pantothenic acid	
		Blood pantothenic acid[a]	
Folate		Serum folates[a]	FIGLU[c] after histidine load[a,c]
		RBC folates[a]	
		Leukocyte folates	Urocanic acid after histidine load[c]
		Liver folates	
Vitamin B_{12}		Serum vitamin B_{12}[a]	FIGLU[d]
		RBC vitamin B_{12}	Methylmalonic acid[a]

[a]Most useful parameter.
[b]Relative dose–response test.
[c]A single large oral dose.
[d]FIGLU, Formiminoglutamic acid.

needs, seasonal effects related to the physical environment[7] or food availability,[8] use of parenteral feeding solutions,[9] use of vitamin supplements,[10] smoking,[11] and so on (Table 20-5).

III. Vitamin Status of Human Populations

Reserve Capacities of Vitamins

Nutritional status, with respect to the vitamins, refers to the reserve capacity provided by the amounts of vitamins in tissue. The reserve capacities of the vitamins vary; each is affected by the history of vitamin intake, the metabolic needs for the vitamin, and the general health status of the individual. Typical reserve capacities of a healthy, adequately nourished human adult are as follows (these are expressed in terms of time-equivalents based on abilities to meet normal metabolic needs):

- *4–10 days*   Thiamin, biotin, and pantothenic acid
- *2–6 weeks*   Vitamins D, E, K, and C; riboflavin, niacin, and vitamin B_6

Table 20-5. Interpretive guidelines for assessing vitamin status

| Vitamin | Parameter | Age group | Values, by category of status (risk)[a] | | |
			Deficient (high risk)	Low (moderate risk)	Acceptable (low risk)
Vitamin A	Plasma[b] retinol (µg/dl)	<5 months	<10	10–19	>20
		0.5–17 years	<20	20–29	>30
		Adult	<10	10–19	>20
Vitamin D	Plasma[b] 25-(OH)-D_3[c] (ng/ml)	All ages	<3	3–10	>10
	Plasma[b] alkaline phosphatase[c] (U/ml)	Infants	>390	298–390	99–298
		Adults	<40	40–56	57–99
Vitamin E	Plasma[b] α-tocopherol (mg/dl)	All ages	<0.35	0.35–0.80	>0.80
Vitamin K	Clotting time (min)	All ages	>10	About 10	
	Prothrombin time (min)	—[d]	—[d]	—[d]	
Vitamin C	Plasma[b] ascorbic acid (mg/dl)	All ages	<0.20	0.20–0.30	>0.30
	Leukocyte ascorbic acid (mg/dl)	All ages	<8	8–15	>15
	Whole blood ascorbic acid (mg/dl)	All ages	<0.30	0.30–0.50	>0.50
Thiamin	Urinary thiamin (µg/g creatinine)	1–3 years	<120	120–175	>175
		4–6 years	<85	85–120	>120
		7–9 years	<70	70–180	>180

[7] For example, individuals living in northern latitudes typically show peak plasma levels of 25-hydroxyvitamin D_3 (25-OH-D_3) around September and low levels around February, with inverse patterns of plasma parathyroid hormone (PTH) concentrations, owing to the seasonal variation in exposure to solar ultraviolet light.

[8] For example, residents of Finland showed peak plasma ascorbic acid levels in August–September and lowest levels in November–January, owing to seasonal differences in the availability of vitamin C-rich fruits and vegetables.

[9] Individuals supported by total parenteral nutrition (TPN) have frequently been found to be of low status with respect to biotin (owing to their abnormal intestinal microflora) and the fat-soluble vitamins (owing to absorption by the plastic bags and tubing, and to destruction by UV light used to sterilize TPN solutions).

[10] The First National Health and Nutrition Examination Survey (NHANESI) showed that more than 51% of Americans over 18 years of age used vitamin/mineral supplements, with 23.1% doing so on a daily basis. Furthermore, the National Ambulatory Medical Care Survey (1981) showed that 1% of office visits to physicians (in particular, general and family practitioners) involved a prescription or recommendation for multivitamins. Multivitamins appear to be the most commonly used supplements, followed by vitamin C, calcium, vitamin E, and vitamin A. The use of vitamin supplements has been found to have greater impact than that of vitamin-fortified food on both the mean and coefficient of variation (CV) of estimates of vitamin intake in free-living populations.

[11] Smokers have been found to have abnormally low plasma levels of ascorbic acid (with a corresponding increase in dehydroascorbic acid), pyridoxal, and pyridoxal phosphate.

Table 20-5. Interpretive guidelines for assessing vitamin status—Cont'd

Vitamin	Parameter	Age group	Deficient (high risk)	Low (moderate risk)	Acceptable (low risk)
Thiamin —(Cont'd)		10–12 years	<60	60–180	>180
		13–15 years	<50	50–150>150	
		Adults	<27	27–65	>65
		Pregnant			
		Second trimester	<23	23–55	>55
		Third trimester	<21	21–50	>50
	Urinary thiamin				
	μg/24 hr	Adults	<40	40–100	>100
	μg/6 hr	Adults	<10	10–25	>25
	Urinary thiamin after load[e] (μg/4 hr)	Adults	<20	20–80	>80
	RBC transketolase stimulated by TPP[f,g] (%)	Adults	>25	15–25	<15
Riboflavin	Urinary riboflavin (μg/g creatinine)	1–3 years	<150	150–500	>500
		4–6 years	<100	100–300	>300
		7–9 years	<85	85–270	>270
		10–15 years	<70	70–200	>200
		Adults	<27	27–80	>80
		Pregnant			
		Second trimester	<39	39–120	>120
		Third trimester	<30	30–90	>90
	Urinary riboflavin (μg/24 hr)	Adults	<40	40–120	>120
	Urinary riboflavin (μg/6 hr)	Adults	<10	10–30	>30
	Urinary riboflavin load[h] (μg/4 hr)	Adults	<1000	1000–1400	>1400
	RBC riboflavin (μg/day)	Adults	<10.0	10.0–14.9	>14.9
	RBC glutathione reductase FAD stimulation (%)	Adults	>40	20–40	<20
Niacin	Urinary N'-methylnicotinamide μg/g creatinine	Adults	<0.5	0.5–1.6	>1.6
		Pregnant			
		Second trimester	<0.6	0.6–2.0	>2.0
		Third trimester	<0.8	0.8–2.5	>2.5
	μg/6 hr	Adults	<0.2	0.2–0.6	>0.6
	Urinary 2-pyridone[j]:N'-methyl nicotinamide	All ages	—[k]	<1.0	≥1.0
Vitamin B$_6$	Plasma PalP[l] (nM)	All ages	—[k]	<60[m]	≥60[m]
	Urinary vitamin B$_6$ (μg/g creatinine)	1–3 years	—[k]	<90[m]	≥90[m]
		4–6 years	—[k]	<75[m]	≥75[m]
Vitamin B$_6$	Urinary vitamin B$_6$ (μg/g creatinine)	7–9 years	—[k]	<50[m]	≥50[m]
		10–12 years	—[k]	<40[m]	≥40[m]
		13–15 years	—[k]	<30[m]	≥30[m]
		Adults	—[k]	<20[m]	≥20[m]
	Urinary 4-pyridoxic acid (mg/24 hr)	Adults	<0.5[m]	0.5–0.8[m]	>0.8[m]

(Continued)

Table 20-5. Interpretive guidelines for assessing vitamin status—Cont'd

Vitamin	Parameter	Age group	Deficient (high risk)	Low (moderate risk)	Acceptable (low risk)
			Values, by category of status (risk)[a]		
Vitamin B$_6$ —(Cont'd)	Urinary xanthurenic acid after tryptophan load[h] (mg/24 hr)	Adults	>50[m]	25–50[m]	<25[m]
	Urinary 3-OH-kynurenine after tryptophan load[h] (mg/24 hr)	Adults	>50[m]	25–50[m]	<25[m]
	Urinary kynurenine after tryptophan load[h] (mg/24 hr)	Adults	>50[m]	10–50[m]	<10[m]
	Quinolinic acid after tryptophan load[h] (mg/24 hr)	Adults	>50[m]	25–50[m]	<25[m]
	Erythrocyte alanine aminotransferase stimulation by PalP[l] (%)	Adults	—[k]	>25[m]	≤25[m]
	Erythrocyte aspartate aminotransferase stimulation by PalP[l] (%)	Adults	—[k]	>50[m]	≤50[m]
Biotin	Urinary biotin (μg/24 hr)	Adults	<10[m]	10–25[m]	>25[m]
	Whole blood biotin (ng/ml)	Adults	<0.4[m]	0.4–0.8[m]	>0.8[m]
Pantothenic acid	Plasma[b] pantothenic acid (μg/dl)	Adults	—[k]	<6[m]	≥6[m]
	Blood pantothenic acid (μg/dl)	Adults	—[k]	<80[m]	≥80[m,n]
	Urinary pantothenic acid (mg/24 hr)	Adults	—[k]	<1[m]	≥1[m,o]
Folate	Plasma[b] folates (ng/ml)	All ages	<3	3–6	>6
	RBC folates (ng/ml)	All ages	140	140–160	>160
	Leukocyte folates (ng/ml)	All ages	—[k]	<60	>60
	Urinary FIGLU[p] after histidine load[q] (mg/8 hr)	Adults	>50[m]	5–50	<5[r]
Vitamin B$_{12}$	Plasma[b] vitamin B$_{12}$ (pg/ml)	All ages	100	100–150	>150[s]
	Urinary methylmalonic acid after valine load[t] (mg/24 hr)	Adults	≥300	2–300	≤2
	Urinary excretion of a radiolabeled vitamin B$_{12}$ dose after vitamin B$_{12}$ flushing dose[u] (%)	Adults	<3	3–8	>8

[a]*Sources:* ICNND. (1963). *Manual for Nutrition Surveys,* 2nd ed. U.S. Government Printing Office, Washington, DC.; ICNND. (1974). *Laboratory Tests for the Assessment of Nutritional Status.* CRC Press, Cleveland, Ohio; and Gibson, R. S. (1990). *Principles of Nutritional Assessment.* Oxford University Press, New York.

[b]Or serum.

[c]Subject to effects of season and sex.

[d]Results vary according to assay conditions; most assays are designed such that normal prothrombin times are 12–13 sec, with greater values indicating suboptimal vitamin K status.

[e]Single oral 2-mg dose.

[f]TPP, Thiamin pyrophosphate.

[g]The *TPP effect.*

[h]Single oral 2-g dose.

[i]FAD, flavin adenine dinucleotide, reduced form, 1–3 μM.

[j]N′-Methyl-2 pyridone-5-carboxamide.

[k]Database is insufficient to support a guideline.

[l]PalP, Pyridoxal phosphate.

[m]These values have only a small database and, therefore, are considered as tentative.

[n]Normal values are about 100 μg/dl.

[o]Normal values are 2–4 mg/24 hr.

[p]FIGLU, Formiminoglutamic acid.

[q]Single oral 2- to 20-mg dose.

[r]Normal adults excrete 5–20 mg/8 hr.

[s]Most healthy individuals show 200–900 pg/ml.

[t]Single oral 5- to 10-g dose.

[u]This is the Schilling test; it involves measurement of labeled vitamin B$_{12}$ excreted from a 0.5- to 2-μg tracer dose after a large flushing dose (e.g., 1 mg) given 1 hr after the tracer.

- *3–4 months*   Folate
- *1–2 years*   Vitamin A
- *3–5 years*   Vitamin B$_{12}$

Differences in reserve capacities reflect differential abilities to retain and store the vitamins and lead, therefore, to differential sensitivities to vitamin deprivation. For example, individuals with histories of generally adequate vitamin nutriture can be expected to sustain longer periods of deprivation of vitamins A or B$_{12}$ than they could of thiamin, biotin, or pantothenic acid. Similarly, metabolic and physiologic lesions caused by deficiencies of thiamin, biotin, or pantothenic acid can be expected to appear much sooner than those of vitamins A or B$_{12}$, which may remain occult. Because nutritional intervention is typically most efficacious and cost-effective in earlier stages of vitamin deficiencies, the early detection of occult deficiencies is important for designing effective therapy and prophylaxis programs.

National Nutrition Studies

Several national studies have been conducted, mostly in the United States, to evaluate the nutritional adequacy of the food supply and/or the nutritional status of people (Table 20-6). These have included efforts to obtain information on most of the high-risk vitamins (e.g., vitamins A, E, C, B$_6$, and B$_{12}$, thiamin, riboflavin, and niacin).

Apparent Increases in Vitamins in U.S. Food Supply

Historical records of the American food supply would indicate general increases in the amounts of most of the vitamins available for consumption (Table 20-7). Whether such increases have been reflected in the actual intakes of vitamins, or whether they have been distributed democratically across the American population is not indicated by such gross evaluations of the food supply. The results of the 1977–1978 Nationwide Food Consumption Survey indicate that the average consumption of most vitamins was generally adequate, the exception being that of pyridoxine, which was low in most age groups. In general, however, it is clear that people with low incomes tend to consume less food, although their food tends to have greater nutritional value per calorie than that consumed by people with greater incomes. Although differences in diet quality due to income status appear to be small on average, variation in nutrient intake within groups of individuals appears to be very large.

Table 20-6.   National surveys of dietary intake and nutritional status in North America

Survey	Description
USDA historical data on U.S. food supply	Tracking since 1909 of foods available to the American public by disappearance to wholesale and retail markets
U.S. Nationwide Food Consumption Surveys	USDA studies (conducted at about 10-year intervals since 1935) of dietary intakes and food use patterns of American households and individuals
Ten-State Nutrition Survey	NIH study (1968–1970) of nutritional status of >60,000 individuals in 10 U.S. states (California, Kentucky, Louisiana, Maine, Mississippi, South Carolina, Texas, Wisconsin, New York, and West Virginia) selected to include low-income groups
Total Diet Study	FDA study of average intakes of certain essential mineral elements (iodine, iron, sodium, potassium, copper, manganese, zinc), pesticides, toxicants, and radionuclides, based on analyses of foods purchased in grocery stores across the United States
Nutrition Canada	Canadian study conducted in the early 1970s of the nutritional status of >19,000 individuals
National Health and Nutrition Examination Surveys	USDA studies conducted to monitor the overall nutritional status of the U.S. population; four studies to date: NHANESI (1971–1974); NHANESII (1976–1980); Hispanic HANES (HHANES, 1982–1984); NHANESIII (1988–1994)

Table 20-7. Vitamins available for consumption[a] by Americans

Vitamin	1909–1913	1947–1949	1967–1969	1977–1979	1985
Vitamin A (IU)	7200	8100	7300	9100	9900
Vitamin E (mg)[b]	11.2	12.5	14.3	16.0	17.6
Vitamin C (mg)	101	110	98	108	114
Thiamin (mg)	1.6	2.0	2.0	2.1	2.2
Riboflavin (mg)	1.8	2.3	2.3	2.3	2.4
Niacin (mg)	19	20	23	25	26
Vitamin B_6 (mg)	2.2	1.9	1.9	2.0	2.1
Vitamin B_{12} (µg)	7.9	8.6	9.2	9.0	8.8

[a]Per person per day.
[b]α-Tocopherol equivalents.
Source: Marston, R. M., and Raper, K. C. (1987). *Natl. Food Rev.* **36**, 18–23.

On average, at least, the vitamin intake of Americans would appear to be generally adequate (Table 20-8). However, it is clear that substantial variations occur among individuals in the actual intake of several vitamins, owing to both qualitative and quantitative differences in intake. More recent studies by the USDA have shown that the vitamin intakes of many Americans may not meet the Recommended Dietary Allowances (RDAs) (Table 20-9).

Impacts of Trends in Food Intake Patterns

The desire to reduce the number of preventable deaths, particularly to heart disease and cancer, is

Table 20-8. Estimated daily vitamin intakes[a] by Americans of all ages

Vitamin	Vegetarians	Nonvegetarians
Vitamin A	163	132
Vitamin C	176	147
Thiamin	117	113
Riboflavin	136	124
Niacin[b]	114	124
Vitamin B_6	76	75
Vitamin B_{12}	156	176

[a]As a percentage of 1980 RDAs.
[b]Preformed niacin only.
Source: 1977–1978 Nationwide Food Consumption Survey; based on 3-day intakes.

Table 20-9. Frequency of low vitamin intake by American women and children

Vitamin	Percentage with intakes <100% RDA			Percentage with intakes <70% RDA (women)
	Women	Children 1–3 years of age	4–5 years of age	
Vitamin A	55	—	—	35
Vitamin E	70	—	—	40
Vitamin C	45	—	—	30
Vitamin B_6	95	20	55	75
Folate	100	5	60	85

Source: USDA data.

driving efforts to alter American diets. The etiologies of these diseases are now seen as affected by diet. It is estimated that at least a fifth of heart disease and a third of all cancers could be prevented by improving the American diet,[12] specifically by increasing the consumption of fruits and vegetables and reducing intakes of saturated and total fat. The most visible effort of this type has been the 5-A-Day for Better Health Program initiated in 1991 by the U.S. National Cancer Institute with joint support from American food industry groups.[13]

Despite an emerging picture of health benefits of diets richer in fruits and vegetables, surveys have

---

[12] Committee on Diet and Health. (1989). *Diet and Health. Implications for Reducing Chronic Disease Risk*. National Academy of Sciences, Washington, DC.

[13] This program has been implemented at the state level under various names (e.g., 5-A-Day, High Five, Gimme 5).

shown that the regular intake of fruits and vegetables of many Americans continues to fall far short of the 5-A-Day goals (Tables 20-10, 20-11). At the start of the 5-A-Day program, only 23% of American adults were consuming that level of fruits and vegetables,[14] and several groups were found to consume particularly low amounts of these foods: men tended to eat one fewer serving than women (3 versus 3.7 servings per day, respectively); Hispanics ate fewer servings than either whites or blacks (3 versus 3.4 versus 3.4 servings per day, respectively); and younger people ate fewer servings than older people (3 versus 3.4 versus 3.6 versus 4.1 servings per day for 18–34 years, 35–49 years, 50–64 years, and 65+ years, respectively). During the last decade these intakes have increased by nearly 29% for vegetables and 38% for noncitrus fruits.[15] However, the list of most frequently consumed fruits and vegetables continues to be short (Table 20-11), with lowest consumption observed among lower socioeconomic groups and among individuals unaware of the health benefits attached to fruits and vegetables.

It is generally accepted that vegetarian, but not fruitarian, diets can be nutritionally adequate if sensibly selected. It is also clear that problems can

Table 20-11. The 10 fruits and vegetables most frequently consumed by Americans

Fruit/vegetable	Median intake (servings/week)
Green salad	2.0
Orange or grapefruit juice	2.0
Fried potatoes	1.0
Other potatoes	1.0
Beans, peas, or corn	1.0
Tomatoes	1.0
Bananas or plantains	0.8
Apples or applesauce	0.6
Tomato sauce or salsa	0.6
Other fruit juices	0.5

Source: Subar, A. F., Heimendinger, J., Krebbs-Smith, S. M., Patterson, B. H., Kessler, R., and Pironka, E. (1992). *5 A Day for Better Health: A Baseline Study of American's Fruit and Vegetable Consumption.* NCI, Rockville, MD.

arise in any type of diet that restricts the variety of food, particularly the consumption of dairy products. Therefore, important questions must be raised concerning the impacts of an emphasis on fruits and vegetables on vitamin and overall nutrient intakes, particularly in the context of reduced intakes of meats (vitamins A, B_6, and B_{12}, thiamin, and niacin) and replacement of vegetable oils (important sources of vitamin E) with reduced- and no-fat substitutes. Such diet changes may increase intakes of vitamins A and C, but they may also reduce intakes of several of the B vitamins.

Nutritional Assessment Reveals Vitamin Deficiencies

The preceding measures of general nutrient supplies and average nutrient consumption are necessary for national food and health policy planning. At the same time they yield no information useful in addressing questions of the nutritional status of individuals within populations. To produce such data, the Ten-State Nutrition Survey, Nutrition Canada, and HANES were conducted.

Table 20-10. Percentages of New Yorkers eating less than the recommended numbers of servings from major food groups

Recommended servings	Percentage below target
Adults (18–64 years)	
Three vegetables	75
Two fruits	48
Two dairy products	73
Six cereal and grain products	80
Two meats, legumes, eggs	41
Older adults (≤65 years)	
Four vegetables plus fruits	95
Two dairy products	50
Four cereal and grain products	98
Two meat, legumes, eggs	56

Source: Campbell, C. (1992). *New York State Nutrition.* Cornell University, Ithaca, NY.

---

[14] Subar et al. (1992). *5 A Day for Better Health: A Baseline Study of American's Fruit and Vegetable Consumption.* NCI, Rockville, MD.

[15] This may reflect such trends as the emergence of salad bars in restaurants, the development of new varieties, increases in imports, and improvements in consumer selection year-round.

- *The Ten-State Nutrition Survey* Results revealed few severe nutritional deficiencies in its study population. However, it showed that people in the lowest groupings by income and education had poorer nutrition in virtually every respect than those in higher income/education groups. The most frequently observed nutritional problems concerned deficiencies of iron in all age groups (especially among blacks), vitamin A (assessed by serum retinol level) among teenagers and Hispanics of all age groups, and riboflavin, particularly among blacks.

- *Nutrition Canada* Results showed the highest incidence of poor nutritional status among lowest income groups, particularly among middle-aged women and older men. Low-income groups showed the greatest frequencies of low blood levels of ascorbic acid and folates. Low blood thiamin levels were observed among teenagers and middle-aged adults. Obesity was widespread, especially among middle-aged adults.

- *NHANESI* Results revealed deficiencies of protein, calcium, vitamin A (assessed by serum retinol level), and iron, especially among low-income groups and more frequently among blacks than whites. Low vitamin A status was found among low-income white teenagers, young adult women, and teenage blacks of all income groups.

- *NHANESII* Results showed low vitamin A status in 2–3% of all subjects examined. In addition, it revealed low blood thiamin levels in 14% of whites and 29% of blacks, low serum riboflavin levels in 3% of whites and 8% of blacks, and low transferrin saturation in 5–15% of whites and 18–27% of blacks. The apparent consumption of vitamin B_6 was less than the 1980 RDAs for 71% of males and 90% of females. The prevalence of low serum and erythrocyte folate levels was greatest in the 20- to 44-year age group (women, 15 and 13%, respectively; men, 18 and 8%, respectively). The prevalence of low plasma ascorbic acid level

was 3% nationally, but was more common in poor adults, with the greatest prevalence (16%) among 55- to 74-year-old black males.

- *NHANESIII*[16] The results of the third National Health and Nutrition Examination Survey are presented in Tables 20-12A and 20-12B.

International Studies Reveal "Hidden Hunger"

Under the auspices of national programs, bilateral programs, and international agencies, many nutrition surveys have been conducted, particularly in developing countries where problems of malnutrition are of the most severe proportions, to assess the nutritional status of high-risk populations. These have shown that malnutrition continues to affect nearly half of the world's population:[17]

More than 800 million people are estimated not to have access to enough food to meet their basic daily needs. More than one-third of the world's children are stunted,[18] owing to diets inadequate in quantity and quality. Some 2 billion people live at risk of diseases resulting from deficiencies of vitamin A, iodine, and iron; most of them are women and children living in the less-developed countries of sub-Saharan Africa, the eastern Mediterranean, southern and Southeast Asia, Latin America, the Caribbean, and the western Pacific. Nearly 13 million young children died in developing countries in 1993[19]; half are estimated to have died because of malnutrition and its potentiating effects on infectious disease.

It is clear that the view that malnutrition results mainly from insufficient supplies of macronutrients (i.e., energy and protein) has underestimated real problems with deficiencies of critical micronutrients (i.e., vitamins and trace elements), problems now being referred to as **hidden hunger**. At least three micronutrient deficiencies are recognized as being prevalent on a global scale: vitamin A deficiency,

---

[16] The NHANESIII included a representative sample of 40,000 noninstitutionalized people 2 years of age and older. It oversampled children, older adults, black Americans, and Mexican Americans and was also designed as a longitudinal study.

[17] Such widespread malnutrition exists despite impressive gains in global agricultural production. In the last two decades cereal yields have doubled, and per capita supplies of food energy are at all-time high levels—totaling some 15% more than present global needs. However, the newly developed, high-yielding, *green revolution* varieties of major staple grains, being much more profitable than traditional crops (including pulses), have displaced the latter and have led to substantial reductions in the diversity of cropping systems. This appears to have contributed to micronutrient malnutrition while increasing caloric output.

[18] That is, below the third height-for-age percentile.

[19] This is 10 times the number of child deaths in developed countries in the same year.

Table 20-12A. Fiftieth and twenty-fifth percentile dietary intakes of vitamins compared to RDAs (parentheses) for Americans, NHANESIII data, 1988–1994

Sex/age group	Vitamin A (μg RE/day)	Vitamin E (mg/day)	Vitamin E (μg/day)	Vitamin K (mg/day)	Vitamin C (mg/day)
Fiftieth Percentile					
Children					
4–8 yrs	829 (400)	5.6 (7)	55 (55)[a]	103 (25)	1.55 (0.6)
Males					
9–13 yrs	859 (600)	6.4 (11)	61 (60)	105 (45)	1.66 (0.9)
14–18 yrs	870 (900)	7.7 (15)	75 (75)	119 (75)	1.86 (1.2)
19–30 yrs	914 (900)	8.5 (15)	98 (120)	114 (90)	1.78 (1.2)
31–50 yrs	949 (900)	8.4 (15)	117 (120)	108 (90)	1.75 (1.2)
51–70 yrs	1012 (900)	7.5 (15)	109 (120)	103 (90)	1.63 (1.2)
>70 yrs	1047 (900)	6.5 (15)	89 (120)	99 (90)	1.56 (1.2)
Females					
9–13 yrs	776 (600)	5.6 (11)	56 (60)	100 (45)	1.54 (0.9)
14–18 yrs	610 (700)	5.6 (11)	60 (75)	89 (65)	1.55 (1.0)
19–30 yrs	668 (700)	6.1 (15)	82 (90)	79 (75)	1.95 (1.1)
31–50 yrs	764 (700)	6.4 (15)	88 (90)	85 (75)	1.41 (1.1)
51–70 yrs	913 (700)	5.6 (15)	85 (90)	97 (75)	1.38 (1.1)
>70 yrs	954 (700)	5.2 (15)	79 (90)	100 (75)	1.38 (1.1)
Pregnant	861 (750–770)	n.a.[b] (15)	80 (75–90)	119 (80–85)	1.68 (1.2)
Twenty-Fifth Percentile					
Children					
4–8 yrs	719 (400)	5.2 (7)	44 (55)	87 (25)	1.35 (0.6)
Males					
9–13 yrs	628 (600)	4.4 (11)	49 (60)	82 (45)	1.42 (0.9)
14–18 yrs	629 (900)	5.3 (15)	60 (75)	89 (75)	1.52 (1.2)
19–30 yrs	638 (900)	5.9 (15)	77 (120)	85 (90)	1.44 (1.2)
31–50 yrs	652 (900)	5.9 (15)	91 (120)	81 (90)	1.43 (1.2)
51–70 yrs	713 (900)	5.1 (15)	82 (120)	76 (90)	1.33 (1.2)
>70 yrs	750 (900)	4.3 (15)	67 (120)	76 (90)	1.31 (1.2)
Females					
9–13 yrs	587 (600)	3.9 (11)	41 (60)	82 (45)	1.33 (0.9)
14–18 yrs	450 (700)	3.8 (15)	45 (75)	68 (65)	1.31 (1.0)
19–30 yrs	490 (700)	4.2 (15)	56 (90)	61 (75)	1.21 (1.1)
31–50 yrs	565 (700)	4.4 (15)	63 (90)	65 (75)	1.19 (1.1)
51–70 yrs	664 (700)	3.9 (15)	60 (90)	74 (75)	1.13 (1.1)
>70 yrs	710 (700)	3.7 (15)	55 (90)	81 (75)	1.18 (1.1)
Pregnant	648 (750–770)	n.a.[b] (15)	59 (75–90)	93 (80–85)	1.35 (1.2)

[a]Adequate intake (AI) indicated; RDA has not been set.
[b]Estimate not available.

Table 20-12B. Fiftieth and twenty-fifth percentile dietary intakes of vitamins compared to RDAs (parentheses) for Americans, NHANESIII data, 1988–1994

Sex/age group	Thiamin (mg/day)	Riboflavin (mg/day)	Niacin (mg/day)	Vitamin B$_6$ (mg/day)	Folate (µg/day)	Vitamin B$_{12}$ (µg/day)
			Fiftieth Percentile			
Children						
6–8 yrs	1.55 (0.6)	1.99 (0.6)	18.62 (8)	1.58 (0.6)	244 (200)	3.78 (1.2)
Males						
9–13 yrs	1.66 (0.9)	2.07 (0.9)	19.98 (12)	1.63 (1.0)	255 (300)	4.55 (1.8)
14–18 yrs	1.86 (1.2)	2.20 (1.3)	23.68 (16)	1.86 (1.3)	274 (400)	5.34 (2.4)
19–30 yrs	1.78 (1.2)	2.09 (1.3)	25.30 (16)	2.02 (1.3)	277 (400)	5.22 (2.4)
31–50 yrs	1.75 (1.2)	2.03 (1.3)	25.52 (16)	1.96 (1.3)	282 (400)	5.20 (2.4)
51–70 yrs	1.63 (1.2)	1.87 (1.3)	25.56 (16)	1.77 (1.7)	283 (400)	5.10 (2.4)
>70 yrs	1.56 (1.2)	1.84 (1.3)	20.79 (16)	1.72 (1.7)	269 (400)	4.99 (2.4)
Females						
9–13 yrs	1.54 (0.9)	1.84 (0.9)	18.70 (12)	1.56 (1.0)	234 (300)	3.87 (1.8)
14–18 yrs	1.55 (1.0)	1.72 (1.0)	18.81 (14)	1.49 (1.2)	232 (400)	4.06 (2.4)
19–30 yrs	1.45 (1.1)	1.63 (1.1)	19.69 (14)	1.54 (1.3)	223 (400)	4.77 (2.4)
31–50 yrs	1.41 (1.1)	1.60 (1.1)	19.84 (14)	1.53 (1.3)	226 (400)	4.84 (2.4)
51–70 yrs	1.38 (1.1)	1.58 (1.1)	19.20 (14)	1.51 (1.5)	246 (400)	4.80 (2.4)
>70 yrs	1.38 (1.1)	1.60 (1.1)	18.74 (14)	1.53 (1.5)	252 (400)	4.74 (2.4)
Pregnant	1.68 (1.4)	1.54 (1.4)	21.55 (18)	1.76 (1.9)	258 (600)	5.05 (2.6)
			Twenty-Fifth Percentile			
Children						
6–8 yrs	1.35 (0.6)	1.69 (0.6)	16.81 (8)	1.41 (0.6)	204 (200)	3.17 (1.2)
Males						
9–13 yrs	1.42 (0.9)	1.70 (0.9)	17.41 (12)	1.43 (1.0)	204 (300)	3.60 (1.8)
14–18 yrs	1.52 (1.2)	1.68 (1.3)	18.75 (16)	1.47 (1.3)	204 (400)	4.05 (2.4)
19–30 yrs	1.44 (1.2)	1.62 (1.3)	20.42 (16)	1.60 (1.3)	219 (400)	4.81 (2.4)
31–50 yrs	1.43 (1.2)	1.61 (1.3)	20.73 (16)	1.57 (1.3)	225 (400)	4.81 (2.4)
51–70 yrs	1.33 (1.2)	1.52 (1.3)	18.53 (16)	1.48 (1.7)	222 (400)	4.77 (2.4)
>70 yrs	1.31 (1.2)	1.49 (1.3)	17.31 (16)	1.35 (1.7)	213 (400)	4.69 (2.4)
Females						
9–13 yrs	1.33 (0.9)	1.56 (0.9)	16.37 (12)	1.33 (1.0)	191 (300)	3.14 (1.0)
14–18 yrs	1.31 (1.0)	1.35 (1.0)	15.63 (14)	1.19 (1.2)	170 (400)	3.26 (2.4)
19–30 yrs	1.21 (1.1)	1.31 (1.1)	16.46 (14)	1.24 (1.3)	183 (400)	4.53 (2.4)
31–50 yrs	1.19 (1.1)	1.32 (1.1)	16.89 (14)	1.25 (1.3)	189 (400)	4.60 (2.4)
51–70 yrs	1.17 (1.1)	1.28 (1.1)	16.06 (14)	1.24 (1.5)	196 (400)	4.58 (2.4)
>70 yrs	1.18 (1.1)	1.32 (1.1)	15.82 (14)	1.24 (1.5)	200 (400)	4.53 (2.4)
Pregnant	1.35 (1.4)	1.52 (1.4)	18.19 (18)	1.43 (1.9)	205 (600)	4.70 (2.6)

iron deficiency, and iodine deficiency.[20] Two of these involve suboptimal status with respect to vitamins:

- *Vitamin A deficiency*   It is estimated that more than 250 million children worldwide are at risk of vitamin A deficiency. In 1991, nearly 14 million preschool children (three-quarters from southern Asia) were estimated to have clinical eye disease (xerophthalmia) due to the deficiency, which is thought to cause blindness in 250,000–500,000 children each year. Two-thirds of affected children die within 6 months of going blind, owing to their increased susceptibility to infections also caused by the deficiency. Even subclinical vitamin A deficiency increases child mortality.
- *Anemia*   An estimated 42% of the world's women are anemic.[21] While anemia can have multiple causes (including malaria, and intestinal parasitism), it is thought that at least half of the anemia worldwide is due to nutritional iron deficiency. The prevalence of anemia may underestimate that of low iron status, which

affects more than 2.1 billion people, particularly women of reproductive age and preschool children living in tropical and subtropical zones, as well as school-aged children and working men in many areas. Iron deficiency can reduce work capacity, impair learning ability, increase susceptibility to infections, and increase risk of death associated with pregnancy and childbirth.[22]

It is bitterly ironic that iron, the fourth most abundant element in the Earth's crust, is so widely deficient in many diets. This results from the very low bioavailability of inorganic and most plant forms of the element,[23] which comprise the major sources of iron in the diets of the world's poor. For this reason it has been said that anemia may better be described as a vitamin C deficiency disease, for the presence of ascorbic acid in the lumen of the gut is known to markedly improve the bioavailability of dietary iron. Vitamin A has also been shown to affect iron utilization, and deficiencies of vitamin E, folate, and vitamin B_{12} also cause anemias.[24]

Study Questions and Exercises

1. List the tests and measurements that might be useful in assessing the vitamin status of (i) a food, (ii) a meal, (iii) a national food supply, (iv) an individual, and (v) a population.

2. Devise a system of biochemical measurements that could be performed on a 7-ml sample of fresh blood to yield as much information as possible about the vitamin status of the donor. (Assume enzyme activities can be assayed using no more than 50 µl of plasma or erythrocyte lysate and other biochemical

measurements can be made using no more than 500 µl each.)

3. Give an example of a situation wherein a particular biochemical test may be necessary for the diagnosis of a vitamin-related disorder detected by clinical examination.

4. In general, what are the relationships of biochemical tests and clinical examination in the assessment of vitamin status? In general terms, discuss the advantages and disadvantages of the various types of biochemical tests used in assessing vitamin status (e.g., functional tests, load tests, urinary excretion tests, circulating metabolite tests).

---

[20] An estimated 1600 million people live in iodine-deficient areas. The most prevalent outcome of iodine deficiency is goiter, affecting some 200 million people. In addition, some 6 million infants born annually to iodine-deficient mothers develop severe mental and neurological impairment known as *cretinism* (half of this number is in southern Asia). The deficiency also increases the rates of stillbirths, abortions, and infant deaths.

[21] This ranges from a high in southern Asia (64%) to the lowest but still surprisingly high rates (< 20%) in industrialized countries.

[22] It is estimated that a fifth of maternal mortality is due to the direct (heart failure) or indirect (inability to tolerate hemorrhage) effects of anemia; severe anemia is responsible for nearly one-third of fatalities among children who are not given immediate transfusions.

[23] These nonheme sources of iron are typically absorbed at less than 5–15% efficiency. In plants, much of this can be bound to phytic acid, which, being indigestible by most monogastric animals, further reduces iron bioavailability. In contrast, some 25–30% of heme iron in animal products is absorbed by monogastrics.

[24] The anemia produced by iron deficiency is easily distinguishable from anemia produced by other vitamin deficiencies. Iron deficiency anemia is normocytic and hypochromic; vitamin E deficiency is characterized by a hemolytic anemia with reticulocytosis; and folate or vitamin B_{12} deficiency anemias are macrocytic and normochromic.

Recommended Reading

Briefel, R. R. (1996). Nutrition monitoring in the United States. In *Present Knowledge in Nutrition* (E. E. Ziegler and L. J. Filer, Jr., eds.), pp. 517–529. ILSI Press, Washington, DC.

Combs, G. F., Jr., Welch, R. M., Duxbury, J. M., Uphoff, N. T., and Nesheim, M. C. (1996). *Food-Based Approaches to Preventing Micronutrient Malnutrition: An International Research Agenda.* Cornell University, Ithaca, NY.

Committee on Diet and Health, Food and Nutrition Board, National Research Council. (1989). Dietary intake and nutritional status: Trends and assessment. In *Diet and Health, Implications for Reducing Chronic Disease Risk*, pp. 41–84. National Academy Press, Washington, DC.

Dwyer, J. T. (1991). Nutritional consequences of vegetarianism. *Annu. Rev. Nutr.* **11,** 61–91.

Gary, P. J., and Koehler, K. M. (1990). Problems in interpretation of dietary and biochemical data from population studies. In *Present Knowledge in Nutrition* (M. Brown, ed.), 6th ed., pp. 407–414. International Life Science Institute-Nutritional Foundation, Washington, DC.

Gibson, R. S. (1990). *Principles of Nutritional Assessment.* Oxford University Press, New York.

Heimberger, D., and Winsier, R. (1997). *Handbook of Clinical Nutrition*, 3rd ed. Mosby, NY.

Interdepartmental Committee on Nutrition for National Defense. (1963). *Manual for Nutrition Surveys*, 2nd ed. U.S. Government Printing Office, Washington, DC.

Life Sciences Research Office, FASEB. (1989). *Nutrition Monitoring in the United States.* DHHS Pub. No. 89-1255. U.S. Government Printing Office, Washington, DC.

Livingston, G. E. (ed.). (1989). *Nutritional Status Assessment of the Individual.* Food and Nutrition Press, Trumbull, CT.

Pao, E. M., and Cypel, Y. S. (1996). Estimation of dietary intake. In *Present Knowledge in Nutrition* (E. E. Ziegler and L. J. Filer, Jr., eds.), pp. 498–507. ILSI Press, Washington, DC.

Pike, R. L., and Brown, M. L. (1984a). Determination of nutrient needs: Vitamins. In *Nutrition: An Integrated Approach*, pp. 795–831. John Wiley & Sons, New York.

Pike, R. L., and Brown, M. L. (1984b). Nutrition surveys in *Nutrition: An Integrated Approach*, pp. 832–851. John Wiley & Sons, New York.

Sauberlich, H. E., Skala, J. H., and Dowdy, R. P. (1974). *Laboratory Tests for the Assessment of Nutritional Status.* CRC Press, Cleveland, Ohio.

Swan, P. B. (1983). Food consumption by individuals in the United States: Two major surveys. *Annu. Rev. Nutr.* **3,** 413–432.

Woteki, C. E., and Fanelli-Kuczmarski, M. T. (1990). The national nutrition monitoring system. In *Present Knowledge in Nutrition* (M. Brown, ed.), 6th ed., pp. 415–429. International Life Science Institute-Nutritional Foundation, Washington, DC.

Yeatley, E., and Johnson, C. (1987). Nutritional applications of the health and nutrition examination surveys (NANES). *Annu. Rev. Nutr.* **7,** 441–463.

Quantifying Vitamin Needs

21

There is not always agreement on the criteria for deciding when a requirement has been met. If the requirement is considered to be the minimal amount that will maintain normal physiological function and reduce the risk of impairment of health from nutritional inadequacy to essentially zero, we are left with questions such as: "What is normal physiological function?," "What is health?," and "What degree of reserve or stores of the nutrient is adequate?" Differences in judgment on such issues are to be expected.

— A. E. Harper

I.	Dietary Standards	485
II.	Determining Dietary Standards for Vitamins	486
III.	Factors Affecting Vitamin Requirements	487
IV.	Vitamin Allowances for Humans	494
V.	Vitamin Allowances for Animals	498
	Study Questions and Exercises	502
	Recommended Reading	502

Anchoring Concepts

1. The vitamins have many metabolic role(s) essential to normal physiological function; these roles can be compromised by quantitatively insufficient or temporarily irregular vitamin intakes.
2. Vitamin needs can be determined by monitoring responses of parameters related to the metabolic functions and/or body reserves of the vitamins.
3. Quantitative information is available concerning the vitamin contents of many common foods and feedstuffs.

Learning Objectives

1. To understand the concepts of minimum requirement, optimal requirement, and allowance as used with respect to vitamins.
2. To understand the methods available for estimating minimal and optimal vitamin requirements of animals and humans.
3. To understand the basis for establishing allowances for vitamins in human and animal feeding.
4. To be familiar with the sources of information concerning vitamin requirements and allowances.

Vocabulary

Adequate Intake (AI)
Average estimated requirement (EAR)
Dietary recommendations
Dietary Reference Intake (DRI)
Dietary standards
Estimated Average Requirement (EAR)
Estimated Safe and Adequate Daily Dietary Intake (ESADDI)
Food and Agriculture Organization (FAO)
Food and Nutrition Board
Margin of safety
Metabolic profiling
Minimum requirement
National Academy of Sciences
National Research Council
Nutrient allowances
Nutrient requirements
Nutritional essentiality
Protective Nutrient Intake
Recommended Dietary Allowance (RDA)
Recommended Dietary Intake (RDI)
Recommended Nutrient Intake (RNI)
World Health Organization (WHO)

I. Dietary Standards

Purposes of Dietary Standards

The need to formulate healthy diets for both humans and animals has stimulated the translation of current nutrition knowledge into a variety of **dietary standards** for the intake of specific nutrients. As these standards are typically developed by committees of experts reviewing the pertinent scientific literature, they are frequently referred to as **dietary recommendations**. Formally, they may be called **Recommended Dietary Allowances (RDAs)** or **Recommended Dietary Intakes (RDIs)**.

Differences between Allowances and Requirements

Regardless of hour they may be named, dietary standards differ from nutrient requirements, although they are derived from the requirements. Dietary standards are relevant to populations; they describe the average amounts of particular nutrients that should satisfy the needs of almost all healthy individuals in defined groups. In contrast, **nutrient requirements** are relevant to individuals; they describe the amounts of particular nutrients that satisfy certain criteria related to the metabolic activity of those nutrients or to general physiological function. Because recommended allowances and intakes are designed to satisfy the needs of groups of individuals whose nutrient requirements vary, they, by definition, exceed the average requirement.

II. Determining Dietary Standards for Vitamins

Determining Nutrient Requirements

The nutrient requirement is a theoretical construct that describes the intake of a particular nutrient that supports a body pool of the nutrient and/or its metabolically active forms adequate to maintain normal physiological function. In practice, it is generally used in reference to the lowest intake that supports normal function, that is, the **minimum requirement**. Minimum requirements, though seemingly physiologically relevant, are difficult to define and impossible to measure with any reasonable precision. They can vary according to the criteria by which they are defined. This problem is illustrated by the widely varying estimates of the vitamin A requirement for calves; various estimates may be derived by different criteria (Table 21-1).

Therefore, in order to be relevant to the overall health of the typical individual, estimates of minimum nutrient requirements must be based on responses of obvious physiological importance. For many nutrients (e.g., the indispensable amino acids) it

Table 21-1. Estimates of vitamin A requirements of calves, based on different criteria

Criterion	Estimated requirement (IU/day)
Prevention of nyctalopia	20
Normal growth	32
Normal serum retinol levels	40
Moderate hepatic retinyl ester reserves	250
Substantial hepatic retinyl ester reserves	1024

Source: Marks, J. (1968). *The Vitamins in Health and Disease: A Modern Reappraisal*, p. 32. Churchill, London.

may thus be appropriate to define minimum requirements on the basis of a fairly nonspecific parameter such as growth. For vitamins, however, it is appropriate to define minimum requirements on the basis of parameters that are more specifically related to their metabolic functions, such as enzyme activities and tissue concentrations, because these can reflect changes at the earlier stages of vitamin deficiencies. The most useful parameters of vitamin status are those that respond early to deprivation of the vitamin, for those can be used to detect suboptimal vitamin status at the early and most easily corrected stages.

Quantifying the minimum requirement, even with the use of an appropriate parameter, is not straightforward. It generally requires an experimental approach in which the test animals are fed a basal diet constructed to be deficient in the nutrient of interest but otherwise adequate with respect to all known nutrients, with this diet being supplemented with known amounts of the nutrient of interest. This may necessitate the use of uncommon feedstuffs such that the diet bears little similarity to those used in practice; it usually means that the test nutrient is provided largely in free form, which may not resemble its form in practical foods and feedstuffs. Even with these caveats in mind, the level of nutrient intake to be identified as the minimum requirement is not always clear, as the desired value for that parameter is usually a matter of judgment.

Most responses of specific nutrient-depleted animals to input of the same nutrient appear to be curvilinear (Fig. 21-1, right panel); however, in most nutrient requirement experiments, both rectilinear and curvilinear models usually fit equally well. For this reason, many investigators have used rectilinear models to impute requirements (e.g., the x value of the intercept of the two linear regressions of the

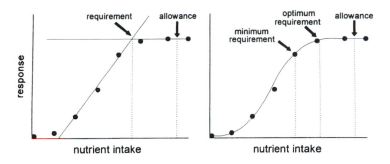

Fig. 21-1. Requirements and allowances for nutrients are determined from the responses of physiologically meaningful parameters to the level of nutrient intake.

observed data in broken-line regression analyses;[1] Fig. 21-1, left panel). Others, however, have used curvilinear models, which consider the variations in the experimental population of both the measured response and the nutrient need for maintenance (usually related to body size). From the proposition of curvilinearity, it follows that no value can be properly described as the "requirement" of the test populations. Nevertheless, the approach can be used to determine the risk of not fully satisfying the nutrient requirement for given proportions of the experimental population. The intake associated with acceptable risk of deficiency (a matter of judgment) is frequently called the optimum requirement or level of optimum intake. In public health, such levels are determined on the basis of assumptions regarding putative health risks and in consideration of interindividual variation. In livestock production, where the cost of feeding accounts for a substantial portion of the total cost of production, optimum intakes of the more costly nutrients (protein, limiting amino acids, energy) are necessary to optimize economic efficiency.

III. Factors Affecting Vitamin Requirements

Many factors can affect nutrient requirements (Tables 21-2 and 21-3), such that those of individuals with the same general characteristics can vary substantially. For most nutrients the requirements of individuals in given populations appear to be normally distributed. For this reason, in the absence of clear information, it is reasonable to assume that the variations in vitamin requirements are similar to those typically observed in biological systems, that is, normally distributed with a coefficients of variation of 10–15%.

Developing Vitamin Allowances

Because nutrient requirements, even for the best cases, are quantitative estimates based on data of uncertain precision derived from a limited number of subjects, those values have limited practical usefulness. In practice, **nutrient allowances**, or recommended intakes, are far more useful. They are selected to meet the needs of those individuals with the greatest requirements. That is, an allowance is set at the right-hand tail of the natural distribution of requirements. An allowance exceeds the **average estimated requirement (EAR)** for the population by an increment sometimes referred to as a **margin of safety**. Allowances for vitamins, particularly in livestock feeding, have often been set on the basis of practical experience; however, rational approaches are available and have been used for establishing official nutrient allowances for both animals and humans. Nutrient allowances are generally described in statistical terms relating to the proportion of the target population, the requirements of which would be met by the recommended level of intake (see Fig. 21-2). For example, committees of the **Food and Nutrition Board** and WHO/FAO[2] have set allowances at 2 standard deviations (SD) above the EAR, in order to meet the needs of

---

[1] This approach offers the advantage of rendering a requirement value that is derived mathematically from the observed data; however, that value tends to be in the region of greatest variation in the input–response curve.

[2] **World Health Organization** and **Food and Agriculture Organization**, respectively, of the United Nations.

Table 21-2. Factors affecting vitamin requirements

Factor	Examples
Physiological determinants	Active growth
	Pregnancy
	Lactation
	Aging
	Intraindividual variation
	Level of physical activity
Hereditary conditions	Vitamin-dependent diseases
Conditions of maldigestion/malabsorption	Pancreatitis
	Gastric resection
	Endocrine disorders (for example, diabetes mellitus, hypoparathyroidism, Addison's disease)
	Hepatobiliary disease
	Intestinal resection/bypass
	Pernicious anemia
	Regional ileitis
	Radiation injury
	Kwashiorkor
	Pellagra
	Gluten sensitivity enteropathy
	Intestinal parasitism (for example, hookworm, *Strongyloides, Giardia lamblia, Dibothriocephalus latus*)
	Acute enteritis
	Cystic fibrosis
	Certain drug treatments
	Hypermetabolic states
	Thyrotoxicosis
	Pyrexial disease
	Infections
Conditions causing decreased nutrient utilization	Chronic liver disease
	Chronic renal disease
Conditions involving increased cell turnover	Congenital or acquired hemolytic anemias
	Sickle cell disease
Conditions increasing nutrient turnover/loss	Extensive burns
	Bullous dermatoses
	Enteropathy
	Nephrosis
	Surgery
	Hemodialysis
	Smoking

Table 21-3. Physiologically significant drug–vitamin interactions

Vitamin	Drugs
Vitamin A	Diuretic: spironolactone Bile acid sequestrant: cholestyramine, colestipol Laxative: phenolphthalein, mineral oil (laxative)
Vitamin D	Antibacterial: isoniazid Anticonvulsant: phenytoin, diphenylhydantoin, primidone Bile acid sequestrant: colestipol Laxative: phenolphthalein, mineral oil
Vitamin E	Smoking
Vitamin K	Anticoagulant: warfarin Anticonvulsant: phenytoin, diphenylhydantoin, primidone Bile acid sequestrant: colestipol Immunosuppressant: cyclosporins Laxative: mineral oil, phenolphthalein
Vitamin C	Antiinflammatant: aspirin Oral contraceptives Smoking
Thiamin	Ethanol
Riboflavin	Antibacterial: boric acid Tranquilizer: chlorpromazine
Niacin	Antibacterial: isoniazid Antiinflammatant: phenylbutazone
Vitamin B_6	Analytical reagent: thiosemicarbazide Antibacterial: isoniazid Anticholinergic, anti-Parkinsonian: L-dopa Antihypertensive: hydralazine Chelating agent, antiarthritic: penicillamine Ethanol Oral contraceptives Smoking
Biotin	None reported
Pantothenic acid	None reported
Folate	Antacid: sodium bicarbonate, aluminum hydroxide Antibacterial: sulfasalazine, trimethoprim Anticonvulsant: phenytoin Antiinflammatant: sulfasalazine, aspirin Antimalarial: pyrimethamine Antineoplastic: methotrexate Bile acid sequestrant: cholestyramine, colestipol Diuretic: triamterene Ethanol Oral contraceptives
Vitamin B_{12}	Analytical reagent: biquanides Antibacterials: p-aminosalicylic acid, neomycin Antihistaminic: cimetidine, ranitidine Antiinflammatant, gout suppressant: colchicine Bile acid sequestrant: cholestyramine, colestipol

approximately 97.5% of the population.[3] This method has yielded satisfactory results, likely due in part to the generous estimates of EARs generally made by expert committees.

Allowances, therefore, are derived from estimates of EARs (of typical individuals) made from actual biological data, usually from nutritional experiments. Because they are used as standards for populations, allowances are developed in consideration of risk of nutrient deficiency. Therefore, allowances are relevant to specified populations, with their characteristic food habits and inherent variations in nutrient requirements. For example, the Recommended Dietary Allowances established by the U.S. Food and Nutrition Board are implicitly intended to relate to the U.S. population. These recommendations were originally developed to facilitate the wartime planning of food supplies, but have become a key source of information for making food and health policy in the United States and elsewhere (Table 21-4).

Understanding the Difference between Requirements and Allowances

Confusion surrounds the allowances for the vitamins (and other nutrients) that have been developed by various expert committees. Some questions arise, particularly concerning dietary recommendations

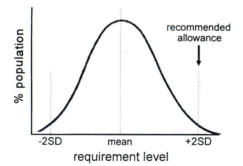

Fig. 21-2. The "mean plus 2 SD" conversion algorithm for determining recommended dietary allowances.

for livestock, because the rationale for such values is frequently not presented. A fairly common example is the mistaken impression, on the part of formulators of animal feeds, that vitamin allowances are requirements; this mistake can lead to overfortification of those feed vitamins. Other questions arise over the publication of differing recommendations by different committees of experts, all of whom consider the same basic data in their respective reviews of the pertinent literature. This situation results from the paucity of clear and compelling data on nutrient requirements; differences in environmental conditions and food supplies; and the lack of consensus on such issues as criteria for defining requirements, appropriate margins of safety, and whether standards should be based on intakes of food as consumed or as purchased. These considerations make the variable factor of scientific judgment important in estimating the nature of nutrient requirements. Thus, dietary recommendations are revised periodically[4] as new information becomes available.

Applications of RDAs

Questions about nutrient allowances for humans arise, owing to the application of those values to purposes for which they were not intended. Although the RDAs were originally developed for use in planning food supplies for groups of people,[5] today they are used for many other purposes: evaluating the nutritional adequacy of diets; evaluating results of dietary surveys; setting standards for food assistance programs, institutional feeding programs, and food and nutrition regulations; developing food and nutrition education programs; and formulating new food products and special dietary foods. Many of these uses have fostered criticism of the RDAs for not dealing with associations of diet and chronic and degenerative diseases, for not including guidelines for appropriate intakes of fat, cholesterol, and fiber, and for not providing guidance for food selection and prevention of obesity. These problems stem from fundamental misunderstandings

---

[3] A notable exception is in the setting of allowances for energy; these are typically set at the estimated average requirements of classes of individuals, for the reason that, unlike other nutrients, both intake and expenditure of energy appear to be regulated such that free-living individuals with free access to food maintain (at least very nearly) energy balance.

[4] As available information bases improve, expert committees typically have reduced the levels of their recommendations for nutrient allowances. This likely reflects the basically conservative nature of the committee system used for these purposes, whereby the paucity of data tends to be handled by generously estimating quantitative needs.

[5] The RDAs were originated in 1941 for use in planning U.S. food policy during World War II.

Table 21-4. History of the recommended daily allowances (RDAa) for vitamins[a]

	1941	1948	1957	1968	1976	1980	1989	1997–2001
Vitamin A (mg RE)	1000	1000	1000	1000	1000	1000	1000	900
Vitamin D (IU/μg)	—	—	—	400 IU	400 IU	5 μg	5 μg	[10][b]
Vitamin E (IU/mg)	—	—	—	30 IU	15 IU	10 IU	10 IU	15 mg
Vitamin K (μg)	—	—	—	—	—	—	80	[120][b]
Vitamin C (mg)	75	75	70	60	45	60	60	90
Thiamin (mg)	2.3	1.5	0.9	1.3	1.4	1.4	1.5	1.2
Riboflavin (mg)	3.3	1.8	1.3	1.7	1.6	1.6	1.7	1.3
Niacin (mg)	23	15	15	17	18	18	19	16
Vitamin B$_6$ (mg)	—	—	—	2.0	2.0	2.2	2.0	1.7
Pantothenic acid	—	—	—	—	—	—	—	[5][b]
Biotin	—	—	—	—	—	—	—	[30][b]
Folate (μg)	—	—	—	400	400	400	200	400
Vitamin B$_{12}$ (μg)	—	—	—	3.0	3.0	5.0	2.0	2.4

[a]Values shown are for males, 25–50 years of age.
[b]RDAs not available for these vitamins; values shown are Adequate Intakes (AIs).

that, although the RDAs may be used in certain programs to implement sound public health policy, they are not intended to be policy recommendations per se. Actually, RDAs cannot serve as general dietary guidelines; by definition, they are reference standards dealing with nutrients, whereas dietary guidelines deal primarily with foods. The RDAs are standards on which sound dietary guidelines are to be based.

The RDAs, like other nutrient allowances, are intended to relate to intakes of nutrients as part of the normal diets[6] of specified populations. They are intended to be average daily intakes based on periods as short as 3 days (for nutrients with fast turnover rates) to several weeks or months (for nutrients with slower turnover rates).

Changes in the RDA Concept

In one sense, the RDA construct is somewhat archaic in that it fails to pertain to biological functions of nutrients that may be nonspecific or nontraditional, in the context of being outside the known functions of nutrients. The conceptual framework on which the RDA was derived is being replaced by a new, more individualistic view of nutrition that relates more broadly to health. This view is the basis of problems that have become apparent concerning the RDA. To retain the practical utility of the RDA, it will be necessary to reconstruct it; such reconstruction must be based on new paradigms for nutritional science that, informed by the "genomics revolution," explicitly consider individual metabolic characteristics.

The RDA was developed to facilitate food planning for the U.S. population. It is a child of the central concept of the field of nutrition, **nutritional essentiality**, which has been used to describe those factors in the external chemical environment that are specifically required for normal metabolic functions and, accordingly, those exogenous sources on which organisms depend for normal physiologic functions (e.g., growth, reproductive success, survival, and freedom from certain clinical/metabolic disorders). The vitamins are among the more than 40 such factors generally considered to be nutritionally essential, that is, indispensable in the diets of animals and humans. Deprivation

---

6 The RDA subcommittee emphasized that the RDAs can typically be met or closely approximated by diets that are based on the consumption of a variety of foods from diverse food groups that contain adequate energy.

of any one of these vitamins is made manifest by clinical signs that are usually specific in nature. Nutritional essentiality has been based on empirical findings that nutrients function to prevent ill health in very specific ways. Under this paradigm, nutrient deficiency diseases have played important roles in developing our knowledge of nutrition: their specific prevention has been used both to define nutrient essentiality and to quantify nutrient needs. Indeed, a nutrient has not been considered essential unless a clinical disease has been related specifically to its deprivation. Therefore, as the term has been used, nutritional essentiality clearly connotes the specific prevention of deficiency disease. This connotation is expressed in the quantitative estimation of population-based nutrient needs, the RDAs. But it now serves to limit the essentiality paradigm as a conceptual framework in modern nutrition, which is cast in a different context—one in which optimum health is more broadly conceptualized.

These limitations have produced a number of major questions concerning RDAs:

- Which level of nutrient need should define a requirement? Should this be the level that supports all/some dependent enzymes at 50, 80, or 100% of maximal activity?
- Can a nutrient be conditionally essential (e.g., glutamine for surgical patients)?
- How can varying individual nutrient requirements be described (e.g., effects of infection)?
- Can nutrients be said to be required for their nonspecific effects (e.g., antioxidants)?
- Can a nonnutrient be required (e.g., dietary fiber)?

The specific deficiency disease connotation of the RDA is, perhaps, most troublesome in dealing with issues of diet and health, for the essentiality paradigm does not pertain to functions of nutrients that are either nonspecific or nontraditional, that is, outside the known functions of nutrients.

Considering Nontraditional Functions of Nutrients

For some dietary factors, functions influencing the risk of chronic disease have been suggested by epidemiological and experimental animal model studies and, to a lesser extent, clinical trials. Reduced risks of several chronic diseases have been associated with increased intakes and/or status of several vitamins. The metabolic bases of these linkages remain to be elucidated; indeed, these areas are among the most active in contemporary nutritional science:

- *Cancer* and foods containing vitamin A[7,8,9,10] or vitamin C,[8,9,10,11] intakes of riboflavin,[12] and plasma levels or intakes of α-tocopherol,[8,9,13] carotenoids,[7,8,14] and 25-OH-vitamin D.[15]
- *Cardiovascular disease* and intakes of vitamin C,[16,17,18,19] vitamin E,[16,17,18,20] and β-carotene.[16,17]
- *Neural tube defects* and periconceptual folate intake.[21]
- *Diabetes* and *multiple sclerosis* and plasma 25-OH-vitamin.[15]

The case of the apparent effects of antioxidants illustrates the limitation of the present RDA conceptualization. Current thinking is that antioxidant nutrients (vitamins E and C, selenium, and, perhaps,

[7] Ziegler, R. J. (1988). *Nutr.* **119,** 116–122.

[8] Doll, R. (1990). *Proc. Nutr. Soc.* **49,** 119–131.

[9] Byers, T., and Perry, G. (1994). *Annu. Rev. Nutr.* **12,** 139–159.

[10] Willett, W. C. (1994). *Am. J. Clin. Nutr.* **59** (Suppl.), 1162S.

[11] Block, G. (1991). *Am. J. Clin. Nutr.* **53** (Suppl.), 270S.

[12] Key, T. (1994). *Proc. Nutr. Soc.* **53,** 605–614.

[13] Knekt, P. (1991). *Ann. Med.* **23,** 3–10.

[14] Kinsky, N. I. (1989). *J. Nutr.* **119,** 123–130.

[15] Whiting, S. J., and Calvo, M. S. (2005). *J. Nutr.* **135,** 304–309.

[16] Simon, J. A. (1992). *J. Am. Coll. Nutr.* **11,** 107–114.

[17] Hennig, B., and Toborek, M. (1993). *J. Optimal Nutr.* **2,** 213–221.

[18] Gaziano, J. M. et al. (1992). *Ann. N.Y. Acad. Sci.* **669,** 249–273.

[19] Reimersma, R. A. (1994). *Proc. Nutr. Soc.* **53,** 59–65.

[20] Anonymous. (1993). *Nutr. Rev.* **51,** 333–345.

[21] Rush, D. (1994). *Am. J. Clin. Nutr.* **59** (Suppl.), 511S–516S.

β-carotene) participate in a system of protection against the deleterious metabolic effects of free radicals.

Because many diseases are thought to involve enhanced free-radical production, protection from oxidative stress is thought to be critical to normal physiologic function. According to this hypothesis, antioxidants would be expected to suppress radical-induced DNA damage involved in the initiation of carcinogenesis, to inhibit the oxidation of cholesterol in low-density lipoproteins (LDLs) in atherosclerosis, and to inhibit the oxidation of lens proteins in cataracts. Antioxidant nutrients have been shown to enhance immune functions, which may also contribute to reduced risks of cancer as well as infectious disease. Many of these antioxidant effects do not appear to have the specificity connoted by the essentiality paradigm. For example, the complementary natures of the antioxidant functions of vitamins E and C and selenium suggest that any one may spare needs for the others in protecting against subcellular free-radical damage and LDL oxidation. It is likely that, through such biochemical mechanisms, the antioxidant nutrients may be modifiers of disease risk rather than primary agents in disease etiologies. However nonspecific they may be, such effects raise legitimate questions concerning nutrient need—questions not easily addressed under the essentiality paradigm or translated into RDAs as they have been conceived.

New Paradigms for Nutrition

The term *essentiality* has become rather elastic in its application. Nutrients have come to be described as being "required" or "essential" for particular functions. Some are called "dispensable" or "indispensable" under specific conditions; several are recognized as "beneficial" at levels greater than those that are considered to be "required." Indeed, the translation of nutritional knowledge into dietary guidance requires such language. However, the emergence of this sort of terminology indicates that the essentiality paradigm is, being displaced by a new conceptualization of nutrition.

It is likely that new paradigms of nutrition will encompass an individualized view of organisms that recognizes both endogenous and exogenous conditions as determinants of the nature and amounts of factors available from the external chemical environment that must be obtained to support definable health outcomes. Accordingly, such factors will be considered as nutrients *if* and *when* their activities, in the metabolism of the host and/or the associated microflora, are beneficial to those outcomes. This view will recognize a variety of outcomes as being appropriate for various individuals, both within and between a species/population. Thus, freedom from overt physiological dysfunction as well as reduced risk of chronic diseases will be important outcomes in human nutrition, whereas such outcomes as maximal growth rate, optimal efficiency of feed utilization, and minimal susceptibility to infection will be priorities in livestock nutrition.

The old paradigm is being outgrown at an increasing pace with the development of the modern field of molecular biology. It has now become clear that some nutrients function as gene regulators and that predisposition to disease can have genetic bases. The mapping of the human genome and, soon, the genomes of associated human microorganisms have led to the development of powerful tools to study individual metabolic characteristics. As **metabolic profiling** becomes more feasible, it will become possible to address individuals' nutritional needs on the basis of their respective genetic and metabolic characteristics. Not only clinicians but also dieticians will be able to ask such questions as whether an individual has sodium-sensitive hypertension, a cystathionine ß-synthase mutation, or the methylenetetrahydrofolate reductase (MTHFR) C677T/C genotype. The time is quickly approaching when it will be possible to identify disease predisposition, metabolic characteristics, and specific dietary needs of individuals based on rapid, genomic/metabolomic analyses. As that becomes practicable, the population-based paradigm will lose its value.

Reconstructing the RDA

This crisis in conceptualization became manifest in the lively discussion concerning the need for new approaches to the development of dietary recommendations that preceded the development of the **Dietary Reference Intakes (DRIs)** in the 1990s. The challenge was to re-create the RDA as a useful construct under this emerging paradigm that addressed both the prevention of overt nutritional deficiencies and the maintenance of health.

The DRIs also needed to accommodate the possibility that a nutrient can have beneficial action at levels above those previously thought to be "required" for normal physiologic function. To do this, it is necessary to convey information concerning three levels of nutrient activity:[22]

- The amount of nutrient required to prevent overt deficiency disease
- If applicable, the amount of nutrient that may provide other health benefits
- The amount of nutrient that may carry specific health hazards

IV. Vitamin Allowances for Humans

Several Standards

The first nutrient allowances were published 50 years ago by the U.S. **National Academy of Sciences**. Based on available information, those Recommended Dietary Allowances (RDAs) have since been revised periodically. Since the first publication of RDAs, similar dietary standards have been produced by several countries and international organizations. For the reasons mentioned previously, the various recommendations tend to be similar but not always identical. For example, most are based on food as consumed; however, some (those of Germany) are based on food as purchased, making them appear higher than those of other countries.

The RDAs

The RDAs are probably the most widely referenced of the dietary standards and the most comprehensive with respect to the vitamins. The RDAs for vitamins are still not complete; that is, quantitative recommendations on some (e.g., vitamin D, vitamin K, biotin, pantothenic acid) have not been made owing to a still-insufficient information base. In 1980, this problem of dealing with nutrients known to be essential for humans but for which insufficient data are available was handled by including provisional recommendations. The ninth and tenth editions of the RDAs present **Estimated Safe and Adequate Daily Dietary Intake (ESADDI)** ranges of daily dietary intakes for such nutrients. This terminology is no longer used. Instead, estimates of **Adequate Intakes (AIs)** are now used in cases where available data are judged to be insufficient for developing RDAs.

The setting of dietary allowances is an exercise of experts who evaluate published literature. Different expert panels can reach different conclusions from the same body of published data, as evidenced by the differences in national dietary allowances. That the growing body of relevant data also changes over time is evidence of the changes seen in the RDAs over the history of that institution (Table 21-4). For example, only in 1968 were RDAs established for vitamins D, E, C, and B_{12}, and folate. In 1989, an RDA for vitamin K was first set; however, that value, as well as that for vitamin D, were replaced with AI values in the most recent version (2000). Clearly, the setting of dietary allowances is a continuing process.

The DRIs

The most recent (1997–2001) edition of dietary allowances (Table 21-5) produced by the Food and Nutrition Board was preceded by a series of workshops that addressed the conceptual framework on which that work was based. This resulted

---

[22] The need for a trilevel allowance is perhaps best illustrated by the impending situation concerning the essential trace element, selenium. The RDA for selenium was established in 1989, largely on the basis of the amount judged sufficient to support maximal activities of the selenium-dependent glutathione peroxidase in the plasma of young men: adult women, 50 µg; adult men, 70 µg. These levels may even be high, a point that is of little importance to the U.S. population, which probably has regular selenium intakes in the range of 80–200 µg/day. What is particularly important, however, is that clinical intervention trials have confirmed a large body of animal tumor model studies in showing cancer-chemopreventive activity of selenium at intakes substantially greater than those sufficient to support maximal activities of selenium enzymes. In a decade-long, double-blind trial involving a cohort of older Americans, our group [Clark, L. C., et al. (1996). *J. Am. Med. Assoc.* **276**, 1957–1963] found that the use of a daily oral supplement of selenium (200 µg, i.e., about twice the normal dietary selenium intake) was associated with significant reductions in risks of total cancer and all leading cancers (lung, colorectal, prostate) in that population.

Table 21-5. Food and Nutrition Board recommended daily allowances (RDAs) for vitamins

Age (years) or conditions	Vitamin A (µg[a])	Vitamin D (µg)	Vitamin E (mg[b])	Vitamin K (µg)	Vitamin C (mg)	Thiamin (mg)	Riboflavin (mg)	Niacin (mg[c])	Vitamin B$_6$ (µg)	Pantothenic acid (µg)	Biotin (µg)	Folate (µg[d])	Vitamin B$_{12}$ (µg)
Infants													
0–6 monts	[400]e	5	4	[2.0]e	[40]e	[0.2]e	[0.3]e	[2c]e	[0.1]e	[1.7]e	[5]e	[65]e	[0.4]e
7–11 months	[500]e	5	5	[2.5]e	[50]e	[0.3]e	[0.4]e	[4]e	[0.3]e	[1.8]e	[6]e	[80]e	[0.5]e
Children													
1–3 yrs.	300	5	6	[30]e	15	0.5	0.5	6	0.5	2	[8]e	[150]e	0.9
4–86 yrs.	400	5	7	[55]e	25	0.6	0.6	8	0.6	3	[12]e	[200]e	1.2
Males													
9–13 yrs.	600	5	11	[60]e	45	0.9	0.9	12	1.0	4	[20]e	[300]e	1.8
14–18 yrs.	900	5	15	[75]e	75	1.2	1.3	16	1.3	5	[25]e	[400]e	2.4
19–30 yrs.	900	5	15	[120]e	90	1.2	1.3	16	1.3	5	[30]e	[400]e	2.4
31–50 yrs.	900	5	15	[120]e	90	1.2	1.3	16	1.3	5	[30]e	[400]e	2.4
51–70 yrs.	900	10	15	[120]e	90	1.2	1.3	16	1.7	5	[30]e	[400]e	2.4
>70 yrs.	900	15	15	[120]e	90	1.2	1.3	16	1.7	5	[30]e	[400]e	2.4
Females													
9–13 yrs.	600	5	11	[60]e	45	0.9	0.9	12	1.0	4	[20]e	[300]e	1.8
14–18 yrs.	700	5	15	[75]e	65	1.0	1.0	14	1.2	5	[25]e	[400]e	2.4
19–30 yrs.	700	5	15	[90]e	75	1.1	1.1	14	1.3	5	[30]e	[400]e	2.4
31–50 yrs.	700	5	15	[90]e	75	1.1	1.1	14	1.3	5	[30]e	[400]e	2.4
51–70 yrs.	700	10	15	[90]e	75	1.1	1.1	14	1.5	5	[30]e	[400]e	2.4
>70 yrs.	700	15	15	[90]e	75	1.1	1.1	14	1.5	5	[30]e	[400]e	2.4
Pregnancy													
=18 yrs.	750	5	15	[75]e	80	1.4	1.4	18	1.9	6	[30]e	[600]e	2.6
19–30 yrs.	770	5	15	[90]e	85	1.4	1.4	18	1.9	6	[30]e	[600]e	2.6
31–50 yrs.	770	5	15	[90]e	85	1.4	1.4	18	1.9	6	[30]e	[600]e	2.6
Lactation													
=18 yrs.	1200	5	19	[75]e	115	1.4	1.6	17	2.0	7	[35]e	[550]e	2.8
19–30 yrs.	1300	5	19	[90]e	120	1.4	1.6	17	2.0	7	[35]e	[550]e	2.8
31–50 yrs.	1300	5	19	[90]e	120	1.4	1.6	17	2.0	7	[35]e	[550]e	2.8

[a]Retinol equivalents.
[b]α-tocopherol.
[c]Niacin equivalents.
[d]Folate equivalents.
[e]RDA has not been set; AI is given instead.

Sources: Food and Nutrition Board (1997). *Dietary Reference Intakes for Calcium, Phosphorus, Magnesium, Vitamin D and Fluoride.* National Academy Press, Washington, DC, 432 pp.
Food and Nutrition Board (2000). *Dietary Reference Intakes for Thiamin, Riboflavin, Niacin, Vitamin B$_6$, Folate, Vitamin B$_{12}$, Pantothenic Acid, Biotin and Choline.* National Academy Press, Washington, DC 564 pp.; Food and Nutrition Board (2000). *Dietary Reference Intakes for Vitamin C, Vitamin E, Selenium and Carotenoids.* National Academy Press, Washington, DC, 506 pp.; Food and Nutrition Board (2001). *Dietary Reference Intakes for Vitamin A, Vitamin K, Arsenic, Boron, Chromium, Copper, Iodine, Iron, Manganese, Molybdenum, Nickel, Silicon, Vanadium and Zinc.* National Academy Press, Washington, DC, 773 pp.

in an expansion of the former RDAs with a system of Dietary Reference Intakes (DRIs[23]). This system involved four types of reference values (Fig. 21-3):

- *Estimated Average Requirements (EARs)* Intakes that are estimated by expert panels to meet the requirements of half the healthy individuals in each age–sex specific demographic subgroup of the American population.
- *Recommended Daily Allowances (RDAs)* Average daily intake levels sufficient to meet the requirements of nearly all (97%) of the healthy individuals in a each age–sex specific demographic subgroup. The RDA is calculated from the EAR:

$$RDA = EAR + 2SD_{EAR}$$

where SD_{EAR} is the standard deviation of the EAR.

While the RDA resembles that construct used previously, it is different in that it assumes the SD_{EAR} to be 10% of the EAR, whereas a value to 15% had been used previously. For this reason many of the new RDAs are lower than earlier ones.

- *Adequate Intakes (AIs)* Values based on observed and/or experimentally determined approximations of nutrient intakes of groups of healthy individuals and extrapolated to each age–sex demographic subgroup. These values are to be used when data are judged by expert panels to be insufficient for the estimation of an EAR and subsequent calculation of an RDA.

- *Tolerable Upper Intake Limits (ULs)* The highest level of daily intake that is likely to pose no risk of adverse health effects to almost all healthy individuals in each age–sex specific demographic subgroup. Use of ULs will facilitate the development of recommendations of nutrient intakes at what might be called "supra-nutritional" levels when such intakes have been shown to have health benefits. Pertinent to this consideration is the emerging understanding of the roles of at least several vitamins in reducing chronic disease risk.

This approach to the development of dietary allowances presumes the availability of empirical data for the distribution of individual nutrient requirements, necessary for calculating both the EAR and the SD_{EAR}. However, such data are available for very few nutrients. Thus, the DRI process involved a consensus opinion to assume that the distributions of individual nutrient requirements are each normal with a coefficient of variation (CV) of 10%, with only two exceptions: for vitamin A, CV = 20%; for niacin, CV = 15%.

International Standards

The FAO and WHO have established standards for energy, protein, calcium, iron, and vitamins (Table 21-6). This system of recommendations is intended for international use and thus to be relevant to varied population groups. It includes reference values similar to those used by the Food and Nutrition Board: Requirements similar to EARs, **Recommended Nutrient Intakes (RNIs),** similar to RDA; and Upper Tolerable Nutrient Intake Levels similar to the ULs. In addition, the FAO/WHO system provides a value applicable for nutrients that

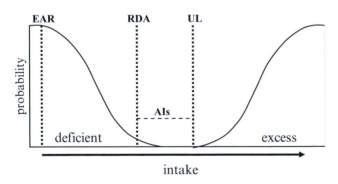

Fig. 21-3. Conceptual basis for DRIs.

---

[23] Questions concerning the means of developing consistent and reliable standards led the Tenth RDA Committee to review the scientific basis of the entire RDA table. The Committee recommended a lower RDA for vitamins A (reducing the RDA for men 1000 to 700 IU, and that for women from 800 to 600 IU and 600 IU) and vitamin C (reducing the RDA for men from 60 to 40 mg, that for women from 60 to 30 mg, and that for infants from 35 to 25 mg). It was reported that these reductions were resisted by the Food and Nutrition Board, which had been advised by another subcommittee to increase the intakes of these nutrients based on cancer risk reduction potential. In an unexpected move, the Board elected not to accept the recommendations of the RDA Committee. This move prompted lively discussion in the nutrition community, ultimately resulting in a rethinking of the RDA construct and the development of the DRIs.

Table 21-6. FAO/WHO recommended nutrient intakes (RNIs) for vitamins

Age (years) or conditions	Vitamin A (µg)[a]	Vitamin D (µg)	Vitamin E (mg)	Vitamin K (µg)	Vitamin C (mg)	Thiamin (mg)	Riboflavin (mg)	Niacin (mg)[b]	Vitamin B$_6$ (µg)	Pantothenic acid (µg)	Biotin (µg)	Folate (µg)[d]	Vitamin B$_{12}$ (µg)
Infants													
0–6 monts	375	5	2.7	5	25	.2	.3	2[c]	0.1	1.7	5	80	0.4
7–11 months	400	5	2.7	10	30	0.3	0.4	4	0.3	1.8	6	80	0.5
Chidlren													
1–3 yrs	400	5	5	15	30	0.5	0.5	6	0.5	2	8	160	0.9
4–6 yrs	450	5	5	20	30	0.6	0.6	8	0.6	3	12	200	1.2
7–9 yr	500	5	7	25	35	0.9	0.9	12	1.0	4	20	300	1.8
Adolescents, 10–18 yrs													
Males	600	5	10	35–65	40	1.2	1.3	16	1.3	5	25	400	2.4
Females	600	5	7.5	35–55	40	1.1	1.0	16	1.2	5	25	400	2.4
Adults													
Males 19–65 yrs	600	5[d], 10[e]	10	65	45	1.2	1.3	16	1.3[d], 1.7[e]	5	30	400	2.4
Females: 19–50 yrs	500	5	7.5	55	45	1.1	1.1	14	1.3	5	30	400	2.4
51–65 yrs	500	10	7.5	55	45	1.1	1.1	14	1.5	5	30	400	2.4
Older adults, 65+ yrs													
Men[c]	600	15	10	65	45	1.2	1.3	16	1.7	5	–	400	2.4
Women[c]	600	15	7.5	55	45	1.1	1.1	14	1.5	5	–	400	2.4
Pregnancy	800	5	–	55	55	1.4	1.4	18	1.9	6	30	600	2.6
Lactation	850	5	–	55	70	1.5	1.6	17	2.0	7	35	500	2.8

[a]Retinol equivalents.
[b]Niacin equivalents.
[c]Pre-formed niacin.
[d]19–50 yrs.
[e]50+ yrs.

Source: Joint WHO/FAO Expert Consultation (2001). *Human Vitamin and Mineral Requirements,* Food and Agriculture Organization, Rome, 286 pp.

may be protective against a specified nutritional or health risk of publish health relevance, **Protective Nutrient Intakes.**

Other dietary standards have been established by several countries; not surprisingly, these have shown considerable variation (Table 21-7).

V. Vitamin Allowances for Animals

Public and Private Information

The development of livestock production enterprises for the economical production of human food and fiber has superimposed practical needs on the formulation of animal feeds that do not exist in the area of human nutrition. Most notably, this involves access to current information on nutrient requirements and feedstuff nutrient composition. Often, it is the availability of such accurate data that enables commercial

Table 21-7. Variations in recommended dietary allowances for vitamins by 30 national or international organizations

Vitamin	Recommended daily allowance[a]	
	Median	Range
Vitamin A (μg)[b]	800	360–1650
Vitamin D$_3$ (μg)	5	2.5–20
Vitamin E (mg)[c]	10	5–50
Vitamin K (mg)	140	30–3000
Vitamin C (mg)	60	15–100
Thiamin (mg)	1.2	0.5–2.2
Riboflavin (mg)	1.6	0.8–3.2
Niacin (mg)	18	5.5–22
Vitamin B$_6$ (mg)	2	1–4
Biotin (μg)	200	100–400
Pantothenic acid (mg)	7	3–14
Folate (mg)	2.1	1–20
Vitamin B$_{12}$ (μg)	2	1–5

[a]For moderately active men.
[b]Retinol equivalents.
[c]α-Tocopherol equivalents.
Source: Brubacher, G. (1989). Estimation of daily requirements for vitamins. In *Elevated Dosages of Vitamins* (P. Walter, G. Brubacher, and H. Stähelin, eds.), pp. 3–11. Hans Huber Publishers, Toronto, Ontario, Canada.

animal nutritionists to formulate nutritionally balanced feeds, using computerized linear programming techniques, that maintain cost competitiveness in a context wherein the cost of feeding can be the largest cost of production.[24] Thus, while recent expansion of understanding in human nutrition has come from discoveries made in public-sponsored research, research in food animal nutrition has, over the past few decades, moved progressively out of the public sector and into the research divisions of agribusinesses with immediate interests in generating such data. The result is that a diminishing proportion of practical animal nutrition data (particularly in the area of amino acid nutrition) remains in the public sector and is thus available to the scrutiny of experts. As a consequence, two types of dietary standards are in use. The first is the standard developed by review of open data available in the scientific literature; the second is the standard developed through in-house testing and/or practical experience by animal producers. Whereas the former data are in the public domain, the latter usually are not.

Public information on nutrient allowances is reviewed by expert committees in the United States, the United Kingdom, and several other countries under programs charged with the responsibility of establishing nutrient recommendations on the basis of the best available data. Perhaps the most widely used source of such recommendations is the Committee on Animal Nutrition of the U.S. **National Research Council** (Table 21-8). Through expert subcommittees, each dedicated to a particular species, the NRC maintains the periodic review of nutrient standards, many of which serve as the bases of recommendations for animal feed formulation throughout the world. Currently, many gaps remain in our knowledge of vitamin requirements. This is particularly true for ruminant species, for which the substantial rumenal destruction of vitamins appears to be compensated by adequate microbial synthesis, and for several nonruminant species that are not widely used for commercial purposes. Therefore, many of the standards for vitamins and other nutrients are imputed from available data on related species; partly for this reason, the requirements for some nutrients (e.g., selenium) appear to be very similar among many species.

---

[24] For example, the feed costs for broiler chickens can account for 60–70% of the total cost of producing poultry meat.

Table 21-8. Estimated vitamin requirements of domestic and laboratory animals

Species	Vitamin A (IU)	Vitamin D (IU)	Vitamin E (mg)[a]	Vitamin K (µg)[b]	Vitamin C (mg)	Thiamin (mg)	Riboflavin (mg)	Niacin (mg)	Vitamin B6 (mg)	Folate (mg)	Pantothenic acid (mg)	Biotin (µg)	Vitamin B12 (µg)	Choline (g)
Vitamin, units per kg of diet														
Birds														
Chickens														
Growing chicks	1,500	200	10	0.5		1.8	3.6	27	2.5–3	0.55	10	0.1–0.15	3–9	0.5–1.3
Laying hens	4,000	500	5	0.5		0.8	2.2	10	3	0.25	2.2	0.1	4	
Breeding hens	4,000	500	10	0.5		0.8	3.8	10	4.5	0.25	10	0.15	4	
Ducks														
Growing	4,000	220		0.4			4	55	2.6		11			
Breeding	4,000	500		0.4			4	40	3		11			
Geese														
Growing	1,500	200				2.5–4		35–55			15			
Breeding	4,000	200				4	20							
Pheasants							3.5	40–60			10			1–1.5
Quail														
Growing bobwhite							3.8	30			13			1.5
Breeding bobwhite							4	20			15			1.0
Growing coturnix	5,000	1,200	12	1		2	4	40	3	1	10	0.3	3	2.0
Breeding coturnix	5,000	1,200	25	1		2	4	20	3	1	15	0.15	3	1.5
Turkeys														
Growing poults	4,000	900	12	0.8–1		2	3.6	40–70	3–4.5	0.7–1	9–11	0.1–0.2	3	0.8–1.9
Breeding hens	4,000	900	25	1		2	4	30	4	1	16	0.15	3	1.0
Cats	10,000	1,000	80			5	5	45	4	1	10	0.5	20	2.0
Cattle														
Dry heifers	2,200	300												
Dairy bulls	2,200	300												
Lactating cows	3,200	300												

(Continued)

Table 21-8. Estimated vitamin requirements of domestic and laboratory animals—Cont'd

Vitamin, units per kg of diet

Species	Vitamin A (IU)	Vitamin D (IU)	Vitamin E (mg)[a]	Vitamin K (μg)[b]	Vitamin C (mg)	Thiamin (mg)	Riboflavin (mg)	Niacin (mg)	Vitamin B6 (mg)	Folate (mg)	Pantothenic acid (mg)	Biotin (μg)	Vitamin B12 (μg)	Choline (g)
Beef cattle	2,200	300												
Dogs	5,000	275	50			1	2.2	11.4	1	0.18	10	22	0.1	1.25
Fishes														
Bream							7	28	5-6		30-50		1	4.0
Carp	10,000	1,000	300						5-6		10-20			
Catfish	2,000	2,400	30		60	1	9	14	3	5	40	20	1	3.0
Coldwater spp.	2,500		30	10	100	10	20	150	10					
Foxes	2,440					1	5.5	9.6	1.8	0.2	7.4			
Goats	60[c]	12.9[c]												
Guinea pigs	23,333	1,000	50	5	200	2	3	10	3	4	20	10	0.3	1.0
Hamsters	3,636	2,484	3	4		20	15	90	6	2	40	20	0.6	2.0
Horses														
Ponies	25[c]													
Pregnant mares	50[c]													
Lactating mares	55-65[c]													
Yearlings	40[c]													
2-year olds	30[c]													
Mice	500	150	20	3		5	7	10	1	0.5	10	10	0.2	0.6
Mink	5,930		27			1.3	1.6	20	1.6	0.5	8	32.6	0.12	
Primates[d]	15,000	2,000	50		0.1		5	50	2.5	0.2	10		0.1	
Rabbits														
Growing	580		40					180	39					1.2
Pregnant	>1,160		40	0.2										
Lactating			40											
Rats	4,000	1,000	30	0.5		4	3	20	6	1	8	50		1.0

Sheep

Ewes													
Early pregnancy	26[c]		5.6[c]										
Late pregnancy/lactating	35[c]		5.6[c]										
Rams	43[c]		5.6[c]										
Lambs													
Early weaned	35[c]		6.6[c]										
Finishing	26[c]		5.5[c]										
Shrimps			10			120			120	120			0.6
Swine													
Growing	2,200	200	11	2	1.3	2.2–3	10–22	1.5	0.6	11–13	0.1	22	0.4–1.1
Bred gilt/sow	4,000	200	10	2		3	10	1	0.6	12	0.1	15	1.25
Lactating gilt/sow	2,000	200	10	2		3	10	1	0.6	12	0.1	15	1.25
Boars	4,000	200	10	2		3	10	1	0.6	12	0.1	15	1.25

[a]α-Tocopherol.

[b]Menadione.

[c]Unlike almost all of the other values in this table, this requirement is expressed in international units (IU) per kilogram body weight.

[d]Nonhuman species.

Sources: National Research Council. (1984). *Nutrient Requirements of Poultry*, 8th ed. (rev.) National Academy Press, Washington, DC; National Research Council. (1978). *Nutrient Requirements of Cats* (rev.). National Academy Press, Washington, DC; National Research Council. (1978). *Nutrient Requirements of Dairy Cattle*, 5th ed. (rev.). National Academy Press, Washington, DC; National Research Council. (1984). *Nutrient Requirements of Beef Cattle*, 6th ed. (rev.). National Academy Press, Washington, DC; National Research Council. (1985). *Nutrient Requirements of Dogs* (rev.). National Academy Press, Washington, DC; National Research Council. (1983). *Nutrient Requirements of Warmwater Fishes and Shellfishes* (rev.). National Academy Press, Washington, DC; National Research Council. (1981). *Nutrient Requirements of Coldwater Fishes*. National Academy Press, Washington, DC; National Research Council. (1982). *Nutrient Requirements of Mink and Foxes* 2nd ed. (rev.). National Academy Press, Washington, DC; National Research Council. (1981). *Nutrient Requirements of Goats: Angora, Dairy and Meat Goats in Temperate and Tropical Countries*. National Academy Press, Washington, DC; National Research Council. (1982). *Nutrient Requirements of Mink and Foxes* 2nd ed. (rev.). National Academy Press, Washington, DC; National Research Council. (1978). *Nutrient Requirements of Nonhuman Primates*. National Academy Press, Washington, DC; National Research Council. (1978). *Nutrient Requirements of Laboratory Animals*, 3rd ed. (rev.). National Academy Press, Washington, DC; National Research Council. (1978). *Nutrient Requirements of Horses* 4th ed. (rev.). National Academy Press, Washington, DC; National Research Council. (1977). *Nutrient Requirements of Rabbits*, 2nd ed. (rev.). National Academy Press, Washington, DC; National Research Council. (1975). *Nutrient Requirements of Sheep*, 5th ed. (rev.). National Academy Press, Washington, DC; National Research Council. (1979). *Nutrient Requirements of Swine*, 8th ed. (rev.). National Academy Press, Washington, DC.

Study Questions and Exercises

1. Prepare a concept map illustrating the relationships of the concepts of minimal and optimal nutrient requirements and nutrient allowances to the concepts of physiological function and health.

2. What issues relate to the application of dietary allowances, as they are currently defined, to individuals?

3. What issues relate to the consideration of nutritional status in such areas as immune function or chronic and degenerative diseases in the development of dietary standards?

Recommended Reading

Beaton, G. H. (2005). When is an individual an individual vs. a member of a group? An issue in application of the Dietary Reference Intakes. *Nutr. Rev.* **64**, 211–225.

Chan, L. N. (2006). Drug-nutrient interactions, Chapter 97 in *Modern Nutrition in Health and Disease*, 10th ed. (M. E. Shils, M. Shike, B. Caballero, and R. Cousins, eds.), pp. 1539–1553. Lippincott, New York.

Dwyer, J. T. (2006). Dietary guidelines: National perspectives, Chapter 105 in *Modern Nutrition in Health and Disease*, 10th ed. (M. E. Shils, M. Shike, B. Caballero, and R. Cousins, eds.), pp. 1673–1686. Lippincott, New York.

Food and Nutrition Board. (1997). *Dietary Reference Intakes for Calcium, Phosphorus, Magnesium, Vitamin D and Fluoride.* National Academy Press, Washington, DC, 432 pp.

Food and Nutrition Board. (2000). *Dietary Reference Intakes for Thiamin, Riboflavin, Niacin, Vitamin B_6, Folate, Vitamin B_{12}, Pantothenic Acid, Biotin and Choline.* National Academy Press, Washington, DC, 564 pp.

Food and Nutrition Board. (2000). *Dietary Reference Intakes for Vitamin C, Vitamin E, Selenium and Carotenoids,* National Academy Press, Washington, DC, 506 pp.

Food and Nutrition Board. (2001). *Dietary Reference Intakes for Vitamin A, Vitamin K, Arsenic, Boron, Chromium, Copper, Iodine, Iron, Manganese, Molybdenum, Nickel, Silicon, Vanadium and Zinc,* National Academy Press, Washington, DC, 773 pp.

Food and Nutrition Board. (2003). *Dietary Reference Intakes: Applications in Dietary Planning.* National Academy Press, Washington, DC, 237 pp.

Food and Nutrition Board. (2003). *Dietary Reference Intakes: Guiding Principles for Nutrition Labeling and Fortification.* National Academy Press, Washington, DC, 205 pp.

Gonzales, C. A. (2006). Nutrition and cancer: The Current epidemiological evidence. *Br. J. Nutr.* **96**, S42–S45.

Hollis, B. W. (2005). Circulating 25-hydroxyvitamin D levels indicative of vitamin D sufficiency: Implications for establishing a new effective dietary intakes recommendation for vitamin D. *J. Nutr.* **135**, 317–322.

Joint WHO/FAO Consultation. (2002). *Diet, Nutrition and the Prevention of Chronic Diseases.* World Health Organization, Geneva, 149 pp.

Joint WHO/FAO Expert Consultation. (2001). *Human Vitamin and Mineral Requirements.* Food and Agriculture Organization, Rome, 286 pp.

Murphy, S. (2006). Dietary Standards in the United States, Chapter 63 in *Present Knowledge in Nutrition*, 9th ed., vol. II (B. A. Bowman and R. M. Russell, eds.), pp. 859–875, ILSI, Washington, DC.

Murphy, S. (2006). The Recommended Dietary Allowance (RDA) should not be abandoned: An individual is *both* an individual and a member of a group. *Nutr. Rev.* **64,** 313–318.

Taylor, C. L., Albert, J., Weisell, R., and Nishida, C. (2006). International Dietary Standards: FAO and WHO, Chapter 64 in *Present Knowledge in Nutrition*, 9th ed. vol. II (B. A. Bowman and R. M. Russell, eds.), pp. 876–887. ILSI, Washington, DC.

Walter, P., Hornig, D. H., and Moser, U. (eds.) (2001). *Functions of Vitamins Beyond Recommended Daily Allowances.* Karger, Basel, 214 pp.

Weaver, C. M., and Fleet, J. C. (2004). Vitamin D requirements: Current and future. *Am. J. Clin. Nutr.* **80**, 1735S–1739S.

Weaver, C., Nicklas, T., and Britten, P. (2005). The 2005 Dietary Guidelines Advisory Committee report. *Nutr. Today* **40,** 102–107.

Yates, A. A. (2006). Dietary Reference Intakes: Rationale and Applications, Chapter 104 in *Modern Nutrition in Health and Disease*, 10th ed. (M. E. Shils, M. Shike, B. Caballero, and R. Cousins, eds.), pp. 1655–1672. Lippincott, New York.

Yates, A. A. (2006). Which dietary reference intake is best suited to serve as the basis for nutrition labeling for daily values? *J. Nutr.* **136**, 2457–2462.

Vitamin Safety

Nutriment is both food and poison. The dosage makes it either poison or remedy.
—Paracelsus

I.	Uses of Vitamins above Required Levels	503
II.	Hazards of Excessive Vitamin Intakes	504
III.	Signs of Hypervitaminoses	505
IV.	Safe Intakes of Vitamins	510
	Study Questions and Exercises	513
	Recommended Reading	514

Anchoring Concepts

1. Vitamins are typically used in human feeding, in animal diets, and in treating certain clinical conditions at levels in excess of their requirements.
2. Several of the vitamins, most notably vitamins A and D, can produce adverse physiological effects when consumed in excessive amounts.

Learning Objectives

1. To understand the concept of upper safe use level as used with respect to the vitamins.
2. To understand the margins of safety above their respective requirements for intakes of each of the vitamins.
3. To understand the factors affecting vitamin toxicities.
4. To understand the signs/symptoms of vitamin toxicities in humans and animals.

Vocabulary

Carotenodermia
Hypervitaminosis
Lowest observed adverse effect level (LOAEL)
Margin of safety
No observed adverse effect level (NOAEL)
Range of safe intake
Reference dose (R_fD)
Safety index (SI)
Toxic threshold
Tolerable Upper Intake Limit (UL)

I. Uses of Vitamins above Required Levels

Typical Uses Exceed Requirements

Most normal diets that include varieties of foods can be expected to provide supplies of vitamins that meet those levels required to prevent clinical signs of deficiencies. In addition, most intentional uses of vitamins are designed to exceed those requirements for most individuals. Indeed, that is the principle by which vitamin allowances are set. Thus, the formulation of diets, the planning of meals, the vitamin fortification of foods, and the designing of vitamin supplements are all done to provide vitamins at levels contributing to total intakes that exceed the requirements of most individuals by some **margin of safety**. This approach minimizes the probability of producing vitamin deficiencies in populations.

Clinical Conditions Requiring Elevated Doses

Some clinical conditions require the use of vitamin supplements at levels greater than those normally used to accommodate the usual margins of safety.

503

These include specific vitamin deficiency disorders[1] and certain rare inherited metabolic defects.[2] In such cases, vitamins are prescribed at doses that far exceed requirement levels; at such pharmacologic doses, many effects may not involve physiological vitamin functions.

Other Putative Benefits of Elevated Doses

Elevated doses of vitamins are also frequently prescribed by physicians or are taken as over-the-counter supplements by affected individuals in the treatment of certain other pathological states, including neurological pains, psychosis, alopecia, anemia, asthenia, premenstrual tension, carpal tunnel syndrome, and prevention of the common cold. Although the efficacies of vitamin supplementation in most of these conditions remain untested in double-blind clinical trials, vitamin prophylaxis and/or therapy for at least some conditions is perceived as effective by many people in the medical community as well as in the general public. For certain groups, such as athletes, this view supports the widespread use of oral vitamin supplements at dosages greater than 50–100 times the Recommended Daily Allowances (RDAs).[3]

II. Hazards of Excessive Vitamin Intakes

Nonlinear Risk Responses to Vitamin Dosages

The risks of adverse effects (toxicity) of the vitamins, like those of any other potentially toxic compounds, are functions of dose level. In general, the risk–dosage function is curvilinear, indicating a **toxic threshold** for vitamin dosage at some level greater than the requirement for that vitamin. Thus, a dosage increment exists between the level required to prevent deficiency and that sufficient to produce toxicity. That increment, the **range of safe intake**, is

bounded on the low-dosage side by the allowance, and on the high-dosage side by the upper safe limit, each of which is set on the basis of similar considerations of risk of adverse effects within the population (Fig. 22-1).

Factors Affecting Vitamin Toxicity

Several factors can affect the toxicity of any vitamin. These include the route of exposure, the dose regimen (number of doses and intervals between doses), the general health of the subject, and potential effects of food and drugs. For example, parenteral routes of vitamin administration may increase the toxic potential of high vitamin doses, as the normal routes of controlled absorption and hepatic first-pass metabolism may be circumvented. Large single doses of the water-soluble vitamins are rarely toxic, as they are generally rapidly excreted, thus minimally affecting tissue reserves; however, repeated multiple doses of these compounds can produce adverse effects. In contrast, single large doses of the fat-soluble vitamins can produce large tissue stores that can steadily release toxic amounts of the vitamin thereafter. Some disease states, such as those involving malabsorption, can reduce the potential for vitamin toxicity; however, most increase that

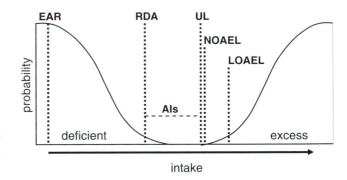

Fig. 22-1. Vitamin safety follows a biphasic dose–response curve: just as very low intakes of vitamins can produce deficiency disorders, very high intakes can produce adverse effects.

---

[1] The most commonly encountered vitamin deficiency disorders, particularly in the developing world, are xerophthalmia, rickets, scurvy, beriberi, pellagra, and disorders related to excessive alcohol consumption (polyneuritis, encephalopathy).

[2] Examples are vitamin B_6-responsive cystathionase deficiency, vitamin B_{12}-responsive transcobalamin II deficiency, and biotin-responsive biotinidase deficiency. Other examples are given in Chapter 4.

[3] Several studies have shown that athletes and their coaches generally believe that athletes require higher levels of vitamins than do nonathletes. This attitude appears to affect their behavior, as athletes use vitamin (and mineral) supplements with greater frequency than the general population. One study found that 84% of international Olympic competitors used vitamin supplements. Despite this widespread belief, it remains unclear whether any of the vitamins at levels of intake greater than RDAs can affect athletic performance.

potential by compromising the subject's ability to metabolize and excrete the vitamin,[4] or by rendering the subject particularly susceptible to **hypervitaminosis**.[5] Foods and some drugs can reduce the absorption of certain vitamins, thus reducing their toxicities.

III. Signs of Hypervitaminoses

The signs of intoxication for each vitamin vary with the species affected and the time-course of overexposure (Tables 22-1 and 22-2). Nevertheless, certain signs or syndromes are characteristic for each vitamin:

(Text Continues on Page 508)

Table 22-1. Signs and symptoms of vitamin toxicities in humans

Vitamin	Children	Adults
Vitamin A	*Acute toxicity:* Anorexia, bulging fontanelles, lethargy, high intracranial fluid pressure, irritability, nausea, vomiting	*Acute toxicity:* Abdominal pain, anorexia, blurred vision, lethargy, headache, hypercalcemia, irritability, muscular weakness, nausea, vomiting, peripheral neuritis, skin desquamation
	Chronic toxicity: Alopecia, anorexia, bone pain, bulging fontanelles, cheilitis, craniotabes, hepatomegaly, hyperostosis, photophobia, premature epiphyseal closure, pruritus, skin desquamation, erythema	*Chronic toxicity:* Alopecia, anorexia, ataxia, bone pain, cheilitis, conjunctivitis, diarrhea, diplopia, dry mucous membranes, dysuria, edema, high CSF pressure, fever, headache, hepatomegaly, hyperostosis, insomnia, irritability, lethargy, menstrual abnormalities, muscular pain and weakness, nausea, vomiting, polydypsia, splenomegaly, weight loss
Vitamin D	Anorexia, diarrhea, hypercalcemia, irritability, lassitude, muscular weakness, neurological abnormalities, polydypsia, polyuria, poor weight gain, renal impairment	Anorexia, bone demineralization, constipation, hypercalcemia, muscular weakness and pain, nausea, vomiting, polyuria, renal calculi
Vitamin E	No adverse effects reported	Mild gastrointestinal distress, some nausea, coagulopathies in patients receiving anticonvulsants
Vitamin K[a]	No adverse effects reported	No adverse effects reported
Vitamin C	No adverse effects reported	Gastrointestinal distress, diarrhea, oxaluria
Thiamin[b]	No adverse effects reported	Headache, muscular weakness, paralysis, cardiac arrhythmia, convulsions, allergic reactions
Riboflavin	No adverse effects reported	No adverse effects reported
Niacin	No adverse effects reported	Vessel dilation, itching, headache, anorexia, liver damage, jaundice, cardiac arrhythmia
Vitamin B$_6$	No adverse effects reported	Neuropathy, skin lesions
Pantothenic acid	No adverse effects reported	Diarrhea[c]
Biotin	No adverse effects reported	No adverse effects reported
Folate	No adverse effects reported	Allergic reactions[c]
Vitamin B$_{12}$	No adverse effects reported	Allergic reactions[c]

[a]Adverse effects observed only for menadione; phylloquinone and the menaquinones appear to have negligible toxicities.
[b]Adverse effects have been observed only when the vitamin was administered parenterally; none have been observed when it has been given orally.
[c]This sign has been observed in only a few cases.

---

[4] For example, individuals with liver damage (e.g., alcoholic cirrhosis, viral hepatitis) have increased plasma levels of free (unbound) retinol and a higher incidence of adverse reactions to large doses of vitamin A.

[5] For example, patients with nephrocalcinosis are particularly susceptible to hypervitaminosis D.

Table 22-2. Signs of vitamin toxicities in animals

Vitamin	Sign	Species
Vitamin A	Alopecia	Rat, mouse
	Anorexia	Cat, cattle, chicken, turkey
	Cartilage abnormalities	Rabbit
	Convulsions	Monkey
	Elevated heart rate	Cattle
	Fetal malformations	Hamster, monkey, mouse, rat
	Hepatomegaly	Rat
	Gingivitis	Cat
	Irritability	Cat
	Lethargy	Cat, monkey
	Reduced CSF pressure	Cattle, goat, pig
	Poor growth	Chicken, pig, turkey
	Skeletal abnormalities	Cat, cattle, chicken, dog, duck, mouse, pig, rabbit, rat, turkey, horse
Vitamin D[a]	Anorexia	Cattle, chicken, fox, pig, rat
	Bone abnormalities	Pig, sheep
	Cardiovascular calcinosis	Cattle, dog, fox, horse, monkey, mouse, pig, rat, sheep, rabbit
	Renal calcinosis	Cattle, chicken, dog, fox, horse, monkey, mouse, pig, rat, sheep, turkey
	Cardiac dysfunction	Cattle, pig
	Hypercalcemia	Cattle, chicken, dog, fox, horse, monkey, mouse, pig, rat, sheep, trout
	Hyperphosphatemia	Horse, pig
	Hypertension	Dog
	Myopathy	Fox, pig
	Poor growth, weight loss	Catfish, chicken, horse, mouse, pig, rat
	Lethality	Cattle
Vitamin E	Atherosclerotic lesions	Rabbit
	Bone demineralization	Chicken, rat
	Cardiomegaly	Rat
	Hepatomegaly	Chicken
	Hyperalbuminemia	Rat
	Hypertriglyceridemia	Rat
	Hypocholesterolemia	Rat
	Impaired muscular function	Chicken
	Increased hepatic vitamin A	Chicken, rat
	Increased prothrombin time	Chicken
	Reduced adrenal weight	Rat
	Poor growth	Chicken
	Increased hematocrit	Rat
	Reticulocytosis	Chicken
	Splenomegaly	Rat
Vitamin K[b,c]	Anemia[c]	Dog
	Renal failure[c]	Horse
	Lethality	Chicken,[c,d] mouse,[c,d] rat[c]

Table 22-2.   Signs of vitamin toxicities in animals—Cont'd

Vitamin	Sign	Species
Vitamin C	Anemia	Mink
	Bone demineralization	Guinea pig
	Decreased circulating thyroid hormone	Rat
	Liver congestion	Guinea pig
	Oxaluria	Rat
Thiamin	Respiratory distress[e]	Rat
	Cyanosis[e]	Rat
	Epileptiform convulsions[e]	Rat
Riboflavin	No adverse effects reported for oral doses	
	Lethality[f]	Rat
Niacin	Impaired growth	Chicken (embryo)
	Developmental abnormalities	Chicken (embryo), mouse (fetus)
	Liver damage	Mouse
	Mucocutaneous lesions	Chicken
	Myocardial damage	Mouse
	Decreased weight gain[g]	Chicken
	Lethality	Chicken (embryo),[f] mouse[f,h]
Vitamin B$_6$	Anorexia	Dog
	Ataxia	Dog, rat
	Convulsions	Rat
	Lassitude	Dog
	Muscular weakness	Dog
	Neurologic impairment	Dog
	Vomiting	Dog
	Lethality[h]	Mouse, rat
Pantothenic acid	No adverse effects reported for oral doses	
	Lethality[d]	Rat
Biotin	No adverse effects reported for oral doses	
	Irregular estrus[e]	Rat
	Fetal resorption[e]	Rat
Folate	No adverse effects reported for oral doses	
	Epileptiform convulsions[e]	Rat
	Renal hypertrophy[e]	Rat
Vitamin B$_{12}$	No adverse effects reported for oral doses	
	Irregular estrus[e]	Rat
	Fetal resorption[e]	Rat
	Reduced fetal weights[e]	Rat

[a]Vitamin D$_3$ is much more toxic than vitamin D$_2$.
[b]Only menadione produces adverse effects; phylloquinone and the menaquinones have negligible toxicities.
[c]These effects observed after parenteral administration of the vitamin.
[d]These effects observed after oral administration of the vitamin.
[e]These signs have been observed only when the vitamin was administered parenterally.
[f]Lethality has been reported for parenterally administered doses of the vitamin.
[g]Nicotinamide is more toxic than nicotinic acid.
[h]Lethality has been reported for orally administered doses of the vitamin.

Vitamin A

The potential for vitamin A intoxication is greater than the potentials for other hypervitaminoses, as its range of safe intake is relatively small. For humans, intakes as low as 25 times the RDA are thought to be potentially intoxicating, although actual cases of hypervitaminosis A have been very rare[6] at chronic doses less than about 9000 μg of retinol equivalents (RE) per day. The consumption of 25,000–50,000 IU/day for periods of several months has been associated with multiple adverse effects. Infants appear to be especially susceptible to hypervitaminosis A, signs of which have been reported in individuals consuming 2100 IU/100 kcal (three to eight times the RDA). The prophylaxis and treatment of xerophthalmia with large doses of vitamin A (100,000 IU for children under 1 year of age and 200,000 IU for others) administered semiannually has been found to produce side effects (mild nausea, vomiting, headaches) in 1–4% of cases. Acute hypervitaminosis A can occur in adults after ingestion of ≥ 500,000 IU (100 times the RDA). In animals, chronic intakes exceeding the requirement levels by 100- to 1000-fold have produced clear intoxication, and some adverse effects have been reported at intakes as low as 10 times the RDA. Ruminants appear to tolerate high intakes of vitamin A better than nonruminants, apparently owing to substantial destruction of the vitamin by the rumen microflora. The most frequently observed signs are loss of appetite, loss of weight or reduced growth, skeletal malformations, spontaneous fractures, and internal hemorrhages; most signs of hypervitaminosis A can be reversed by discontinuing excess exposure to the vitamin.

That retinoids can be toxic to maternally exposed embryos raises concerns about the safety of high-level vitamin A supplementation for pregnant animals and humans. This is especially true for 13-*cis*-retinoic acid, which can cause severe disruption of cephalic neural crest cell activity that results in birth defects characterized by craniofacial, central nervous system, cardiovascular, and thymus malformations. Similar effects have been induced in animals by high doses of retinol, all-*trans*-retinoic acid, or 13-*cis*-retinoic acid. Fetal malformations have been reported in cases of oral use of all-*trans*-retinoic acid in treating *acne vulgaris* and of regular prenatal vitamin A supplements

in humans; these have generally been linked to daily exposures at or above 20,000–25,000 IU. A retrospective epidemiologic study reported an increased risk of birth defects associated with an apparent threshold exposure of about 10,000 IU of preformed vitamin A per day. However, the elevated risk of birth defects was observed in a small group of women whose average intake of the vitamin exceeded 21,000 IU/day.

The toxicities of carotenoids are considered low, and circumstantial evidence suggests that for β-carotene intakes of as much as 30 mg/day are without side effects other than **carotenodermia**, the accumulation of the carotenoid in the skin. While a regular daily dose of 20 mg of β-carotene was found to increase lung cancer mortality among smokers, it is not clear whether that effect was due to toxic properties of the carotenoid per se.

Vitamin D

Because they are stored in adipose tissue, vitamins D_2 and D_3 have relatively high potentials for producing systemic toxicity after single overdoses. Intakes as low as 50 times the RDA have been reported to be toxic to humans. Children appear to be particularly sensitive to hypervitaminosis; cases of toxicity have been reported resulting from the use of large doses of the vitamin for prophylaxis or treatment of rickets. Studies with animals indicate that vitamin D_3 is 10 to 20 times more toxic than vitamin D_2,[7] apparently because it is more readily metabolized than the latter vitamer to 25-hydroxyvitamin D (25-OH-D), which is thought to produce the lesions that characterize hypervitaminosis D. Those lesions (hypercalcemia, calcinosis) suggest that hypervitaminosis D involves extremes of the normal physiologic functions of calcium homeostasis for which vitamin D is essential. Accordingly, hypervitaminosis D can be exacerbated by high intakes of calcium and phosphorus, and reduced by intakes of low calcium levels or of calcium-chelating agents.

Vitamin E

The toxic potential of vitamin E is very low; intakes of 100 (or more) times the typical allowance levels are tolerated without adverse reactions by all species

---

[6] According to Bendich (*Am. J. Clin. Nutr.* [1989]. **49**, 358), fewer than 10 cases per year were reported in 1976–1987. Several of those occurred in individuals with concurrent hepatic damage due to drug exposure, viral hepatitis, or protein-energy malnutrition.

[7] That is, vitamin D_3 can produce effects comparable to those of vitamin D_2 at doses representing only 5–10% of vitamin D_2.

tested. Substantial clinical experience has shown that daily intakes of up to 2 g for several years or as much as 3.5 g for several months have produced few or no ill effects in healthy people. Studies with animals indicate that excessive dosages of tocopherols exert most, if not all, of their adverse effects by antagonizing the utilization of the other fat-soluble vitamins, probably at the level of their common micelle-dependent absorption. The scant data available indicate that vitamin E is safe for most animals at dietary levels up to 100 times their typical dietary allowances.

Vitamin K

The toxic potential of the naturally occurring forms of vitamin K are negligible. Phylloquinone exhibits no adverse effects when administered to animals in massive doses by any route; the menaquinones are similarly thought to have little, if any, toxicity. The synthetic vitamer menadione, when administered parenterally, can produce fatal anemia, hyperbilirubinemia, and severe jaundice; however, its toxic threshold appears to be at least 1000 times the allowance levels. The horse appears to be particularly vulnerable to menadione toxicity. Parenteral doses of 2–8 mg/kg have been found to be lethal in that species, whereas the parenteral LD_{50}[8] values for most other species are an order of magnitude greater than that.

Vitamin C

Although it is often cited as a concern, there is no solid evidence for so-called systemic conditioning or rebound scurvy, that is, the induction of ascorbic acid degradation sufficient to lead to a deficiency after stopping the administration of high-level doses of the vitamin. In fact, the only adverse effects of large doses of vitamin C that have been consistently observed in humans are gastrointestinal disturbances and diarrhea occurring at levels of intake nearly 20–80 times the RDAs. Such intakes have been shown to produce slight increases in urinary oxalic acid excretion. However, it is not clear whether such low-magnitude effects, which are still within normal variation, are associated with increased risks of forming urinary calculi.[9] Concern has also been expressed that excess

ascorbic acid may be prooxidative or may enhance iron absorption and ferritin synthesis, which has been associated with increased risk of heart disease in men; such effects are not supported by clinical trial results. Dietary vitamin C concentrations 100–1000 times the allowance levels appear safe for most species.

Thiamin

The toxic potential of thiamin appears to be low, particularly when it is administered orally. Parenteral doses of the vitamin at 100–200 times the RDAs have been reported to cause intoxication in humans, characterized by headache, convulsions, muscular weakness, paralysis, cardiac arrhythmia, and allergic reactions. The few animal studies to date indicate that thiamin HCl, administered parenterally at doses 1000 times the allowance levels, can suppress the respiratory center of the brain, producing dyspnea, cyanosis, and epileptiform convulsions.

Riboflavin

High oral doses of riboflavin are very safe, probably owing to the relatively poor absorption of the vitamin at high levels. No adverse effects in humans have been reported. Studies with animals indicate that doses as great as 100 times the allowance levels have negligible risks of toxicity.

Niacin

In humans, small doses (10 mg) of nicotinic acid (but not nicotinamide) can cause flushing, particularly if taken on an empty stomach, although this effect is not associated with other seriously adverse reactions. At high dosages (2–4 g/day), nicotinic acid can cause vasodilation, itching, nausea, vomiting, headaches, and, less frequently, skin lesions; nicotinamide, on the other hand, only rarely produces these reactions. The higher dosage form of the vitamin, therefore, is recommended for medical use. Many patients have taken daily oral doses of 200 mg to 10 g of nicotinamide for periods of years with only occasional side effects at the higher dosages (skin rashes, hyperpigmentation, reduced glucose tolerance in diabetics, some liver dysfunction). Nicotinamide

---

[8] The LD_{50} value is a useful parameter indicative of the degree of toxicity of a compound. It is defined as the lethal dose for 50% of a reference population and is calculated from experimental dose–survival data using the probit analysis.

[9] There is also some question as to whether oxalate may have been produced artifactually by the analytical procedure used in these reports.

doses 50–100 times the RDAs have not been associated with these effects and can therefore be considered safe for most people. Available information on the tolerances of animals for niacin is scant but suggests that daily doses greater than 350–500 mg of nicotinic acid equivalents per kilogram body weight can be toxic.

Vitamin B$_6$

Daily doses as great as 500 mg of vitamin B$_6$ have been used for humans (treatment of premenstrual tension in women) for periods of several months without significant adverse effects.[10] However, larger dosages (500 mg to 6 g per day) have produced reversible sensory neuropathies after chronic use. It would appear, therefore, that most people can safely use levels as great as 100 times the RDAs. Substantial information concerning the safety of large doses of vitamin B$_6$ in animals is available for only the dog and the rat. That information indicates that doses less than 1000 times the allowance levels are safe for those species and, by inference, for other animal species.

Pantothenic Acid

Pantothenic acid is generally regarded as being nontoxic. No ill effects have been reported for any species given the vitamin orally, although parenteral administration of very large amounts (e.g., 1 g per kg body weight) of the calcium salt have been shown to be lethal to rats.[11] A very few reports indicate diarrhea occurring in humans consuming 10–20 g of the vitamin per day. Thus, it appears that pantothenic acid is safe for humans at doses at least 100 times the RDAs; for animals, doses as great as 1000 times the allowance levels can be considered safe.

Biotin

Biotin is generally regarded as being nontoxic. Adverse effects of large doses of biotin have not been reported in humans or animals given the vitamin orally. Limited data suggest that biotin is safe for most people at doses as great as 500 times the RDAs and for animals at probably more than 1000 times allowance levels.

Folate

Folate is generally regarded as being nontoxic. Adverse reactions to large doses of it have not been observed in animals. Other than a few cases of apparent allergic reactions, the only proposed adverse effect in humans (interference with the enteric absorption of zinc) is not supported with adequate data. Dosages of 400 mg of folate per day for several months have been tolerated without side effects in humans, indicating that levels at least as great as 2000 times the RDAs are safe. Because no adverse effects of folate in animals have ever been reported, it would appear that similarly wide ranges of intakes are also safe for animals. Nevertheless, concern has been expressed that the use of folate may mask pernicious anemia, thus allowing vitamin B$_{12}$ deficiency to go undetected in its early stages during the progression of neurologic disease; this effect appears to be significant at doses exceeding about 5 mg.

Vitamin B$_{12}$

Vitamin B$_{12}$ is generally regarded as being nontoxic.[12] A few cases of apparent allergic reactions have been reported in humans; otherwise no adverse reactions have been reported for humans or animals given high levels of the vitamin. Upper safe limits of vitamin B$_{12}$ use are, therefore, highly speculative; it appears that doses at least as great as 1000 times the RDAs/allowances are safe for humans and animals.

IV. Safe Intakes of Vitamins

Ranges of Safe Intakes

The vitamins fall into four categories of relative toxicity at levels of exposure above typical allowances:

- *Greatest toxic potential*   Vitamin A, vitamin D
- *Moderate toxic potential*   Niacin
- *Low toxic potential*   Vitamin E, vitamin C, thiamin, riboflavin, vitamin B$_6$
- *Negligible toxic potential*   Vitamin K, pantothenic acid, biotin, folate, vitamin B$_{12}$, carotenes

Under circumstances of vitamin use at levels appreciably greater than the standard allowances (RDAs for humans, or recommended use levels for animals), prudence dictates giving special consideration to those vitamins with greatest potentials for toxicity (those in the first two or three categories). In practice, it may only be necessary to consider the most potentially toxic vitamins of the first category (vitamins A and D).

---

[10] A transient dependency condition was reported.

[11] Ten times that level (i.e., 10 g/kg body weight) produced no adverse effects in rats.

[12] Indeed, low toxicity would be predicted for this vitamin on the basis of its poor absorption.

Quantifying Safe Intakes

There is no standard algorithm for quantifying the ranges of safe intakes of vitamins, but an approach developed for environmental substances that cause systemic toxicities has recently been employed for this purpose with nutritionally essential inorganic elements. This approach involves the imputation of an acceptable daily intake (ADI)[13] based on the application of a safety factor (SF)[14] to an experimentally determined highest **no observed adverse effect level (NOAEL)** of exposure to the substance. In the absence of sufficient data to ascertain an NOAEL, an experimentally determined **lowest observed adverse effect level (LOAEL)** is used:

$$ADI = \frac{LOAEL}{SF}$$

An extension of this approach is to express the comparative safety of nutrients using a **safety index (SI)**. This index is analogous to the therapeutic index (TI) used for drugs; it is the ratio of the minimum toxic dose and the recommended intake (RI) derived from the RDA:

$$SI = \frac{LOAEL}{RI}$$

Hathcock[15] used this approach to express quantitatively the safety limits of four vitamins for humans (Table 22-3).

The Dietary Reference Intakes (DRIs) of the Food and Nutrition Board (1997–2001) addressed the safety of high doses of essential nutrients with the **Tolerable Upper Intake Limit (UL).** The UL is defined as the highest level of daily intake that is likely to pose *no* risks of adverse health effects to almost all healthy individuals in a each age–sex specific demographic subgroup. In this context, "adverse effect" is defined as any significant alteration in structure or function. It should be noted that the Food and Nutrition Board chose to use the term *tolerable intake* to avoid implying possible beneficial effects of

Table 22-3. Use of a safety index to quantitate the toxic potentials of selected vitamins for humans

Parameter	Vitamin A	Vitamin C	Niacin	Vitamin B$_6$
RDI^a	3,300 IU	60 mg	20 mg	2 mg
Tentative LOAEL	25,000 IU	2,000 mg	500 mg	50 mg
SI	7.58	33.3	25	25

^{a}The greatest RDA for individuals ≥4 years of age, excluding pregnant and lactating women.
Source: Hathcock, J. (1993). *J. Nutr. Rev.* **51**, 278–285.

intakes greater than the RDA.[16] The ULs are based on chronic intakes.

The ULs are derived through a multistep process of hazard identification and dose–response evaluation:

1. *Hazard identification* involving the systematic evaluation of all information pertaining to adverse effects of the nutrient
2. *Dose–response assessment* involving the determination of the relationship between level of nutrient intake and incidence/severity of adverse effects
3. *Intake assessment* involving the evaluation of the distribution of nutrient intakes in the general population
4. *Risk characterization* involving the expression of conclusions from the previous steps in terms of the fraction of the exposed population having nutrients in excess of the estimated UL.

In practice, ULs are set at less than the respective LOAELs and no greater than the NOAELs (Fig. 22-2) from which they are derived, subject to uncertainty factors (UFs) used to characterize the level of uncertainty associated with extrapolating from observed data to the general population.[17] The ULs for the vitamins are presented in Table 22-4. Recommended upper safe intakes for vitamins by animals are present in Table 22-5.

---

[13] The U.S. Environmental Protection Agency has replaced the ADI with the **reference dose (R$_f$D),** a name the agency considers to be more value neutral, that is, avoiding any implication that the exposure is completely safe or acceptable.

[14] SF values are selected according to the quality and generalizability of the reported data in the case selected as the reference standard. Higher values (e.g., 100) may be used if animal data are extrapolated to humans, whereas lower values (e.g., 1 or 3) may be used if solid clinical data are available.

[15] Hathcock, J. (1993). *Nutr. Rev.* **51**, 278–285.

[16] See Food and Nutrition Board (1998). *Dietary Reference Intakes: A Risk Assessment Model for Establishing Upper Intake Levels for Nutrients*, National Academy Press, Washington, DC, 71 pp.

[17] Small UFs (close to 1) are used in cases where little population variability is expected for the adverse effects, where extrapolation from primary data is not believed to underpredict the average human response, and where a LOAEL is available. Larger UFs (as high as 10) are used in cases where the expected variability is great, where extrapolation is necessary from primary animal data, and where a LOAEL is not available and a NOAEL value must be used.

Table 22-4. Food and nutrition board tolerable upper intake limits (ULs) for vitamins

Age (years) or conditions	Vitamin A (μg^a)	Vitamin D (μg)	Vitamin E (mg^b)	Vitamin K (μg)	Vitamin C (mg)	Thiamin (mg)	Riboflavin (mg)	Niacin (mg^c)	Vitamin B$_6$ (μg)	Pantothenic acid (μg)	Biotin (μg)	Folate (μg^d)	Vitamin B$_{12}$ (μg)
Infants													
0–11 monts	600	25	–^{e}	–^{e}	–^{e}	–^{e}	–^{e}	–^{e}	–^{e}	–^{e}	–^{e}	–^{e}	–^{e}
Children													
1–3 yrs	600	50	200	–^{e}	400	–^{e}	–^{e}	10	–^{e}	–^{e}	–^{e}	300	–^{e}
4–8 yrs	600	50	300	–^{e}	650	–^{e}	–^{e}	15	–^{e}	–^{e}	–^{e}	400	–^{e}
Males													
9–13 yrs	1700	50	600	–^{e}	1200	–^{e}	–^{e}	20	–^{e}	–^{e}	–^{e}	600	–^{e}
14–18 yrs	2800	50	800	–^{e}	1800	–^{e}	–^{e}	30	–^{e}	–^{e}	–^{e}	800	–^{e}
19+ yrs	3000	50	1000	–^{e}	2000	–^{e}	–^{e}	35	–^{e}	–^{e}	–^{e}	1000	–^{e}
Females													
9–13 yrs	1700	50	600	–^{e}	1200	–^{e}	–^{e}	20	–^{e}	–^{e}	–^{e}	600	–^{e}
14–18 yrs	2800	50	800	–^{e}	1800	–^{e}	–^{e}	30	–^{e}	–^{e}	–^{e}	800	–^{e}
19+ yrs	3000	50	1000	–^{e}	2000	–^{e}	–^{e}	35	–^{e}	–^{e}	–^{e}	1000	–^{e}
Pregnancy													
=18 yrs	2800	50	800	–^{e}	1800	–^{e}	–^{e}	30	–^{e}	–^{e}	–^{e}	800	–^{e}
19+ yrs	2800	50	1000	–^{e}	2000	–^{e}	–^{e}	35	–^{e}	–^{e}	–^{e}	1000	–^{e}
Lactation													
=18 yrs	2800	50	800	–^{e}	1800	–^{e}	–^{e}	30	–^{e}	–^{e}	–^{e}	800	–^{e}
19+ yrs	3000	50	1000	–^{e}	2000	–^{e}	–^{e}	35	–^{e}	–^{e}	–^{e}	1000	–^{e}

^{a}Retinol equivalents.
^{b}α-tocopherol.
^{c}Niacin equivalents.
^{d}Folate equivalents.
^{e}UL not established.

Sources: Food and Nutrition Board (1997). *Dietary Reference Intakes for Calcium, Phosphorus, Magnesium, Vitamin D and Fluoride.* National Academy Press, Washington, DC, 432 pp.
Food and Nutrition Board (2000). *Dietary Reference Intakes for Thiamin, Riboflavin, Niacin, Vitamin B$_6$, Folate, Vitamin B$_{12}$, Pantothenic Acid, Biotin and Choline.* National Academy Press, Washington, DC, 564 pp.; Food and Nutrition Board (2000), *Dietary Reference Intakes for Vitamin C, Vitamin E, Selenium and Carotenoids,* National Academy Press, Washington, DC, 506 pp.; Food and Nutrition Board (2001). *Dietary Reference Intakes for Vitamin A, Vitamin K, Arsenic, Boron, Chromium, Copper, Iodine, Iron, Manganese, Molybdenum, Nickel, Silicon, Vanadium and Zinc,* National Academy Press, Washington, DC, 773 pp.

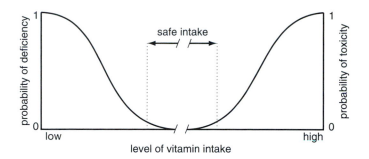

Fig. 22-2. Conceptual basis for tolerable upper intake limit (UL) in DRI system.

Table 22-5. Recommended upper safe intakes of the vitamins for animals

Vitamin	× allowance[a]
High toxic potential	
Vitamin A	10^b–30^c
Vitamin D	10–20^d
Moderate toxic potential	
Niacin[e]	50–100
Low toxic potential	
Vitamin E	100
Vitamin C	100–1000
Thiamin	500
Riboflavin	100–500
Vitamin B_6	100–1000
Negligible toxic potential	
Vitamin K[f]	1000
Pantothenic acid	1000
Biotin	1000
Folate	1000
Vitamin B_{12}	1000

[a]Based on the Estimated Vitamin Requirements of Domestic and Laboratory Animals (from National Research Council reports); see Chapter 21.
[b]For nonruminant species.
[c]For ruminant species.
[d]Vitamin D_3 is more toxic than vitamin D_2.
[e]Nicotinamide is more toxic than nicotinic acid.
[f]Only menadione has significant (low) toxicity.

Study Questions and Exercises

1. Which vitamins are most likely to present potential for hazards for humans?

2. For each vitamin, determine the range of safe intakes (which satisfy needs without risking toxicity) for humans or animals, and identify the most useful parameters by which that safety can be ascertained.

3. Identify treatments that can reduce the manifestations of vitamin toxicities.

4. Use specific examples to discuss the relationship of the toxic potential of vitamins to their absorption and metabolic disposition.

Recommended Reading

Food and Nutrition Board. (1997). *Dietary Reference Intakes for Calcium, Phosphorus, Magnesium, Vitamin D and Fluoride*. National Academy Press, Washington, DC, 432 pp.

Food and Nutrition Board. (1998). *Dietary Reference Intakes: A Risk Assessment Model for Establishing Upper Intake Levels for Nutrients*. National Academy Press, Washington, DC, 71 pp.

Food and Nutrition Board. (2000). *Dietary Reference Intakes for Thiamin, Riboflavin, Niacin, Vitamin B_6, Folate, Vitamin B_{12}, Pantothenic Acid, Biotin and Choline*. National Academy Press, Washington, DC, 564 pp.

Food and Nutrition Board. (2000). *Dietary Reference Intakes for Vitamin C, Vitamin E, Selenium and Carotenoids*. National Academy Press, Washington, DC, 506 pp.

Food and Nutrition Board. (2001). *Dietary Reference Intakes for Vitamin A, Vitamin K, Arsenic, Boron, Chromium, Copper, Iodine, Iron, Manganese, Molybdenum, Nickel, Silicon, Vanadium and Zinc*. National Academy Press, Washington, DC, 773 pp.

Food and Nutrition Board. (2003). *Dietary Reference Intakes: Applications in Dietary Planning*. National Academy Press, Washington, DC, 237 pp.

Hathcock, J. N. (1997). Vitamins and minerals: Efficacy and safety. *Am. J. Clin. Nutr.* **66,** 427–437.

Hollis, B. W. (2005). Circulating 25-hydroxyvitamin D levels indicative of vitamin D sufficiency: Implications for establishing a new effective dietary intakes recommendation for vitamin D. *J. Nutr.* **135,** 317–322.

Joint WHO/FAO Consultation. (2002). *Diet, Nutrition and the Prevention of Chronic Diseases*. World Health Organization, Geneva, 149 pp.

Joint WHO/FAO Exepert Consultation. (2001). *Human Vitamin and Mineral Requirements*. Food and Agriculturel Organization, Rome, 286 pp.

Subcommittee on Vitamin Tolerance, Committee on Animal Nutrition, National Research Council. (1987). *Vitamin Tolerance in Animals*. National Academy Press, Washington, DC.

Walter, P., Brubacher, G., and Stähelin, H. (1989). *Elevated Dosages of Vitamins: Benefits and Hazards*. Hans Huber Publishers, Toronto, Ontario, Canada.

Yates, A. A. (2006). Dietary Reference Intakes: Rationale and Applications, Chapter 104 in *Modern Nutrition in Health and Disease*, 10th ed. (M. E. Shils, M. Shike, B. Caballero, and R. Cousins, eds.), pp. 1655–1672. Lippincott, New York.

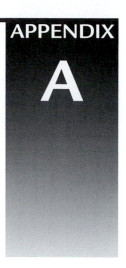

Vitamin Terminology: Past and Present

APPENDIX

A

THE NATURE of vitamin research has been such that a confusing array of names has been used in the past; many of these terms are still encountered today. In the following table, which surveys vitamin terminology, those words appearing in boldface are currently in accepted use.

Table A-I. Current and obsolete designations of vitamins and vitamin-like factors

Term	Explanation
Aneurin	Infrequently used synonym for thiamin
A-N factor	Obsolete term for the *antineuritic factor* (thiamin)
Bios factors	Obsolete terms for yeast growth factors now known to include biotin
Citrovorum factor	Infrequently used term for a naturally occurring form of folic acid (N^5-formyl-S,6,7,8-tetrahydropteroylmonoglutamic acid) that is required for the growth of *Leuconostoc citrovorum*
Extrinsic factor	Obsolete term for the antianemic activity in liver, now called vitamin B_{12}
Factor R	Obsolete term for chick antianemic factor, now known as a form of folate
Factor U	Obsolete term for chick antianemic factor, now known as a form of folate
Factor X	Obsolete term used at various times to designate the rat fertility factor, now called *vitamin E,* and the rat growth factor, now called *vitamin B_{12}*
Filtrate factor	Obsolete term for the anti-black tongue disease activity, now known to be niacin, that could be isolated from the B_2 complex by filtration through fuller's earth; also used to describe the chick antidermatitis factor, now known to be pantothenic acid, isolated from acid solutions of the B_2 complex by filtration through Fuller's earth
Flavin	Term originally used to describe the water-soluble fluorescent rat growth factors isolated from yeast and animal tissues; now a general term for isoalloxazine derivatives, including riboflavin and its active forms, FMN and FAD
Hepatoflavin	Obsolete term for the water-soluble rat growth factor, now known to be riboflavin, isolated from liver
Lactoflavin	Obsolete term for the water-soluble rat growth factor, now known to be riboflavin, isolated from whey
LLD factor	Obsolete term for the activity in liver that promoted the growth of *Lactobacillus lactis* Dorner, now known to be vitamin B_{12}
Norit eluate	Obsolete term for *Lactobacillus casei* growth promotant, a factor now known as folic acid, that could be isolated from liver and yeasts by adsorption on Norit
Ovoflavin	Obsolete term for the water-soluble rat growth factor, now known to be riboflavin, isolated from egg white

(Continued)

515

Table A-I. Current and obsolete designations of vitamins and vitamin-like factors—Cont'd

Term	Explanation
P-P factor	Obsolete term for the thermostable pellagra-preventive component, now known to be niacin, of the water-soluble B activity of yeast
Rhizopterin	Obsolete synonym for the *SLR factor,* that is, a factor from *Rhizobium* species fermentation that stimulated the growth of *Streptococcus lactis* R. (now called *S. faecalis),* which is now known to be a folate activity
SLR factor	Obsolete term for the *Streptococcus lactis* R. (now called *S. faecalis*) growth promotant later called *rhizopterin* and now known to be a folate activity
Streptogenin	A peptide, present in liver and in enzymatic hydrolysates of casein and other proteins, that promotes growth of mice and certain microorganisms (hemolytic streptococci and lactobacilli); not considered a vitamin
Vitamin A	Accepted designation of retinoids that prevent xerophthalmia and nyctalopia, and are essential for epithelial maintenance
Vitamin B	Original antiberiberi factor; now known to be a mixture of factors and designated the *vitamin B complex*
Vitamin B complex	Term introduced when it became clear that *water-soluble B* contained more than one biologically active substance (such preparations were subsequently found to be mixtures of thiamin, niacin, riboflavin, pyridoxine, and pantothenic acid); the term has contemporary lay use as a nonspecific name for all of the B-designated vitamins
Vitamin B_1	Synonym for thiamin
Vitamin B_2	Synonym for riboflavin
Vitamin B_2	Obsolete term for the thermostable second nutritional factor in yeast, which was found to be a mixture of niacin, riboflavin, pyridoxine, and pantothenic acid
Vitamin B_3	Infrequently used synonym for pantothenic acid; was also used for nicotinic acid
Vitamin B_4	Unconfirmed activity preventing muscular weakness in rats and chicks; believed to be a mixture of arginine, glycine, riboflavin, and pyridoxine
Vitamin B_5	Unconfirmed growth promotant for pigeons; probably niacin
Vitamin B_6	Synonym for pyridoxine
Vitamin B_7	Unconfirmed digestive promoter for pigeons; may be a mixture; also called *vitamin I*
Vitamin B_8	Adenylic acid; no longer classified as a vitamin
Vitamin B_{10}	Growth promotant for chicks; likely a mixture of folic acid and vitamin B_{12}
Vitamin B_{11}	Apparently the same as vitamin B_{10}
Vitamin B_{12}	Accepted designation of the cobalamins (cyano- and aquacobalamins) that prevent pernicious anemia and promote growth in animals
Vitamin B_{12a}	Synonym for aquacobalamin
Vitamin B_{12b}	Synonym for hydroxocobalamin
Vitamin B_{12c}	Synonym for nitritocobalamin
Vitamin B_{13}	Synonym for orotic acid, an intermediate of pyrimidine metabolism; not considered a vitamin
Vitamin B_{l4}	Unconfirmed growth factor
Vitamin B_{15}	Synonym for pangamic acid; no proven biological value
Vitamin B_{17}	Synonym for laetrile, a cyanogenic glycoside with unsubstantiated claims of anticarcinogenic activity; not considered a vitamin
Vitamin B_c	Obsolete term for pteroylglutamic acid
Vitamin B_p	Activity preventing perosis in chicks; replaceable by choline and manganese

Table A-I. Current and obsolete designations of vitamins and vitamin-like factors—Cont'd

Term	Explanation
Vitamin B_c	Activity promoting insect growth; identified as carnitine
Vitamin B_t	Activity associated with pantothenic acid and p-aminobenzoic acid
Vitamin C	Accepted designation of the antiscorbutic factor, ascorbic acid
Vitamin C_2	Unconfirmed antipneumonia activity; also called *vitamin J*
Vitamin D	Accepted designation of the antirachitic factor (the calciferols)
Vitamin D_2	Accepted designation for ergocalciferol (a vitamin D-active substance derived from plant sterols)
Vitamin D_3	Accepted designation for cholecalciferol (a vitamin D-active substance derived from animal sterols)
Vitamin E	Accepted designation for tocopherols active in preventing myopathies and certain types of infertility in animals
Vitamin F	Obsolete term for essential fatty acids; also an abandoned term for thiamin activity
Vitamin G	Obsolete term for riboflavin activity; also an abandoned term for the pellagra-preventive factor (niacin)
Vitamin H	Obsolete term for biotin activity
Vitamin I	Mixture also formerly called *vitamin B_7*
Vitamin J	Postulated antipneumonia factor also formerly called *vitamin C_2*
Vitamin K	Accepted designation for activity preventing hypoprothrombinemic hemorrhage; shared by related naphthoquinones
Vitamin K_1	Accepted designation for phylloquinones (vitamin K-active substances produced by plants)
Vitamin K_2	Accepted designation for prenylmenaquinones (vitamin K-active substances synthesized by microorganisms and produced from other vitamers K by animals)
Vitamin K_3	Accepted designation for menadione (synthetic vitamin K-active substance not found in nature)
Vitamin L_1	Unconfirmed liver filtrate activity, probably related to anthranilic acid, proposed as necessary for lactation
Vitamin L_2	Unconfirmed yeast filtrate activity, probably related to adenosine, proposed as necessary for lactation
Vitamin M	Obsolete term for antianemic factor in yeast, now known to be pteroylglutamic acid
Vitamin N	Obsolete term for a mixture proposed to inhibit cancer
Vitamin P	Activity reducing capillary fragility, related to citrin; it is no longer classified as a vitamin
Vitamin Q	Unused designation (the letter was used to designate coenzyme Q)
Vitamin R	Obsolete term for folic acid; from Norris's chick antianemic *factor R*
Vitamin S	Chick growth activity related to the peptide streptogenin; the term was also applied to a bacterial growth activity probably related to biotin
Vitamin T	Unconfirmed group of activities isolated from termites, yeasts, or molds and reported to improve protein utilization in rats
Vitamin U	Unconfirmed activity isolated from cabbage; proposed to cure ulcers and promote bacterial growth, and may have folic acid activity
Vitamin V	Tissue-derived activity promoting bacterial growth; probably related to NAD
Wills factor	Obsolete term for the antianemic factor in yeast; now known to be a form of folate
Zoopherin	Obsolete term for a rat growth factor now known to be vitamin B_{12}

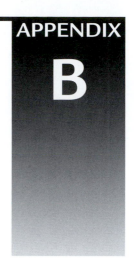

Original Reports for Case Studies

FOR THOSE researching the history of vitamins, the following reports—presented in the text as case studies—should be of interest.

Chapter 5	*Case 1*
	McLaren, D. S., Ahirajian, E., Tchalian, M., and Koury, G. (1965). Xerophthalmia in Jordan. *Am. J. Clin. Nutr.* **17,** 117–130.
	Case 2
	Wechsler, H. L. (1979). Vitamin A deficiency following small-bowel bypass surgery for obesity. *Arch. Dermatol.* **115,** 73–75.
	Case 3
	Sauberlich, H. E., Hodges, R. E., Wallace, D. L., Kolder, H., Canham, J. E., Hood, H., Racia, N., Jr., and Lowry, L. K. (1974). Vitamin A metabolism and requirements in the human studied with the use of labeled retinol. *Vitam. Horm.* **32,** 251–275.
Chapter 6	Marx, S. J., Spiegel, A. M., Brown, E. M., Gardner, D. G. R., Downs, W., Jr., Attie, M., Hamstra, A. J., and DeLuca, H. F. (1978). *J. Clin. Endocrinol. Metab.* **47,** 1303–1310.
Chapter 7	*Case 1*
	Boxer, L. A., Oliver, J. M., Spielberg, S. P., Allen, J. M., and Schulman, J. D. (1979). Protection of granulocytes by vitamin E in glutathione synthetase deficiency. *N. Engl. J. Med.* **301,** 901–905.
	Case 2
	Harding, A. E., Matthews, S., Jones, S., Ellis, C. J. K., Booth, I. W., and Muller, D. P. R. (1985). Spinocerebellar degeneration associated with a selective defect in vitamin E absorption. *N. Engl. J. Med.* **313,** 32–35.
Chapter 8	*Case 1*
	Colvin, B. T., and Lloyd, M. J. (1977). Severe coagulation defect due to a dietary deficiency of vitamin K. *J. Clin. Pathol.* **30,** 1147–1148.
	Case 2
	Corrigan, J., and Marcus, F. I. (1974). Coagulopathy associated with vitamin E ingestion. *J. Am. Med. Assoc.* **230,** 1300–1301.
Chapter 9	*Case 1*
	Hodges, R. E., Hood, J., Canham, J. E., Sauberlich, H. E., and Baker, E. M. (1971). Clinical manifestations of ascorbic acid deficiency in man. *Am. J. Clin. Nutr.* **24,** 432–443.
	Case 2
	Dewhurst, K. (1954). A case of scurvy simulating a gastric neoplasm. *Br. Med. J.* **2,** 1148–1150.
Chapter 10	*Case 1*
	Burwell, C. S., and Dexter, L. (1947). Beriberi heart disease. *Trans. Assoc. Am. Physiol.* **60,** 59–64.

Case 2

Blass, J. P., and Gibson, G. E. (1977). Abnormality of a thiamin-requiring enzyme in patients with Wernicke–Korsakoff syndrome. *N. Engl. J. Med.* **297,** 1367–1370.

Chapter 11   Dutta, P., Gee, M., Rivlin, R. S., and Pinto, J. (1988). Riboflavin deficiency and glutathione metabolism in rats: Possible mechanisms underlying altered responses to hemolytic stimuli. *J. Nutr.* **118,** 1149–1157.

Chapter 12   Vannucchi, H., and Moreno, F. S. (1989). Interaction of niacin and zinc metabolism in patients with alcoholic pellagra. *Am. J. Clin. Nutr.* **50,** 364–369.

Chapter 13   *Case 1*

Barber, G. W., and Spaeth, G. L. (1969). The successful treatment of homocystinuria with pyridoxine. *J. Pediatr.* **75,** 463–478.

Case 2

Schaumberg, H., Kaplan, J., Windebank, A., Vick, N., Rasmus, S., Pleasure, D., and Brown, M. J. (1983). Sensory neuropathy from pyridoxine abuse. *N. Engl. J. Med.* **309,** 445–448.

Chapter 14   Mock, D. M., DeLorimer, A. A., Liebman, W. M., Sweetman, L., and Baker, H. (1981). Biotin deficiency: An unusual complication of parenteral alimentation. *N. Engl. J. Med.* **304,** 820–823.

Chapter 15   Lacroix, B., Didier, E., and Grenier, J. F. (1988). Role of pantothenic and ascorbic acid in wound healing processes: *In vitro* study on fibroblasts. *Int. J. Vitam. Nutr. Res.* **58,** 407–413.

Chapter 16   Freeman, J. M., Finkelstein, J. D., and Mudd, S. H. (1975). Folate-responsive homocystinuria and schizophrenia. A defect in methylation due to deficient 5,10-methylenetetrahydrofolic acid reductase activity. *N. Engl. J. Med.* **292,** 491–496.

Chapter 17   Higginbottom, M. C., Sweetman, L., and Nyhan, W. L. (1978). A syndrome of methylmalonic aciduria, homocystinuria, megaloblastic anemia and neurological abnormalities of a vitamin B_{12}-deficient breast-fed infant of a strict vegetarian. *N. Engl. J. Med.* **299,** 317–323.

A Core of Current Vitamin Research Literature

The following tables list journals publishing original research and reviews about the vitamins, as well as Web site and reference books useful to those interested in the field.

Table C-1. Journals presenting original research reports

Title	Publisher/URL[a,b]
American Journal of Clinical Nutrition	American Society for Nutrition http:www.ajcn.org
American Journal of Public Health	American Public Health Association http://www.ajph.org/
Annals of Internal Medicine	American College of Physicians http://www.annals.org/
Annals of Nutrition and Metabolism	S. Karger, Basel http://content.karger.com/ProdukteDB/produkte.asp?Aktion =JournalHome&ProduktNr=223977
Archives of Internal Medicine	American Medical Association, http://archinte.ama-assn.org/
Australian Journal of Nutrition and Dietetics	Dietetics Association of Australia http://blackwellpublishing.com/journal.asp?ref=1446–6368
Biofactors	ILR Press, Oxford http://www.iospress.nl/loadtop/load.php?isbn=09516433
British Journal of Nutrition	Nutrition Society http://www.cabi-publishing.org/Journals.asp?SubjectArea=&PID=63
British Medical Journal	BMJ Publishing Group, London http://bmj.bmjjournals.com/
Cell	Cell Press http://www.cell.com/
Clinical Chemistry	American Association of Clinical Chemists http://www.clinchem.org/
Ernährungsforschung	Taylor & Francis Sciences, New York http://journalsonline.tandf.co.uk/openurl.asp?genre=issue&issn =0071–1179&issue=current
European Journal of Clinical Nutrition	Stockton Press, London http://www.nature.com/ejcn/index.html
Gastroenterology	American Gastroenterology Association Institute http://www.gastrojournal.org/

(Continued)

Table C-1. Journals presenting original research reports—Cont'd

Title	Publisher/URL[a,b]
International Journal of Food Science and Nutrition	Taylor & Francis, New York http://www.tandf.co.uk/journals/titles/09637486.asp
International Journal for Vitamin and Nutrition Research	Hogrefe & Huber Publishers, Berne verlag.hanshuber.com/ezm/index/VIT
Journal of the American Dietetics Association	American Dietetics Association http://www.adajournal.org/
Journal of the American Medical Association	American Medical Association http://jama.ama-assn.org/
Journal of Biological Chemistry	American Society of Biological Chemists http://www.jbc.org/
Journal of Clinical Biochemistry and Nutrition	Institute of Applied Biochemistry http://www.jstage.jst.go.jp/browse/jcbn/
Journal of Food Composition and Analysis	Elsevier, Amsterdam http://www.elsevier.com/wps/find/journaldescription.cws_home/622878/description#description
Journal of Immunology	American Association of Immunologists http://www.jimmunol.org/
Journal of Lipid Research	American Society for Biochemistry and Molecular Biology http://www.jlr.org/
Journal of Nutrition	American Society for Nutrition www.nutrition.org
Journal of Nutritional Biochemistry	Elsevier, Amsterdam http://www.elsevier.com/wps/find/journaldescription.cws_home/525013/description#description
Journal of Nutritional Science and Vitaminology	Society of Nutrition and Food Science and the Vitamin Society of Japan http://ci.nii.ac.jp/vol_issue/nels/AA00703822_en.html
Journal of Parenteral and Enteral Nutrition	American Society of Parenteral and Enteral Nutrition http://jpen.aspenjournals.org/
Journal of Pediatric Gastroenterology and Nutrition	Lippincott Williams & Wilkins, New York http://www.jpgn.org/pt/re/jpgn/home.htm;jsessionid=FGLN1Qr58pXJDjB6n0vYQjD3LKtV-vM06y1YBt2crTL29RpYzMg5r!-136204674!-949856145!8091&-1
Lipids	American Oil Chemists Society http://www.aocs.org/press/jtoc.asp?journal=2
Nutrition and Food Science	Forbes Publications, London http://www.emeraldinsight.com/info/journals/nfs/nfs.jsp
Nutrition Journal	BioMed Central, Lessburg, Virginia http://www.nutritionj.com/
Nutritional Biochemistry	Elsevier, Amsterdam http://www.us.elsevierhealth.com/product.jsp?isbn=09552863
Proceedings of the National Academy of Sciences	National Academy of Sciences (US) http://www.pnas.org/
Proceedings of the Nutrition Society	Nutrition Society http://www.cabi-publishing.org/Journals.asp?SubjectArea=&PID=66
Proceedings of the Society for Experimental Biology and Medicine	Society for Experimental Biology and Medicine www.sebm.org

[a]URL, uniform resource locator.
[b]Sites accessed November 1, 2006.

Table C-2.   Publications presenting reviews

Title	Publisher/URL[a,b]
American Journal of Clinical Nutrition	American Society for Nutrition www.ajcn.org
Annual Review of Biochemistry	Annual Review, Inc., Palo Alto, California http://arjournals.annualreviews.org/loi/biochem
Annual Review of Nutrition	Annual Review, Inc., Palo Alto, California http://arjournals.annualreviews.org/loi/nutr
Biofactors	ILR Press, Oxford http://www.iospress.nl/loadtop/load.php?isbn=09516433
British Journal of Nutrition	Nutrition Society www.cabi-publishing.org/bjn

Critical Reviews in Biochemistry and Molecular Biology	Taylor & Francis, New York
	http://journalsonline.tandf.co.uk/(0pg0i3epoy0ix4vjbtigihvi)/app/
	    home/journal.asp?referrer=parent&backto=linkingpublicationresults,
	    1:104766,1&linkin=

Critical Reviews in Food Science and Nutrition	Taylor & Francis, New York
	http://journalsonline.tandf.co.uk/(eu5blh55xodkpg3gpqmxry3)/app/
	    home/journal.asp?referrer=parent&backto=linkingpublicationresults,
	    1:106795,1&linkin=

Current Nutrition and Food Science	Bentham Science, San Francisco http://www.bentham.org/cnfs
Journal of Nutrition	American Society for Nutrition www.nutrition.org
Nutrition Abstracts and Reviews Series A (human, experimental)	Aberdeen University Press, Aberdeen, United Kingdom http://www.cabi-publishing.org/AbstractDatabases. asp?SubjectArea=&PID=79
Nutrition Abstracts and Reviews Series B (feeds, feeding)	Aberdeen University Press, Aberdeen, United Kingdom http://www.cabi-publishing.org/AbstractDatabases. asp?SubjectArea=&PID=80
Nutrition in Clinical Care	International Life Sciences Institute, Washington, DC http://www.ilsi.org/Publications/NCC/
Nutrition Research Reviews	The Nutrition Society, London, United Kingdom http://journals.cambridge.org/action/displayJournal?jid=NRR
Nutrition Reviews	International Life Sciences Institute, Washington, DC http://www.ilsi.org/Publications/NutritionReviews/
Nutrition Today	Lippincott Williams & Wilkins, Hagerstown, Maryland www.nutritiontodayonline.com
Proceedings of the Nutrition Society	Nutrition Society http://www.cabi-publishing.org/Journals.asp?SubjectArea=&PID=66

[a]URL, uniform resource locator.
[b]Sites accessed November 1, 2007.

Table C-3.   Some useful Web sites

Programs/Information	URL[a,b]
United Nations	
Food and Agriculture Organization (FAO)	http://www.fao.org/
Codex Alimentarius Commission[c]	http://www.codexalimentarius.net/web/index_en.jsp
UN University	http://www.unu.edu/
INFOODS[d] project	http://www.fao.org/infoods/index_en.stm
World Health Organization (WHO)	http://www.who.int/en/
United States Government	
Department of Agriculture (USDA)	http://www.usda.gov/wps/portal/usdahome
Dietary Guidelines for Americans, 2005	http://www.health.gov/dietaryguidelines/dga2005/document/
Food and Nutrition Information Center	http://www.nal.usda.gov/fnic/topics_a-z.shtml
Food and Nutrition Information Service (FNIS)	http://www.fns.usda.gov/nutritionlink/
Food and Nutrition Service Assistance Program	http://www.fns.usda.gov/fns/
MyPyramid Dietary Guidance System	http://www.mypyramid.gov/
National Agricultural Library	http://www.nal.usda.gov/
National Nutrient Data Laboratory	http://www.ars.usda.gov/main/site_main.htm?modecode=12354500
National Nutrient Database, release 19	http://www.ars.usda.gov/Services/docs.htm?docid=8964
Department of Health and Human Services	http://www.hhs.gov/
Center for Disease Control and Prevention	http://www.cdc.gov/about/default.htm
physical activity portal	http://www.cdc.gov/nccdphp/dnpa/physical/index.htm
Food and Drug Administration (FDA)	http://www.fda.gov/
Center for Food Safety and Applied Nutrition (CSFAN)	http://www.cfsan.fda.gov/
National Institutes of Health (NIH)	http://www.nih.gov/
National Library of Medicine	http://www.nlm.nih.gov/
University On-Line Resources	
Cornell University: "Cornell Nutrition Works"	http://www.nutritionworks.cornell.edu/home/index.cfm
Harvard University: "The Nutrition Source"	http://www.hsph.harvard.edu/nutritionsource/index.html
Johns Hopkins School of Public Health: "Johns Hopkins Public Health"	http://magazine.jhsph.edu/2006/Spring/
Tufts University: "Health and Nutrition Newsletter"	http://healthletter.tufts.edu/
University of California, Davis: "Maternal and Infant Nutrition Briefs"	http://nutrition.ucdavis.edu/briefs/
Information on specific topics	
anemia	http://www.4woman.gov/faq/anemia.htm
diabetes	http://www.fda.gov/diabetes/
food safety	http://www.foodsafety.gov/
general nutrition	http://www.nutrition.gov/
heart and vascular disease	http://www.nhlbi.nih.gov/health/public/heart/index.htm#chol
hypertension	http://www.nhlbi.nih.gov/health/public/heart/index.htm#hbp
	http://www.nhlbi.nih.gov/health/dci/Diseases/Hbp/HBP_WhatsI.html

Table C-3. Some useful Web sites—Cont'd

Programs/Information	URL[a,b]
neural tube defects	http://www.nlm.nih.gov/medlineplus/neuraltubedfects.html#preventionscreening
obesity and weight management	http://www.nhlbi.nih.gov/health/public/heart/index.html#obesity
	http://www.nhlbi.nih.gov/health/public/heart/obesity/lose_wt/index.htm
	http://www.win.niddk.nih.gov
osteoporosis	http://www.fda.gov/fdac/features/796_bone.html

[a]URL, uniform resource locator.
[b]Sites accessed November 1, 2007.
[c]Joint program of FAO and WHO.
[d]International Network of Food Data Systems.

Table C-4. Some useful general reference books

Ball, G. F. M. (1998). *Bioavailability and Analysis of Vitamins in Foods.* Chapman & Hall, New York, 569 pp.

Bender, D. A. (2003). *Nutritional Biochemistry of the Vitamins,* 2nd ed., Cambridge University Press, Cambridge, 488 pp.

Berdanier, C. D., and Moutaid-Moussa, N. (eds.) (2004). *Genomics and Proteomics in Nutrition.* Marcel Dekker, New York, 507 pp.

Bowman, B. A., and Russell, R. M. (eds.) (2006). *Present Knowledge in Nutrition,* 9th ed., ILSI Press, Washington, D.C., Vols. I and II, 967 pp.

Brody, T. (1999). *Nutritional Biochemistry,* 2nd ed., Academic Press, New York, 1006 pp.

Eitenmiller, R. R., and Landen, W. O., Jr. (1999). *Vitamin Analyses for the Health and Food Sciences.* CRC Press, New York, 518 pp.

Food and Nutrition Board. (1997). *Dietary Reference Intakes for Calcium, Phosphorus, Magnesium, Vitamin D and Fluoride.* National Academy Press, Washington, DC, 432 pp.

Food and Nutrition Board. (2000). *Dietary Reference Intakes for Thiamin, Riboflavin, Niacin, Vitamin B$_6$, Folate, Vitamin B$_{12}$, Pantothenic Acid, Biotin and Choline.* National Academy Press, Washington, DC, 564 pp.

Food and Nutrition Board. (2000). *Dietary Reference Intakes for Vitamin C, Vitamin E, Selenium and Carotenoids.* National Academy Press, Washington, DC, 506 pp.

Food and Nutrition Board. (2001). *Dietary Reference Intakes for Vitamin A, Vitamin K, Arsenic, Boron, Chromium, Copper, Iodine, Iron, Manganese, Molybdenum, Nickel, Silicon, Vanadium and Zinc.* National Academy Press, Washington, DC, 773 pp.

Food and Nutrition Board. (2003). *Dietary Reference Intakes: Applications in Dietary Planning.* National Academy Press, Washington, DC, 237 pp.

Food and Nutrition Board. (2003). *Dietary Reference Intakes: Guiding Principles for Nutrition Labeling and Fortification.* National Academy Press, Washington, DC, 205 pp.

Gibson, R. S. (1990). *Principles of Nutritional Assessment.* Oxford University Press, New York, 525 pp.

Insel, P., Turner, R. E., and Ross, D. (2001). *Nutrition.* Jones and Bartlett, Boston, 730 pp.

Leeson, S., and Summers, J. D. (2001). *Scott's Nutrition of the Chicken,* 4th ed., University Press, Toronto, 535 pp.

Mahan, L. K., and Escott-Stump, S. (2000). *Krause's Food, Nutrition, & Diet Therapy.* 10th ed., W. B. Saunders, Philadelphia, 1194 pp.

Pond, W. G., Church, D. C., Pond, K. R., and Schokneckt, P. A. (2005). *Basic Animal Nutrition and Feeding,* 5th ed., John Wiley & Sons, New York, 580 pp.

Rucker, R. B., Suttie, J. W., McCormick, D. B., and Machlin, L. J. (eds.) (2001). *Handbook of Vitamins,* 3rd ed., Marcel Dekker, New York, 600 pp.

Sauberlich, H. E. (1999). *Laboratory Tests for the Assessment of Nutritional Status,* 2nd ed., CRC Press, New York, 486 pp.

Shils, M. E., Shike, M., Ross, A. C., Caballero, B., and Cousins, R. J. (eds.) (2006). *Modern Nutrition in Health and Disease,* 10th ed., Lippincott Williams & Wilkins, New York, 2069 pp.

Vitamin Contents of Foods

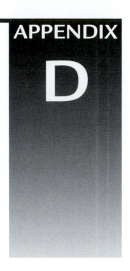

THE FOLLOWING table was derived from the National Nutrition Database. It may be used to determine the vitamin contents of many common foods. The following abbreviations are used in the table, which begins on page 528.

- Bkd, Baked
- Bld, Boiled
- Bnless, Boneless
- Bns, Beans
- Brld, Broiled
- Brsd, Braised
- Btld, Bottled
- Choc, Chocolate
- Chs, Cheese
- Ckd, Cooked
- Cnd, Canned
- Conc, Concentrate
- Cttnsd, Cottonseed
- Dehyd, Dehydrated
- Dk, Dark
- Drnd, Drained

- Drsg, Dressing
- Enr, Enriched
- Ex, Extra
- Flr, Flour
- Fort, Fortified
- Frsh, Fresh
- Frz, Frozen
- Hydr, Hydrogenated
- Incl, Including
- Lofat, Low fat
- Ln, Lean
- Lt, Light
- Mxd, Mixed
- Parbld, Parboiled
- Pdr, Powder
- Pk, Packed

- Pln, Plain
- Prepd, Prepared
- Reg, Regular
- Rstd, Roasted
- RTE, Ready to eat
- RTS, Ready to serve
- Sfflwr, Safflower
- Skn, Skin
- Sol, Solids
- Sp, Species
- Stmd, Steamed
- Stwd, Stewed
- Veg, Vegetable
- Vit, Vitamin
- Whl, Whole

Table D-I.   Vitamin contents of foods: units per 100-g edible portion

Food, by major food group	Vitamin											
	A (IU)	D (IU)	E (mg TE)[a]	K (mg)	C (mg)	Thiamin (mg)	Riboflavin (mg)	Niacin (mg)	B$_6$ (mg)	Pantothenic acid (mg)	Folate (µg)	B$_{12}$ (µg)
Cereals												
Barley, pearled, cooked	7		0.05		0	0.083	0.062	2.063	0.115	0.135	16	0
Buckwheat groats, rstd, ckd	0		0.236		0	0.04	0.039	0.94	0.077	0.359	14	0
Bulgur, cooked	0		0.029		0	0.057	0.028	1	0.083	0.344	18	0
Corn flr, whole-grain, yellow	469		0.25		0	0.246	0.08	1.9	0.37	0.658	25	0
Cornmeal, whole-grain, yellow	469		0.67		0	0.385	0.201	3.632	0.304	0.425	25.4	0
Couscous, cooked	0		0.013		0	0.063	0.027	0.983	0.051	0.371	15	0
Hominy, canned, white	0		0.05		0	0.003	0.006	0.033	0.005	0.154	1	0
Hominy, canned, yellow	110		0		0	0.003	0.006	0.033	0.005	0.154	1	0
Macaroni, cooked, enriched	0		0.03		0	0.204	0.098	1.672	0.035	0.112	7	0
Millet, cooked	0		0.18		0	0.106	0.082	1.33	0.108	0.171	19	0
Noodles, Chinese, chow mein	85		0.16		0	0.578	0.421	5.95	0.11	0.533	22	0
Noodles, egg, ckd, enr	20		0.05		0	0.186	0.083	1.487	0.036	0.145	7	0.09
Noodles, egg, spinach, ckd, enr	103		0.05		0	0.245	0.123	1.474	0.114	0.233	21	0.14
Noodles, Japanese, soba, ckd	0		0		0	0.094	0.026	0.51	0.04	0.235	7	0
Noodles, Japanese, somen, ckd	0		0		0	0.02	0.033	0.097	0.013	0.172	2	0
Oat bran, cooked	0		0		0	0.16	0.034	0.144	0.025	0.217	6	0
Oats	0		0.7		0	0.763	0.139	0.961	0.119	1.349	56	0
Rice, brown, long-grain, ckd	0		0.72		0	0.096	0.025	1.528	0.145	0.285	4	0

Rice, white, glutinous, ckd	0	0.03	0	0.02	0.013	0.29	0.026	0.215	1	0
Rice, white, long-grain, parbld, ckd, enr	0	0.05	0	0.25	0.018	1.4	0.019	0.324	4	0
Rice, white, long-grain, reg, ckd	0	0.05	0	0.163	0.013	1.476	0.093	0.39	3	0
Rye flour, medium	0	1.33	0	0.287	0.114	1.727	0.268	0.492	19	0
Semolina, enriched	0	0.06	0	0.811	0.571	5.99	0.103	0.58	72	0
Sorghum	0	0	0	0.237	0.142	2.927	0	0	0	0
Spaghetti, enr, ckd	0	0.06	0	0.204	0.098	1.672	0.035	0.112	7	0
Spaghetti, spinach, ckd	152	0	0	0.097	0.103	1.53	0.096	0.183	12	0
Spaghetti, whole-wheat, ckd	0	0.05	0	0.108	0.045	0.707	0.079	0.419	5	0
Tapioca, pearl, dry	0	0	0	0.004	0	0	0.008	0.135	4	0
Wheat bran, crude	0	2.32	0	0.523	0.577	13.58	1.303	2.181	79	0
Wheat flour, white, all-purpose, enr, bleached	0	0.06	0.6	0.785	0.494	5.904	0.044	0.438	26	0
Wheat flour, whole-grain	0	1.23	0	0.447	0.215	6.365	0.341	1.008	44	0
Wheat germ, crude	0	0	0	1.882	0.499	6.813	1.3	2.257	281	0
Wild rice, cooked	0	0.23	0	0.052	0.087	1.287	0.135	0.154	26	0
Breads, cakes, and pastries										
Bagels, pln, enr	0	0.033	0	0.463	0.305	4.415	0.049	0.254	17	0
Biscuits, pln/buttermilk	2	2.875	0	0.427	0.292	3.352	0.047	0.3	7	0.14
Bread, banana, w/veg shortening	92	0	1.7	0.173	0.198	1.458	0.151	0.261	11	0.09
Bread, cornbread, w/2% milk	277	0	0.3	0.291	0.294	2.254	0.113	0.339	19	0.15
Bread, cracked-wheat	0	0.564	0	0.358	0.24	3.671	0.304	0.512	39	0.03
Bread, French/Vienna/sourdough	0	0.236	0	0.52	0.329	4.749	0.043	0.387	31	0
Bread, Irish soda	194	1.057	0.8	0.298	0.269	2.405	0.083	0.25	10	0.05

(Continued)

Table D-I. Vitamin contents of foods: units per 100-g edible portion—Cont'd

Food, by major food group	A (IU)	D (IU)	E (mg TE)[a]	K (mg)	C (mg)	Thiamin (mg)	Riboflavin (mg)	Niacin (mg)	B6 (mg)	Pantothenic acid (mg)	Folate (µg)	B12 (µg)
Bread, Italian	0		0.277		0	0.473	0.292	4.381	0.048	0.378	30	0
Bread, mixed-grain	0		0.615		0.3	0.407	0.342	4.365	0.333	0.512	48	0.07
Bread, oat bran	5		0.395		0	0.504	0.346	4.831	0.04	0.159	25	0
Bread, oatmeal	16		0.343		0.4	0.399	0.24	3.136	0.068	0.341	27	0.02
Bread, pita, white, enriched	0		0.038		0	0.599	0.327	4.632	0.034	0.397	24	0
Bread, pita, whole-wheat	0		0.934		0	0.339	0.08	2.84	0.231	0.548	35	0
Bread, pumpernickel	0		0.507		0	0.327	0.305	3.091	0.126	0.404	34	0
Bread, raisin, enriched	2		0.758		0.5	0.339	0.398	3.466	0.069	0.387	34	0
Bread, rye	4		0.552		0.2	0.434	0.335	3.805	0.075	0.44	51	0
Bread, wheat bran	0		0.674		0	0.397	0.287	4.402	0.176	0.536	25	0
Bread, wheat	0		0.546		0	0.418	0.28	4.124	0.097	0.436	41	0
Bread, wheat germ	1		0.87		0.3	0.369	0.375	4.498	0.098	0.313	55	0.07
Bread, white	0		0.286		0	0.472	0.341	3.969	0.064	0.39	34	0.02
Bread, whole-wheat	0		1.036		0	0.351	0.205	3.837	0.179	0.552	50	0.01
Cake, angelfood	0		0		0	0.102	0.491	0.883	0.031	0J98	3	0.07
Cake, Boston cream pie	80		1.064		0.1	0.408	0.27	0.191	0.026	0.301	8	0.16
Cake, fruitcake	78		3.12		0.4	0.05	0.099	0.791	0.046	0.226	3	0.06
Cake, gingerbread	55		1.372		0.1	0.189	0.186	1.562	0.038	0.224	10	0.07
Cake, pound	606		0		0.1	0.137	0.229	1.311	0.035	0.341	11	0.18
Cake, shomake, biscuit-type	72		0		0.2	0.311	0.272	2.573	0.03	0.248	10	0.07
Cake, sponge	154		0.45		0	0.243	0.269	1.932	0.052	0.478	13	0.24
Cake, white, w/o frosting	56		1.825		0.2	0.186	0.242	1.533	0.021	0.184	7	0.08
Cake, yellow, w/o frosting	139		2.056		0.2	0.183	0.233	1.456	0.036	0.31	10	0.16

Cheesecake	1.05	552		0.6	0.028	0.193	0.195	0.052	0.571	15	0.17
Cookies, animal crackers	1.827	0		0	0.35	0.326	3.47	0.022	0.376	14	0.05
Cookies, brownies	2.134	69		0.1	0.255	0.21	1.721	0.035	0.547	12	0.15
Cookies, butter, enr	0.464	600		0	0.37	0.335	3.19	0.036	0.488	6	0.25
Cookies, choc chip, low fat	0	3		0.3	0.289	0.266	2.767	0.262	0.146	6	0
Cookies, choc sandwich, w/creme filling	3.03	1		0	0.079	0.179	2.074	0.019	0.172	5	0.02
Cookies, fig bars	0.702	44		0.2	0.158	0.217	1.874	0.075	0.364	10	0.02
Cookies, fortune	0.344	10		0	0.182	0.13	1.84	0.013	0.297	10	0.05
Cookies, gingersnaps	1.488	1		0	0.2	0.293	3.235	0.183	0.339	6	0
Cookies, graham crackers	1.907	0		0	0.222	0.314	4.122	0.065	0.537	17	0
Cookies, molasses	2.08	1		0	0.355	0.264	3.031	0.241	0.425	7	0
Cookies, oatmeal	2.822	16		0.4	0.267	0.23	2.227	0.054	0.207	7	0
Cookies, peanut butter	3.516	29		0	0.17	0.18	4.27	0.07	0.437	32	0.05
Cookies, raisin, soft-type	1.543	41		0.3	0.216	0.206	1.967	0.054	0.31	9	0.1
Cookies, vanilla wafers	0	1		0	0.361	0.209	2.976	0.026	0.31	8	0.05
Crackers, cheese	1.012	162		0	0.57	0.428	4.671	0.553	0.526	25	0.46
Crackers, chs, w/peanut butter filling	4.419	319		0	0.403	0.344	6.52	1.492	0.51	25	0.01
Crackers, matzo	0.402	0		0	0.387	0.291	3.892	0.115	0.443	14	0
Crackers, melba toast	0.234	0		0	0.413	0.273	4.113	0.098	0.693	26	0
Crackers, rusk toast	0	46		0	0.404	0.399	4.625	0.038	0.406	64	0.07
Crackers, rye	1.362	0		0	0.243	0.145	1.04	0.21	0.676	22	0
Crackers, rye, wafers	1.999	23		0.1	0.427	0.289	1.581	0.271	0.569	45	0
Crackers, saltines	1.653	0	2	0	0.565	0.462	5.249	0.038	0.456	31	0
Crackers, wheat	4.012	0		0	0.505	0.327	4.961	0.136	0.522	18	0
Croissants, butter	0.43	539		0.2	0.388	0.241	2.188	0.058	0.861	28	0.3
Croutons, plain	0	0		0	0.623	0.272	5.439	0.026	0.429	22	0
Danish pastry, cheese	2.583	203		0.1	0.19	0.26	2	0.044	0.27	25	0.24
Danish pastry, fruit, enr	1.759	52		3.9	0.263	0.22	1.992	0.028	0.634	16	0.09

(Continued)

Table D-I.　Vitamin contents of foods: units per 100-g edible portion—Cont'd

Food, by major food group	A (IU)	D (IU)	E (mg TE)[a]	K (mg)	C (mg)	Thiamin (mg)	Riboflavin (mg)	Niacin (mg)	B$_6$ (mg)	Pantothenic acid (mg)	Folate (µg)	B$_{12}$ (µg)
Doughnuts, cake-type, pln	57		3.457		0.2	0.222	0.24	1.853	0.056	0.276	8	0.23
Doughnuts, cake-type, pln, sugared/glazed	10		0		0.1	0.233	0.198	1.512	0.027	0.353	12	0.2
English muffins, pln, enr	0		0.126		0.1	0.384	0.275	3.799	0.042	0.315	29	0.04
English muffins, wheat	2		0.31		0	0.431	0.292	3.356	0.09	0.302	39	0
French toast, w/lofat (2%) milk	484		0		0.3	0.204	0.321	1.628	0.074	0.549	23	0.31
Hush puppies	142		1.05		0.2	0.352	0.332	2.782	0.102	0.357	20	0.19
Muffins, blueberry	34		1.049		1.1	0.14	0.12	1.1	0.022	0.335	16	0.58
Muffins, corn	208		1.224		0.1	0.273	0.326	2.037	0.084	0.444	34	0.19
Muffins, pln, w/lofat (2%) milk	140		0		0.3	0.284	0.301	2.308	0.042	0.351	13	0.15
Pancakes, blueberry	199		0		2.2	0.195	0.272	1.524	0.049	0.395	12	0.2
Pancakes, plain	196		0		0.3	0.201	0.281	1.567	0.046	0.405	12	0.22
Pie, apple, enr flour	124		1.649		3.2	0.028	0.027	0.263	0.038	0.119	4	0
Pie, banana cream	261		1.472		1.6	0.139	0.207	1.054	0.133	0.388	11	0.25
Pie, cherry	237		1.408		0.7	0.023	0.029	0.2	0.041	0.319	8	0
Pie, chocolate creme	2		2.387		0.3	0.036	0.107	0.678	0.02	0.393	7	0.04
Pie, coconut creme	90		1.607		0	0.05	0.08	0.2	0.068	0.315	5	0.19
Pie, lemon meringue	175		1.429		3.2	0.062	0.209	0.649	0.03	0.793	8	0.15
Pie, peach	105		1.722		1	0.061	0.033	0.2	0.023	0.094	4	0
Pie, pecan	175		2.53		1.1	0.091	0.122	0.249	0.021	0.424	6	0.08
Pie, pumpkin	4,515		1.608		1.5	0.055	0.153	0.187	0.057	0.507	15	0.39
Rolls, dinner, pln	0		0.776		0.1	0.493	0.319	4.034	0.054	0.505	30	0.03
Rolls, dinner, wheat	0		1.041		0	0.433	0.273	4.072	0.085	0.154	15	0
Rolls, French	4		0.361		0	0.523	0.3	4.352	0.041	0.222	33	0
Rolls, hamburger/ hot dog, pln	0		0.462		0	0.484	0.312	3.933	0.047	0.529	27	0.02

Rolls, hard (incl kaiser)	0	0.181		0	0.478	0.336	4.239	0.055	0.222	15	0
Strudel, apple	30	1.78		1.7	0.04	0.025	0.33	0.043	0.181	6	0.15
Sweet rolls, cinnamon w/raisins	215	2.857		2	0.324	0.265	2.384	0.107	0.338	24	0.12
Taco shells, baked	350	3.033		0	0.228	0.053	1.35	0.368	0.47	6	0
Waffles, pln	228	0		0.4	0.263	0.347	2.073	0.056	0.485	15	0.25
Wonton wrappers	14	0.082		0	0.519	0.378	5.424	0.03	0.025	17	0.02
Breakfast cereals											
All-bran	2,500	1.843	2	50	1.3	1.4	16.7	1.7	1.734	300	5
Corn cereal, extruded circles	4,167	0.687		50	1.25	1.42	16.67	1.67	0.077	333	0
Corn cereal, extruded waffle-type	504	0.25		53	1.3	0.24	17.6	1.8	0.163	353	5.3
Corn flakes	2,500	0.125	0.04	50	1.3	1.4	16.7	1.7	0.329	353	0
Corn grits, ckd w/H_2O	0	0.05		0	0.1	0.06	0.81	0.024	0.064	1	0
Cream of rice, ckd w/H_2O	0	0.02		0	0	0	0.4	0.027	0.076	3	0
Cream or wheat, ckd w/H_2O	0	0.013		0	0.1	0	0.6	0.014	0.075	4	0
Farina, ckd w/H_2O	0	0.013		0	0.08	0.05	0.55	0.01	0.056	2	0
Granola (oats, wheat germ)	37	12.875		1.4	0.74	0.28	2.05	0.32	0.603	86	0
Mixed bran (wheat, barley)	0	2.32		95	2.4	2.7	31.7	3.2	1.93	71	9.5
Oat bran	1,531	0.662		30.6	0.765	0.867	10.2	1.02	0.747	278	0
Oatmeal, w/o fort, ckd w/H_2O	16	0.1	3	0	0.11	0.02	0.13	0.02	0.2	4	0
Puffed rice	0	0.101	0.08	0	0.41	0.05	6.25	0	0.34	10	0
Puffed wheat	0	0	2	0	2.6	1.8	35.3	0.17	0.518	32	0
Raisin bran	1,364	0.912		0	0.7	0.8	9.1	0.9	0.66	200	2.7
Rice cereal, crispy style	2,500	0.125		50	1.3	1.4	16.7	1.7	0.976	353	0
Rice cereal, extruded, check-style	60	0.13		53	1.3	0.03	17.6	1.8	0.353	353	5.3
Shredded wheat	0	0.53	0.7	0	0.28	0.28	4.57	0.253	0.814	50	0

(Continued)

Table D-I. Vitamin contents of foods: units per 100-g edible portion—Cont'd

Food, by major food group	A (IU)	D (IU)	E (mg TE)[a]	K (mg)	C (mg)	Thiamin (mg)	Riboflavin (mg)	Niacin (mg)	B$_6$ (mg)	Pantothenic acid (mg)	Folate (µg)	B$_{12}$ (µg)
Wheat flakes	2,500		1.231		50	1.25	1.42	16.67	1.67	0.796	333	0
Wheat germ, toasted	0		18.14		6	1.67	0.82	5.59	0.978	1.387	352	0
Vegetables												
Alfalfa seeds, sprouted, raw	155	0	0.02		8.2	0.076	0.126	0.481	0.034	0.563	36	0
Amaranth leaves, ckd, bld, drnd	2,770	0	0	800	41.1	0.02	0.134	0.559	0.177	0.062	56.8	0
Artichokes, ckd, bld, drnd	177	0	0.19		10	0.065	0.066	1.001	0.111	0.342	51	0
Asparagus, ckd, bld, drnd	539	0	0.38		10.8	0.123	0.126	1.082	0.122	0.161	146	0
Balsam-pear (bitter gourd), tips, bld, drnd	1,733	0	0.5		55.6	0.147	0.282	0.995	0.76	0.06	87.6	0
Bamboo shoots, ckd, bld, drnd	0	0	0		0	0.02	0.05	0.3	0.098	0.066	2.3	0
Beans, navy, sprouted, ckd, bld, drnd	4	0	0		17.3	0.381	0.235	1.263	0.198	0.854	106.3	0
Beans, pinto, immature seeds, frz, ckd, bld, drnd	0	0	0		0.7	0.274	0.108	0.632	0.194	0.258	33.5	0
Beans, snap, green, ckd, bld, drnd	666	0	0.14	38	9.7	0.074	0.097	0.614	0.056	0.074	33.3	0
Beans, snap, yel, ckd, bld, drnd	81	0	0.29		9.7	0.074	0.097	0.614	0.056	0.074	33.3	0
Beet greens, ckd, bld, drnd	5,100	0	0.3		24.9	0.117	0.289	0.499	0.132	0.329	14.3	0
Beets, ckd, bld, drnd	35	0	0.3		3.6	0.027	0.04	0.331	0.067	0.145	80	0
Beets, pickled, canned, ckd, solids and liquids	11	0	0		2.3	0.01	0.048	0.251	0.05	0.137	26.5	0

Food												
Broadbeans, immature seeds, ckd, bld, drnd	0	270	0	0		19.8	0.128	0.09	1.2	0.029	0.066	57.8	0
Broccoli, ckd, bld, drnd	0	1,388	0	1.69	205	74.6	0.055	0.113	0.574	0.143	0.508	50	0
Broccoli, raw	0	1,542	0	1.66	270	93.2	0.065	0.119	0.638	0.159	0.535	71	0
Cabbage, Chinese (bok choy), ckd, bld, drnd	0	2,568	0	0.12		26	0.032	0.063	0.428	0.166	0.079	40.6	0
Cabbage, ckd, bld, drnd	0	132	0	0.105	145	20.1	0.057	0.055	0.282	0.113	0.139	20	0
Cabbage, raw	0	133	0	0.105		32.2	0.05	0.04	0.3	0.096	0.14	43	0
Cabbage, red, ckd, bld, drnd	0	27	0	0.12		34.4	0.034	0.02	0.2	0.14	0.22	12.6	0
Cabbage, savoy, ckd, bld, drnd	0	889	0			17	0.051	0.02	0.024	0.152	0.159	46.3	0
Carrots, baby, raw	0	15,010	0	0		8.4	0.031	0.05	0.885	0.077	0.229	33	0
Carrots, ckd, bld, drnd	0	24,554	0	0.42	18	2.3	0.034	0.056	0.506	0.246	0.304	13.9	0
Carrots, frz, ckd, bld, drnd	0	17,702	0	0.42		2.8	0.027	0.037	0.438	0.129	0.161	10.8	0
Carrots, raw	0	28,129	0	0.46	5	9.3	0.097	0.059	0.928	0.147	0.197	14	0
Cassava, raw	0	25	0	0.19		20.6	0.087	0.048	0.854	0.088	0.107	27	0
Catsup	0	1,016	0	1.465		15.1	0.089	0.073	1.367	0.175	0.143	15	0
Cauliflower, ckd, bld, drnd	0	17	0	0.04	10	44.3	0.042	0.052	0.41	0.173	0.508	44	0
Cauliflower, raw	0	19	0	0.04	10	46.4	0.057	0.063	0.526	0.222	0.652	57	0
Celery, raw	0	134	0	0.36	12	7	0.046	0.045	0.323	0.087	0.186	28	0
Chard, Swiss, ckd, bld, drnd	0	3,139	0	1.89	660	18	0.034	0.086	0.36	0.085	0.163	8.6	0
Chives, raw	0	4,353	0	0.21	190	58.1	0.078	0.115	0.647	0.138	0.324	105	0
Cilantro, raw	0	6,130	0	2.041		35.3	0.063	0.182	1.306	0.132	0.57	62	0
Collards, ckd, bld, drnd	0	3,129	0	0.88		18.2	0.04	0.106	0.575	0.128	0.218	93	0
Coriander, raw	0	2,767	0	2.5	310	10.5	0.074	0.12	0.73	0.105	0.185	10.3	0
Corn, sweet, yel, canned, solids and liquids	0	152	0	0		5.5	0.026	0.061	0.939	0.037	0.522	38.1	0
Corn, sweet, yellow, ckd, bld, drnd	0	217	0	0.09		6.2	0.215	0.072	1.614	0.06	0.878	46.4	0
Corn, sweet, yellow, raw	0	281	0	0.09	0.5	6.8	0.2	0.06	1.7	0.055	0.76	45.8	0

(Continued)

Table D-I. Vitamin contents of foods: units per 100-g edible portion—Cont'd

Food, by major food group	A (IU)	D (IU)	E (mg TE)[a]	K (mg)	C (mg)	Thiamin (mg)	Riboflavin (mg)	Niacin (mg)	B₆ (mg)	Pantothenic acid (mg)	Folate (µg)	B₁₂ (µg)
Cowpeas (blackeyes), ckd, bld, drnd	791	0	0.22		2.2	0.101	0.148	1.403	0.065	0.154	127	0
Cucumber, with peel, raw	215	0	0.079	19	5.3	0.024	0.022	0.221	0.042	0.178	13	0
Dandelion greens, raw	14,000	0	2.5		35	0.19	0.26	0.806	0.251	0.084	27.2	0
Eggplant, ckd, bld, drnd	64	0	0.03		1.3	0.076	0.02	0.6	0.086	0.075	14.4	0
Endive, raw	2,050	0	0.44		6.5	0.08	0.075	0.4	0.02	0.9	142	0
Garlic, raw	0	0	0.01		31.2	0.2	0.11	0.7	1.235	0.596	3.1	0
Ginger root, raw	0	0	0.26		5	0.023	0.029	0.7	0.16	0.203	11.2	0
Gourd, calabash, ckd, bld, drnd	0	0	0		8.5	0.029	0.022	0.39	0.038	0.144	4.3	0
Hearts of palm, canned	0	0	0		7.9	0.011	0.057	0.437	0.022	0.126	39	0
Kale, ckd, bld, drnd	7,400	0	0.85	650	41	0.053	0.07	0.5	0.138	0.049	13.3	0
Kohlrabi, ckd, bld, drnd	35	0	1.67		54	0.04	0.02	0.39	0.154	0.16	12.1	0
Leeks, ckd, bld, drnd	46	0	0	11	4.2	0.026	0.02	0.2	0.113	0.072	24.3	0
Lemon grass (citronella), raw	11	0	0		2.6	0.065	0.135	1.101	0.08	0.05	75	0
Lettuce, butterhead, raw	970	0	0.44	122	8	0.06	0.06	0.3	0.05	0.18	73.3	0
Lettuce, cos or romaine, raw	2,600	0	0.44		24	0.1	0.1	0.5	0.047	0.17	135.7	0
Lettuce, iceberg, raw	330	0	0.28		3.9	0.046	0.03	0.187	0.04	0.046	56	0
Lettuce, looseleaf, raw	1,900	0	0.44	210	18	0.05	0.08	0.4	0.055	0.2	49.8	0
Lima beans, ckd, bld, drnd	370	0	0.14		10.1	0.14	0.096	1.04	0.193	0.257	26.3	0
Lotus root, ckd, bld, drnd	0	0	0.01		27.4	0.127	0.01	0.3	0.218	0.302	7.9	0
Mung beans, sprouted, ckd, stir-fried	31	0	0		16	0.14	0.18	1.2	0.13	0.559	69.6	0

Mushrooms, cloud fungus, dried	0	0			0	0.015	0.844	6.267	0.112	0.481	38	0
Mushrooms, oyster, raw	48	0			0	0.055	0.36	3.579	0.122	1.291	47	0
Mushrooms, cnd, drnd sol	0	0.12			0	0.085	0.021	1.593	0.061	0.811	12.3	0
Mushrooms, raw	0	0.12	0.02	76	3.5	0.102	0.449	4.116	0.097	2.2	21.1	0
Mushrooms, shiitake, dried	0	0.12		1,660	3.5	0.3	1.27	14.1	0.965	21.879	163.2	0
Mushrooms, straw, cnd, drnd sol	0	0			0	0.013	0.07	0.224	0.014	0.412	38	0
Mustard greens, ckd, bld, drnd	3,031	2.01		130	25.3	0.041	0.063	0.433	0.098	0.12	73.4	0
New Zealand spinach, ckd, bld, drnd	3,622	0			16	0.03	0.107	0.39	0.237	0.256	8.3	0
Okra, ckd, bld, drnd	575	0.69			16.3	0.132	0.055	0.871	0.187	0.213	45.7	0
Onions, ckd, bld, drnd	0	0.13		2	5.2	0.042	0.023	0.165	0.129	0.113	15	0
Onions, raw	0	0.13		540	6.4	0.042	0.02	0.148	0.116	0.106	19	0
Parsley, raw	5,200	1.79			133	0.086	0.098	1.313	0.09	0.4	152	0
Parsnips, ckd, bld, drnd	0	1			13	0.083	0.051	0.724	0.093	0.588	58.2	0
Peas, edible-podded, ckd, bld, drnd	131	0.39		20	47.9	0.128	0.076	0.539	0.144	0.673	29.1	0
Peas, edible-podded, raw	145	0.39		25	60	0.15	0.08	0.6	0.16	0.75	41.7	0
Peas, green, ckd, bld, drnd	597	0.39			14.2	0.259	0.149	2.021	0.216	0.153	63.3	0
Peas, green, raw	640	0.39		36	40	0.266	0.132	2.09	0.169	0.104	65	0
Peppers, banana, raw	340	0.69			82.7	0.081	0.054	1.242	0.357	0.265	29	0
Peppers, chili, grn, cnd	126	0			34.2	0.01	0.03	0.627	0.12	0.084	54	0
Peppers, Hungarian, raw	140	0			92.9	0.079	0.055	1.092	0.517	0.205	53	0
Peppers, jalapeño, raw	215	0.473			44.3	0.144	0.057	1.117	0.508	0.228	47	0
Peppers, sweet, green, raw	632	0.69		17	89.3	0.066	0.03	0.509	0.248	0.08	22	0
Peppers, sweet, red, raw	5,700	0.69			190	0.066	0.03	0.509	0.248	0.08	22	0
Pickles, cucumber, sweet	126	0.16			1.2	0.009	0.032	0.174	0.015	0.12	1	0

(Continued)

Table D-I. Vitamin contents of foods: units per 100-g edible portion—Cont'd

Food, by major food group	Vitamin											
	A (IU)	D (IU)	E (mg TE)[a]	K (mg)	C (mg)	Thiamin (mg)	Riboflavin (mg)	Niacin (mg)	B6 (mg)	Pantothenic acid (mg)	Folate (µg)	B12 (µg)
Pickles, cucumber, dill	329	0	0.16	26	1.9	0.014	0.029	0.06	0.013	0.054	1	0
Pigeonpeas, ckd, bld, drnd	130	0	0.17		28.1	0.35	0.166	2.153	0.053	0.63	100	0
Pimento, canned	2,655	0	0.69		84.9	0.017	0.06	0.615	0.215	0.01	6	0
Potatoes, au gratin, prepd w/butter	264	0	0		9.9	0.064	0.116	0.993	0.174	0.387	8.1	0
Potatoes, bkd, flesh	0	0	0.04		12.8	0.105	0.021	1.395	0.301	0.555	9.1	0
Potatoes, cnd, drnd	0	0	0.05		5.1	0.068	0.013	0.915	0.188	0.354	6.2	0
Potatoes, french fries, frz, oven heated	0	0	0.19	5	10.1	0.113	0.028	2.088	0.308	0.337	12	0
Potatoes, hashed brown	0	0	0.19		5.7	0.074	0.02	2.001	0.278	0.499	7.7	0
Potatoes, mashed, prepared w/whole milk and margarine	169	0	0.3		6.1	0.084	0.04	1.079	0.224	0.57	7.9	
Potatoes, microwaved, cooked in skin, flesh	0	0	0		15.1	0.129	0.025	1.625	0.319	0.597	12.4	0
Potatoes, scalloped, prepared w/butter	135	0	0		10.6	0.069	0.092	1.053	0.178	0.514	8.7	0
Pumpkin, canned	22,056	0	1.06	16	4.2	0.024	0.054	0.367	0.056	0.4	12.3	0
Radishes, raw	8	0	0.001	0.1	22.8	0.005	0.045	0.3	0.071	0.088	27	0
Rutabagas, ckd, bld, drnd	561	0	0.15		18.8	0.082	0.041	0.715	0.102	0.155	15	0
Sauerkraut, cnd, sol and liquids	18	0	0.1	25	14.7	0.021	0.022	0.143	0.13	0.093	23.7	0
Shallots, raw	1,190	0	0		8	0.06	0.02	0.2	0.345	0.29	34.2	0
Soybeans, grn, ckd, bld, drnd	156	0	0.01		17	0.26	0.155	1.25	0.06	0.128	111	0
Spinach, ckd, bld, drnd	8,190	0	0.955		9.8	0.095	0.236	0.49	0.242	0.145	145.8	0
Spinach, raw	6,715	0	1.89	400	28.1	0.078	0.189	0.724	0.195	0.065	194.4	0

Squash, acorn, ckd, bkd	428	0	0		10.8	0.167	0.013	0.881	0.194	0.504	18.7	0
Squash, butternut, ckd, bkd	7,001	0	0		15.1	0.072	0.017	0.969	0.124	0.359	19.2	0
Squash, hubbard, ckd, bkd	6,035	0	0		9.5	0.074	0.047	0.558	0.172	0.447	16.2	0
Squash, spaghetti, ckd, bld, drnd/bkd	110	0	0.12		3.5	0.038	0.022	0.81	0.099	0.355	8	0
Squash, summer, ckd, bld, drnd	287	0	0.12		5.5	0.049	0.049	0.513	0.094	0.137	20.1	0
Squash, zucchini, ckd, bld, drnd	240	0	0.12		4.6	0.041	0.041	0.428	0.078	0.114	16.8	0
Succotash (corn and limas), ckd, bld, drnd	294	0	0		8.2	0.168	0.096	1.327	0.116	0.567	32.8	0
Sweet potato leaves, ckd, stmd	916	0	0.96		1.5	0.112	0.267	1.003	0.16	0.2	48.8	0
Sweet potato, ckd, bkd in skn	21,822	0	0.28	4	24.6	0.073	0.127	0.604	0.241	0.646	22.6	0
Taro, cooked	0	0	0.44		5	0.107	0.028	0.51	0.331	0.336	19.2	0
Taro leaves, ckd, stmd	4,238	0	0		35.5	0.139	0.38	1.267	0.072	0.044	48.3	0
Taro shoots, ckd	51	0	0		18.9	0.038	0.053	0.81	0.112	0.076	2.6	0
Tomato juice, cnd	556	0	0.91	4	18.3	0.047	0.031	0.673	0.111	0.25	19.9	0
Tomato paste, cnd	2,445	0	4.3		42.4	0.155	0.19	3.223	0.38	0.753	22.4	0
Tomato sauce, cnd	979	0	1.4	7	13.1	0.066	0.058	1.149	0.155	0.309	9.4	0
Tomatoes, green, raw	642	0	0.38		23.4	0.06	0.04	0.5	0.081	0.5	8.8	0
Tomatoes, red, ripe, cnd, stwd	541	0	0.38		11.4	0.046	0.035	0.714	0.017	0.114	5.4	0
Tomatoes, red, ripe, raw	623	0	0.38	6	19.1	0.059	0.048	0.628	0.08	0.247	15	0
Turnip grns, ckd, bld, drnd	5,498	0	1.721	200	27.4	0.045	0.072	0.411	0,18	0.274	118.4	0
Turnips, ckd, bld, drnd	0	0	0.03	0.06	11.6	0.027	0.023	0.299	0.067	0.142	9.2	0
Waterchestnuts, Chinese, cnd	4	0	0.5		1.3	0.011	0.024	0.36	0.159	0.221	5.8	0
Watercress, raw	4,700	0	1	250	43	0.09	0.12	0.2	0.129	0.31	9.2	0

(*Continued*)

Table D-I. Vitamin contents of foods: units per 100-g edible portion—Cont'd

Food, by major food group	A (IU)	D (IU)	E (mg TE)[a]	K (mg)	C (mg)	Thiamin (mg)	Riboflavin (mg)	Niacin (mg)	B$_6$ (mg)	Pantothenic acid (mg)	Folate (µg)	B$_{12}$ (µg)
Winged bns, ckd, bld, drnd	88	0	0		9.8	0.086	0.072	0.652	0.082	0.041	35.1	0
Yams, ckd, bld, drnd, bkd	0	0	0.16		12.1	0.095	0.028	0.552	0.228	0.311	16	0
Yardlong beans, ckd, bld, drnd	450	0	0		16.2	0.085	0.099	0.63	0.024	0.051	44.5	0
Fruits and fruit juices												
Apple juice, cnd/btld, w/o vit C	1	0	0.01	0.1	0.9	0.021	0.017	0.1	0.03	0.063	0.1	0
Apples, raw, w/skin	53	0	0.32		5.7	0.017	0.014	0.077	0.048	0.061	2.8	0
Applesauce, cnd, w/o vit C	29	0	0.01	0.5	1.2	0.013	0.025	0.188	0.026	0.095	0.6	0
Apricot nectar, cnd, w/o vit C	1,316	0	0.08	5	0.6	0.009	0.014	0.26	0.022	0.096	1.3	0
Apricots, dehyd	12,669	0	0		9.5	0.043	0.148	3.58	0.52	1.067	4.4	0
Apricots, raw	2,612	0	0.89		10	0.03	0.04	0.6	0.054	0.24	8.6	0
Avocados, raw	612	0	1.34	40	7.9	0.108	0.122	1.921	0.28	0.971	61.9	0
Bananas, raw	81	0	0.27	0.5	9.1	0.045	0.1	0.54	0.578	0.26	19.1	0
Blackberries, raw	165	0	0.71		21	0.03	0.04	0.4	0.058	0.24	34	0
Blueberries, raw	100	0	1	6	13	0.048	0.05	0.359	0.036	0.093	6.4	0
Cantaloupes, raw	3,224	0	0.15	1	42.2	0.036	0.021	0.574	0.115	0.128	17	0
Casaba melons, raw	30	0	0.15		16	0.06	0.02	0.4	0.12	0	17	0
Cherries, sour, red, raw	1,283	0	0.13		10	0.03	0.04	0.4	0.044	0.143	7.5	0
Cherries, sweet, raw	214	0	0.13		7	0.05	0.06	0.4	0.036	0.127	4.2	0
Crabapples, raw	40	0	0	0.005	8	0.03	0.02	0.1	0	0	0	0
Cranberries, raw	46	0	0.1		13.5	0.03	0.02	0.1	0.065	0.219	1.7	0
Cranberry sauce, cnd	20	0	0.1		2	0.015	0.021	0.1	0.014	0	1	0

Currants, European black, raw	230	0	0.1		181	0.05	0.05	0.3	0.066	0.398	0	0
Custard apple (bullock's-heart), raw	33	0	0		19.2	0.08	0.1	0.5	0.221	0.135	0	0
Dates, domestic, dried	50	0	0.1		0	0.09	0.1	2.2	0.192	0.78	12.6	0
Elderberries, raw	600	0	1		36	0.07	0.06	0.5	0.23	0.14	6	0
Figs, dried, uncooked	133	0	0		0.8	0.071	0.088	0.694	0.224	0.435	7.5	0
Figs, raw	142	0	0.89		2	0.06	0.05	0.4	0.113	0.3	6	0
Fruit cocktail, cnd, H$_2$Opk, solids and liquids	250	0	0.29	0.8	2.1	0.016	0.011	0.363	0.052	0.062	2.7	0
Gooseberries, raw	290	0	0.37		27.7	0.04	0.03	0.3	0.08	0.286	6	0
Grape juice, cnd/btld, w/o vit C	8	0	0	0.2	0.1	0.026	0.037	0.262	0.065	0.041	2.6	0
Grapefruit juice, cnd	7	0	0.05	0.2	29.2	0.042	0.02	0.231	0.02	0.13	10.4	0
Grapefruit, raw, pink/red/white	124	0	0.25	0.02	34.4	0.036	0.02	0.25	0.042	0.283	10.2	0
Grapes, adherent skn type, raw	73	0	0.7	3	10.8	0.092	0.057	0.3	0.11	0.024	3.9	0
Guavas, raw	792	0	1.12		183.5	0.05	0.05	1.2	0.143	0.15	14	0
Honeydew melons, raw	40	0	0.15		24.8	0.077	0.018	0.6	0.059	0.207	6	0
Jackfruit, raw	297	0	0.15		6.7	0.03	0.11	0.4	0.108		14	0
Kiwi fruit, raw	175	0	1.12	25	98	0.02	0.05	0.5	0.09	0	38	0
Kumquats, raw	302	0	0.24		37.4	0.08	0.1	0.5	0.06	0	16	0
Lemon juice, cnd/btld	15	0	0.09		24.8	0.041	0.009	0.197	0.043	0.091	10.1	0
Lemons, raw, w/o peel	29	0	0.24		53	0.04	0.02	0.1	0.08	0.19	10.6	0
Lime juice, cnd/btld	16	0	0.07		6.4	0.033	0.003	0.163	0.027	0.066	7.9	0
Litchis, raw	0	0	0.7		71.5	0.011	0.065	0.603	0.1	0	14	0
Mangos, raw	3,894	0	1.12		27.7	0.058	0.057	0.584	0.134	0.16	14	0
Nectarines, raw	736	0	0.89		5.4	0.017	0.041	0.99	0.025	0.158	3.7	0
Olives, ripe, cnd	403	0	3		0.9	0.003	0	0.037	0.009	0.015	0	0
Orange juice, chilled, incl from cone	78	0	0.19	0.1	32.9	0.111	0.021	0.28	0.054	0.191	18.1	0
Oranges, raw	205	0	0.24	0.1	53.2	0.087	0.04	0.282	0.06	0.25	30.3	0

(Continued)

Table D-I. Vitamin contents of foods: units per 100-g edible portion—Cont'd

Food, by major food group	A (IU)	D (IU)	E (mg TE)[a]	K (mg)	C (mg)	Thiamin (mg)	Riboflavin (mg)	Niacin (mg)	B$_6$ (mg)	Pantothenic acid (mg)	Folate (µg)	B$_{12}$ (µg)
Papayas, raw	284	0	1.12		61.8	0.027	0.032	0.338	0.019	0.218	38	0
Passion fruit, purple, raw	700	0	1.12		30	0	0.13	1.5	0.1	0	14	0
Peaches, cnd, H$_2$O pk, solids and liquids	532	0	0.89		2.9	0.009	0.019	0.521	0.019	0.05	3.4	0
Peaches, raw	535	0	0.7	3	6.6	0.017	0.041	0.99	0.018	0.17	3.4	0
Pears, cnd, H$_2$O pk, solids and liquids	0	0	0.5	0.5	1	0.008	0.01	0.054	0.014	0.022	1.2	0
Pears, raw	20	0	0.5		4	0.02	0.04	0.1	0.018	0.07	7.3	
Pineapple, cnd, H$_2$O pk, solids and liquids	15	0	0.1		7.7	0.093	0.026	0.298	0.074	0.1	4.8	0
Pineapple, raw	23	0	0.1	0.1	15.4	0.092	0.036	0.42	0.087	0.16	10.6	0
Plantains, cooked	909	0	0.14		10.9	0.046	0.052	0.756	0.24	0.233	26	0
Plums, raw	323	0	0.6	12	9.5	0.043	0.096	0.5	0.081	0.182	2.2	0
Pomegranates, raw	0	0	0.55		6.1	0.03	0.03	0.3	0.105	0.596	6	0
Prickly pears, raw	51	0	0.01		14	0.014	0.06	0.46	0.06	0	6	0
Prunes, cnd, hvy syrup pk, solids and liquids	797	0	0		2.8	0.034	0.122	0.866	0.203	0.1	0.1	0
Prunes, dehyd, stwd	523	0	0		0	0.046	0.03	0.985	0.191	0.108	0.2	0
Prunes, dehyd, unckd	1,762	0	0		0	0.118	0.165	2.995	0.745	0.418	1.9	0
Quinces, raw	40	0	0.55		15	0.02	0.03	0.2	0.04	0.081	3	0
Raisins, golden seedless	44	0	0.7		3.2	0.008	0.191	1.142	0.323	0.14	3.3	0
Raisins, seedless	8	0	0.7		3.3	0.156	0.088	0.818	0.249	0.045	3.3	0
Raspberries, raw	130	0	0.45		25	0.03	0.09	0.9	0.057	0.24	26	0
Rhubarb, frz, ckd	69	0	0.2		3.3	0.018	0.023	0.2	0.02	0.05	5.3	0
Strawberries, cnd, hvy syrup, solids and liquids	26	0	0.14		31.7	0.021	0.034	0.057	0.049	0.179	28	0
Strawberries, raw	27	0	0.14		56.7	0.02	0.066	0.23	0.059	0.34	17.7	0
Tangerines, raw	920	0	0.24		30.8	0.105	0.022	0.16	0.067	0.2	20.4	0
Watermelon, raw	366	0	0.15		9.6	0.08	0.02	0.2	0.144	0.212	2.2	0

Beans and peas

Food												
Black beans, ckd, bld	6	0	0		0	0.244	0.059	0.505	0.069	0.242	148.8	0
Broad beans (fava), ckd, bld	15	0	0.09		0.3	0.097	0.089	0.711	0.072	0.157	104.1	0
Chickpeas, ckd, bld	27	0	0.35		1.3	0.116	0.063	0.526	0.139	0.286	172	0
Cowpeas (blackeyes), ckd, bld	15	0	0.28		0.4	0.202	0.055	0.495	0.1	0.411	207.9	0
Falafel	13	0	0		1.6	0.146	0.166	1.044	0.125	0.292	77.6	0
French beans, ckd, bld	3	0	0		1.2	0.13	0.062	0.546	0.105	0.222	74.7	0
Great northern beans, ckd, bld	1	0	0		1.3	0.158	0.059	0.681	0.117	0.266	102.2	0
Hummus, raw	25	0	1		7.9	0.092	0.053	0.411	0.398	0.288	59.4	0
Kidney beans, ckd, bld	0	0	0.21		1.2	0.16	0.058	0.578	0.12	0.22	129.6	0
Lentils, ckd, bld	8	0	0.11		1.5	0.169	0.073	1.06	0.178	0.638	180.8	0
Lima beans, large, ckd, bld	0	0	0.18		0	0.161	0.055	0.421	0.161	0.422	83.1	0
Lupins, ckd, bld	7	0	0		1.1	0.134	0.053	0.495	0.009	0.188	59.3	0
Mung beans, ckd, bld	24	0	0.51		1	0.164	0.061	0.577	0.067	0.41	158.8	0
Navy beans, ckd, bld	2	0	0		0.9	0.202	0.061	0.531	0.164	0.255	139.9	0
Peanut butter, smooth style	0	0	10		0	0.083	0.105	13.4	0.454	0.806	74	0
Peanuts, ckd, bld	0	0	3.17		0	0.259	0.063	5.259	0.152	0.825	74.6	0
Peanuts, dry-roasted	0	0	7.41		0	0.438	0.098	13.53	0.256	1.395	145.3	0
Peanuts, oil-roasted	0	0	7.41		0	0.253	0.108	14.28	0.255	1.39	125.7	0
Peas, split, ckd, bld	7	0	0.39		0.4	0.19	0.056	0.89	0.048	0.595	64.9	0
Pigeon peas (red gram), ckd, bld	3	0	0		0	0.146	0.059	0.781	0.05	0.319	110.8	0
Pinto beans, ckd, bld	2	0	0.94		2.1	0.186	0.091	0.4	0.155	0.285	172	0
Refried beans, canned	0	0	0		6	0.027	0.016	0.315	0.143	0.097	11	0
Soybeans, rstd	200	0	1.95	37	2.2	0.1	0.145	1.41	0.208	0.453	211	0
Soy flour, full-fat, rstd	110	0	0		0	0.412	0.941	3.286	0.351	1.209	227.4	0
Soy milk	32	0	0.01	3	0	0.161	0.07	0.147	0.041	0.048	1.5	0

(Continued)

Table D-I. Vitamin contents of foods: units per 100-g edible portion—Cont'd

Food, by major food group	A (IU)	D (IU)	E (mg TE)ᵃ	K (mg)	C (mg)	Thiamin (mg)	Riboflavin (mg)	Niacin (mg)	B₆ (mg)	Pantothenic acid (mg)	Folate (µg)	B₁₂ (µg)
Tempeh	686	0	0		0	0.131	0.111	4.63	0.299	0.355	52	1
Tofu, raw	85	0	0.01		0.1	0.081	0.052	0.195	0.047	0.068	15	0
Winged beans, ckd, bld	0	0	0	2	0	0.295	0.129	0.83	0.047	0.156	10.4	0
Yardlong beans, ckd, bld	16	0	0		0.4	0.212	0.064	0.551	0.095	0.398	145.7	0
Nuts												
Acorns, dried	0	0	0		0	0.149	0.154	2.406	0.695	0.94	114.6	0
Almonds, dry-roasted, unblanched	0	0	5.55		0.7	0.13	0.599	2.817	0.074	0.254	63.8	0
Brazil nuts, dried, unblanched	0	0	7.6		0.7	1	0.122	1.622	0.251	0.236	4	0
Butternuts, dried	124	0	3.5		3.2	0.383	0.148	1.045	0.56	0.633	66.2	0
Cashew nuts, dry-roasted	0	0	0.57		0	0.2	0.2	1.4	0.256	1.217	69.2	0
Chestnuts, European, rstd	24	0	1.2		26	0.243	0.175	1.342	0.497	0.554	70	0
Coconut meat, dried, flaked	0	0	0.73		0	0.03	0.02	0.3	0.261	0.696	7.8	0
Coconut meat, raw	0	0	0.73		3.3	0.066	0.02	0.54	0.054	0.3	26.4	0
Coconut milk, cnd	0	0	0		1	0.022	0	0.637	0.028	0.153	13.5	0
Coconut water	0	0	0		2.4	0.03	0.057	0.08	0.032	0.043	2.5	0
Filberts (hazelnuts), dry-roasted	69	0	23.9		1	0.213	0.213	2.772	0.635	1.19	74.5	0
Hickory nuts, dried	131	0	5.21		2	0.867	0.131	0.907	0.192	1.746	40	0
Macadamia nuts, oil-roasted	9	0	0.41		0	0.213	0.109	2.02	0.198	0.442	15.9	0
Pecans, dry-roasted	133	0	3.1		2	0.317	0.106	0.922	0.195	1.774	40.7	0
Pine nuts, pifton, dried	29	0	0		2	1.243	0.223	4.37	0.111	0.21	57.8	0
Pistachio nuts, dry-roasted	238	0	5.21	70	7.3	0.423	0.246	1.408	0.255	1.212	59.1	0

Food											
Pumpkin and squash seeds, whl, rstd	62	0	0	0.3	0.034	0.052	0.286	0.037	0.056	9	0
Sunflower kernels, dried	50	0	50.27	1.4	2.29	0.25	4.5	0.77	6.745	227.4	0
Tahini, from roasted and toasted sesame kernels	67	0	2.27	0	1.22	0.473	5.45	0.149	0.693	97.7	0
Walnuts, black, dried	296	0	2.62	3.2	0.217	0.109	0.69	0.554	0.626	65.5	0
Poultry											
Chicken, dk meat, meat and skn, fried w/batter	103		0	0	0.117	0.218	5.607	0.25	0.953	9	0.27
Chicken, dk meat, meat and skn, rstd	201		0	0	0.066	0.207	6.359	0.31	1.111	7	0.29
Chicken, giblets, simmrd	7,431		1.302	8	0.087	0.953	4.103	0.34	2.959	376	10.14
Chicken, lt meat, meat and skn, fried w/batter	79		0	0	0.113	0.147	9.156	0.39	0.794	6	0.28
Chicken, lt meat, meat and skn, rstd	110		0	0	0.06	0.118	11.13	0.52	0.926	3	0.32
Chicken, liver, simmrd	16,375		1.44	15.8	0.153	1.747	4.45	0.58	5.411	770	19.39
Duck, meat only, rstd	77		0.7	0	0.26	0.47	5.1	0.25	1.5	10	0.4
Duck, meat and skn, rstd	210		0.7	0	0.174	0.269	4.825	0.18	1.098	6	0.3
Goose, meat only, rstd	40		0	0	0.092	0.39	4.081	0.47	1.834	12	0.49
Turkey, breast, meat and skn, rstd	0		0	0	0.057	0.131	6.365	0.48	0.634	6	0.36
Turkey, dk meat, rstd	0		0.64	0	0.063	0.248	3.649	0.36	1.286	9	0.37
Turkey, meat only, rstd	0		0.329	0	0.062	0.182	5.443	0.46	0.943	7	0.37
Turkey, meat and skn, rstd	0		0.339	0	0.057	0.177	5.086	0.41	0.858	7	0.35
Beef											
Brisket, whl, ln, 1/4 fat, brsd	0		0.14	0	0.07	0.22	3.71	0.29	0.36	8	2.6
Chuck, arm pot rst, 1/4 fat, brsd	0		0.22	0	0.07	0.24	3.18	0.28	0.33	9	2.95
Chuck, blade rst, 1/4 fat, brsd	0		0.2	0	0.07	0.24	2.42	0.26	0.31	5	2.28

(*Continued*)

Table D-I. Vitamin contents of foods: units per 100-g edible portion—Cont'd

Food, by major food group	A (IU)	D (IU)	E (mg TE)[a]	K (mg)	C (mg)	Thiamin (mg)	Riboflavin (mg)	Niacin (mg)	B$_6$ (mg)	Pantothenic acid (mg)	Folate (μg)	B$_{12}$ (μg)
Corned beef, cnd	0	0	0.15		0	0.02	0.147	2.43	0.13	0.626	9	1.62
Dried beef, cured	0	0	0.14		0	0.083	0.2	5.451	0.35	0.611	11	2.66
Hank, brsd	0	0	0		0	0.14	0.18	4.42	0.35	0.37	9	3.3
Ground, ln, bkd, med	0	0	0		0	0.05	0.19	4.28	0.2	0.27	9	1.77
Ground, reg, bkd, med	0	0	0		0	0.03	0.16	4.75	0.23	0.22	9	2.34
Rib, eye, sml cnd (ribs 10–12), one-quarter fat, brld	0	0	0		0	0.09	0.19	4.22	0.35	0.31	7	3.01
Rib, whl (ribs 6–12), 1/4 fat, brld	0	0	0.236			0.08	0.17	3.25	0.27	0.32	6	2.87
Round, bottom round, 1/4 fat, brsd	0	0	0.19		0	0.07	0.24	3.73	0.33	0.38	10	2.35
Round, eye of round, 1/4 fat, rstd	0	0	0.179		0	0.08	0.16	3.49	0.35	0.42	7	2.1
Round, full cut, 1/4 fat, brld	0	0	0.19		0	0.09	0.21	3.99	0.38	0.38	9	3.01
Round, top round, 1/4 fat, brld	0	0	0.15		0	0.11	0.26	5.71	0.53	0.46	11	2.42
Short loin, porterhouse steak, 1/4 fat, brld	0	0	0.217		0	0.09	0.21	3.89	0.34	0.3	7	2.11
Short loin, top loin, 1/4 fat, brld	0	0	0.021		0	0.08	0.18	4.7	0.37	0.33	7	1.94
Tenderloin, 1/4 fat, brld	0	0	0.19		0	0.11	0.26	3.52	0.39	0.34	6	2.41
Top sirloin, 1/4 fat, brld	0	0	0.18		0	0.11	0.27	3.93	0.41	0.36	9	2.69
Pork												
Bacon, Canadian-style, grilled	0		0.26		0	0.824	0.197	6.915	0.45	0.52	4	0.78
Bacon, ckd, brld/pan-fried/rstd	0		0.54		0	0.692	0.285	7.322	0.27	1.055	5	1.75

Cured ham, bnless, ex ln (5% fat), rstd	0		0.26	0	0.754	0.202	4.023	0.4	0.403	3	0.65
Cured ham, bnless, reg (11% fat), rstd	0		0.26	0	0.73	0.33	6.15	0.31	0.72	3	0.7
Cured ham, ex ln (4% fat), cnd	0		0.26	0	0.836	0.23	5.302	0.45	0.492	6	0.82
Cured ham, reg (13% fat), cnd	0		0.26	0	0.963	0.231	3.218	0.48	0.394	5	0.78
Leg (ham), whl, ln, rstd	9		0.26	0.4	0.69	0.349	4.935	0.45	0.67	12	0.72
Loin, blade (chops), bone-in, ln and fat, brsd	8		0.26	0.6	0.476	0.232	3.59	0.297	0.562	2	0.65
Loin, tenderloin, ln, rstd	7		0.26	0.4	0.94	0.39	4.709	0.42	0.687	6	0.55
Loin, top loin (chop), bnless, ln and fat, brsd	7		0	0.3	0.552	0.256	4.54	0.329	0.638	4	0.46
Loin, top loin (roast), bnless, ln and fat, rstd	8		0	0.4	0.614	0.296	5.129	0.373	0.545	8	0.55
Loin, whl, ln, brld	7		0.26	0.7	0.923	0.338	5.243	0.492	0.729	6	0.72
Shoulder, arm picnic, ln, rstd	7		0	0.3	0.578	0.357	4.314	0.41	0.592	5	0.78
Shoulder, whl, ln, rstd	7		0.26	0.6	0.628	0.37	4.26	0.317	0.651	5	0.86
Spareribs, ln and fat, brsd	10		0.26	0	0.408	0.382	5.475	0.35	0.75	4	1.08
Sausages and luncheon meats											
Bologna, beef	0	28	0.19	0	0.05	0.109	2.407	0.15	0.28	5	1.42
Bologna, pork	0	56	0.26	0	0.523	0.157	3.9	0.27	0.72	5	0.93
Bologna, turkey	0		0.53	0	0.055	0.165	3.527	0.22	0.7	7	0.27
Bratwurst, cooked, pork	0	44	0.25	1	0.505	0.183	3.2	0.21	0.32	2	0.95
Chicken roll, light meat	82	82	0.265	0	0.065	0.13	5.291	0.21	0.39	2	0.15
Frankfurter, beef	0	36	0.19	0	0.051	0.102	2.415	0.12	0.29	4	1.54
Frankfurter, beef and pork	0	36	0.25	0	0.199	0.12	2.634	0.13	0.35	4	1.3
Frankfurter, chicken	130		0.215	0	0.066	0.115	3.089	0.32	0.83	4	0.24

(Continued)

Table D-I. Vitamin contents of foods: units per 100-g edible portion—Cont'd

Food, by major food group	Vitamin A (IU)	D (IU)	E (mg TE)a	K (mg)	C (mg)	Thiamin (mg)	Riboflavin (mg)	Niacin (mg)	B6 (mg)	Pantothenic acid (mg)	Folate (µg)	B12 (µg)
Frankfurter, turkey	0		0.617		0	0.041	0.179	4.132	0.23	0.72	8	0.28
Ham, chopped, canned	0		0.25		2	0.535	0.165	3.2	0.32	0.28	1	0.7
Ham, sliced, ex ln (5% fat)	0		0.29		0	0.932	0.223	4.838	0.46	0.47	4	0.75
Ham, sliced, reg (11% fat)	0		0.29		0	0.863	0.252	5.251	0.34	0.45	3	0.83
Italian sausage, ckd, pork	0		0.25		2	0.623	0.233	4.165	0.33	0.45	5	1.3
Kielbasa, pork, beef and nonfat dry milk	0		0.22		0	0.228	0.214	2.879	0.18	0.82	5	1.61
Knockwurst, pork and beef	0		0.57		0	0.342	0.14	2.734	0.17	0.32	2	1.18
Olive loaf, pork	200	44	0.25		0	0.295	0.26	1.835	0.23	0.77	2	1.26
Pastrami, turkey	0		0.216		0	0.055	0.25	3.527	0.27	0.58	5	0.24
Polish sausage, pork	0		0		1	0.502	0.148	3.443	0.19	0.45	2	0.98
Salami, beef	0	36	0.19		0	0.103	0.189	3.238	0.18	0.95	2	3.06
Salami, beef and pork	0		0.22		0	0.239	0.376	3.553	0.21	0.85	2	3.65
Smoked link sausage, pork	0	52	0.25		2	0.7	0.257	4.532	0.35	0.78	5	1.63
Smoked link sausage, pork and beef	0	28	0.22		0	0.26	0.17	3.227	0.17	0.44	2	1.51
Turkey breast meat	0		0.09		0	0.04	0.107	8.322	0.36	0.59	4	2.02
Turkey ham	0		0.64		0	0.052	0.247	3.527	0.24	0.85	6	0.24
Turkey roll, light meat	0		0.134		0	0.089	0.226	7	0.32	0.42	4	0.24
Vienna sausage, cnd, beef and pork	0		0.22		0	0.087	0.107	1.613	0.12	0.35	4	1.02
Fish and seafood												
Abalone, mxd species, fried	5	0		18	1.8	0.22	0.13	1.9	0.15	2.87	5.4	0.69
Anchovy, cnd in oil, drnd sol	70	5			0	0.078	0.363	19.9	0.203	0.909	12.5	0.88

Carp, cooked, dry heat	32	0		1.6	0.14	0.07	2.1	0.219	0.87	17.3	1.471
Catfish, channel, breaded and fried	28	0		0	0.073	0.133	2.282	0.19	0.73	16.5	1.9
Caviar, black and red	1,868	7	232	0	0.19	0.62	0.12	0.32	3.5	50	20
Clam, mxd species, breaded and fried	302	0	4	10	0.1	0.244	2.064	0.06	0.43	18.2	40.269
Cod, Atlantic, ckd, dry heat	46	0.3		1	0.088	0.079	2.513	0.283	0.18	8.1	1.048
Cod, Atlantic, dried and salted	141	0.6		3.5	0.268	0.24	7.5	0.864	1.675	24.7	10
Crab, Alaska king, ckd, moist heat	29	0		7.6	0.053	0.055	1.34	0.18	0.4	51	11.5
Crab, blue, ckd, moist heat	6	1		3.3	0.1	0.05	3.3	0.18	0.43	50.8	7.3
Crayfish, mxd sp, wild, ckd, moist heat	50	1.5		0.9	0.05	0.085	2.28	0.076	0.58	44	2.15
Eel, mxd species, ckd, dry heat	3,787	5.1		1.8	0.183	0.051	4.487	0.077	0.28	17.3	2.885
Flatfish (flounder/sole), ckd, dry heat	38	1.89		0	0.08	0.114	2.179	0.24	0.58	9.2	2.509
Gefiltefish	89	0		0.8	0.065	0.059	1	0.08	0.2	2.8	0.844
Haddock, ckd, dry heat	63	0		0	0.04	0.045	4.632	0.346	0.15	13.3	1.387
Halibut, ckd, dry heat	179	1.09		0	0.069	0.091	7.123	0.397	0.38	13.8	1.366
Herring, ckd, dry heat	102	1.34		0.7	0.112	0.299	4.124	0.348	0.74	11.5	13.141
Herring, kippered	128	1		1	0.126	0.319	4.402	0.413	0.88	13.7	18.701
Herring, pickled	861	1	680	0	0.036	0.139	3.3	0.17	0.081	2.4	4.27
Lobster, northern, ckd, moist heat	87	1		0	0.007	0.066	1.07	0.077	0.285	11.1	3.11
Mackerel, ckd, dry heat	180	0		0.4	0.159	0.412	6.85	0.46	0.99	1.5	19
Mackerel, jack, cnd, drnd, sol	434	1.4	228	0.9	0.04	0.212	6.18	0.21	0.305	5	6.94
Mussel, blue, ckd, moist heat	304	0		13.6	0.3	0.42	3	0.1	0.95	75.6	24
Ocean perch, ckd, dry heat	46	0		0.8	0.13	0.134	2.436	0.27	0.42	10.4	1.154

(Continued)

Table D-I.   Vitamin contents of foods: units per 100-g edible portion—Cont'd

Food, by major food group	A (IU)	D (IU)	E (mg TE)[a]	K (mg)	C (mg)	Thiamin (mg)	Riboflavin (mg)	Niacin (mg)	B$_6$ (mg)	Pantothenic acid (mg)	Folate (µg)	B$_{12}$ (µg)
Oyster, breaded and fried	302		0		3.8	0.15	0.202	1.65	0.064	0.27	13.6	15.629
Oyster, canned	300		0.85		5	0.15	0.166	1.244	0.095	0.18	8.9	19.133
Oyster, raw	100		0.85	0.1	3.7	0.1	0.095	1.38	0.062	0.185	10	19.46
Perch, ckd, dry heat	32		0		1.7	0.08	0.12	1.9	0.14	0.87	5.8	2.2
Pike, northern, ckd, dry heat	81		0		3.8	0.067	0.077	2.8	0.135	0.87	17.3	2.3
Pollock, walleye, ckd, dry heat	76		0.2		0	0.074	0.076	1.65	0.069	0.16	3.6	4.2
Roe, mixed species, raw	263		7		16	0.24	0.74	1.8	0.16	1	80	10
Salmon, Chinook, smoked	88		1.35		0	0.023	0.101	4.72	0.278	0.87	1.9	3.26
Salmon, coho, wild, ckd, moist heat	108		0		1	0.115	0.159	7.779	0.556	0.834	9	4.48
Salmon, pink, cnd, sol w/bone and liquid	55	624	1.35		0	0.023	0.186	6.536	0.3	0.55	15.4	4.4
Salmon, sockeye, ckd, dry heat	209		0		0	0.215	0.171	6.67	0.219	0.7	5	5.8
Sardine, cnd in oil, drnd sol	224	272	0.3		0	0.08	0.227	5.245	0.167	0.642	11.8	8.94
Scallop, mxd sp, breaded and fried	75		0		2.3	0.042	0.11	1.505	0.14	0.2	18.2	1.318
Sea bass, mxd sp, ckd, dry heat	213		0		0	0.13	0.15	1.9	0.46	0.87	5.8	0.3
Shark, mxd sp, battered and fried	180		0		0	0.072	0.097	2.783	0.3	0.62	5.2	1.211
Shrimp, mxd sp, breaded and fried	189		0		1.5	0.129	0.136	3.07	0.098	0.35	8.1	1.87
Shrimp, mxd sp, ckd, moist heat	219	152	0.51		2.2	0.031	0.032	2.59	0.127	0.34	3.5	1.488

Food												
Smelt, rainbow, ckd, dry heat	58			0	0	0.01	0.146	1.766	0.17	0.74	4.6	3.969
Snapper, mxd sp, ckd, dry heat	115			0	1.6	0.053	0.004	0.346	0.46	0.87	5.8	3.5
Squid, mxd sp, fried	35			0	4.2	0.056	0.458	2.602	0.058	0.51	5.3	1.228
Surimi	66			0	0	0.02	0.021	0.22	0.03	0.07	1.6	1.6
Swordfish, ckd, dry heat	137			0	1.1	0.043	0.116	11.79	0.381	0.38	2.3	2.019
Trout, rainbow, wild, ckd, dry heat	50			0	2	0.152	0.097	5.77	0.346	1.065	19	6.3
Tuna, frsh, bluefin, ckd, dry heat	2,520			0	0	0.278	0.306	10.54	0.525	1.37	2.2	10.878
Tuna, lt, cnd in H2O, drnd sol	56	236		0.53	0	0.032	0.074	13.28	0.35	0.214	4	2.99
Whiting, mxd sp, ckd, dry heat	114			0.3	0	0.068	0.06	1.67	0.18	0.25	15	2.6
Dairy products and eggs												
Butter	3,058	56	7	1.58	0	0.005	0.034	0.042	0.003	0.11	3	0.125
Cheese, American	1,209.6			0.46	0	0.027	0.353	0.069	0.071	0.482	7.8	0.696
Cheese, blue	721			0.64	0	0.029	0.382	1.016	0.166	1.729	36.4	1.217
Cheese, Brie	667			0.655	0	0.07	0.52	0.38	0.235	0.69	65	1.65
Cheese, Camembert	923	12		0.655	0	0.028	0.488	0.63	0.227	1.364	62.2	1.296
Cheese, cheddar	1,059	12		0.36	0	0.027	0.375	0.08	0.074	0.413	18.2	0.827
Cheese, colby	1,034		3	0.35	0	0.015	0.375	0.093	0.079	0.21	18.2	0.826
Cheese, cottage, 1% fat	37			0.11	0	0.021	0.165	0.128	0.068	0.215	12.4	0.633
Cheese, cottage, crmd	163			0.122	0	0.021	0.163	0.126	0.067	0.213	12.2	0.623
Cheese, cream	1,427			0.941	0	0.017	0.197	0.101	0.047	0.271	13.2	0.424
Cheese, cream, fat free	930			0.03	0	0.05	0.172	0.16	0.05	0.194	37	0.55
Cheese, Edam	916	36		0.751	0	0.037	0.389	0.082	0.076	0.281	16.2	1.535
Cheese, feta	447			0.03	0	0.154	0.844	0.991	0.424	0.967	32	1.69
Cheese, Gouda	644			0.35	0	0.03	0.334	0.063	0.08	0.34	20.9	1.535
Cheese, Gruyère	1,219			0.35	0	0.06	0.279	0.106	0.081	0.562	10.4	1.6
Cheese, Monterey	950			0.34	0	0.015	0.39	0.093	0.079	0.21	18.2	0.826

(Continued)

Table D-I. Vitamin contents of foods: units per 100-g edible portion—Cont'd

Food, by major food group	A (IU)	D (IU)	E (mg TE)[a]	K (mg)	C (mg)	Thiamin (mg)	Riboflavin (mg)	Niacin (mg)	B$_6$ (mg)	Pantothenic acid (mg)	Folate (µg)	B$_{12}$ (µg)
Cheese, mozzarella, skm milk	584		0.43		0	0.018	0.303	0.105	0.07	0.079	8.8	0.817
Cheese, mozzarella, whl milk	792		0.35		0	0.015	0.243	0.084	0.056	0.064	7	0.654
Cheese, Muenster	1,120		0.465		0	0.013	0.32	0.103	0.056	0.19	12.1	1.473
Cheese, Parmesan	701	28	0.8		0	0.045	0.386	0.315	0.105	0.527	8	1.4
Cheese, provolone	815		0.35		0	0.019	0.321	0.156	0.073	0.476	10.4	1.463
Cheese, ricotta, skm milk	432		0.214		0	0.021	0.185	0.078	0.02	0.242	13.1	0.291
Cheese, ricotta, whl milk	490		0.35		0	0.013	0.195	0.104	0.043	0.213	12.2	0.338
Cheese, Swiss	845	44	0.5		0	0.022	0.365	0.092	0.083	0.429	6.4	1.676
Cream, half and half	434		0.11		0.86	0.035	0.149	0.078	0.039	0.289	2.5	0.329
Cream, lt, coffee/table	633		0.15		0.76	0.032	0.148	0.057	0.032	0.276	2.3	0.22
Cream, sour	790		0.566	1	0.86	0.035	0.149	0.067	0.016	0.36	10.8	0.3
Egg, white, dried	0	0	0		0	0.005	2.53	0.865	0.036	0.775	18	0.18
Egg, white, raw, fresh	0	0	0	0.01	0	0.006	0.452	0.092	0.004	0.119	3	0.2
Egg, whole, fried	857	32	1.64		0	0.057	0.523	0.077	0.143	1.224	38	0.92
Egg, whole, hard-boiled	560		1.05		0	0.066	0.513	0.064	0.121	1.398	44	1.11
Egg, whole, raw	635	52	1.05	2	0	0.062	0.508	0.073	0.139	1.255	47	1
Egg, yolk, raw	1,945		3.16		0	0.17	0.639	0.015	0.392	3.807	146	3.11
Milk, buttermilk, from skim milk	33		0.06		0.98	0.034	0.154	0.058	0.034	0.275	5	0.219
Milk, cnd, evap, whl, w/o vit A	243		0.18		1.88	0.047	0.316	0.194	0.05	0.638	7.9	0.163
Milk, dry, skim, non-fat sol, reg, w/o vit A	36		0.021		6.76	0.415	1.55	0.951	0.361	3.568	50.1	4.033
Milk, goat	185	12	0.09		1.29	0.048	0.138	0.277	0.046	0.31	0.6	0.065

Food												
Milk, human	241	4	0.9		5	0.014	0.036	0.177	0.011	0.223	5.2	0.045
Milk, lofat, 1% fat, w/vit A	205	40	0.04		0.97	0.039	0.167	0.087	0.043	0.323	5.1	0.368
Milk, lofat, 2% fat, w/vit A	205	40	0.07		0.95	0.039	0.165	0.086	0.043	0.32	5.1	0.364
Milk, skim, w/vit A	204	40	0.04	0.02	0.98	0.036	0.14	0.088	0.04	0.329	5.2	0.378
Milk, whole, 3.3% fat	126	40	0.1	0.3	0.94	0.038	0.162	0.084	0.042	0.314	5	0.357
Yogurt, pin, whl milk	123		0.088		0.53	0.029	0.142	0.075	0.032	0.389	7.4	0.372
Fats and oils												
Fat, chicken	0		2.7		0	0	0	0	0	0	0	0
Lard	0		1.2		0	0	0	0	0	0	0	0
Margarine, hard, corn (hydr and reg)	3,571	0	USA		0.16	0.01	0.037	0.023	0.009	0.084	1.18	0.095
Margarine, hard, corn, soy, and cttnsd (hydr)	3,571	0	0	51	0.16	0.01	0.037	0.023	0.009	0.084	1.18	0.095
Margarine, soft, corn (hydr and reg)	3,571	0	0		0.141	0.009	0.032	0.02	0.008	0.075	1.05	0.084
Margarine, soft, sfflwr, cttnsd and pnut (hydr)	3,571	0	0		0.141	0.009	0.032	0.02	0.008	0.075	1.05	0.084
Margarine, soft, soybn (hydr and reg)	3,571	0	0		0.141	0.009	0.032	0.02	0.008	0.075	1.05	0.084
Mayonnaise	220		4	81	0	0.013	0.024	0.004	0.017	0.243	6.28	0.208
Oil, canola	0	0	20.95	141	0	0	0	0	0	0	0	0
Oil, cocoa butter	0	0	0		0	0	0	0	0	0	0	0
Oil, coconut	0	0	0.28		0	0	0	0	0	0	0	0
Oil, cod liver	100,000	16,700	0	3	0	0	0	0	0	0	0	0
Oil, corn		0	0		0	0	0	0	0	0	0	0
Oil, mustard	0	0	0		0	0	0	0	0	0	0	0
Oil, olive	0	0	12.4	49	0	0	0	0	0	0	0	0
Oil, palm	0	0	21.76		0	0	0	0	0	0	0	0
Oil, peanut	0	0	12.92	0.7	0	0	0	0	0	0	0	0
Oil, rice bran	0	0	0		0	0	0	0	0	0	0	0
Oil, sesame	0	0	4.09	10	0	0	0	0	0	0	0	0

(Continued)

Table D-I. Vitamin contents of foods: units per 100-g edible portion—Cont'd

Food, by major food group	A (IU)	D (IU)	E (mg TE)[a]	K (mg)	C (mg)	Thiamin (mg)	Riboflavin (mg)	Niacin (mg)	B$_6$ (mg)	Pantothenic acid (mg)	Folate (μg)	B$_{12}$ (μg)
Oil, soybean	0	0	18.19	193	0	0	0	0	0	0	0	0
Oil, sunflower	0	0	0	9	0	0	0	0	0	0	0	0
Oil, wheat germ	0	0	192.44		0	0	0	0	0	0	0	0
Salad dressing, Thousand Island	320		1.14		0	0.013	0.024	0.004	0.017	0.243	6.28	0.208
Salad dressing, Thousand Island, lofat	320		1.19		0	0.011	0.021	0.003	0.015	0.216	5.58	0.185
Salad dressing, French, lofat	1,300		1.19		0	0	0	0	0	0	0	0
Salad dressing, Italian, lofat	0		1.5		0	0	0	0	0	0	0	0
Salad dressing, Russian	690		10.2		6	0.05	0.05	0.6	0.03	0.4	10.4	0.3
Salad dressing, Russian, lofat	56		0.76		6	0.007	0.013	0.002	0.009	0.135	3.49	0.116
Shortening, soybn and cttnsd (hydr)	0	0	8.28		0	0	0	0	0	0	0	0
Tallow	0	0	2.7		0	0	0	0	0	0	0	0
Spices												
Allspice	540	0	1.03		39	0.101	0.063	2.86	0.34	0	36	0
Anise seed	311	0	1.03		21	0.34	0.29	3.06	0.34	0.797	10	0
Basil	9,375	0	1.69		61	0.148	0.316	6.948	1.21	0	274	0
Bay leaf	6,185	0	1.786		47	0.009	0.421	2.005	1	0	180	0
Caraway seed	363	0	2.5		21	0.383	0.379	3.606	0.34	0	10	0
Cardamom	0	0	0		21	0.198	0.182	1.102	0	0	0	0
Celery seed	52	0	1.03		17.1	0.34	0.29	3.06	0.34	0	10	0
Chili powder	34,927	0	1.03		64	0.349	0.794	7.893	1.87	0	100	0
Cinnamon	260	0	0.01		28	0.077	0.14	1.3	0.25	0	29	0
Cloves	530	0	1.69		81	0.115	0.267	1.458	1.29	0	93	0

Coriander leaf, dried	5,850	0	1.03	567	1.252	1.5	10.71	1.21	0	274	0
Coriander seed	0	0	0	21	0.239	0.29	2.13	0	0	0.032	0
Cumin seed	1,270	0	1.03	7.7	0.628	0.327	4.579	0.34	0	10	0
Curry powder	986	0	0.3	11.4	0.253	0.281	3.467	0.68	0	154	0
Dill seed	53	0	1.03	21	0.418	0.284	2.807	0.34	0	10	0
Dill weed, dried	5,850	0	0	50	0.418	0.284	2.807	1.461	0	0	0
Fennel seed	135	0	0	21	0.408	0.353	6.05	0	0	0	0
Garlic powder	0	0	0.01	18	0.466	0.152	0.692	2.7	0	2	0
Ginger	147	0	0.28	7	0.046	0.185	5.155	1.12	0	39	0
Mace	800	0	2.5	21	0.312	0.448	1.35	0.3	0	76	0
Marjoram, dried	8,068	0	1.69	51	0.289	0.316	4.12	1.21	0	274	0
Mustard seed, yellow	62	0	2.5	3	0.543	0.381	7.89	0.3	0	76	0
Nutmeg	102	0	2.5	3	0.346	0.057	1.299	0.3	0	76	0
Oregano	6,903	0	1.69	50	0.341	0.32	6.22	1.21	0	274	0
Paprika	60,604	0	0.69	71	0.645	1.743	15.32	2.06	1.78	106	0
Pepper, black	190	0	1.03	21	0.109	0.24	1.142	0.34	0	10	0
Pepper, red/cayenne	41,610	0	4.8	76	0.328	0.919	8.701	2.06	0	106	0
Pepper, white	0	0	2.5	21	0.022	0.126	0.212	0.34	0	10	0
Peppermint, fresh	4,248	0	0.34	31.8	0.082	0.266	1.706	0.129	0.338	114	0
Poppy seed	0	0	2.72	3	0.849	0.173	0.976	0.444	0	58	0
Rosemary, dried	3,128	0	0	61	0.514	0	1	0	0	0	0
Saffron	530	0	1.69	81	0.115	0.267	1.46	1.3	0	93	0
Sage	5,900	0	1.69	32.3	0.754	0.336	5.72	1.21	0	274	0
Savory	5,130	0	0	50	0.366	0	4.08	0	0	0	0
Spearmint, fresh	4,054	0	0.34	13	0.078	0.175	0.948	0.158	0.25	105	0
Tarragon	4,200	0	1.69	50	0.251	1.339	8.95	1.21	0	274	0
Thyme	3,800	0	1.69	50	0.513	0.399	4.94	1.21	0	274	0
Turmeric	0	0	0.07	26	0.152	0.233	5.14	1.8	0	39	0
Vanilla extract	0	0	0	0	0.011	0.095	0.425	0.026	0.035	0	0
Soups											
Bean w/pork, cnd	662	0	0.285	1.2	0.065	0.025	0.421	0.031	0.07	23.7	0.03
Black bean, cnd	445	0	0.058	0.2	0.042	0.039	0.41	0.07	0.16	20	0

(Continued)

Table D-I. Vitamin contents of foods: units per 100-g edible portion—Cont'd

Food, by major food group	A (IU)	D (IU)	E (mg TE)[a]	K (mg)	C (mg)	Thiamin (mg)	Riboflavin (mg)	Niacin (mg)	B$_6$ (mg)	Pantothenic acid (mg)	Folate (µg)	B$_{12}$ (µg)
Chicken broth, cnd	0		0.028		0	0.006	0.046	2.23	0.02	0.04	4	0.2
Chicken gumbo, cnd	108		0.031		4	0.2	0.3	0.53	0.05	0.16	5	0.02
Chicken noodle, cnd	532		0.051		0	0.052	0.054	1.228	0.021	0.14	1.8	0.13
Chicken w/rice, cnd	539		0.043		0.1	0.014	0.02	0.918	0.02	0.14	0.9	0.13
Clam chowder, Manhattan, cnd	767		0.581		3.2	0.024	0.032	0.65	0.08	0.15	8	3.23
Clam chowder, New England, cnd	8		0.066		1.9	0.016	0.03	0.74	0.06	0.26	2.9	7.82
Cream of asparagus, cnd	355		0.5		2.2	0.043	0.062	0.62	0.01	0.11	19	0.04
Cream of celery, cnd	244		0.15		0.2	0.023	0.039	0.265	0.01	0.92	1.9	0.04
Cream of chicken, cnd	446		0.13		0.1	0.023	0.048	0.653	0.013	0.17	1.3	0.07
Cream of mushroom, cnd	0		1.04		0.9	0.024	0.066	0.645	0.01	0.2	3	0.1
Cream of onion, cnd	236		0.68		1	0.04	0.06	0.4	0.02	0.24	5.7	0.04
Cream of potato, cnd	230		0.06		0	0.028	0.029	0.43	0.03	0.7	2.4	0.04
Gazpacho, cnd, RTS	1,067		0.19		2.9	0.02	0.01	0.38	0.06	0.07	4	0
Lentil w/ham, cnd, RTS	145		0		1.7	0.07	0.045	0.545	0.09	0.14	20	0.12
Minestrone, cnd	1,908		0.6		0.9	0.044	0.036	0.77	0.08	0.28	13.1	0
Oyster stew, cnd	58		0		2.6	0.017	0.029	0.19	0.01	0.1	2	1.79
Pea, green, cnd	153	0	0.099		1.3	0.082	0.052	0.943	0.04	0.1	1.4	0
Pea, split w/ham, cnd	331	0	0		1.1	0.11	0.056	1.098	0.05	0.2	1.9	0.2
Tomato, cnd	555		2.02		53	0.07	0.04	1.13	0.09	0.12	11.7	0
Tomato rice, cnd	588		0.6		11.5	0.048	0.039	0.822	0.06	0.1	11	0
Turkey noodle, cnd	233		0.047		0.1	0.059	0.051	1.112	0.03	0.14	1.8	0.13
Vegetable beef, cnd	1,508		0		1.9	0.029	0.039	0.823	0.06	0.28	8.4	0.25
Vegetarian vegetable, cnd	2,453	0	0.26		1.2	0.044	0.037	0.747	0.045	0.28	8.6	0

Beverages

Beer, reg	0	0	0		0	0.006	0.026	0.453	0.05	0.058	6	0.02
Clam and tomato juice, cnd	215	0	0		4.1	0.04	0.03	0.19	0.084	0.251	15.9	30.6
Cocoa mix, w/o added nutrients, pdr	14	0	0.15		1.8	0.096	0.565	0.586	0.114	0.893	0	1.32
Coffee, brewed, espresso	0	0	0		0.2	0.001	0.177	5.207	0.002	0.028	1	0
Coffee, brewed, regular	0	0	0		0	0	0	0.222	0	0.001	0.1	0
Distilled (gin/rum/vodka/whiskey), 80 proof	0	0	0	10	0	0.006	0.004	0.013	0.001	0	0	0
Sodas, ginger ale/grape/orange	0	0	0		0	0	0	0	0	0	0	0
Sodas, lemon-lime	0	0	0		0	0	0	0.015	0	0	0	0
Tea, brewed	0	0	0	0.05	0	0	0.014	0	0	0.011	5.2	0
Wine, table	0	0	0	0.005	0	0.004	0.016	0.074	0.024	0.028	1.1	0.01

Snack foods and desserts

Banana chips	83	0	5.4	0	6.3	0.085	0.017	0.71	0.26	0.62	14	0
Candies, caramels	32	0	0.463	0	0.5	0.01	0.181	0.25	0.035	0.592	5	0
Candies, gumdrops	0	0	0	0	0	0	0.002	0.002	0	0.006	0	0
Candies, hard	0	0	0	0	0	0.004	0.003	0.007	0.003	0.008	0	0
Candies, jellybeans	0	0	0	0	0	0	0	0	0	0	0	0
Candies, marshmallows	1	0	0	0	0	0.001	0.001	0.078	0.002	0.005	1	0
Candies, milk chocolate	185	0	1.24	0	0.4	0.079	0.301	0.324	0.042	0.424	8	0.39
Candies, semisweet choc	21	0	1.19	0	0	0.055	0.09	0.427	0.035	0.105	3	0
Frosting, vanilla, creamy, RTE	746	0	2.016		0	0	0.006	0.011	0	0.002	0	0
Gelatins, prepd w/H$_2$O	0	0	0	0	0	0	0.003	0.001	0.002	0.002	0	0
Ice milk, vanilla	165	0	0		0.8	0.058	0.265	0.09	0.065	0.505	6	0.67
Jams and preserves	12	0	0	0	8.8	0	0.022	0.036	0.02	0.02	33	0
Jellies	17	0	0	0	0.9	0.001	0.026	0.036	0.02	0.197	1	0
Marmalade, orange	47	0	0	0	4.8	0.005	0.006	0.052	0.014	0.015	36	0
Molasses	0	0	0	0	0	0.041	0.002	0.93	0.67	0.804	0	0
Popcorn, air-popped	196	0	0.12	0	0	0.203	0.283	1.944	0.245	0.42	23	0

(*Continued*)

Table D-I. Vitamin contents of foods: units per 100-g edible portion—Cont'd

Food, by major food group	Vitamin									Pantothenic		
	A (IU)	D (IU)	E (mg TE)[a]	K (mg)	C (mg)	Thiamin (mg)	Riboflavin (mg)	Niacin (mg)	B$_6$ (mg)	acid (mg)	Folate (µg)	B$_{12}$ (µg)
Popcorn, cakes	72	0	0.12		0	0,075	0.178	6.006	0.181	0.434	18	0
Popcorn, caramel-coated, w/pnuts	64	0	1.5		0	0.051	0.126	1.99	0.185	0.23	16	0
Popcorn, oil-popped	154	0	0.12		0.3	0.134	0.136	1.55	0.209	0.305	17	0
Potato chips, barbecue	217	0	5	10	33.9	0.215	0.215	4.692	0.622	0.617	83	0
Potato chips, plain	0	0	4.88	10	31.1	0.167	0.197	3.827	0.66	0.402	45	0
Pretzels, hard, salted	0	0	0.21	1	0	0.461	0.623	5.251	0.116	0.288	83	0
Pudding, choc, prepd w/2% milk	185	0	0		0.6	0.03	0.139	0.128	0.034	0.26	4	0.23
Pudding, choc, w/whl milk	107		0.06		0.9	0.033	0.141	0.096	0.038	0.269	4	0.3
Pudding, lemon, prepd w/2% milk	170		0		0.8	0.033	0.137	0.072	0.036	0.267	4	0.3
Pudding, rice, w/whl milk	107		0		0.7	0.075	0.139	0.445	0.034	0.285	4	0.24
Pudding, tapioca, prepd w/whl milk	109		0		0.7	0.03	0.141	0.073	0.038	0.274	4	0.25
Rice cakes, brown rice, pln	46	0	0.72		0	0.061	0.165	7.806	0.15	1	21	0
Sugar, brown	0	0	0		0	0.008	0.007	0.082	0.026	0.111	1	0
Sugar, granulated	0	0	0	0	0	0	0.019	0	0	0	0	0
Syrup, choc, fudge-type	90	0	0		0.5	0.03	0.22	0.2	0.035	0.306	4	0.3
Syrup, corn	0	0	0		0	0.011	0.009	0.02	0.009	0.023	0	0
Syrup, maple	0	0	0		0	0.006	0.01	0.03	0.002	0.036	0	0
Syrup, sorghum	0	0	0		0	0.1	0.155	0.1	0.67	0.804	0	0
Tortilla chips, plain	196	0	1.36		0	0.075	0.184	1.279	0.286	0.788	10	0
Tortilla chips, taco flavor	905	0	0		0.9	0.242	0.204	1.999	0.297	0.29	21	0

American fast foods

Biscuit, w/egg, chs, and bacon	450		0	1.1	0.21	0.3	1.6	0.07	0.82	26	0.73
Biscuit, w/ham	118		1.984	0.1	0.45	0.28	3.08	0.12	0.36	7	0.03
Burrito, w/bns and chs	672		0	0.9	0.12	0.38	1.92	0.13	0.86	44	0.48
Burrito, w/bns and meat	275		0	0.8	0.23	0.36	2.34	0.16	0.97	32	0.75
Cheeseburger, single patty, w/condmnt	409	12	0.47	1.7	0.22	0.2	3.29	0.1	0.28	16	0.83
Chicken fillet sndwch, w/chs	272		0	1.3	0.18	0.2	3.98	0.18	0.59	20	0.2
Chicken, breaded and fried (breast/wing)	118		0	0	0.09	0.18	7.35	0.35	1.59	5	0.41
Chicken, breaded and fried (drumstk/thigh)	150		0	0	0.09	0.29	4.87	0.22	1.66	6	0.56
Chili con carne	657		0	0.6	0.05	0.45	0.98	0.13	1.42	12	0.45
Croissant, w/egg, chs, and ham	297		0	7.5	0.34	0.2	2.1	0.15	0.82	24	0.66
Enchilada, w/chs and bf	591		0	0.7	0.05	0.21	1.31	0.14	0.75	100	0.53
English muffin, w/egg, chs, and Canadian bacon	428		0.621	1.3	0.361	0.327	2.434	0.107	0.653	32	0.49
French toast	32		2.81	0	0.16	0.18	2.1	0.18	0.4	95	0.05
Hamburger, single patty, w/condiment	70	12	0.012	2.1	0.274	0.222	3.69	0.111	0.263	49	1.03
Hot dog, plain	0		0	0.1	0.24	0.28	3.72	0.05	0.52	30	0.52
Hot dog, w/chili	51		0	2.4	0.19	0.35	3.28	0.04	0.48	44	0.26
Hot dog, w/corn flr coating (corndog)	118		0	0	0.16	0.4	2.38	0.05	0.77	34	0.25
Hush puppies	120		0	0	0	0.03	2.6	0.13	0.28	27	0.22
Nachos, w/chs	495		0	1.1	0.17	0.33	1.36	0.18	1.16	9	0.73
Onion rings, breaded and fried	10		0.4	0.7	0.1	0.12	1.11	0.07	0.24	14	0.15
Pizza w/cheese, meat, and veg	663		0	2	0.27	0.22	2.48	0.12	1.05	34	0.46

(Continued)

Table D-I. Vitamin contents of foods: units per 100-g edible portion—Cont'd

Food, by major food group	A (IU)	D (IU)	E (mg TE)[a]	K (mg)	C (mg)	Thiamin (mg)	Riboflavin (mg)	Niacin (mg)	B$_6$ (mg)	Pantothenic acid (mg)	Folate (µg)	B$_{12}$ (µg)
Pizza w/cheese	607		0		2	0.29	0.26	3.94	0.07	0.35	93	0.53
Pizza w/pepperoni	397		0		2.3	0.19	0.33	4.29	0.08	0.35	74	0.26
Potato salad	100		0		1.1	0.07	0.11	0.27	0.15	0.37	25	0.12
Potato, bkd and topped w/chs, sau, and bacon	210		0		9.6	0.09	0.08	1.33	0.25	0.43	10	0.11
Potato, bkd and topped w/chs, sau, and broccoli	500		0		14.3	0.08	0.08	1.06	0.23	0.42	18	0.1
Potato, mashed	41		0		0.4	0.09	0.05	1.2	0.23	0.48	8	0.05
Potatoes, hashed brown	25		0.17		7.6	0.11	0.02	1.49	0.23	0.47	11	0.02
Roast beef sandwich, pln	151		0		1.5	0.27	0.22	4.22	0.19	0.6	29	0.88
Salad, taco	297		0		1.8	0.05	0.18	1.24	0.11	0.68	20	0.32
Salad, tossed, w/o drsng, w/turkey, ham, and chs	323		0		5	0.12	0.12	1.83	0.13	0.28	31	0.26
Salad, tossed, w/o drsng, w/chick	429		0		8	0.05	0.06	2.7	0.2	0.27	31	0.09
Salad, tossed, w/o drsng, w/chs and egg	379		0		4.5	0.04	0.08	0.45	0.05	0.24	39	0.14
Salad, tossed, w/o drsng	1136		0		23.2	0.03	0.05	0.55	0.08	0.12	37	0
Submarine sandwich, w/cold cuts	186		0		5.4	0.44	0.35	2.41	0.06	0.39	24	0.48
Submarine sandwich, w/rst beef	191		0		2.6	0.19	0.19	2.76	0.15	0.36	21	0.84
Submarine sandwich, w/tuna salad	73		0		1.4	0.18	0.13	4.43	0.09	0.73	22	0.63
Taco	500		0		1.3	0.09	0.26	1.88	0.14	0.99	14	0.61
Tostada, w/bns, beef, and chs	567		0		1.8	0.04	0.22	1.27	0.11	0.83	43	0.5

[a] TE, α-Tocopherol equivalents.

Sources: Nutrient Data Laboratory, Agricultural Research Service, U.S. Department of Agriculture; USDA Nutrient Database for Standard Reference, Release 11-1 (http://www.nal.usda.gov/fnic/food-com/Data/SRII-1/srII-1.html); Provisional Table on the Vitamin D Content of Foods, revised 1991 (http://www.nal.usda.gov/fnic/foodcom/Data/Other/vitd.dat); Provisional Table on the Vitamin K Content of Foods, revised 1994 (http://www.nal.usda.gov/fnic/foodcom/Data/Other/vitk2.dat).

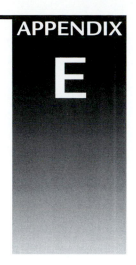

Vitamin Contents of Feedstuffs

THE FOLLOWING table is used with the permission of M. L. Scott, M. C. Nesheim, and R. J. Young (Cornell University, Ithaca, New York), and was derived from their table of feed composition [Scott, M. L., Nesheim, M. C., and Young, R. J. (1982). *Nutrition of the Chicken,* 3rd ed., pp. 490–493. M. L. Scott and Associates, Ithaca, New York]. It is a useful reference to the vitamin contents of common feedstuffs. The table begins on page 562.

Table E-1. Vitamin contents of feedstuffs: units per kilogram

Feedstuff	E (IU)	Riboflavin (mg)	Niacin (mg)	B$_6$ (mg)	Biotin (mg)	Pantothenic acid (mg)	Folate (mg)	B$_{12}$ (µg)	Choline (mg)
Alfalfa leaf meal, dehydrated	140	15	55	11	0.35	33	4		1,600
Alfalfa meal, dehydrated	120	13	46	10	0.33	27	3.5		1,600
Alfalfa meal, sun-cured	66	11	40	9	0.3	20	3.3		1,500
Bakery product, dehydrated	25	0.8	50	4.4	0.07	9	0.15		660
Barley	36	2	57	2.9	15	6.6	0.5		1,100
Beans, field	1	1.8	24	0.3	0.11	3.1	1.3		
Blood meal	0	4.2	29	0		5.3			280
Brewers' dried grains	26	1.5	44	0.66		8.8	9.7		1,600
Buckwheat		11	18			5.9			13,000
Buttermilk, dried	6.3	30	9	2.4	0.3	30	0.4	20	1,800
Casein, purified		1.5	1.3	0.4		2.6	0.4		200
Citrus pulp, dried		2.2	22			13			900
Coconut oil	35	0	0	0	0	0	0	0	0
Coconut oil meal (copra meal)		3.5	24	4.4		6.6	0.3		1,100
Corn and cob meal	20	1.1	20	5	0.05	5	0.3		550
Corn germ meal	87	3.7	42		3	3.3	0.7		1,540
Corn gluten feed	24	2.2	66		0.3	0.5	0.2		1,100
Corn gluten meal	42	1.5	50	8	0.15	10	0.7		330
Corn gluten meal, 60% protein	50	1.8	60	9.6	0.2	12	0.84		400
Corn oil	280	0	0	0	0	0	0	0	0
Corn, dent, No. 2, yellow	22	1.3	22	7	0.06	5.7	0.36		620
Cottonseed meal, dehulled		5.7	51	7	0.1	15	1.1		3,300
Cottonseed meal, hydraulic/expeller	40	4	5	5.3	0.1	11	1		2,800
Cottonseed meal, solvent	15	5	44	6.4	0.1	13	1		2,900
Crab meal		5.9	44		0.7	6.6		330	2,000
Distillers' dried grains (corn)	30	3.1	42			5.9			1,900
Distillers' dried grains w/solubles (corn)	40	8.6	66		1.1	11	0.9		2,500
Distillers' dried solubles (corn)	55	17	115	10	1.5	22	2.2		4,800

Ingredient									
Feathers, poultry, hydrolyzed	3.4	2	24		44	11	0.22	70	900
Fish meal, anchovetta	27	6.6	64	3.5	0.26	8.8	0.2	100	3,700
Fish meal, herring	9	9	89	3.7	0.42	11	0.24	240	4,000
Fish meal, menhaden	9	4.8	55	3.5	0.26	8.8	0.2	88	3,500
Fish meal, pilchard	9	9.5	55	3.5	0.26	9	0.2	100	2,200
Fish meal, redfish waste	6			3.3	0.08		0.2	100	3,500
Fish meal, whitefish waste	9	9	70	3.3	0.08	8.8	0.2	100	2,200
Fish oils, stabilized	70	0	0	0	0	0	0	0	0
Fish solubles, dried	6	7.7	230		0.26	45		400	5,300
Hominy feed, yellow		2.2	44	11	0.13	7.7	0.28		1,000
Lard, stabilized	23	0	0	0	0	0	0	0	0
Liver and glandular meal		40	160	5	0.8	105	4	440	10,500
Meat and bone meal, 45% protein	1	5.3	38	2.3	0.1	2.4	0.05	44	2,000
Meat and bone meal, 50% protein	1	4.4	49	2.5	0.14	3.7	0.05	44	2,200
Meat meal, 55% protein	1	5.3	57	3	0.26	4.8	0.05	44	2,200
Milk, dried skim		20	11	4.9	0.33	33	0.02	60	1,400
Milo (grain sorghum)	12	1.2	40	4	0.18	11	0.24		680
Molasses, beet		0.4	40	5.4	88	66	0.2		880
Molasses, cane	5	2.5	100	4.4	100	58	0.04		880
Oat mill by-product		1.5	10			3.3			440
Oatmeal feed	24	1.8	13	2.2	0.22	15	0.35		1,200
Oats, heavy	20	1.1	18	1.3	0.11	13	0.3		1,100
Olive oil	125								
Peanut meal, dehulled, solvent	3	12	180	10	0.39	60	0.36		2,100
Peanut meal, solvent	3	11	170	10	0.39	53	0.36		2,000
Peanut oil	280	0	0	0	0	0	0	0	0
Peas, field dry		1.8	37	1	0.18	10	0.36		
Potato meal, white, dried		0.7	33	14	0.1	20	0.6		2,600
Poultry byproduct meal	2	11	40		0.3	8.8	1		6,000
Poultry offal fat, stabilized	30	0	0	0	0	0	0	0	0
Rapeseed meal	19	3.7	155			9			6,600
Rice bran	420								

(Continued)

Table E-1. Vitamin contents of feedstuffs: units per kilogram—Cont'd

Feedstuff	E (IU)	Riboflavin (mg)	Niacin (mg)	B$_6$ (mg)	Biotin (mg)	Pantothenic acid (mg)	Folate (mg)	B$_{12}$ (µg)	Choline (mg)
Rice bran	60	2.6	300		0.42	23			1,300
Rice polishings	90	1.8	530		0.62	57			1,300
Rice, rough	14	0.5	37			3.3	0.25		800
Rice, white, polished	3.6	0.6	14	0.4		3.3	0.15		900
Safflower meal	1	4	6		1.4	4	0.44		2,600
Safflower oil	500	0	0	0	0	0	0	0	0
Sesame meal		3.3	30	12.5		6			1,500
Sesame oil	250	0	0	0	0	0	0	0	0
Soybean meal	2	3.3	27	8	0.32	14.5	3.6		2,700
Soybean meal, dehulled	3.3	3.1	22	8	0.32	14.5	3.6		2,700
Soybean oil	280	0	0	0	0	0	0	0	0
Soybean, isolated protein	0	1.25	4.9	1.3		0.63			
Soybeans, full-fat, processed	50	2.6	22	11	0.37	15	2.2		2,800
Sunflower oil	350	0	0	0	0	0	0	0	0
Sunflower seed meal, dehulled, solvent	20	7.2	106	16		40			4,200
Sunflower seed meal, solvent	11	6.4	91	16		10			2,900
Tallow, stabilized	13	0	0	0	0	0	0	0	0
Tomato pomace, dried		6.2							
Wheat bran	17	3.1	200	10	0.48	29	0.78		1,000
Wheat germ meal	130	5	50	13	0.22	12	2.4		3,300
Wheat middlings	44	2	100	11	0.37	20	1.1		1,100
Wheat shorts	57	2	95	11	0.37	8	1.1		930
Wheat, hard, northern U.S. and Canada	11	1.1	60	4	0.11	13	0.4		1,000
Wheat, hard, south–central U.S.	11	2	60	4	0.11	13	0.35		1,000
Wheat, soft	11	1.1	60	4	0.11	13	0.3		1,000
Whey product, dried		40	15	3.2	0.28	60	0.8	40	260
Whey, dried		30	11	2.5	0.25	47	0.58	0.3	200
Yeast, brewers', dried	0	35	450	3.3	1.3	110	12		3,900
Yeast, torula, dried	0	44	500		2	83	21		2,900

Source: Data derived, with permission, from Scott, M. L., Nesheim, M. C., and Young, R. J. (1982). *The Nutrition of the Chicken*, 3rd ed., pp. 490–493. M. L. Scott and Associates, Ithaca, NY.

Index

Page numbers followed by f, t, or n indicate figures, tables and footnotes respectively.

Abetalipoproteinemia, 103, 187n15, 207
Absorption
  biotin, 334
  calcium, 161
  carnitine, 408
  of carotenoids, 99–100
  choline, 402–404
  folate, 358–360
  myo-inositol, 415–416
  niacin, 298, 298f
  pantothenic acid, 347
  phosphate, 161
  of retinoids, 99
  riboflavin, 283–284
  thiamin, 268–269
  of ubiquinones, 421
  vitamin A, 99–102
  vitamin B_6, 316
  vitamin B_{12}, 383–384
  vitamin C, 239–240
  vitamin D, 150
  vitamin E, 184–185, 186f
  vitamin K, 216–217
  of vitamins/vitamers, 37–41t, 64–65, 66t
Accessory factors, 4
  disease prevention through, 17
  fat-soluble A, 17, 17t, 19
  Hopkins on, 15–16
  in milk, 15, 16, 16f
  vitamine theory and, 15–18
  vitamines as, 17
  vitamins as, 399
  water-soluble B, 17, 17t, 20–21
p-Acetaminobenzoylglutamate, 364, 365
Acetylcholine, 403, 405
Acetyl-CoA, 248, 300
  carboxylase, 337–338
  metabolism and, 351f
Achlorhydria, 79, 83t
Achromotrichia, 80t, 339, 339t
ACP. *See* Acyl-carrier protein

Acrodynia, 80t, 88t, 323
ACS. *See* α-Amino-β-carboxymuconic-ε-semialdehyde
Active transport, of phylloquinones, 217
Acylcarnitine esters, 409, 411
Acyl-carrier protein (ACP), 345, 349
Acyl-CoA
  dehydrogenase, 288
  synthase, 352
Acyl-CoA: retinol acyltransferase (ARAT), 101, 102, 103
Adenosylcobalamin, 41t, 60, 70t, 384, 385, 386t
  generation of, 386
Adequate Intakes (AIs), 491t, 494, 496
Adipose tissue, vitamin A in, 109
Adrenal necrosis, 84t
Adrenodoxin reductase, 289t
Age pigments, 82t, 197
Aging
  free-radical theory of, 197
  vitamin E and, 196–197
AIs. *See* Adequate Intakes
Alcohol dehydrogenase, 101
Alcohol/drugs/, vitamin B_6 and, 318
Aldehyde dehydrogenase (NAD+), 318
Aldehyde (pyridoxal) oxidase, 318
Alkaline phosphatase, 283
Alkaline phosphatases, 317–318
Alkylation, vitamin K and, 218
Allowances, nutrient, 487. *See also* Recommended Dietary Allowances
Alopecia, 80t, 89t, 91t, 338, 339t
Alzheimer's disease, thiamin and, 277
Americans
  fruits/vegetables consumed by, 479t
  vitamin availability for, 477, 478t
  vitamin intakes by, 478, 478t
Amine, vital, 4, 16
α-Amino-β-carboxymuconic-ε-semialdehyde (ACS), 300

p-Aminobenzoic acid, 31t, 401, 429
  folate and, 429
γ-Aminobutyric acid (GABA), 273, 325
α-Aminomuconic-semialdehyde, 300
Amphipaths, 36n1
Analysis methods, for vitamins, 61–62, 63t
Anemia, 25, 81t, 82t, 87t, 88t, 89t, 90t, 91t
  hemolytic, 206, 210
  hidden hunger and, 483
  hypoplastic, 291
  iron deficiency and, 483
  macrocytic, 356, 366, 376, 376t
  megaloblastic, 90t, 91t, 390, 391, 392
  normocytic hypochromic, 291
  pernicious, 28, 91t, 357, 375, 377, 381, 389–390
  sideroblastic, 326
  vitamin A and, 120t
  vitamin B_{12} and, 382
  yeast growth and, 27
Animal(s)
  biotin deficiencies in, 339
  flavoproteins of, 289t
  folate deficiencies in, 376
  niacin deficiencies in, 304–305
  nutrient requirements and, 486, 487, 487f
  PAC in, 301t
  pantothenic acid deficiencies in, 352
  polyneuritis in, 274–276
  protein factors, 28–29, 29t
  pyridine nucleotide-dependent enzymes of, 304t
  pyridoxal phosphate-dependent enzymes of, 320t
  riboflavin deficiencies in, 291
  toxicity of vitamins in, 506–507t
  transgenic, 103, 112
  ULs for, 513t
  vitamin allowances for, 498, 499–501t

Animal(s) (*Continued*)
  vitamin B_6 deficiencies in, 323–324
  vitamin B_{12} deficiencies in, 391–392
  vitamin C deficiency in, 256
  vitamin D and osteoporosis in, 174
  vitamin D and tibial
    dyschondroplasia in, 174
  vitamin D deficiencies in, 173–174
  vitamin deficiencies and, 79
  vitamin K in livers of, 217t
Animal models, 8, 13, 13n5
  for beriberi, 13–14
  for pellagra, impact of, 22–23
  vitamin C and, 18–19
Anorexia, 77, 78, 274
Antagonists
  biotin, 338
  folate, 59, 361
  niacin, 55
  pantothenic acid, 352
  riboflavin, 54
  thiamin, 267–268
  vitamin A, 121
  vitamin K, 220–221
Anthranilic acid, 302
Anthropometric evaluation, 470
Antialopecia factor, 413
Antianemia factors, 26
Antiberiberi. *See also* Beriberi
  factor, 14–15
  vitamine, 16
Antiestrogenic effects, of
  soy isoflavones, 424–425
Antihemorrhagic factor, as
  vitamin K, 25
Antihistamine reactions, ascorbic acid
    and, 249
Antioxidants, 191n33
  ascorbic acid as, 243–245
  carotenoids as, 126–127, 126t
  definition, 191n33
  flavonoids as, 423–424
  lipids and, in human LDLs, 200, 200t
  lipoic acid as, 429
  RDAs and, 492–493
  ubiquinones as, 420
  vitamin A as, 126–127
  vitamin E and, 194–196, 195f, 196t
  vitamin E as biological, 181, 191–192
  vitamins as, 72, 72t
Antipellagra vitamine, 16
Antirickets vitamine, 16
Antiscurvy vitamine, 16
Antixerophthalmic factor, 17, 19, 30
Apocarboxylases, 337
ApoE. *See* Apolipoprotein E
Apolipoprotein E (apoE), 187
  genotype and tocopherols, 187t
Apoptosis, 197, 198
Apo-RBP, 104, 105

Aquocobalamin, 384
Arachidonic acid, 416, 417
ARAT. *See* Acyl-CoA: retinol
    acyltransferase
Arteriosclerosis, 78n5, 82t, 88t
Ascorbate polyphosphate, 237
Ascorbic acid, 5, 5n4, 6t, 38t, 51, 52.
    See also Vitamin C
  antihistamine reactions and, 249
  antioxidant functions of, 243–245
  biopotency of, 52, 52t
  biosynthesis of, 237–238, 238f, 238t
  blood pressure and, 251, 251f
  cancer and, 254
  concentrations, of human tissues,
    240, 241t
  CVD and, 250–252
  discovery of, 18–19
  drug/steroid metabolism and, 247
  enzyme co-substrate functions of,
    245–247, 246t
  enzymes and, 245, 246t
  excretion of, 242–243, 243t
  health effects of, 249–254
  immune function and, 249–250
  inflammation and, 250, 251t
  iron and, 248, 249
  neurologic function and, 252–253
  nonenzymatic functions of, 247–249
  prooxidant potential of, 245
  pulmonary function and, 253–254
  redox cycle, 240, 240f
  regeneration of, 240f, 242
  skin health and, 253
  smoking and level of, 244, 244f,
    245f
  transport of, to plasma, 240
  vitamin C and, 61t, 62t
  vitamin C intake and, 241, 241f
  vitamin C-active derivatives of, 238t
L-Ascorbic acid 2-sulfate, 242
Ascorbyl free radical, 241
Ash, 4, 9
Assessment, vitamin status, 469–484
  approaches, 471
  biochemical methods for, 470,
    471–474, 472t, 473t
  human populations and, 474–483
  interpretive guidelines for, 472,
    474–476t
Ataxia, 85t, 87t, 88t, 89t, 188, 207, 274
Atherocalcin, 226. *See also* Gla
    proteins
Atherogenesis prevention, vitamin E
    and, 201, 201f
Atherosclerosis, vitamin K in, 226
ATPase, 268
Autoimmune diseases, vitamin D and,
    166–167
Avidin, 332, 335n11

Bacteria, menaquinones and enteric,
    216t
Beriberi, 9, 10, 12t, 80t, 81t, 83t, 85t,
    86t, 90t, 276. *See also* Eijkman,
    Christian
  animal model for, 13–14
  cardiac, 276
  factor for anti-, 14–15
  infantile, 276
  in Javanese prisons, 14, 14t
  neuritic, 276
  shoshin, 276
  thiamin and, 266
  vitamine for anti-, 16
  wet, 276
Betaine, 365n30, 379t
Betaine aldehyde dehydrogenase, 404
Betaine: homocysteine
    methyltransferase, 404
Binding proteins, vitamin, 67t, 68,
    69, 70t. *See also specific binding
    proteins*
Bioavailability
  biopotency and, 64t
  biotin, 332–333
  biotin, in feedstuffs, 334t
  folate, 357–358, 358t
  niacin, 296–297
  pantothenic acid, 347
  vitamin, 44, 64, 64t, 448–449, 448t
  vitamin B_6, 314–315
  vitamin B_{12}, 383
  vitamin C, 236–237
  vitamin K, 216
Biochemical lesions, vitamin
    deficiencies and, 86–91
Biochemical methods, for assessing
    vitamin status, 471–474, 472t, 473t
Biochemistry, 7. *See also* Chemistry
Biocytin, 332, 334
Bioflavonoids, 5n5, 31t, 401
Biological functions, of vitamins, 90t
Biopotency
  ascorbic acid, 52, 52t
  bioavailability and, 64t
  β-Carotene, 44, 44t
  of tocopherols, 183t
  of tocotrienols, 183t
  vitamin A, 44–45, 44t
  vitamin C, 52, 52t
  vitamin D, 46–47, 47t
  vitamin E, 49, 49t
  vitamin K, 50–51
  vitamin K vitamers, 214–215
Bios IIb, 26, 26n40
  biotin from, 26, 26t
Biosynthesis
  ascorbic acid, 237–238, 238f, 238t
  biotin, 333–334
  carnitine, 407–408, 407f

choline, 5, 403–404, 404f
CoA, 348–349
of *myo*-inositol, glucose and, 414
niacin, 5, 69t, 299–302
of ubiquinones, 420
vitamin C, 5, 69t
vitamin D, 5
vitamin D₃, 69, 69t, 147–149, 149f
of vitamins, 69, 69t
Biotechnology, vitamin contents and, 447
Biotin, 331–344
  absorption of, 334
  antagonists, 338
  bioavailability of, 332–333
  bioavailability of, in feedstuffs, 334t
  from bios IIb, 26, 26t
  biosynthesis of, 333–334
  case study, 341–343
  catabolism of, 336
  chemical structure, 56
  chemistry, 56
  congenital disorders and, 341, 341t, 342t
  d-, 39t
  deficiencies, 331, 338–341
  deficiencies, in animals, 339
  deficiency signs, 89t, 339t
  definition of, 331
  discovery of, 26, 29t, 331
  distribution in food, 332, 333t
  excretion of, 336
  factors leading to discover of, 26, 26t
  gene expression and, 338
  holoenzyme synthetase, 335, 337
  metabolic functions of, 331, 336–338
  metabolism of, 335–336
  nomenclature, 56
  physical properties of, 39t
  physiological function of, 6t
  RDA, 495t
  RDA, history, 491t
  RNI, 497t
  significance of, 331–332
  sources of, 332–334
  sulfoxide, 333
  tissue distribution of, 335
  toxicity and, 341, 510
  transport of, 334–335
Biotin-binding proteins, 332, 335
Biotinidase, 332, 335
Biotinyl 5′-adenylate, 337
Bishop, Katherine, 24
Bisnorbiotin, 334, 336
Bitot's spots, 96, 121n69, 123n70, 131, 132, 134t, 135, 136t
Black tongue disease, 22, 23, 295, 305n26. *See also* Pellagra
  pellagra and, 295
Bleaching, 114, 127

Bloch, Konrad, 30t
Blood clotting, vitamin K and, 222–224, 223f
Blood pressure, ascorbic acid and, 251, 251f
Bone health, vitamin D and, 164
Bone lesions, 145
Bone metabolism, vitamin A and, 119–120
Bone mineral turnover, vitamin D and, 162
Bone mineralization, vitamin K and, 225–226
Boron, vitamin D and, 163–164
Bradycardia, 88t, 275
Branched chain α-keto acid dehydrogenase, 271
Brown bowel disease, 83t
Brown fat disease, 84t
Burning feet syndrome, 353n32
γ-Butyrobetai ne hydroxylase, 407, 411

C677T/C genotype, MTHFR, 493
CA²⁺ channel, 417
CaBP. *See* Calcium-binding protein
Cage layer fatigue, 86t, 174
Calbindins, 160
Calcidiol, 154, 155
Calcification proteins, 224–225
Calcified tissues, vitamin K dependent proteins in, 224–225
Calcinosis, 157, 175
Calcipotriol, 167n87
Calcisomes, 417
Calcitonin (CT), 156, 159t, 160, 163
Calcitriol, 155
Calcitroic acid, 155
Calcium, 146
  homeostasis, 162–163, 163f
  renal absorption of, 161
  vitamin D and metabolism of, 160–163
Calcium-binding protein (CaBP), 160
Calmodulin, 161
Calves, vitamin A requirements for, 486t
Cancer
  ascorbic acid and, 254
  β-carotene, retinol and, 129–130, 129t, 130t
  carotenoids and, 492
  choline and, 406
  folate and, 371–372
  riboflavin and, 492
  α-tocopherol and, 492
  vitamin A and, 127–130, 492
  vitamin B₁₂ and, 394
  vitamin C and, 492
  vitamin D and, 168–169, 168f
  25-OH-vitamin D and, 492

vitamin E and, 197–198
vitamin K and, 227
Canthaxanthin, 100, 130, 425f
Capillary fragility, 82t, 88t
α-Carboxyethylchromanol, 190
Carboxyglutamate (Gla), 221. *See also* Gla proteins
Carboxylase deficiencies, multiple, 341
Cardiac beriberi, 276
Cardiac hypertrophy, 275
Cardiomyopathy, 81t, 88t
Cardiovascular disease (CVD)
  ascorbic acid and, 250–252
  β-carotene and, 492
  folate and, 369
  vitamin C and, 492
  vitamin D and, 167
  vitamin E and, 198–201, 199t, 492
Cardiovascular function, carnitine and, 412–413
Carnitine, 31t, 406–413
  absorption of, 408
  biosynthesis of, 407–408, 407f
  cardiovascular function and, 412–413
  chemical structure, 407
  children/infants and, 411–412, 411t
  diabetes and, 412
  excretion of, 409
  exercise and, 413
  food sources of, 408, 408t
  health effects of, 411
  hepatic function of, 412
  insects and, 410
  male reproductive function and, 413
  metabolic function of, 409–410
  need for, 410–411
  renal function of, 412
  synthesis, 246t, 247
  thyroid function and, 413
  transport of, 408–409
Carnitine acyltransferases I and II, 409
β-Carotene, 6t, 37t, 43, 44, 62t, 67t
  15,15′-dioxygenase, 100
  biopotency of, 44, 44t
  cancer, retinol and, 129–130, 129t, 130t
  CVD and, 492
  iron solubility and, 121f
  plant iron and, 122t
  as provitamin, 19
  smoking and, 130t
Carotenodermia, 138, 508
Carotenoids, 43, 44, 45, 61t, 64, 64t, 97–98
  absorption of, 99–100
  as antioxidants, 126–127, 126t
  cancer and, 492
  contents, in corn, 447t
  in lipoproteins, 102t

Carotenoids (*Continued*)
metabolism of, 100–101
micelle-dependent passive diffusion and, 95, 99–100
non-protovitamin A, 425–428
toxicity of, 138–139
transport of, 102–103
Casal's collar, 305n28
Case studies
biotin, 341–343
folate, 378–379
niacin, 309–310
pantothenic acid, 353
riboflavin, 293
thiamin, 278–279
vitamin A, 139–141
vitamin B_6, 327–328
vitamin B_{12}, 395–397
vitamin C, 260–262
vitamin D, 176–177
vitamin E, 210–211
vitamin K, 230–232
Castle, W. B., 381
Catabolism
biotin, 336
CoA, 349–350
folate, 364–365
histamine, 365
menadione and, 219–220
menaquinones and, 220
niacin, 302
phylloquinones and, 220
retinoic acid, 111f
riboflavin, 286
thiamin, 270
vitamin, 3
vitamin B_6 and, 318
vitamin B_{12}, 386–387
vitamin D, 155
vitamin K, 219–220
Catalase, 195, 195f, 204
Cataracts
tryptophan and, 201, 292
vitamin C and, 253, 253t
vitamin deficiency and, 84t, 87t
vitamin E and, 201
Catecholamine synthesis, 246, 246t, 247f
CDP-choline. *See* Cytidine diphosphorylcholine
Cellular antioxidation, 247–248
Cellular retinal-binding protein. *See* CRALBP
Cellular retinoic acid-binding protein. *See* CRABP
Cellular uptake, of vitamin E, 187–188
Cervical paralysis, 85t, 376
cGMP phosphodiesterase, 114, 115
Chastek paralysis, 268n3
Cheilosis, 83t, 88t, 292, 324

Chelates, 415
Chemical structure
biotin, 56
carnitine, 407
choline, 402
folate, 57
myo-inositol, 413–414
niacin, 54–55
pantothenic acid, 56–57
PQQ, 418
riboflavin, 53
thiamin, 52
ubiquinones, 420
vitamin A, 42–43
vitamin B_6, 55–56
vitamin B_{12}, 59–60
vitamin C, 51
vitamin D, 45
vitamin E, 47–48
vitamin K, 49
Chemical/physiological properties, of vitamins, 37–73. *See also specific vitamins*
Chemistry
biotin, 56
folate, 58–59
niacin, 55
pantothenic acid, 57
riboflavin, 54
thiamin, 53
vitamin A, 43–44
vitamin B_6, 56
vitamin B_{12}, 60
vitamin C, 51–52
vitamin D, 46
vitamin E, 48–49
vitamin K, 50
Chickens, polyneuritis in, 17, 18
Chicks
antidermatitis factor, 21, 24, 24t
encephalomalacia in vitamin E-deficient, 209f
nutritional muscular dystrophy in vitamin E-deficient, 209f
with rickets, 174f
Children. *See also* Infants; Neonates
carnitine and, 411–412, 411t
with rickets, 172f
toxicity of vitamins in, 505t
vitamin A and measles in, 124t
vitamin A and mortality in, 124t, 125t
vitamin A deficiency and retinol in, 136t
xerophthalmia in, 97t, 120, 120t, 123t
Chloro-K, 221
Cholecalciferol. *See* Vitamin D_3
Cholesterol 7α-hydroxylase, 247
Cholesteryl ester transfer protein, 102

Choline, 31t, 401–406
absorption of, 402–404
acetyltransferase, 405
biosynthesis of, 5, 403–404, 404f
cancer and, 406
CDP-, 404
chemical structure, 402
dehydrogenase, 404
distribution in foods/feedstuffs, 402, 402t
health effects of, 406
kinase, 404
metabolic functions of, 405–406
metabolism of, 404–405
oxidase, 404
phosphotransferase, 404
toxicity and, 406
Chondrodystrophy, 86t
6-Chromanol nucleus, 47, 48
Chylomicra, 65–66, 65n30, 67t
remnants, 102, 103
vitamin A and, 102, 103
vitamin D and, 151
vitamin E and, 185, 186
Cirrhosis, 83t
Clinical evaluation, 470
Clinical signs
symptoms *v.*, 77n2
of vitamin deficiencies, 76, 77, 77t, 87–89t
Clubbed down, 82t
CoA. *See* Coenzyme A
Coagulopathies, 227
Cobalamins, 6t, 40t, 60, 70t, 71t, 384
in plasma, 386t
Cobalt, 383, 386
Cocarboxylase, 266, 270–271
Coenzyme A (CoA), 57, 61t, 66t, 67t, 69n32, 70t, 72t, 271n17
biosynthesis of, 348–349
catabolism of, 349–350
malonyl, 348
metabolic functions, 350–351
Coenzyme Q_{10} (CoQ$_{10}$), 420, 421
Coenzymes, 69n32
folate as, 355, 366t
lipoic acid as, 429
niacin as, 303
PQQ, 418
R, 26, 26t
riboflavin as, 287
vitamin A as, 118–119
vitamin B_{12} as, 387–388
vitamins as, 72–73t
Cognitive function, folate and, 372
Colds, vitamin C and, 257–258, 258t
Collagen
fibers, 222
synthesis, 245–246, 246t
Color, of vitamins/vitamers, 37–41t

Committee on Animal Nutrition, 498
Confabulation, 277
Congenital disorders
 biotin and, 341, 341t, 342t
 vitamin B_6 and, 325, 325t
 vitamin B_{12} and, 395, 395t
Conjugated diene, 192
Conjugation, of retinol, 110
Conjunctival impression cytology, 131, 132
Convulsions, 88t
Coprophagy, 216, 217n5
CoQ_{10}. *See* Coenzyme Q_{10}
Core foods, for vitamins, 438, 440t, 441
Corn, carotenoid contents in, 447t
Corneal ulceration, 9, 12
Corneal xerosis, 131, 132, 139
Cornification, 81t, 87t
Corrin nucleus, 59, 60, 381
Corrinoids, 381. *See also* Vitamin B_{12}
Coumarin-based drugs, 214
CRABP (cellular retinoic acid-binding protein), 105, 106t, 107, 112, 113t, 117, 118
 II (type 2), 106t, 113t, 118
CRALBP (cellular retinal-binding protein), 105, 106t, 107, 112, 113t
Cryptoxanthin, 6t
β-Cryptoxanthin, 126
CT. *See* Calcitonin
Curled-toe paralysis, 85t, 291
CVD. *See* Cardiovascular disease
Cyanide metabolism, 388
Cyanocobalamin, 40t, 59, 60, 61t, 384
Cyanogenic glycoside, 431
Cystathionuria, 325t
Cysteine, 193n39, 206n96, 210n111
Cytidine diphosphorylcholine (CDP-choline), 404
Cytochrome P450, 190, 192

Dam, Henrik, 25, 30t
Davis, Marguerite, 17, 30
DBPs. *See* Vitamin D-binding proteins
Dealkylation, vitamin K and, 218
Deficiencies
 enzyme, vitamin C and, 238–239
 FIVE, 188, 208
 iron, anemia and, 483
 multiple carboxylase, 341
Deficiencies, vitamin, 75–92, 76, 86
 animals and, 79, 173–174
 biochemical lesions and, 86–91
 biotin, 89t, 331, 338–341, 339, 339t
 cascade of effects in, 76, 77t
 cataracts and, 84t, 87t
 causes of, 78–79
 clinical manifestations of, 79, 80–86t
 clinical signs of, 76, 77, 77n2, 77t, 87–89t

definition of, 76
dermatologic disorders from, 80t
diseases from, 86–91
emotional disorders from, 86t
folate, 89t, 355, 375–377, 376–377, 376t
folate, in animals, 376
folate, vitamin B_{12} and, 374–375
Funk on, 75
gastrointestinal disorders from, 83t
high-risk groups for, 79
intervention and, 77–78
muscular disorders from, 81t
nervous disorders from, 85t
niacin, 89t, 295, 304–307, 305t
niacin, in animals, 304–305
nutritional assessment and, 479–480
ocular disorders from, 84t
pantothenic acid, 89t, 345, 352–353, 352t, 353
pantothenic acid, in animals, 352
primary, 78, 79
psychological disorders from, 86t
reproductive disorders from, 81–82t
riboflavin, 88t, 281, 288, 290–292, 290t, 291–292
riboflavin, in animals, 291
risk factors for, 470–471, 470t
secondary, 78, 79
skeletal disorders from, 86t
smoking and risk of, 79
stages of, 76–77, 77t
thiamin, 88t, 265, 274–278
vascular disorders from, 82t
vital organ disorders from, 83–84t
vitamin A, 87t, 120t, 131–134, 132f, 133f, 134t, 135, 135f, 136t, 483
vitamin B_6, 88t, 313, 323–325, 324t
vitamin B_6, in animals, 323–324
vitamin B_{12}, 89t, 381, 388–395
vitamin B_{12}, folate and, 374–375
vitamin B_{12}, in animals, 391–392
vitamin C, 88t, 235, 254–257, 255t
vitamin C, in animals, 256, 256f
vitamin D, 87t, 169–174, 170f, 172t, 173t, 174f
vitamin D, in animals, 173–174
vitamin E, 87t, 181, 206–207, 208t
vitamin K, 87t, 213, 225t, 227–228, 227–229
vitamin-responsive inborn metabolic lesions in, 91t
Defined diets, 13, 15
Dehydroascorbic acid, 6t, 51, 52, 52t, 61t, 72t, 239, 240f
 reductase, 240f, 242
7-Dehydrocholesterol, 147, 148, 149
DeLuca, H.F., 145
Dental health, vitamin C and, 253
Dephospho-CoA kinase, 349

Dermatitis, 20, 22, 80t, 87t, 89t, 90t. *See also* Pellagra
 in rodents, 20, 23
Dermatologic hemorrhage, 225t
Dermatology
 disorders, from vitamin deficiencies, 80t
 disorders, retinoids and, 125–126
 vitamin A and, 125
Desquamation, 80t
Diabetes
 carnitine and, 412
 lipoic acid and, 430
 tocopherol status influenced by, 202, 202t
 vitamin C and, 252, 252f
 vitamin D and insulin-dependent, 166–167
 vitamin D and noninsulin dependent, 165–166, 166f
 25-OH-vitamin D and, 492
 vitamin E and, 201–202, 202t
Dicumarol, 214, 220
3,4-Didehydroretinol, 134
Diet(s)
 of defined composition, 13, 15
 diseases linked with, 9–12, 12t
 monotonous, 471
 purified, 8, 13, 15, 24, 27
 vitamins in human, 454–457
Dietary essential nutrients, disease and, 3
Dietary evaluation, 470
Dietary recommendations, 486. *See also* Recommended Dietary Allowances
Dietary Reference Intakes (DRIs), 511
 as dietary standard, 494, 496
Dietary standards, 485–486
 DRI as, 494, 496
 international, 496, 498, 498t
 nutrient requirements *v.*, 486
 purposes of, 485–486
 RDA as, 494
 for vitamins, 486–487
Digestion, of NAD(H)/NADP(H), 298
7,8-Dihydrofolate reductase, 362
Dihydrofolic acid (FH_2), 357, 362
1, 25-Dihydroxyvitamin D_3 (1, 25-$[OH]_2$-vitamin D_3), 147, 156, 158
Dimethylglycine, 404, 430
Discovery, of vitamins, 7–33
Diseases. *See also* Deficiencies, vitamin; Health; *specific diseases*
 accessory factors and prevention of, 17
 definition of, 75
 diet and associated, 9–12, 12t
 dietary essential nutrients and, 3
 flavonoids and chronic, 424

Diseases (*Continued*)
from vitamin deficiencies, 86–91
vitamin E and prevention of, 196–206, 197t
Disorders. *See specific disorders*
Diuresis, 162
DNA methylation, folate and, 371
Doisy, Edward A., 25, 30t
Dopamine-β-monooxygenase, 246, 247f
DRIs. *See* Dietary Reference Intakes
Drug metabolism
ascorbic acid and, 247
vitamin A and, 126
Drug uses, for vitamins. *See* Pharmacologic uses
Drugs' influence, on folate, 377
Drugs/alcohol, vitamin B$_6$ and, 318
Drug-vitamin interactions, 489t
Drummond, J.C., 16n8, 19
DT-diaphorase, 219
Dyspnea, 276
Dysprothrombinemia, 227
Dystrophy, 81t, 87t

EARs. *See* Estimated average requirements
Edema, 80t, 82t, 88t
EFT. *See* Electron transfer flavoprotein
Egg white injury, 331, 338–339
Eicosanoids, 417
Eijkman, Christian, 9, 13, 14, 15, 16, 18, 30t, 265. *See also* Beriberi
Einstein, Albert, 3
Elastin, 246
Electron transfer flavoprotein (EFT), 289t
Electron transport, vitamin C and, 243
Elevated doses, of vitamins, 503–504. *See also* Hypervitaminosis; Toxicity, vitamin
clinical conditions for, 503–504
hazards of, 504–505
putative benefits of, 503, 504
Embryonic development, vitamin A and, 119
Emotional/psychological disorders, from vitamin deficiencies, 86t
Empirical phase, of vitamin discovery, 7, 8, 9–12, 400
Encephalomalacia, 85t, 207, 208t
in vitamin E-deficient chick, 209f
Encephalopathy, 85t, 87t, 276
Wernicke's, 277
Enteric malabsorption, 471
Environmental stress, vitamin C and, 254, 255t
Enzyme cofactors, vitamins as, 3, 6t

Enzyme co-substrate functions, of ascorbic acid, 245–247, 246t
Enzyme deficiency, vitamin C and, 238–239
Enzyme modulation, flavonoids and, 424
Enzymes, ascorbic acid and, 245, 246t
Epinephrine, 321
Epiphyseal plate, 163n65
Ergocalciferol. *See* Vitamin D$_2$
Ergosterol, 20, 147
Erythrocyte glutathione reductase, 288
Erythrocytes, vitamin E, lipoproteins and, 185–187
Erythropoiesis, folate and, 371
ESADDI. *See* Estimated Safe and Adequate Daily Dietary Intake
Essentiality, 493
nutritional, 491–492, 493
Esterification, of retinol, 109–110
Estimated average requirements (EARs), 487, 496
Estimated Safe and Adequate Daily Dietary Intake (ESADDI), 494
Ethane, 192, 193, 206
Evaluations. *See also* Assessment, vitamin status
anthropometric, 470
biochemical, 470, 471–474, 472t, 473t
clinical, 470
dietary, 470
sociologic, 470
Evans, H. M., 24
Excretion
of ascorbic acid, 242–243, 243t
of biotin, 336
of carnitine, 409
of folate, 365
of niacin, 302
of pantothenic acid, 350
of riboflavin, 286–287
of thiamin, 270
of vitamin A, 113, 113t
of vitamin B$_6$, 318
of vitamin B$_{12}$, 387
of vitamin C, 242–243
of vitamins, 70, 71t, 72
Exercise
carnitine and, 413
vitamin C and, 252
vitamin E and, 202, 202t
Experimental phase, of vitamin discovery, 7, 8, 12–15, 400
Extrinsic clotting system, 222
Extrinsic factors, 28, 29t, 381
Exudative diathesis, 82t, 87t, 195, 208t
Eye lesions, vitamin A deficiency and, 136t

Factor. *See specific factors*
Factor II. *See* Prothrombin

Factor IIa. *See* Thrombin
Factor IX, 222, 230f, 232
Factor R, 27, 28t
Factor U, 27, 28t
Factor VII (proconvertin), 222, 222n18, 223, 227, 230f, 232
Factor X (Stuart factor), 24, 29, 29t, 222, 223, 224, 230f, 232
FAD. *See* Flavin adenine dinucleotide
FAD-pyrophosphatase, 283
FAD-synthase, 285
Familial isolated vitamin E (FIVE) deficiency, 188, 208
FAO. *See* Food and Agriculture Organization
FAO/WHO. *See* WHO/FAO
Fats/oils, vitamin E in, 183–184, 184t
Fat-soluble A, 17, 17t, 42
factors of, 19
vitamin A and, 19
Fat-soluble vitamins, 42
Fatty acid synthase, 351
Fatty liver and kidney syndrome (FLKS), 83t, 84t, 89t, 339
FBPs. *See* Folate-binding proteins
Feedstuffs
biotin availability in, 334t
choline in, 402
vitamins in, 441, 442t, 447, 448, 448t, 461–466
Fescue toxicity, 275
FH$_2$. *See* Dihydrofolic acid
FH$_4$. *See* Tetrahydrofolic acid
Fibrin, 222, 223
Fibrinogen, 222, 223
Filtrate factor, 23, 24, 24t
FIVE deficiency. *See* Familial isolated vitamin E deficiency
Flavanols, 422
Flavin adenine dinucleotide (FAD), 39t, 53, 54, 61t, 66t, 70t, 72t, 73t, 282, 286
Flavin mononucleotide (FMN), 53, 54, 61t, 66t, 70t, 72t, 73t, 282, 286
Flavins, 21–22, 21n26
Flavokinase, 285
Flavonoids, 422–425
as antioxidants, 423–424
chronic diseases and, 424
discovery of, 422
enzyme modulation and, 424
in foods, 423, 423t
health effects of, 423–425
Szent-Györgyi and, 422
Flavonols, 422
Flavoproteins, 288
of animals, 289t
Flemma salada, 11

FLKS. *See* Fatty liver and kidney syndrome
Fluorescence, in vitamins/vitamers, 37–41t
Flushing, 307
FMN. *See* Flavin mononucleotide
FMN-phosphatase, 283
Foam cells, 200, 201f
Folacin, 58
Folate, 3, 355–380
  absorption of, 358–360
  p-Aminobenzoic acid and, 429
  antagonists, 59, 361
  bioavailability, 357–358, 358t
  cancer and, 371–372
  case study, 378–379
  catabolism of, 364–365
  chemical structure, 57
  chemistry, 58–59
  coenzymes, 366t
  cognitive function and, 372
  CVD and, 369
  deficiencies, 355, 375–377
  deficiencies, in animals, 376
  deficiencies, vitamin B_{12} and, 374–375
  deficiency signs, 89t, 376–377, 376t
  definition of, 355
  discovery of, 29t
  distribution in foods, 356, 357t
  DNA methylation and, 371
  drugs' influence on, 377
  erythropoiesis and, 371
  excretion of, 365
  health effects of, 367–375
  immune function and, 372
  metabolic functions of, 365–375, 366t
  metabolism of, 362–365
  neural tube defects and, 369–371, 492
  nomenclature, 58
  nucleotide metabolism and, 366
  pharmacological uses of, 377
  physical properties of, 40t
  RDA, 495t
  RDA, history, 491t
  RNI, 497t
  significance of, 356–357
  single-carbon metabolism and, 366–367
  single-carbon units and, 362f
  sources of, 356–358
  tissue distribution of, 362
  toxicity and, 377–378, 510
  transport of, 360–362
  transporter, 359, 360
  trap of methyl-, 367
  vitamers, 40t
  zinc and, 376

Folate receptor (FR), 360, 361
Folate-binding proteins (FBPs), 359, 361–362
  isoforms, 361t
  in milk, 361
Folic acid, 40t, 58, 59, 356, 356n1, 357
  factors leading to discovery of, 27–28, 28t, 355
  physiological function of, 6t
  vitamers, 6t
Folkers, K., 399
Folyl conjugase, 358
Folyl polyglutamates, 356. *See also* Folate
  hydrolysis of, 358–359
  synthetase, 363
Food and Agriculture Organization (FAO), 487. *See also* WHO/FAO
Food and Nutrition Board, 487, 490. *See also* Recommended Dietary Allowances
Foods. *See also* Sources
  biotin distribution in, 332, 333t
  carnitine in, 408, 408t
  choline distribution in, 402, 402t
  core, for vitamins, 438, 440t, 441
  flavonoids in, 423, 423t
  folate distribution in, 356, 357t
  fortification of, 451–454
  labeling of, vitamins and, 459–461
  lipoic acid in, 429–430
  myo-inositol in, 414–415, 415t
  niacin distribution in, 296, 297t, 298t
  non-protovitamin A carotenoids in, 425, 426t
  orotic acid in, 428
  pantothenic acid distribution in, 346–347, 346t
  PQQ in, 418
  riboflavin in, 282, 283t
  thiamin distribution/stability in, 266–267, 267t
  ubiquinones in, 420–421
  vitamin A distribution in, 97–98, 98t, 99t
  vitamin B_6 distribution in, 314, 315t
  vitamin B_{12} distribution in, 382–383, 382t
  vitamin C contents of uncooked, 237t
  vitamin C distribution/stability in, 236
  vitamin D distribution in, 147, 148t
  vitamin E distribution in, 182–183
  vitamin K contents in, 215–216, 215t
  vitamins in, 437–441, 439t, 440t
5-Formimino-FH_4, 364t, 366t
Forms
  excretory, of vitamins, 70, 71t, 72
  of niacin, 295

  synthetic, of vitamin E, 183
  of vitamin A, 113, 113t
  vitamin B_6, 313
  of vitamins/vitamers, 37–41t, 60, 61t
5-Formyl-FH_4, 356, 358, 359, 364t
10-Formyl-FH_4, 356, 357, 360, 362, 364t
Formylase, 299
Fortification, of foods, 451–454
FR. *See* Folate receptor
Fractures
  osteocalcin and, 225t
  pseudo, 171, 172t
Framingham offspring cohort study, 288, 290, 290t
Free radical scavenging, 193
  of vitamin E, 193–194
Free radicals, 192–194
Free-radical theory of aging, 197
Frölich, Theodor, 18
Fruits/vegetables, American consumption of, 479t
Funk, Casimir, 4, 16, 17
  on vitamin deficiency, 75
  vitamine theory of, 4, 15–18

GABA. *See* γ-Aminobutyric acid
Gas6, 226
Gastric parietal cell, 383
Gastrointestinal disorders, from vitamin deficiencies, 83t
Gastrointestinal hemorrhage, 225t
Gene expression
  biotin and, 338
  pyridoxal phosphate and, 322
Gene transcription
  vitamin A and regulation of, 116–118
  vitamin E and regulation of, 196
  vitamins and, 72
Genes, vitamin D regulation of, 159t
Genetic engineering, 447
Genomic pathways, vitamin D function and, 158–160
Genomic stability
  of niacin, 304
  of vitamin B_{12}, 394
Genotype, MTHFR C677T/C, 493
Genu varum, 176
Geographical tongue, 83t, 292f
Germ theory, 9, 12, 16, 22
Gerovital, 31t, 431
Gizzard myopathy, 81t, 208t
Gla. *See* Carboxyglutamate
Gla proteins
  matrix, 224–225
  proline-rich, 226
  in rat dentine, 225
  renal, 226
  vitamin K-dependent, 221–222, 222t, 226
Glossitis, 83t, 89t, 292, 324

Glucokinase, 338
Gluconeogenesis, 321
Glucose, *myo*-inositol biosynthesis
  from, 414
Glucose tolerance factor, 304
Glucose transporters (GLUTs), 239
Glucuronic acid pathway, 238
Glutathione (GSH), 191
  vitamin C and, 244, 244f
Glutathione peroxidases, 195, 204
Glutathione reductase, 195n44,
  207n98
GLUTs. *See* Glucose transporters
Glycerylphosphorylcholine, 402, 403,
  404
  diesterase, 404
Glycogen phosphorylase, 316, 322
Glycoproteins, 108, 118, 119
Goldberger, Joseph, 20, 21, 22. *See also*
  Pellagra
  on pellagra, 295
*Golden*Rice, 447, 448t
Grains/oil seeds, vitamin E in, 183, 185t
Grant, R., 19n19, 30t
Grijns, Gerrit, 14, 15, 16, 265
GSH. *See* Glutathione
GSSG. *See* Oxidized glutathione
Guinea pigs
  adipose tissue, α-tocopherol in, 189f
  vitamin C and, 238t, 239, 242, 247,
    250, 251, 253, 256, 257
L-Gulonolactone oxidase, 238, 285, 289
György, P., 281

H₂O₂. *See* Hydrogen peroxide
Hale, T. H., 381
Haptocorrin, 385
Harper, A.E., 485
Harris, L.J., 12, 15, 17, 469
Hartline, Haldan K., 19n19, 30t
Hartnup disease, 307
Haworth, Walter N., 19, 30t
HDLs (high-density lipoproteins), 67t,
  68n31, 102, 102t, 103, 104t, 137
H⁺/e⁻ donors/acceptors, vitamins as,
  72, 72t
Health. *See also* Diseases
  ascorbic acid and, 249–254
  carnitine and, 411
  choline and, 406
  flavonoids and, 423–425
  folate and, 367–375
  lipoic acid and, 430
  myo-inositol and, 418
  niacin and, 307
  non-protovitamin A carotenoids
    and, 427–428
  orotic acid and, 428
  pantothenic acid and, 351–352
  ubiquinones and, 421

vitamin B₆ and, 322–323
vitamin E and, 196–206, 197t
Heart disease risk, vitamin A and,
  127
Helicobacter pylori infection, 243, 250,
  390
Hematopoiesis, vitamin A and,
  120–121
Hemodialysis, vitamin E and, 202
Hemoglobin, 316
  synthesis/function, 321
Hemolysis, 183t, 187, 206
Hemolytic anemia, 206, 210
Hemorrhages, 9, 25
  dermatologic, 225t
  gastrointestinal, 225t
  in infants, 229
  intraventricular, 204, 207, 208t
  muscular, 225t
  in neonates, 213, 218
  vitamin K and, 25, 227
Hemorrhagic disease of the newborn,
  229
Hemorrhagic necrosis, 84t
Heparin, 220, 231
Hepatic function, of carnitine, 412
Herpes, 250, 257, 258t, 326
Hexose monophosphate shunt, 271
Hexuronic acid, 18, 19, 51, 235. *See also*
  Vitamin C
Hidden hunger, 480, 483
  anemia and, 483
  vitamin A deficiency and, 483
High-density lipoproteins. *See* HDLs
High-risk groups, for vitamin
  deficiencies, 79
Histamine, 249
  catabolism, 365
  synthesis, 321
HIV transmission, vitamin A and, 123t
HO•. *See* Hydroxyl radical
Holocarboxylases, 336, 342t
Holo-RBP, 104, 105, 107, 137
Holst, Axel, 18, 25
Homocysteine, 365
  MTHFR genotype, folate and, 370t
Homocysteinemia, 367–368, 393, 393t
Homocysteinuria, 320, 325
Homogentisate 1,2-dioxygenase, 247
Hopkins, Frederick G., 9, 10, 30t
  on accessory factors, 15–16
Hormones
  parathyroid, 159t, 169
  thyroid, 115, 116, 117, 118
  vitamin A as, 3, 72t
  vitamin D as, 3, 5, 72t
  vitamin D₃ as steroid, 157–158
  vitamins *v.*, 5
Human populations, vitamin status of,
  474–483

Hydrogen peroxide (H₂O₂), 191, 192,
  195, 210
Hydroperoxide (ROOH), 191f, 192,
  195f
Hydrophilic, 35
  riboflavin, 281
  thiamin, 265
  vitamin C-active substances, 235
Hydrophobic, 35
  vitamin A-active substances, 95
  vitamin D vitamers, 145
  vitamin E vitamers, 181
  vitamin K vitamers, 213
3-Hydroxyanthranilic acid (3-OH-
  AA), 299
3-Hydroxyanthranilic acid oxygenase
  (3-HAAO), 299
3-Hydroxyisovaleric acid, 338, 341
3-Hydroxykynurenine
  (3-OH-Ky), 299
Hydroxyl radical (HO•), 192
Hydroxylations, vitamin D, 154–156
  1-, 155
  24-, 155
  25-, 154
  other, 155–156
Hydroxylysine, 246
4-Hydroxyphenylpyruvate, 243, 246t,
  247
Hydroxyproline, 246
Hydroxyvitamin K, 220
Hypercalcemia, 155, 163, 167, 175
Hyperkeratosis, 80t, 125n73, 140
Hyperoxaluria, 325
Hyperphosphatemia, 155, 170n102
Hypersensitivity, 171, 175
Hypervitaminosis, 128. *See also*
  Toxicity, vitamin
  A, 135–139, 503, 508, 510
  A, embryotoxic potential of,
    137–138
  A, signs of, 137t
  C, 258–260, 509
  D, 175, 503, 508, 510
  D, signs of, 175t
  E, 208–209, 508–509
  K, 509
  signs of, 505–507t, 508–510
Hypoascorbemia, 239
Hypocalcemia, 157, 162, 170, 171
Hypochlorhydria, 390
Hypoparathyroidism, 170, 175n118
  pseudo, 171
Hypophosphatemia, 162
Hypoplastic anemia, 291
Hypoprothrombinemia, 217n6, 221,
  227
Hypotheses, scientific, 7
Hypovitaminosis, 76, 86. *See also*
  Deficiencies, vitamin

ICNND. *See* Interdepartmental Committee on Nutrition for National Defense

IF. *See* Intrinsic factor

IF-vitamin B_{12} complex, 384

Immune function
ascorbic acid and, 249–250
folate and, 372
vitamin B_6 and, 323, 323t

Immunity
vitamin A and, 122–125
vitamin D and, 164–165
vitamin E and, 202–203, 202t

Impaired vitamin retention/utilization, 471

Indian fruit bat, 239

Ineffective factors, vitamins as, 430–431. *See also* Quasi-vitamins

Infantile beriberi, 276

Infants. *See also* Children; Neonates
carnitine and, 411–412, 411t
hemorrhages in, 229
vitamin K-dependent coagulation factors in, 230f

Infections
Helicobacter pylori, 243, 250, 390
vitamin C and, 258, 258t
vitamin E and, 202–203

Inflammation, 80t, 83t, 84t, 88t
ascorbic acid and, 250, 251t

Inflammatory diseases, vitamin E and, 203–204

INH. *See* Isonicotinic acid hydrazide

Inositol 1,4,5-triphosphate (IP_3), 414. *See also* myo-inositol

Insect growth factor, 406–407

Insects, carnitine and, 410

Insulin, 240. *See also* Diabetes
discovery of, 401

Interdepartmental Committee on Nutrition for National Defense (ICNND), 469n1
guidelines for vitamin status assessment, 472, 474–476t

Interdigitation, of PUFAs and tocopherols, 194, 194f

International dietary standards, 496, 498, 498t

Interphotoreceptor retinol-binding proteins (IRBPs), 106, 106t, 107, 108

Intervention, vitamin deficiencies and, 77–78

Intestinal lipodystrophy, 413, 418

Intestinal microbial synthesis, of vitamin K, 216, 216t

Intraventricular hemorrhage, 204, 207, 208t

Intrinsic clotting system, 222

Intrinsic factor (IF), 28, 381, 383–384
receptors, 384

Iodopsins, 113

β-Ionone nucleus, 42, 43

IP_3. *See* Inositol 1,4,5-triphosphate

IRBPs. *See* Interphotoreceptor retinol-binding proteins

Iron
ascorbic acid and, 248, 249
deficiency, anemia and, 483
plant, vitamin A/β-carotene and, 122t
solubility, vitamin A/β-carotene and, 121f
vitamin D and, 163

Ischemia-reperfusion injury, vitamin E and, 204

Isoflavones, 423
soy, 424–425

Isomerizations, retinal and, 111, 112f

Isonicotinic acid hydrazide (INH), 318

Isoprenoid units, 42

Javanese prisons, beriberi in, 14, 14t

Jukes, T.H., 213, 401

Kangaroo gait, 339

Karrer, Paul, 19, 20, 22, 25, 30t

Keratomalacia, 84t, 87t, 90t, 131, 134t, 135f, 136t

α-Keto acid dehydrogenases, 271

α-Ketoglutarate dehydrogenase, 273

King, Charles G., 18, 19, 30t

Kuhn, R., 21, 22, 23, 30t

Kuhn, T.H., 4n3

Kynurenic acid, 300

Kynureninase, 320

Kynurenine 3-hydroxylase, 299

Labeling of foods, vitamins and, 459–461

Labile methyl groups, 404, 405

Lactobacillus
casei, 27, 28t, 430
lactis Dorner, 28, 29, 29t

Lactoflavin, 21

Laetrile (vitamin B_{17}), 31t, 431

Lavoisier, Antoine, 9

LDLs (low-density lipoproteins), 68n31, 102, 103, 104t, 121n79
lipid and antioxidant contents of human, 200, 200t
oxidized, 200
vitamin E and oxidation of, 182

Lead, vitamin D and, 164, 164t

Lecithin, 401, 402. *See also* Phosphatidylcholine

Lecithin-retinol acyltransferase (LRAT), 101, 109, 112, 113t

Lepkovsky, S., 313

Lesions, 86. *See also* Deficiencies, vitamin
biochemical, 86–91
bone, 145
vitamin-responsive inborn metabolic, 91t

Leucine, 306

Leukopenia, 82t, 292, 376

Liebig, Justus von, 9

Lind, James, 10

Lipid peroxidation
mechanism of, 192–193
self-propagating nature of, 193f
vitamin E and, 181, 191, 192–193, 200, 201t

Lipids
and antioxidants, in human LDLs, 200, 200t
metabolism, 321–322
responses, to niacin, 308t

Lipmann, Fritz A., 30t

Lipoamide, 429

Lipofuscinosis, 81t, 83t, 84t, 87t

Lipofuscins, 197

Lipoic acid, 31t, 429–430
as antioxidant, 429
as coenzyme, 429
diabetes and, 430
in foods, 429–430
health effects of, 430
MS and, 430
need for, 430

Lipoprotein lipase, 186, 187

Lipoproteins, 65n30, 67t, 68, 68n31. *See also* HDLs; LDLs; VLDLs
carotenoids in, 102t
vitamin E transferred to erythrocytes and, 185–187
vitamin K transferred to, 217

Lipotrope, 391, 402, 405

Liver(s)
animal, vitamin K in, 217t
necrosis, 83t, 87t, 195, 208t
vitamin A storage in, 103

LLD factor, 28n52, 29t

LOAEL. *See* Lowest observed adverse effect level

Losses, vitamin, 449–451, 449t, 450f, 450t, 451t

Low-calorie intake, 471

Low-density lipoproteins. *See* LDLs

Lowest observed adverse effect level (LOAEL), 511

LRAT. *See* Lecithin-retinol acyltransferase

Lumichrome, 286

Lung disease, vitamin E and, 204

Lunin, Nicholai, 15

Lutein, 425, 426t, 427–428
zeaxanthin and, 427–428

Lycopene, 100, 101, 102, 126, 126t, 425, 426t, 427
Lymphoid necrosis, 84t
Lynen, Feordor, 30t
Lysolecithin, 402, 403
Lysyl hydroxylase, 246
Lysyl oxidase, 419

Macrocytic anemia, 356, 366, 376, 376t
Macular degeneration, 428
Mal de la rosa, 11
Malabsorption, 79, 91t
  enteric, 471
Male reproductive function, carnitine and, 413
Malonyl CoA, 348
Malonyldialdehyde (MDA), 192, 193, 193n37, 197, 206t
Maple syrup urine disease, 271
Marasmus, 129
Margin of safety, 503
Marks, J., 437
Matrix Gla protein, 224–225
McCollum, Elmer, 17, 30
  rat growth factors and, 17, 17t
  vitamin D and, 19, 20
McLaren, D.S., 95
MCT1. *See* Monocarboxylate transporter
MDA. *See* Malonyldialdehyde
Measles, vitamin A and, 124t
Megadose vitamin C, 257–258
Megaloblastic anemia, 90t, 91t, 390, 391, 392
Megaloblastic transformation, 391
Megaloblasts, 376
Melanopsin, 106t, 115
Mellanby, Edward, 19
Melting point, for vitamins/vitamers, 37–41t
Menadione (vitamin K$_3$), 6t, 25, 50, 51t, 61t, 62t, 66t, 67t, 68t, 70t, 71t, 214
  catabolism and, 219–220
Menadione pyridinol bisulfite (MPB), 214
Menadione sodium bisulfite complex, 214
Menaquinones (vitamin K$_2$), 6t, 25, 50, 50t, 51t, 61t, 214
  catabolism and, 220
  enteric bacteria and, 216t
  phylloquinone conversion to, in rats, 218f
Metabolic functions
  biotin, 331, 336–338
  carnitine, 409–410
  choline, 405–406
  CoA, 350–351
  folate, 365–375, 366t
  myo-inositol, 416–417
  niacin, 203–204

orotic acid, 428
pantothenic acid, 345, 350–352
PQQ, 418–419
riboflavin, 287–288
thiamin, 270–274
of ubiquinones, 420
vitamin A, 114–130
vitamin B$_6$, 318–323
vitamin B$_{12}$, 381, 387–388
vitamin C, 243–254
vitamin D, 157–169, 158f
vitamin E, 191–206
vitamin K, 221–227
of vitamins, 72–73, 72–73t
Metabolic profiling, 493
Metabolism
  acetyl-CoA and, 351f
  of biotin, 335–336
  bone, vitamin A and, 119–120
  calcium/phosphorus, vitamin D and, 160–163
  of carotenoids, 100–101
  of choline, 404–405
  cyanide, 388
  drug, ascorbic acid and, 247
  drug, vitamin A and, 126
  drug/steroid, ascorbic acid and, 247
  of folate, 362–365
  of lipids, 321–322
  metal ion, 248–249
  of *myo*-inositol, 416
  of niacin, 299–302, 301f
  of pantothenic acid, 348–350
  regulation, vitamin D and, 156–157
  of retinoids, 101
  of retinol, 101–102, 109–113, 110f
  of riboflavin, 285–287
  sulfatide, vitamin K in, 226
  of thiamin, 269–270
  TTP-enzymes in, 272, 272f
  tyrosine, 247
  of vitamin A, 109–113
  of vitamin A, retinoid-binding proteins and, 112, 112f, 113t
  of vitamin B$_6$, 317–318, 317f
  of vitamin B$_{12}$, 386–387
  of vitamin C, 241–243
  of vitamin D, 154–157, 154f
  of vitamin D$_2$, 157
  of vitamin E, 189–191, 190f
  of vitamin K, 218–221, 219t
  of vitamins, 68–72, 70t
Metal ion metabolism, 248–249
Meta-rhodopsin II, 115
5,10-Methenyl-FH$_4$, 364t, 365
5,10-Methenyl-FH$_4$ reductase (MTHFR), 365, 367, 368
  C677T/C genotype, 373, 493
  folate, homocysteine and, 370t
  polymorphisms, 373–374, 373t

Methionine, 404, 405
  load, 320
  synthase, 365, 373t, 387–388
  synthetase, 363, 366t, 367, 375, 385
Methotrexate, 361t, 363, 377
  therapy, 374
5-Methyl-FH4, 356
1-Methyl-6-pyridone 3-carboxamide, 302
5-Methyl-FH$_4$: homocysteine methyltransferase, 386
Methylcobalamin, 41t, 59, 60, 61t, 67t, 68t, 70t, 384
  generation of, 386
  metabolic role of, 388f
3-Methylcrotonoyl-CoA carboxylase, 338
5,10-Methylene-FH$_4$, 364t
  dehydrogenase, 364t
Methyl-FH$_4$ methyltransferase, 385
Methyl-folate trap, 367, 388, 392
Methylmalonic acid (MMA), 392
Methylmalonic aciduria, 387
Methylmalonyl-CoA mutase, 385
1-Methylnicotinamide, 302
1-Methylnicotinic acid, 297
ω-Methylpantothenic acid, 353
Micellar solubilization
  of vitamin A, 99
  of vitamin K, 216–217
Micelle-dependent passive diffusion
  carotenoids and, 95, 99–100
  vitamin D and, 150
  vitamin E and, 184–185
Micelles, mixed, 36n1, 64t, 65
Mickey Mouse enzyme, 337n15
Milk
  accessory factors in, 15, 16, 16f
  FBPs in, 361
  retinol in, 109
  vitamin K in, 216t
  vitamins in breast, 456–457, 456t
Milk fever, vitamin D and, 174
Minimum nutrient requirements, 486, 487
Minot, George R., 28, 30t
Mitchell, H. K., 355
MMA. *See* Methylmalonic acid
Models, 13
  animal, 8, 13
Modified relative dose-response test. *See* MRDR test
Moeller-Barlow disease, 256
Molecular weight, of vitamins/vitamers, 37–41t
Monoamine oxidase, 286
Monocarboxylate transporter (MCT1), 335
Monodehydroascorbate, 246
  reductase, 243, 246

Monotonous diet, 471
MPB. *See* Menadione pyridinol bisulfite
MRDR (modified relative dose-response) test, 134
MS. *See* Multiple sclerosis
MTHFR. *See* 5,10-Methenyl-FH_4 reductase
Mulberry heart disease, 81t, 208t
Multiple carboxylase deficiencies, 341
Multiple sclerosis (MS), 167
    lipoic acid and, 430
    vitamin B_{12} and, 394
    25-OH-vitamin D and, 492
Murphy, William P., 28, 30t
Muscular disorders, from vitamin deficiencies, 81t
Muscular dystrophy, vitamin E-deficient chick with nutritional, 209f
Muscular function, vitamin D and, 168
Muscular hemorrhage, 225t
Muscular myopathy, 87t
Musculoskeletal pain, vitamin D and, 173
myo-inositol, 31t, 413–418
    absorption of, 415–416
    biosynthesis, from glucose, 414
    chemical structure, 413–414
    in foods, 414–415, 415t
    health effects of, 418
    metabolic functions of, 416–417
    metabolism of, 416
    need for, 417–418
    transport of, 416
Myopathy
    gizzard, 81t, 208t
    muscular, 87t
    skeletal, 81t
MyPyramid, 456f

NA. *See* Nicotinic acid
NAD^+. *See* Aldehyde dehydrogenase
NAD(H), 54, 55, 72, 72t, 295, 296
    digestion of, 298
    sources of, 300
NAD (Nicotinamide adenine dinucleotide), 23, 23n30, 61t, 70t
    redox reactions and, 303
NAD(P)+ glycohydrolase, 298, 302
NAD+ kinase, 300
NAD+ synthetase, 300
NADH dehydrogenase, 288
NADH-cytochrome *P*-450 reductase, 289t
NADP(H), 55, 70t, 72t, 295, 296
    digestion of, 298
    in reduction reactions, 303
    sources of, 300

NADP (Nicotinamide adenine dinucleotide phosphate), 7, 23, 23n30, 61t, 70t
NAm. *See* Nicotinamide
Naphthoquinone nucleus, 49
National Academy of Sciences, 494
National Health and Nutrition Examination Survey (NHANES), 438, 454f, 480
    I, 251, 480
    II, 480
    III, 136, 166, 167, 480, 480n16, 481–482t
National Nutrient Database, 437, 438, 439t, 460
National nutrition studies, 477, 477t
National Research Council, 498
    vitamin allowances for animals from, 499–501t
Necrosis
    adrenal, 84t
    hemorrhagic, 84t
    liver, 83t, 87t, 195, 208t
    lymphoid, 84t
Needs, vitamin, 485–502
Neonates. *See also* Children; Infants
    hemorrhage in, 213, 218
    vitamin K deficiency and, 228–229
Nepal pregnancies, vitamin A and, 122t
Nephritis, 84t, 87t
Nervous disorders, from vitamin deficiencies, 85t
Nervous function, thiamin and, 272–274
Nervous system, vitamin K in, 226–227
Neural tube defects, folate and, 369–371, 492
Neuritic beriberi, 276
Neurodegenerative disorders, vitamin E and, 204–205, 205t
Neurologic function
    ascorbic acid and, 252–253
    carnitine and, 413
    vitamin B_6 and, 322–323
    vitamin B_{12} and, 393–394
Neuropathy, 85t
    peripheral, 85t, 88t, 89t, 382, 391t, 392
Neurotransmitter synthesis, 321
N-Formylkynurenine, 299
NHANES. *See* National Health and Nutrition Examination Survey
Niacin, 295–311
    absorption of, 298, 298f
    antagonists, 55
    bioavailability, 296–297
    biosynthesis of, 5, 69t, 299–302
    case study, 309–310
    catabolism and, 302
    chemical structure, 54–55

chemistry, 55
coenzyme functions of, 303
deficiencies, 295, 304–307
deficiencies, in animals, 304–305
deficiency signs, 89t, 305t
definition of, 295
discovery of, 29t
distribution in foods, 296, 297t, 298t
excretion of, 302
facilitated diffusion of, 298
forms of, 295
genomic stability of, 304
health benefits of, 307
lipid responses to, 308t
metabolic functions of, 203–204
metabolism of, 299–302, 301f
nomenclature, 55
pharmacologic uses of, 307
physical properties of, 39t
physiological function of, 6t
protein turnover and, 300
RDA, 495t
RDA, history, 491t
RNI, 497t
significance of, 296
sources of, 296
toxicity, 309, 509–510
transport of, 298–299
tryptophan conversion to, 299–300, 299f, 320–321
vitamers, 6t, 39t
vitamin B_6 and, 300, 302
Niacytin, 296, 448, 452
Nicotinamide (NAm), 6t, 23, 39t, 55, 61t, 62t, 66t, 67t, 71t, 296
Nicotinamide adenine dinucleotide. *See* NAD
Nicotinamide adenine dinucleotide phosphate. *See* NADP
Nicotinamide methylase, 302n12
Nicotinamide *N*-methyltransferase, 302
Nicotinamide riboside (NR), 298
Nicotinate phosphoribosyltransferase, 300
Nicotinic acid (NA), 6t, 23, 39t, 55, 61t, 62t, 66t, 67t, 70t, 296
Nicotinic acid mononucleotide (NMN), 5, 69t, 298, 300
Night blindness (nyctalopia), 8, 9, 12, 19, 84t, 86, 87t, 90t, 96, 105, 115, 131, 132, 133f, 134t, 135, 136t, 140
5-Nitro-tocopherol, 190, 191t, 206
NLEA. *See* Nutrition Labeling and Education Act
NMN. *See* Nicotinic acid mononucleotide
No observed adverse effect level (NOAEL), 504, 511

NOAEL. *See* No observed adverse effect level

Nobel prizes, for vitamin research, 30t

Nomenclature, vitamin, 42. *See also specific vitamins*

Non-antioxidant functions, of vitamin E, 196

Noncalcified tissue, vitamin D and, 164, 165t

Nonpolar solvents, 36n1, 42, 48

Non-protovitamin A carotenoids, 425–428. *See also* Carotenoids
in foods, 425, 426t
health effects of, 427–428
utilization of, 425–427

Norepinephrine, 321

Normocytic hypochromic anemia, 291

Norris, L. C., 345

Novak, J.D., 7, 17

NR. *See* Nicotinamide riboside

Nuclear receptor proteins, vitamins with, 69, 70t

Nucleotide metabolism, folate and, 366

Nutrient requirements
animals and, 486, 487, 487f
determination of, 486–487
dietary standards *v.*, 486
factors affecting, 487, 488t, 489t, 490
minimum, 486, 487
RDAs *v.*, 490

Nutrients, 3
allowances, 487
dietary essential, 3
nontraditional functions of, 492–493
types of, 4
vitamins *v.* other, 4–5

Nutrilites, 31n56, 355

Nutrition, 7
screening, 470
studies, national, 477, 477t
surveillance, 470
surveys, 470

Nutrition Canada (study), 480

Nutrition Labeling and Education Act (NLEA), 459, 460

Nutritional assessment, 469
general aspects of, 469–471
methods of, 470
systems of, 470
vitamin deficiencies and, 479–480

Nutritional essentiality, 491–492

Nutritional science, 7
emergence of, 8, 13
new paradigms for, 493
scientific discovery process in, 8

Nyctalopia. *See* Night blindness

Nystagmus, 85t, 279

$O_2 \bullet$. *See* Superoxide radical

Ocular disorders, from vitamin deficiencies, 84t

Oil seeds/grains, vitamin E in, 183, 185t

Oils/fats, vitamin E in, 183–184, 184t

Ophthalmoplegia, 277

Opisthotonos, 85t, 88t, 274

Opsins, 113

Ornithine transcarbamylase, 338

Orotic acid (vitamin B_{13}), 31t, 428
in foods, 428
health effects of, 428
metabolic function, 428

Osteoblasts, 153t, 162, 163, 171

Osteocalcin, 159t, 160, 162, 224, 224t
in fracture/nonfracture patients, 225t
vitamin K intake and, 229f

Osteochondrosis, 174

Osteoclasts, 155, 159t, 162, 163, 169

Osteomalacia, 81t, 86t, 87t, 90t, 91t
vitamin D and, 171

Osteons, 163n65

Osteopenia, 171

Osteoporosis, 86t, 146
in animals, vitamin D and, 174
vitamin B_{12} and, 394–395
vitamin D and, 171–173

Otitis media, 139

Ovoflavin, 21, 285n17

Ovolactovegetarians, 389

Oxalic acid, 241, 242, 243

Oxidases, 285

Oxidation, of retinol, 110–111

Oxidative stress, 182
conditions associated with, 196, 197t

Oxidized glutathione (GSSG), 191f, 195, 210

Oxidized LDLs, 200

PAC. *See* Picolinic acid carboxylase

Pancreatic insufficiency, vitamin B_{12} and, 390

Pancreatic nonspecific lipase, 99n7

Pangamic acid (vitamin B_{15}), 5n5, 31, 430–431

Pantetheinase, 347

Pantetheine, 347, 351

Pantothenate kinase, 348

Pantothenic acid (vitamin B_3), 345–354
absorption of, 347
antagonists, 352
bioavailability, 347
case study, 353
chemical structure, 56–57
chemistry, 57
deficiencies, 345, 352–353
deficiencies, in animals, 352
deficiency signs, 89t, 352t, 353
definition of, 345
discovery of, 24, 29t

distribution in foods, 346–347, 346t
excretion of, 350
factors leading to discovery of, 24, 24t
health effects of, 351–352
metabolic functions of, 345, 350–352
metabolism of, 348–350
nomenclature, 57
physical properties of, 39t
physiological function of, 6t
RDA, 495t
RDA, history, 491t
RNI, 497t
significance of, 345–346
sources of, 346–347, 346t
tissue distribution of, 348
toxicity and, 353, 510
transport of, 347–348
vitamers, 39t
from vitamin B_2 complex, 23–24

Paracelsus, 503

Paralysis
cervical, 85t, 376
Chastek, 268n3
curled-toe, 85t, 291

Parathyroid gland, vitamin D functioning and, 169, 169f

Parathyroid hormone (PTH), 159t, 169

Parkinson's disease, thiamin and, 277

Passive diffusion, vitamin K and, 217

Pauling, Linus, 257

Pekalharing, Cornelius, 13, 14, 15

Pellagra, 9, 11–12, 12t, 80t, 83t, 85t, 86t, 90t, 295, 306f
black tongue disease and, 295
Goldberger on, 295
impact of animal model for, 22–23
as noninfectious disease, 22
vitamine for anti-, 16

Pellagra-preventive factor. *See* P-P factor

Pentane, 192, 193, 202t, 206

Pentose phosphate pathway, 274

PEPCK. *See* Phospho*enol*pyruvate carboxykinase

Pepsin, 383

Peptide hormone synthesis, 246–247, 246t

Peptidylglycine α-amidating monooxygenase, 246, 246t, 249

Periodontal disease
vitamin C and, 253, 256
vitamin D and, 167

Peripheral neuropathy, 85t, 88t, 89t, 382, 391t, 392

Pernicious anemia, 28, 91t, 357, 375, 377, 381, 389–390

Perosis, 86t, 89t, 305f, 401, 402

Peroxide tone, 196, 197, 203

Peroxyl radical (ROO•), 192, 194, 200
and oxidation of tocopherols, 194f

Perseveration, 279
Petechiae, 260, 261
Pharmacologic uses
    of folate, 377
    of niacin, 307–309
    of vitamin B$_6$, 326–327
    of vitamin C, 257–258
    of vitamin E, 207–208
Phosphate, vitamin D and, 160–163
    homeostasis, 162–163
    intestinal absorption, 161
    renal absorption, 161
Phosphatidylcholine, 401, 402, 403, 404, 405
    glyceride choline transferase, 404
Phosphatidylethanolamine, 403
    N-methyl transferase, 403, 404
Phosphatidylinositol (PI), 416
Phosphatidylinositol 4-phosphate (PIP), 416, 417
Phosphodiesterase, 298
Phospho*enol*pyruvate carboxykinase (PEPCK), 337
Phospholipases A1, A2, B, C, and D, 402
Phospholipid transfer protein, 187, 188
Phosphopantetheine
    adenyltransferase, 349
4′-Phosphopantetheine, 349, 350
4′-Phosphopantothenic acid, 348, 349
Phosphopantothenylcysteine
    decarboxylase, 349
    synthase, 349
4′-Phosphopantothenylcysteine, 349
Phosphorylase, 271
Phosphorylation
    riboflavin and, 284
    thiamin and, 269–270
    vitamin B$_6$ and, 316
Phosphorylcholine, 402, 404
Photophobia, 84t, 88t
Phthiocol, 213
Phylloquinones (vitamin K$_1$), 6t, 25, 49, 50, 51t, 61t, 65, 66t, 214
    active transport of, 217
    catabolism and, 220
    conversion to menaquinone, in rats, 218f
Physical properties, of vitamins, 37–41t
Physiological utilization, of vitamins, 64–68
Physiological/chemical properties, of vitamins, 35–73. *See also specific vitamins*
Physiology, 7
Phytic acid, 414, 415
Phytoestrogens, 423
PI. *See* Phosphatidylinositol
Picolinic acid, 300

Picolinic acid carboxylase (PAC), 300
    in animals, 301t
PIP. *See* Phosphatidylinositol 4-phosphate
PIVKA. *See* Protein induced by vitamin K absence
Plant breeding, 447
Plasma, cobalamins in, 386t
Plasma retinol homeostasis, 108–109
Plasma thromboplastin, 222
Polar solvents, 36n1, 42, 49, 58
Polioencephalomalacia, 275
Polyglutamyl folacins, 6t
Polyneuritis, 14, 15, 16, 80t, 85t, 90t
    in animals, 274–276
    in chickens, 17, 18
    thiamin and, 266
Poly(ADP-ribose) polymerase, 304, 308
Polyunsaturated fatty acids (PUFAs)
    interdigitation of tocopherols and, 194, 194f
Portomicrons, 65n30, 67t, 68n31
P-P factor (pellagra-preventive factor), 21, 22, 23, 295, 345
PQQ. *See* Pyrroloquinoline quinone
Prediction, of vitamin contents, 441–448
    inaccuracy in, 441, 443, 446–447
Preeclampsia, vitamin E and, 205
Pregnancies
    vitamin A and Nepal, 122t
    vitamin C and outcomes of, 253
Premenstrual syndrome, 327
Premixes
    vitamin, 462, 464t, 465t
    vitamin-mineral, 462
Proconvertin. *See* Factor VII
Prolactin, 159t, 163
Proliferative skin diseases, vitamin D and, 167–168
Proline-rich Gla proteins, 226
Prooxidant capabilities
    of ascorbic acid, 245
    of vitamin E, 196
Propionyl-CoA, 348
    carboxylase, 337t, 338
Proposed vitamins, 5n5, 31t. *See also* Quasi-vitamins
Protective Nutrient Intakes, 498
Protein(s), 9. *See also specific proteins*
    C, 223
    intake, vitamin B$_6$ and, 319t
    M, 223
    nuclear receptor, vitamins with, 69, 70t
    R, 383, 385
    S, 223, 225
    turnover, niacin and, 300
    Z, 223–224

Protein induced by vitamin K absence (PIVKA), 227
Protein-energy malnutrition, 104, 105, 123, 137t
Prothrombin (factor II), 25, 222t, 223, 230f, 232
Provitamins, 5
    β-carotene as, 19
    D, 147, 148
    D$_3$, 148
    vitamin A, 6t, 37t
    vitamin A conversion, to retinal, 100f
Pseudofactors, vitamins v., 31, 31t
Pseudofractures, 171, 172t
Pseudohypoparathyroidism, 171
Psoriasis, 167
Psychological/emotional disorders, from vitamin deficiencies, 86t
Pteridines, 57, 58, 71t, 364
    ring system, 362–363
Pterin ring, 362, 363
Pteroylglutamic acid, 58, 61t, 71t, 356n1. *See also* Folic acid
    derivatives of, 27–28
PTH. *See* Parathyroid hormone
PUFAs. *See* Polyunsaturated fatty acids
Pulmonary function, ascorbic acid and, 253–254
Puppy, with rickets, 174f
Purified
    diets, 8, 13, 15, 24, 27
    vitamins, 451–452
Purine synthesis, 366
Pyridine nucleotide, 296
    -dependent enzymes, in animals, 304t
    in rats, 299t, 300
Pyridine nucleus, 54, 55
Pyridoxal, 6t, 39t, 55, 56, 61t, 62t, 66t, 67t, 68t, 70t, 71t, 314
    dehydrogenase, 318
    kinase, 317
    oxidase, 318
Pyridoxal phosphate, 299
    -dependent enzymes, of animals, 320t
    gene expression and, 322
Pyridoxamine, 6t, 39t, 55, 56, 61t, 66t, 71t, 73t, 314
Pyridoxamine phosphate, 316
Pyridoxamine phosphate oxidase, 318
4-Pyridoxic acid, 318
Pyridoxine, 314
    hydrochloride, 314
    -responsive seizures, 325
    from vitamin B$_2$ complex, 23, 29
Pyridoxol, 6t, 39t, 56, 62t, 66t, 71t, 314
Pyrimidine ring, 52, 53, 268

Pyrithiamin, 271
Pyrroloquinoline quinone (PQQ), 31t, 418–419
  chemical structure, 418
  as coenzyme, 418
  in food, 418
  metabolic function, 418–419
  need for, 419
Pyruvate dehydrogenase, 271

QA. *See* Quinolinic acid
Quantification, of vitamin needs, 485–502
Quasi-vitamins, 5n5, 31t, 399–433
  list of, 401
Quinolinate phosphoribosyltransferase, 300
Quinolinic acid (QA), 300
Quinoproteins, 418, 419

R proteins, 383, 385
Radiation protection, vitamin E and, 205
Range of safe intakes, for vitamins, 504, 508, 510–513
RAREs. *See* Retinoic acid response elements
RARs. *See* Retinoic acid receptors
Rats
  GLA protein in dentine of, 225
  growth factors, McCollum and, 17, 17t
  phylloquinone-menaquinone conversion in, 218f
  pyridine nucleotide in, 299t, 300
  vitamin K and germ-free, 216, 216t
RBPs. *See* Retinol binding proteins
RDAs. *See* Recommended Dietary Allowances
RDIs. *See* Recommended Dietary Intakes
RDR test. *See* Relative dose-response test
RE. *See* Retinol equivalents
Reactive nitrogen species (RNS), 197
Reactive oxygen species (ROS)
  conditions associated with, 196, 197t
  vitamin E and, 192
Recommended Dietary Allowances (RDAs), 504, 510, 511. *See also specific vitamins*
  algorithm for determination of, 490f
  antioxidants and, 492–493
  applications of, 490–491
  changes in concept of, 491–492
  as dietary standard, 494
  questions concerning, 492
  reconstruction of, 493–494
  selenium, 494n22

vitamin/nutrient requirements v., 490
vitamins, Food and Nutrition Board, 495t
vitamins, history of, 491t
Recommended Dietary Intakes (RDIs), 486
Recommended Nutrient Intakes (RNIs), 496. *See also specific vitamins*
  WHO/FAO, for vitamins, 497t
Redox cycle
  ascorbic acid, 240, 240f
  vitamin E, 191, 191f
  vitamin K, 218–219, 219f
Redox reactions, NAD and, 303
Reduction reactions, NADP(H) in, 303
Red-vented bulbul, 239n10
Reference dose (R$_f$D), 511n13
Relative dose-response (RDR) test, 134
Relevance, 13
Renal absorption, of calcium, 161
Renal function, of carnitine, 412
Renal Gla protein, 226
Repeatability, 13
Reproduction
  disorders, from vitamin deficiencies, 81–82t
  vitamin A and, 119
Reserve capacities, of vitamins, 474, 477
Resorption-gestation syndrome, 208
Respiratory burst, 192, 203
Reticulocytopenia, 292
Retinal, 6t, 37t, 43, 44, 61t, 62t, 67t, 70t
  11-*cis*-, 106t, 108, 111, 112, 113, 114
  all-*trans*-, 106, 114, 115
  conversion from provitamin A, 101f
  isomerase, 111
  isomerizations and, 111, 112f
  oxidase, 110
  reductase, 112
Retinaldehyde reductase, 101
Retinen, 19
Retinoic acid, 6t, 43, 44, 61t, 62t, 67t, 70, 70t, 71t
  9-*cis*-, 101, 110, 111
  11-*cis*-, 112
  all-*trans*-, 106t, 111, 113, 116, 117
  catabolism of, 111f
  retinol and, 111
Retinoic acid receptors (RARs), 116, 117, 118
  nuclear, 116t
Retinoic acid response elements (RAREs), 106, 117, 118
Retinoid X receptors (RXRs), 116, 117, 118, 119, 138

Retinoid-binding proteins
  vitamin A metabolism and, 112, 112f, 113t
Retinoids, 43, 44, 70t, 97
  absorption of, 99
  dermatologic diseases and, 125–126
  metabolism of, 101
Retinol, 6t, 20, 37t, 43, 44, 61t, 62t, 66t, 67t, 70t
  cancer, β-Carotene and, 129–130, 129t, 130t
  in children, vitamin A deficiency and, 136t
  conjugation of, 110
  dehydrogenases, 110
  esterification of, 109–110
  metabolism of, 101–102, 109–113, 110f
  in milk, 109
  oxidation of, 110–111
  plasma, homeostasis in, 108–109
  recycling, 108
  retinoic acid and, 111
  transport of, 104–105
Retinol binding proteins (RBPs), 104, 108
Retinol equivalents (RE), 44, 97
Retinyl
  palmitate, 97, 101, 104, 108, 138t
  phosphate, 110, 119
  stearate, 101
Retinyl β-glucuronide, 110, 111, 113
Retinyl esters, 99
  hydrolase, 103, 113t
  hydrolysis, 103
  transport of, 102
Retrolental fibroplasia, 84t, 87t, 88t
RfBPs. *See* Riboflavin-binding proteins
R$_f$D. *See* Reference dose
Rhizobium species, 26, 28t
Rhizopterin, 27, 28t, 30. *See also* Folic acid
Rhodopsin, 106t, 112, 113, 114, 115
Riboflavin, 6t, 281–294
  absorption of, 283–284
  antagonists, 54
  cancer and, 492
  case study, 293
  catabolism of, 286
  chemical structure, 53
  chemistry, 54
  coenzyme functions of, 287
  deficiencies, 281, 288, 290–292
  deficiencies, in animals, 291
  deficiency signs, 88t, 290t, 291–292
  definition of, 281
  discovery of, 21–22, 29t, 281
  excretion of, 286–287
  in food, 282, 283t

hydrophilic, 281
metabolic functions of, 287–288
metabolism of, 285–287
nomenclature, 54
phosphorylation and, 284
physical properties of, 39t
RDA, 495t
RDA, history, 491t
RNI, 497t
significance of, 282
sources of, 282–283
tissue distribution of, 284–285
toxicity, 293, 509
transport of, 284–285
vitamers, 39t
from vitamin B_2 complex, 21–22
Riboflavin-5′-phosphate, 282, 285
Riboflavin-binding proteins (RfBPs), 284
Riboflavinuria, 284
Rickets, 9, 10–11, 12t, 85t, 86t, 87t, 90t
in animals, vitamin D and, 173
chicks with, 174f
child with, 172f
puppy with, 174f
vitamin A and, 19
vitamin D and, 171
vitamin D-dependent, type I, type II, 171
vitamine for anti-, 16
Ringrose, A. T., 345
RNIs. *See* Recommended Nutrient Intakes
RNS. *See* Reactive nitrogen species
Rodents, dermatitis in, 20, 23
ROO•. *See* Peroxyl radical
ROOH. *See* Hydroperoxide
ROS. *See* Reactive oxygen species
RXRs. *See* Retinoid X receptors

L-Saccharoascorbic acid, 242
S-adenosylmethionine (SAM), 365, 388
Safe intakes, of vitamins, 510–513
Safety index (SI), 511, 511t
Safety, vitamin, 503–514
SAM. *See* S-adenosylmethionine
Sarcopenia, 168
Scavenger receptors, 188, 196, 200
Schiff bases, 316
Schilling test, 387
Schizophrenia, 307, 326
Scientific
discovery process, in nutrition, 8
hypotheses, 7
revolution, 4n3
theories, 7
Scurvy, 9–10, 12t, 81t, 82t, 90t
in man, 256f
vitamine for anti-, 16

Seafoods, thiaminase activities in, 268t
Second messenger, 417
Selenium, 182, 195, 196, 198, 206, 207, 208t, 493, 498
RDA for, 494n22
Selenocysteine
β-lyase, 320
γ-lyase, 320
Serine hydroxymethyltransferase, 363, 364, 366t, 367
Serine protease, 222, 223
Serotonin, 321
Short-chain alcohol dehydrogenase/ aldehyde reductase, 117f
Shoshin beriberi, 276
SI. *See* Safety index
Side-chain modification, of vitamin K, 218
Sideroblastic anemia, 326
SIDS. *See* Sudden infant death syndrome
Signal transduction, vitamin E and, 196
Simon's metabolites, 190
Single-carbon metabolism, folate and, 366–367
Single-carbon units, folate and, 362f
Skeletal disorders, from vitamin deficiencies, 86t
Skeletal myopathy, 81t
Skin diseases
vitamin D and proliferative, 167–168
vitamin E and, 205
Skin health, ascorbic acid and, 253
SLR factor, 27, 28, 28t. *See also* Folic acid
Smoking
ascorbic acid level and, 244, 244f, 245f
β-carotene and, 130t
plasma tocopherols and, 190, 191t
vitamin deficiency risks and, 79
vitamin E and, 206, 206t
SMVT. *See* Sodium-dependent vitamin transporter
Snell, E. S., 355
Sociologic evaluation, 470
Sodium-dependent vitamin C transporters (SVCTs), 239, 240
Sodium-dependent vitamin transporter (SMVT), 335
Solubilities, of vitamins/vitamers, 36, 36n1, 37–41t, 42
Sources. *See also* Foods
of biotin, 332–334
of carnitine, 408, 408t
of folate, 356–358
of NAD(H), 300
of NADP(H), 300
of niacin, 296
of pantothenic acid, 346–347, 346t

of riboflavin, 282–283
of thiamin, 266–268
of vitamin A, 97–99, 98t, 99t
of vitamin B_6, 314–316
of vitamin B_{12}, 382–383, 382t
of vitamin C, 236–239
of vitamin D, 147–149
of vitamin E, 182–184
of vitamin K, 214–216
of vitamins, 437–467
Soy isoflavones, antiestrogenic effects of, 424–425
Spectacle eye, 339
Sphingomyelin, 402, 403
Star-gazing, 274
Stearic acid, 416
Steatitis, 83t
Steatorrhea, 207
Stepp, Wilhelm, 15, 17
Steroids, 45, 46, 46n7, 145
hormone, vitamin D_3 as, 157–158
metabolism, ascorbic acid and, 247
Stomatitis, 80t, 83t, 88t, 290t, 324
Stone, Irwin, 257
Streptavidin, 339n21
Streptococcus
faecalis, 27, 28t, 430
lactis R, 355
Stuart factor. *See* Factor X
Succinate dehydrogenase, 286t
Sudden infant death syndrome (SIDS), 340
Sulfa drugs, 376
Sulfate, 268
Sulfatide metabolism, vitamin K in, 226
Sulfites, 267
Superoxide dismutases, 195, 207n97
Superoxide radical (O_2•), 192
Superoxides, 230
Supplements, vitamin, 451–454, 457–459
SVCTs. *See* Sodium-dependent vitamin C transporters
Symptoms, clinical signs *v.*, 77n2. *See also* Clinical signs
Synergists, of vitamin C, 422. *See also* Flavonoids
Synthesis. *See* Biosynthesis
Synthetic forms, of vitamin E, 183
Systemic conditioning, 259, 260
Szent-Györgyi, Albert von, 30t
flavonoids and, 422
on vitamin C, 235

T_3. *See* Thyroid hormone
Tachycardia, 276
Takaki, Kanehiro, 10
Tappel, A. L., 181
TAPs. *See* Tocopherol-associated proteins

TBPs. *See* Thiamin-binding proteins
TC. *See* Transcobalamin
Ten-State Nutrition Survey, 480
Tetrahydrofolate reductase, 362
Tetrahydrofolic acid (FH$_4$), 58, 58t, 70t, 356, 360, 362
Tetrahydrothiophene (thiophane) nucleus, 56
Tetrahymena geleii, 430
Theorell, Hugo, 30t
Theories, scientific, 7
Thermal isomerization, of vitamin D, 46, 47f
Thiamin, 4, 9, 265–280
  absorption of, 268–269
  Alzheimer's disease and, 277
  antagonists, 267–268
  beriberi and, 266
  case studies, 278–279
  catabolism of, 270
  chemical structure, 52
  chemistry, 53
  deficiencies, 265, 274–278
  deficiency signs, 88t
  definition of, 265
  deprivation, 77t
  discovery of, 21, 29t
  disulfide, 268
  excretion of, 270
  in foods, 266–267, 267t
  hydrophilic, 265
  metabolic activation of, 270f
  metabolic functions of, 270–274
  metabolism of, 269–270
  nervous function and, 272–274
  nomenclature, 53
  Parkinson's disease and, 277
  phosphorylation and, 269–270
  physical properties of, 38–39t
  polyneuritis and, 266
  pyrophosphate, 39t, 52, 53, 61t, 67t, 68t, 70t, 71t
  RDA, 495t
  RDA, history, 491t
  RNI, 497t
  significance of, 266
  sources of, 266–268
  tissue distribution of, 269
  toxicity, 278, 509
  transport of, 269
  vitamers, 38–39t
Thiamin monophosphate (TMP), 269
Thiamin pyrophosphate (TPP), 266, 270–271
Thiamin pyrophosphokinase, 268
Thiamin triphosphate (TTP), 269
  -enzymes, in metabolism, 272, 272f
Thiaminases, 267, 268, 275
  in seafoods, 268t
  types of, 268t

Thiamin-binding proteins (TBPs), 269
Thiamin-responsive megaloblastic anemia (TRMA), 278
Thiazole rings, 52, 53, 268
Thiochrome, 270
Thiophane nucleus.
    See Tetrahydrothiophene nucleus
3-HAAO. *See* 3-Hydroxyanthranilic acid oxygenase
3-OH-AA. *See* 3-Hydroxyanthranilic acid
3-OH-Ky. *See* 3-Hydroxykynurenine
Thrombin (factor IIa), 222, 223
Thrombocytopenia, 292
Thromboplastin
  plasma, 222
  tissue, 222
Thymidylate synthesis, 366
Thyroid function, carnitine and, 413
Thyroid hormone (T$_3$), 115, 116, 117, 118
Thyroxine, 285n22
Tibial dyschondroplasia in animals, vitamin D and, 174
Tissue distribution
  of biotin, 335
  of folate, 362
  of pantothenic acid, 348
  of riboflavin, 284–285
  of thiamin, 269
  of ubiquinones, 421
  of vitamin B$_{12}$, 386
  of vitamin C, 240–241
  of vitamin D, 152
  of vitamin K, 217–218
  of vitamins, 68, 68t
Tissue factor, 222
Tissue thromboplastin, 222
TMP. *See* Thiamin monophosphate
Tocol, 5, 5n6, 48
Tocopherol radical tocopheryl quinone, 191
Tocopherol-associated proteins (TAPs), 189
α-Tocopherol, 6t, 25, 61t, 68t, 182–183, 183t
  cancer and, 492
  concentrations in human tissues, 189t
  in guinea pig adipose tissue, 189f
  phosphate, 183
  serum concentrations, in humans, 187t
α-Tocopherol transfer protein (α-TTP), 188
β-Tocopherol, 25, 61t, 183t
δ-Tocopherol, 25, 61t, 183t
γ-Tocopherol, 6t, 25, 61t, 183t

Tocopherols, 24–25, 47, 48, 66t, 67t, 68t, 72t
  apoE gentotype and, 187t
  -binding proteins, 188–189
  biopotencies of, 183t
  coining of term, 24–25
  diabetes and status of, 202, 202t
  interdigitation of PUFAs and, 194, 194f
  oxidation of, peroxyl radicals and, 194f
  smoking and plasma, 190, 191t
α-Tocopheronic acid, 190
α-Tocopheronolactone, 190
All-*rac*-α-tocopheryl polyethylene, 183
α-Tocopheryl hydroquinone, 190
α-Tocopheryl phosphate, 183, 190
All-*rac*-α-tocopherylglycol-succinate, 183, 197, 198
α-Tocotrienol, 183t
β-Tocotrienol, 183t
Tocotrienols, 5, 5n6, 25, 37t, 38t, 47, 48t, 49t
  biopotencies of, 183t
Tolerable Upper Intake Limits (ULs), 511, 512t
  for animals, 513t
  conceptual basis for, 513f
  derivation of, 511
Toxic threshold, 504, 509
Toxicity, vitamin. *See also* Hypervitaminosis
  in animals, 506–507t
  biotin and, 341, 510
  of carotenoids, 138–139
  in children, 505t
  choline, 406
  factors affecting, 504–505
  folate and, 377–378, 510
  niacin, 309, 509–510
  pantothenic acid and, 353, 510
  riboflavin, 293, 509
  risks of, 504, 504f
  thiamin, 509
  vitamin A, 135–139
  vitamin B$_6$, 510
  vitamin B$_{12}$ and, 395, 510
  vitamin C, 258–260
  vitamin D, 175
  vitamin E, 208–209, 510
  vitamin K, 229–230
TPP. *See* Thiamin pyrophosphate
Transaminases, 302, 318, 319, 320
Transcalciferin, 151. *See also* Vitamin D-binding proteins
Transcaltachia, 160, 161n54
Transcarboxylases, 337
Transcobalamin I (TC$_I$), 385
Transcobalamin II (TC$_{II}$), 384, 385
Transcobalamin III (TC$_{III}$), 385

Transcobalamin receptors, 385
Transducin, 115, 116
Transgenic animals, 103, 112
Transhydrogenase, 303
Transketolase, 270, 271–272
Transport
    of ascorbic acid, to plasma, 240
    biotin, 334–335
    carnitine, 408–409
    of carotenoids, 102–103
    electron, vitamin C and, 243
    folate, 360–362
    myo-inositol, 416
    niacin, 298–299
    pantothenic acid, 347–348
    phylloquinones, 217
    retinol, 104–105
    of retinyl esters, 102
    riboflavin, 284–285
    thiamin, 269
    vitamin A, 102–109
    vitamin B_6, 316–317
    vitamin B_{12}, 385–386
    vitamin C, 240–241
    vitamin D, 151–154
    vitamin E, 185–189, 186f
    vitamin K, 217–218, 217t
    of vitamins, 65, 67t, 68
Transporter, folate, 359, 360
Transthyretin, 104, 105, 107
Treatise on Scurvy (Lind), 10
Trigonelline, 297
Trimethylamine, 402, 403
ε-*N*-Trimethyllysine, 407, 411
TRMA. *See* Thiamin-responsive
    megaloblastic anemia
Tropical sprue, 390
Tropoelastin, 246
Trout, vitamin C-deficient, 256f
Tryptophan, 5, 15n6, 22, 69, 69t, 70t, 91t
    cataracts and, 201, 292
    importance of, 298, 298t
    load, 321, 323
    -niacin conversion, 299–300, 299f,
        320–321
    pyrrolase, 299
TTP. *See* Thiamin triphosphate
TTP-ATP phosphoryltransferase, 269
α-TTP. *See* α-Tocopherol transfer
    protein
Tyrosine metabolism, 247

Ubiquinones, 31t, 420–421
    absorption/tissue distribution of, 421
    as antioxidant, 420
    biosynthesis of, 420
    chemical structure, 420
    in food, 420–421
    health effects of, 421
    metabolic function of, 420

need for, 421
reductase, 289t
UGFs. *See* Unidentified growth factors
ULs. *See* Tolerable Upper Intake
    Limits
Ultraviolet light
    vitamin D and, 145, 151t
    vitamin D_3 and, 149, 150f, 151t
Unidentified growth factors (UGFs),
    399, 431. *See also* Quasi-vitamins
Ureido nucleus, 56

Varus deformity, 176, 177
Vascular disorders, from vitamin
    deficiencies, 82t
VDKB. *See* Vitamin K deficiency
    bleeding
VDREs. *See* Vitamin D-responsive
    elements
VDRs. *See* Vitamin D receptors
Vegans, 382, 389t
Vegetables/fruits, American
    consumption of, 479t
Vegetarian diets, vitamin B_{12} and,
    388–389
Vegetarians, 389t
    ovolacto, 389
Verdeman, Adolphe, 14
Very low-density lipoproteins.
        See VLDLs
Vision, vitamin A and, 19–20, 113–115
Visual cycle, vitamin A in, 114f
Vital amine, 4
Vitamers, 5. *See also specific vitamers*
    absorption of, 37–41t
    colors of, 37–41t
    enteric absorption of, 64–65, 66t
    fluorescence in, 37–41t
    forms of, 37–41t, 60, 61t
    list of, 6t, 37–41t
    melting point for, 37–41t
    molecular weight of, 37–41t
    provitamin A, 37t
    solubilities of, 36, 36n1, 37–41t, 42
Vitamin(s). *See also* Deficiencies,
    vitamin; Feedstuffs; Toxicity,
    vitamin
    absorption of, 37–41t
    as accessory factors, 399
    analysis methods, 61–62, 63t
    animals and allowance of, 498,
        499–501t
    as antioxidants, 72, 72t
    assessment of status of, 469–484
    availability, for Americans, 477, 478t
    binding to proteins, 67t, 68, 69, 70t
    bioavailability, 44, 64, 64t, 448–449,
        448t
    biological functions of, 90t
    biosynthesis of, 69, 69t

in breast milk, 456–457, 456t
catabolism, 3
caveats, 5
chemical/physiological properties
    of, 35–73
as coenzymes, 72–73t
colors of, 37–41t
contents, biotechnology and, 447
contents, prediction of, 441–448
contents, variations in, 447–448
core foods for, 438, 440t, 441
definition of, 399
dietary standards for, 486–487
discovery of, 7–33, 400, 401
drug interactions with, 489t
elevated doses of, 503–505
elucidation of, 17–30
enteric absorption of, 64–65, 66t
enzyme cofactors and, 3, 6t
excretory forms of, 70, 71t, 72
fat-soluble, 42
fluorescence in, 37–41t
in foods, 437–441, 439t, 440t
forms of, 37–41t, 60, 61t
as gene transcription elements, 72
general properties, 60–63
as H^+/e^- donors/acceptors, 72, 72t
hormones *v.*, 5
in human diets, 454–457
as ineffective factors, 430–431
intakes, by Americans, 478, 478t
labeling of foods for, 459–461
list of, 6t
losses, 449–451, 449t, 450f, 450t, 451t
melting point for, 37–41t
metabolic functions of, 72–73, 72–73t
metabolism of, 68–72, 70t
-mineral premix, 462
modern history of, 31, 32t
molecular weight of, 37–41t
needs, 485–502
Nobel prizes for research on, 30t
nomenclature, 42
nuclear receptor proteins of, 69, 70t
operating definition of, 4–5
origin of term, 16, 16n8
other nutrients *v.*, 4–5
physical properties of, 37–41t
physiological functions of, 3, 6t
physiological utilization of, 64–68
premixes, 462, 464t, 465t
proposed, 5n5, 31t
pseudofactors *v.*, 31, 31t
purified, 451–452
quantification of needs for, 485–502
quasi-, 5n5, 31t, 399–433
range of safe intakes for, 504, 508,
    510–513
RDAs, history of, 491t
recognized, 5, 6t

Vitamin(s) (*Continued*)
  research foci for, 31, 32t
  reserve capacities of, 474, 477
  -responsive inborn metabolic
      lesions, 91t
  retention/utilization, impaired, 471
  as revolutionary concept, 4
  safe intakes of, 510–513
  safety, 503–514
  solubilities of, 36, 36n1, 37–41t, 42
  sources of, 437–467
  stabilities of, 60–61, 62t
  supplements, 451–454, 457–459
  terminology of, 30
  thoughts on, 3
  tissue distribution of, 68, 68t
  transport, 65, 67t, 68
  ULs for, 511, 512t, 513f
  uses of, 503
  water-soluble, 42
Vitamin A, 95–143
  absorption of, 99–102
  in adipose tissue, 109
  anemia and, 120t
  antagonists, 121
  antioxidant activities of, 126–127
  -binding proteins, 105–108, 106t
  biopotency, 44–45, 44t
  bone metabolism and, 119–120
  cancer and, 127–130, 492
  case studies, 139–141
  chemical structure, 42–43
  chemistry, 43–44
  child mortality and, 124t, 125t
  chylomicrons and, 102, 103
  coenzyme role for, 118–119
  deficiency, calf and, 135f
  deficiency, detection of, 131–134
  deficiency, eye lesions and, 136t
  deficiency, hidden hunger and, 483
  deficiency, progression of, 133f
  deficiency, retinol in children and,
      136t
  deficiency, signs of, 87t, 120t, 134t
  deficiency, treatment of, 135
  deficiency, WHO framework and,
      132f
  definition of, 95
  dermatology and, 124–125
  discovery of, 29t, 95
  distribution in foods, 97–98, 98t, 99t
  drug metabolism and, 126
  embryonic development and, 119
  excretion of, 113
  fat-soluble A and, 19
  functional forms of, 113t
  gene transcription and, 116–118
  heart disease risk and, 127
  hematopoiesis and, 120–121
  high/low intakes of, 134f

  HIV transmission and, 123t
  as hormone, 3, 72t
  hydrophobic, active substances, 95
  immunity and, 121–125
  iron and, 122t
  iron solubility and, 121f
  liver storage of, 103
  measles and, 124t
  metabolic functions of, 114–130
  metabolism of, 109–113
  metabolism of, intestinal, 102f
  metabolism, retinoid-binding
      proteins and, 112, 112f, 113t
  micellar solubilization of, 99
  Nepal pregnancies and, 122t
  nomenclature, 43
  percentage distribution in sera of
      fasted humans, 104t
  physical properties of, 37t
  physiological function of, 6t
  provitamins of, 6t, 37t
  RDA, 495t
  RDA, history, 491t
  -related compounds, biopotency of,
      44t
  reproduction and, 119
  requirements, for calves, 486t
  rickets and, 19
  RNI, 497t
  significance of, 96–97
  sources of, 97–99, 98t, 99t
  systemic functions of, 115
  teratogenicity of, 138t
  toxicity, 135–139
  transport of, 102–109
  vision and, 19–20, 113–115
  in visual cycle, 114f
  vitamers, 6t
Vitamin B
  complex, 30, 458
  vitamine as, 17
Vitamin B$_1$, 21, 265. *See also* Thiamin
  physiological function of, 6t
  vitamer, 6t
Vitamin B$_2$, 21, 345. *See also*
      Riboflavin
  physiological function of, 6t
  vitamer, 6t
Vitamin B$_2$ complex, 21
  components of, 21
  niacin from, 22
  pantothenic acid from, 23–24
  pyridoxine from, 23, 29
  riboflavin from, 21–22
Vitamin B$_3$. *See* Pantothenic acid
Vitamin B$_6$, 313–329
  absorption of, 316
  active form of, 313
  bioavailability, 314–315
  case studies, 327–328

  catabolism and, 318
  chemical structure, 55–56
  chemistry, 56
  congenital disorders and, 325, 325t
  deficiencies, 313, 323–325
  deficiencies, in animals, 323–324
  deficiency signs, 88t, 324–325, 324t
  definition of, 313
  discovery of, 23, 29t
  distribution in foods, 314, 315t
  drugs/alcohol and, 318
  metabolic functions of, 318–323
  metabolic roles of, 319–323, 320t
  metabolism of, 317–318, 317f
  neurologic function and, 322–323
  niacin and, 300, 302
  nomenclature, 56
  pharmacologic uses of, 326–327
  phosphorylation and, 316
  physical properties of, 39t
  physiological function of, 6t
  protein intake and, 319t
  RDA, 495t
  RDA, history, 491t
  RNI, 497t
  significance of, 314
  sources of, 314–316
  toxicity and, 327, 510
  transport of, 316–317
  vitamers, 6t, 39t
  vitamers, in species, 317t
Vitamin B$_{12}$, 29, 381–398
  absorption of, 383–384
  anemia and, 382
  bioavailability of, 383
  cancer and, 394
  case study, 395–397
  catabolism of, 386–387
  chemical structure, 59–60
  chemistry, 60
  coenzyme functions of, 387–388
  coenzyme synthetase, 386
  complex, IF-, 384
  congenital disorders and, 395, 395t
  deficiencies, 381, 388–395
  deficiencies, folate and, 374–375
  deficiencies, in animals, 391–392
  deficiency signs, 89t
  definition of, 381
  discovery of, 28, 29, 29t
  distribution in foods, 382–383, 382t
  distribution in tissues, 386
  excretion of, 387
  factors leading to discovery of, 29,
      29t
  genomic stability and, 394
  metabolic functions, 381, 387–388
  metabolism of, 386–387
  MS and, 394
  neurological function and, 393–394

nomenclature, 60
osteoporosis and, 394–395
pancreatic insufficiency and, 390
physical properties of, 40–41t
physiological function of, 6t
RDA, 495t
RDA, history, 491t
RNI, 497t
significance of, 382
sources of, 382–383, 382t
toxicity and, 395, 510
transport of, 385–386
vegetarian diets and, 388–389
vitamers, 6t, 40–41t
Vitamin B$_{13}$. *See* Orotic acid
Vitamin B$_{15}$ (pangamic acid), 31,
    430–431
Vitamin B$_{17}$ (laetrile), 31t, 431
Vitamin B$_c$, 27, 28, 28t
Vitamin binding proteins, 67t, 68,
    69, 70t. *See also specific binding*
    proteins
Vitamin B$_T$, 406. *See also* Carnitine
Vitamin C, 235–263
    absorption of, 239–240
    -active derivatives, of ascorbic acid,
      238t
    -active substances, 235
    -active substances, biopotency of, 52t
    -active substances, hydrophilic, 235
    animal model and, 18–19
    ascorbic acid and, 61t, 62t
    ascorbic acid and intake of, 240, 241f
    bioavailability, 236–237
    biopotency, 52
    biosynthesis of, 5, 69t
    cancer and, 492
    case studies, 260–262
    cataracts and, 253, 253t
    chemical structure, 51
    chemistry, 51–52
    colds and, 257–258, 258t
    contents, of uncooked foods, 237t
    CVD and, 492
    deficiencies, 235, 254–257
    deficiencies, in animals, 256
    deficiencies, in trout, 256f
    deficiency signs, 88t, 255–256, 255t
    definition of, 235
    dental health and, 253
    diabetes and, 252, 252f
    discovery of, 18–19, 29t
    distribution/stability, in foods, 236
    dopamine-β-monooxygenase and,
      246, 247f
    electron transport and, 243
    environmental stress and, 254, 255t
    enzyme deficiency and, 238–239
    excretion of, 242–243

exercise and, 252
GSH and, 244, 24 4f
guinea pigs and, 238t, 239, 242, 247,
    250, 251, 253, 256, 257
infections and, 258, 258t
megadose, 257–258
metabolic functions of, 243–254
metabolism of, 241–243
oxidation-reduction reactions of,
    241–242, 241f, 242f
periodontal disease and, 253, 256
pharmacologic uses of, 257–258
physical properties of, 38t
physiological function of, 6t
pregnancy outcomes and, 253
RDA, 495t
RDA, history, 491t
RNI, 497t
significance of, 236
sources of, 236–239
synergists of, 422
Szent-Györgyi on, 235
tissue distribution of, 240–241
toxicity, 258–260
transport of, 240–241
vitamers, 6t, 38t
Vitamin D, 145–179
    -active compounds, biopotency of,
      47t
    activities in food, 148t
    analogs, 157, 158t
    autoimmune diseases and, 166–167
    biopotency, 46–47, 47t
    biosynthesis of, 5
    bone health and, 164
    bone mineral turnover and, 162
    boron and, 163–164
    calcium/phosphorus metabolism
      and, 160–163
    cancer and, 168–169, 168f
    cardiovascular disease and, 167
    case studies, 176–177
    catabolism, 155
    chemical structure, 45
    chemistry, 46
    deficiency, causes of, 169–171, 170f
    deficiency, in animals, 173–174
    deficiency, signs of, 87t, 171–174,
      172t, 173t, 174f
    definition of, 145
    diabetes and, 165–166, 166–167, 166f
    discovery of, 19, 20, 29t
    distribution in foods, 147, 148t
    enteric absorption of, 150
    genes regulated by, 159t
    genomic pathways and function of,
      158–160
    healthful intakes of, 169
    as hormone, 3, 5, 72t

hydrophobic, vitamers, 145
1-hydroxylase, 155
24-hydroxylase, 155
25-hydroxylase, 154
hydroxylations and, 154–156
immunity and, 164–165
lead and, 164, 164t
McCollum and, 19, 20
metabolic functions of, 157–169, 158f
metabolism of, 154–157, 154f
metabolism regulation, 156–157
metabolites and vitamin D$_2$, 157t
micelle-dependent passive diffusion
    and, 150
milk fever and, 174
muscular function and, 168
musculoskeletal pain and, 173
nature of, 20
nomenclature, 46
noncalcified tissue and function of,
    164, 165t
nongenomic pathways and function
    of, 160
osteomalacia and, 171
osteoporosis and, 171–173
parathyroid gland and functioning
    of, 169, 169f
periodontal disease and, 167
physical properties of, 37t
physiological function of, 6t
proliferative skin diseases and,
    167–168
RDA, 495t
RDA, history, 491t
-resistance, 171
rickets and, 171
rickets in animals and, 173
RNI, 497t
significance of, 146–147
sources of, 147–149
thermal isomerization of, 46, 47f
tissue distribution of, 152
toxicity, 175
transport of, 151–154
ultraviolet light and, 145, 151t
vitamers, 6t, 20, 37t
zinc and, 163
Vitamin D receptors (VDRs), 152–154
    distribution of nuclear, 153t
Vitamin D$_2$ (ergocalciferol), 6t, 20, 42,
    45, 46, 47t, 61t, 64t
    differential metabolism of, 157
    vitamin D metabolites and, 157t
Vitamin D$_3$ (cholecalciferol), 5, 6t, 45,
    46, 47t, 61t, 64t
    biosynthesis of, 69, 69t, 147–149, 149f
    as steroid hormone, 157–158
    ultraviolet light and, 149, 150f, 151t